ADVANCES IN NEUROLOGY
Volume 34

Advances in Neurology

INTERNATIONAL ADVISORY BOARD

Advances in Neurology
Volume 34

Status Epilepticus
Mechanisms of Brain Damage and Treatment

Editors

Antonio V. Delgado-Escueta, M.D.
Professor of Neurology
UCLA School of Medicine
Director, Comprehensive Epilepsy Program and
Veterans Administration Southwest Regional
Epilepsy Center
Veterans Administration Wadsworth Medical
Center
Los Angeles, California

Claude G. Wasterlain, M.D.
Professor and Vice Chairman
Department of Neurology
UCLA School of Medicine
Chief, Neurology Service
Veterans Administration Medical Center,
Sepulveda
Los Angeles, California

David M. Treiman, M.D.
Assistant Professor of Neurology
UCLA School of Medicine
Director, Veterans Administration Southwest
Regional Epilepsy Center
Veterans Administration Wadsworth Medical
Center
Los Angeles, California

Roger J. Porter, M. D.
Chief, Epilepsy Branch
Neurological Disorders Program
National Institute of Neurological and
Communicative Disorders and Stroke
National Institutes of Health
Bethesda, Maryland

Raven Press ■ New York

Raven Press, 1140 Avenue of the Americas, New York, New York 10036

Great care has been taken to maintain the accuracy of the information contained in the volume. However, Raven Press cannot be held responsible for errors or for any consequences arising from the use of the information contained herein.

Library of Congress Cataloging in Publication Data
Main entry under title:

Status epilepticus, mechanisms of brain damage and
    treatment.

    (Advances in neurology ; v. 34)
    Based on the International Symposium on Status
Epilepticus held in Santa Monica, California, November
17–19, 1980.
    Includes bibliographical references and index.
    1. Epilepsy—Congresses. 2. Brain damage—Congresses.
I. Delgado-Escueta, Antonio V. II. International Sym-
posium on Status Epilepticus (1980 : Santa Monica,
Calif.) III. Series. [DNLM: 1. Status epilepticus.
2. Status epilepticus—Drug therapy. W1 AD684H v. 34/
WL 385 S796]
RC372.S77   1983   616.8′53   80-6214
ISBN 0-89004-623-9

Advances in Neurology Series

Preface

Twenty years have now passed since the Marseille conference on status epilepticus. Perhaps the most important advance from that conference was the extension of the term "status epilepticus" to mean "epileptic seizures that are so frequently repeated or so prolonged as to create a fixed and lasting epileptic condition." Thus, in addition to tonic-clonic status epilepticus and epilepsia partialis continuans, prolonged states of nonconvulsive absence and complex partial seizures have been accepted as forms of status epilepticus. Since then, rapid advances in documentation of prolonged seizures by closed-circuit television and electroencephalography and a new understanding of the cellular and molecular consequences of uncontrolled convulsions have provided a new rationale for the treatment of status epilepticus.

Clinicians have long suspected that extensive neuronal damage may follow uncontrolled seizures, especially in children. This clinical concept has been supported by various studies over the past 30 years. Chief among these was identification of the H. H. E. syndrome (hemiconvulsions, hemiplegia, and epilepsy) by H. Gastaut and collaborators and observations of permanent neurological damage following status epilepticus in children by Aicardi and Chevrie. Moreover, recent studies have shown that prolonged complex partial seizures can produce chronic loss of memory and other symptoms of the Klüver-Bucy syndrome.

These clinical observations have stimulated research on the molecular effects of seizures and status epilepticus. Studies in the 1950s and 1960s, for example, examined the effects of electroshock seizures on ion transport and brain energy utilization. It was soon shown that repeated seizures and status epilepticus impaired protein synthesis. Selective inhibition of peptide chain initiation caused polysomes of mammalian cerebral cortex to break down, whereas corresponding monomers increased acutely. Such events are now considered responsible for the block of memory consolidation frequently observed after convulsive status. A spate of studies on mechanisms of epileptic brain damage followed B. S. Meldrum's report, in 1973, of hippocampal cell damage (Sommer's sector sclerosis) after convulsive status. These studies explored the effects of repeated seizures on glial and synaptic function, biochemical regulators, receptors, amino acid neurotransmitters, and, perhaps most exciting, regional glucose metabolism *in vivo*. The conclusions are examined in the chapters on mechanisms of brain damage in status epilepticus.

Seizures must be arrested as quickly as possible to prevent serious brain damage. Unfortunately, the ideal drug for convulsive status epilepticus has not been developed. In earlier times, phenobarbital or amobarbital was frequently used to stop prolonged seizures, and paraldehyde was the drug of choice for tonic-clonic status. Today, these drugs have been replaced by diazepam, clonazepam, phenytoin, and lorazepam. When these newer drugs cannot be used or have failed to control the seizures, however, paraldehyde or phenobarbital is still often employed, even though little is known about the pharmacological effects of these drugs when administered intravenously. Controlled comparisons of the drugs used to treat convulsive status epilepticus have never been done, and the preferred general anesthetic has never been defined. In this volume, the treatment of status epilepticus is discussed from many different but valid perspectives of investigators who seek the definitive therapy.

We hope that this volume will bring a new level of understanding about status epilepticus to medical students, clinical neurologists, internists, pediatricians, emergency room physicians, and neuroscientists who treat or study the problem. Our knowledge of the disorder is still far from complete, however. For instance, electroclinical documentation of neonatal status epilepticus remains difficult, and debates on the classification of neonatal seizures continue. We do not know if prolonged seizures per se can cause selective brain damage in newborns. Consequently, a rational and generally accepted method of treatment of neonatal status epilepticus is far from a reality. In children and adults, the molecular events that set in motion the fine structural changes of cell damage remain unknown. The cellular and molecular mechanisms that transform a single seizure into the fixed and progressive epileptic state that is status epilepticus are also unknown. Thus, we hope that this work will help bring into focus technical and conceptual advances that will stimulate new research efforts to eventually close the important gaps in our knowledge of status epilepticus.

The Editors

Acknowledgments

The editors are grateful for the help of many diligent and capable people. We especially wish to acknowledge the editorial advice and assistance of B. J. Hessie from the Epilepsy Branch, National Institute of Neurological and Communicative Disorders and Stroke. We thank Janis Rosebrook from the Department of Continuing Education in Health Sciences, UCLA Extension, for helping to organize the International Symposium on Status Epilepticus (Santa Monica, California, November 17–19, 1980) on which this book is based. Also, secretarial assistance and word processing were provided by Patricia Almendarez, Susan Clark, Bob Mitchell, Susan Pietsch, and Teresina Williams.

This project was supported by USPHS grant 1 R13 NS16171–01 SRC, in part by USPHS contract NO1-NS-0-2332 from the National Institute of Neurological and Communicative Disorders and Stroke and by grants-in-aid from Abbott Laboratories and Parke-Davis, Division of Warner-Lambert Company.

Contents

Summary

Contributors

Jean Aicardi, M.D.
Institut National de la Santé et de la Recherche
  Médicale
Hôpital des Enfants Malades
75730 Paris 15, France

Michael Albani, M.D.
University Children's Hospital
D-2000 Hamburg 20, Federal Republic of
  Germany

A. M. Baars
Department of Pharmacy
Sint Radboud Hospital
Catholic University of Nijmegen
Nijmegen, The Netherlands

T. L. Babb, Ph.D.
Adjunct Assistant Professor of Neurology
Mental Retardation Research Center
Brain Research Institute
University of California (Los Angeles) Center
  for the Health Sciences
Los Angeles, California 90024

Nicolás G. Bazán, M.D.
LSU Eye Center
136 S. Roman St.
New Orleans, Louisiana 70112

L. S. Benardo
Department of Neurology
Stanford University School of Medicine
Stanford, California 94305

Harold E. Booker, M.D.
Director
Neurology Service
Department of Medicine and Surgery
Veterans Administration Central Office
Washington, D. C. 20420

W. Jann Brown, M.D.
Professor of Pathology, Psychiatry
Chief, Division of Neuropathology
Mental Retardation Research Center
Brain Research Institute
University of California (Los Angeles) Center
  for the Health Sciences
Los Angeles, California 90024

Thomas R. Browne, M.D.
Assistant Professor of Neurology
Chief, Seizure Unit
Neurology Service
Veterans Administration Medical Center, and
Boston University School of Medicine
Boston, Massachusetts 02130

C. J. Bruton
Department of Neuropathology
Runwell Hospital
Wickford, Essex SS11 7QE, England

M. Bureau
Centre St. Paul
Marseille, France

Gastone G. Celesia, M.D.
Professor and Chief
Department of Neurology
William S. Middleton Memorial Veterans
  Hospital, and
University of Wisconsin Center for Health
  Sciences
Madison, Wisconsin 53705

Astrid G. Chapman
Institute of Psychiatry
De Crespigny Park
Denmark Hill
London SE5 8AF, England

Jean-Jacques Chevrie
Institut National de la Santé et de la Recherche
  Médicale
Hôpital des Enfants Malades
75730 Paris 15, France

Robert C. Collins, M.D.
Associate Professor
Department of Neurology
Washington University School of Medicine
St. Louis, Missouri 63110

B. W. Connors, Ph.D.
Department of Neurology
Stanford University School of Medicine
Stanford, California 94305

J. A. N. Corsellis, M.D.
Professor
Department of Neuropathology
Runwell Hospital
Wickford
Essex SS11 7QE, England

Ronald E. Cranford, M.D.
Assistant Professor
Department of Neurology
University of Minnesota School of Medicine,
* and*
Hennepin County Medical Center
Minneapolis, Minnesota 55101

O. Daniele
Neurological Clinic
University of Palermo School of Medicine
Palermo, Italy

C. Geoffrey Davis
Department of Neurology
University of California (San Francisco) School
* of Medicine*
San Francisco, California 94143

R. Degen
Department of Electroencephalography
Anstalt Bethel
Bielefeld, Federal Republic of Germany

Antonio V. Delgado-Escueta, M.D.
Professor of Neurology
Director, Comprehensive Epilepsy Program and
Southwest Regional Epilepsy Center
Wadsworth VA Medical Center, and
Reed Neurological Research Center
University of California (Los Angeles) School of
* Medicine*
Los Angeles, California 90024

Robert John DeLorenzo, M.D., Ph.D.
Associate Professor
Department of Neurology
Yale University School of Medicine
New Haven, Connecticut 06510

Ivan Diamond, M.D.
Professor
Departments of Neurology, Pediatrics, and
* Pharmacology*
University of California (San Francisco) School
* of Medicine*
San Francisco, California 94143

Marcia Divoll
Division of Clinical Pharmacology
Departments of Psychiatry and Medicine
Tufts University School of Medicine, and
New England Medical Center Hospital
Boston, Massachusetts 02111

Hermann Doose, M.D.
Professor
Neuropediatric Department
University of Kiel, D-2300
Kiel, Federal Republic of Germany

C. Dravet
Centre St. Paul
Marseille, France

Barney E. Dwyer, Ph.D.
Postdoctoral Fellow
Epilepsy Research Laboratory
Veterans Administration Medical Center
Sepulveda, and
Department of Neurology and Brain Research
* Institute*
University of California (Los Angeles) School of
* Medicine*
Los Angeles, California 90024

Yigal H. Ehrlich, Ph.D.
Research Associate Professor
Departments of Psychiatry and Biochemistry
University of Vermont College of Medicine
Burlington, Vermont 05405

Jerome Engel, Jr., M.D., Ph.D.
Professor
Departments of Neurology and Anatomy
Reed Neurological Research Center
University of California (Los Angeles) School of
* Medicine*
Los Angeles, California 90024

F. Enrile-Bacsal, M.D.
Fogarty Scholar
Department of Neurology
University of California (Los Angeles) School of
  Medicine
Los Angeles, California 90024

James A. Ferrendelli, M.D.
Professor and Chief
Division of Clinical Neuropharmacology
Departments of Neurology, Neurological
  Surgery and Pharmacology
Washington University School of Medicine
St. Louis, Missouri 63110

Jaroslava Folbergrová
Institute of Physiology
Czechoslovak Academy of Sciences
Prague, Czechoslovakia

Georges Franck
Professor of Neurology
Chief, Laboratory of Neurochemistry
University of Liege
4020 Liege, Belgium

Patrick N. Friel
Department of Neurological Surgery
University of Washington School of Medicine
Seattle, Washington 98195

Henri Gastaut, M.D.
Professor à la Faculté, Medecin
Chef des Hôpitaux
Service de Neurophysiologie Clinique
Centre Hospitalier et Universitaire de Marseille
Marseille, France

Antonio Giuditta, Ph.D.
International Institute of Genetics and
  Biophysics
80125 Naples, Italy

Gilbert H. Glaser, M.D.
Professor and Chairman
Department of Neurology
Yale University School of Medicine
New Haven, Connecticut 06510

Mark A. Goldberg, M.D., Ph.D.
Professor of Neurology and Pharmacology
University of California (Los Angeles) School of
  Medicine, and
Chairman, Department of Neurology
Harbor–UCLA Medical Center
Torrance, California 90509

Adrienne S. Gordon
Associate Research Biochemist
Departments of Neurology and Pharmacology
University of California (San Francisco) School
  of Medicine
San Francisco, California 94143

David J. Greenblatt, M.D.
Professor and Chief
Division of Clinical Pharmacology
Departments of Psychiatry and Medicine
Tufts University School of Medicine, and
New England Medical Center Hospital
Boston, Massachusetts 02111

Thierry Grisar, M.D.
Assistant Professor of Neurology
Laboratory of Neurochemistry
University of Liege
4020 Liege, Belgium

W. Allen Hauser, M.D.
Associate Professor
Department of Neurology
College of Physicians and Surgeons, and
Associate Director
G. H. Sergievsky Center
Faculty of Medicine
Columbia University
New York, New York 10032

R. W. Homan, M.D.
Assistant Professor
Department of Neurology
University of Texas Health Science Center, and
Chief, Epilepsy Center
Veterans Administration Medical Center
Dallas, Texas 75235

Michael Horan
Predoctoral Student
Neuroscience Training Program
Brain Research Institute
University of California (Los Angeles) School of
  Medicine
Los Angeles, California 90024

David C. Howse, M.D.
Department of Medicine (Neurology)
Queen's University
Kingston, Ontario, Canada K7L 3J7

Richard A. Hrachovy
Section of Neurophysiology
Department of Neurology
Baylor College of Medicine, and
Epilepsy Research Center
The Methodist Hospital
Houston, Texas 77030

Martin Ingvar
Laboratory of Experimental Brain Research
University of Lund Hospital
S-221, 85 Lund, Sweden

Dieter Janz, M.D.
Professor
Department of Neurology
Free University of Berlin
D-1000 Berlin 19, Federal Republic of
*   Germany*

Hannu Kalimo
Department of Pathology
University of Turku
S-20520 Turku, Finland

Peter Kellaway, M.D., Ph.D.
Professor of Neurology and Chief
Section of Neurophysiology
Director, Epilepsy Research Center
Baylor College of Medicine
The Methodist Hospital
Houston, Texas 77030

D. Koch
Department of Anesthesiology and Intensive
*   Care*
Sarepta Hospital
D-4800 Bielefeld 13, Federal Republic of
*   Germany*

Kevin M. Koch
Department of Pharmaceutics
University of Washington School of Pharmacy
Seattle, Washington 98195

Norman R. Kreisman
Department of Physiology
Tulane University School of Medicine
New Orleans, Louisiana 70112

David E. Kuhl
Professor
Division of Nuclear Medicine
University of California (Los Angeles) School of
*   Medicine*
Los Angeles, California 90024

Joseph C. LaManna
Departments of Neurology and
*   Physiology/Biophysics*
University of Miami School of Medicine
Miami, Florida 33101

Ilo E. Leppik, M.D.
Assistant Professor
Department of Neurology
University of Minnesota School of Medicine,
*   and*
St. Paul–Ramsey Medical Center
Minneapolis, Minnesota 55101

René H. Levy, Ph.D.
Professor and Chairman
Department of Pharmaceutics, and
Professor of Neurological Surgery
University of Washington Schools of Pharmacy
*   and Medicine*
Seattle, Washington 98195

Edward Lewin
Professor
Neurology Service
Veterans Administration Medical Center, and
Department of Neurology
University of Colorado Health Sciences Center
Denver, Colorado 80220

Joan S. Lockard, Ph.D.
Research Affiliate
Department of Neurological Surgery, and
Child Development and Mental Retardation
*   Center*
University of Washington School of Medicine
Seattle, Washington 98195

Lawrence A. Lockman, M.D.
Assistant Professor
Division of Pediatric Neurology
Department of Neurology and Pediatrics
University of Minnesota School of Medicine
Minneapolis, Minnesota 55455

Cesare T. Lombroso, M.D.
Professor of Neurology and Chief
Seizure Unit and Division of Neurophysiology
The Children's Hospital Medical Center, and
Department of Neurology, Harvard Medical
  School
Boston, Massachusetts 02115

Eric W. Lothman
Assistant Professor
Department of Neurology
Washington University School of Medicine
St. Louis, Missouri 63110

Paul J. Marangos
Clinical Psychobiology Branch
National Institute of Mental Health
Bethesda, Maryland 20205

Donald O. Maris
Department of Neurological Surgery
University of Washington School of Medicine
Seattle, Washington 98195

M. Marschall
Department of Anesthesiology and Intensive
  Care
Sarepta Hospital
D-4800 Bielefeld 13, Federal Republic of
  Germany

Richard H. Mattson, M.D.
Clinical Professor of Neurology, and
Chief of Neurology Service
Veterans Administration Medical Center
West Haven, and
Department of Neurology
Yale University School of Medicine
New Haven, Connecticut 06510

Hugh B. McIntyre, M.D., Ph.D.
Adjunct Professor
Department of Neurology
University of California (Los Angeles) School of
  Medicine, and
Clinical Neurophysiology Laboratory
Harbor–UCLA Medical Center
Torrance, California 90509

Brian S. Meldrum, M.B., Ph.D.
Senior Lecturer
Department of Neurology
Institute of Psychiatry
De Crespigny Park
Denmark Hill
London SE5 8AF, England

Salvatore Metafora
Laboratory of Molecular Embryology
80072 Arco Felice (Naples), Italy

R. Michelucci, M.D.
Neurological Clinic
University of Bologna School of Medicine
40123 Bologna, Italy

Dale Milfay
Department of Neurology
University of California (San Francisco) School
  of Medicine
San Francisco, California 94143

Susana A. Morelli de Liberti
Instituto de Investigaciones Bioquímicas
Universidad Nacional del Sur
Consejo Nacional de Investigaciones Científicas
  y Técnicas
800 Bahía Blanca, Argentina

Anne M. Morin, Ph.D.
Chief, Neurology Research Laboratory
Veterans Administration Medical Center
Sepulveda, and
Department of Neurology
University of California (Los Angeles) School of
  Medicine
Los Angeles, California 90024

John W. Olney
Professor
Department of Psychiatry
Washington University School of Medicine
St. Louis, Missouri 63110

Yngve Olsson
Neuropathology Laboratory
Institute of Pathology
University of Uppsala
S-751 22 Uppsala, Sweden

A. Opitz
Department of Anesthesiology and Intensive
  Care
Sarepta Hospital
D-4800 Bielefeld 13, Federal Republic of
  Germany

Michael J. Painter, M.D.
Associate Professor
Division of Child Neurology
University of Pittsburgh School of Medicine
Pittsburgh, Pennsylvania 15213

Barbara K. Patrick
Department of Neurology
University of Minnesota School of Medicine,
*   and*
Hennepin County Medical Center
Minneapolis, Minnesota 55101

Steven M. Paul
Clinical Psychobiology Branch
National Institute of Mental Health
Bethesda, Maryland 20205

J. Kiffin Penry, M.D.
Associate Dean for Neuroscience Development
and Professor, Department of Neurology
Bowman Gray School of Medicine
Winston-Salem, North Carolina 27103

Carla Perrone-Capano
International Institute of Genetics and
*   Biophysics*
80125 Naples, Italy

Michael E. Phelps, Ph.D.
Division of Nuclear Medicine
University of California (Los Angeles) School of
*   Medicine*
Center for the Health Sciences
Los Angeles, California 90024

Maurizio Popoli
Clinica Malattie Nervose e Mentali
2ª Facoltà di Medicina
80131 Naples, Italy

Roger J. Porter, M.D.
Chief, Epilepsy Branch
Neurological Disorders Program
National Institute of Neurological and
*   Communicative Disorders and Stroke*
Bethesda, Maryland 20205

D. A. Prince, M.D.
Professor and Chairman
Department of Neurology
Stanford University School of Medicine
Stanford, California 94305

Elena B. Rodríguez de Turco
Instituto de Investigaciones Bioquímicas
Universidad Nacional del Sur
Consejo Nacional de Investigaciones Científic
*   y Técnicas*
8000 Bahía Blanca, Argentina

J. Roger
Centre St. Paul
Marseille, France

Myron Rosenthal
Associate Professor
Departments of Neurology and
*   Physiology/Biophysics*
University of Miami School of Medicine
Miami, Florida 33101

Thomas J. Sick
Departments of Neurology and
*   Physiology/Biophysics*
University of Miami School of Medicine
Miami, Florida 33101

Bo K. Siesjö, Ph.D.
Laboratory of Experimental Brain Research
University of Lund Hospital
S-221 85 Lund, Sweden

Phil Skolnick, Ph.D.
Senior Investigator
Laboratory of Bioorganic Chemistry
National Institute of Arthritis, Diabetes, and
*   Digestive and Kidney Diseases*
Bethesda, Maryland 20205

Birgitta Söderfeldt
Laboratory of Experimental Brain Research
University of Lund Hospital
S-221 85 Lund, Sweden

C. A. Tassinari, M.D.
Neurological Clinic
University of Bologna School of Medicine
40123 Bologna, Italy

David M. Treiman, M.D.
Assistant Professor and Co-Director
Veterans Administration Southwest Regional
*   Epilepsy Center, Wadsworth Medical Center,*
*   and*
Department of Neurology
University of California (Los Angeles) School of
*   Medicine*
Los Angeles, California 90024

F. J. E. Vajda, M.D.
Neurologist and Senior Clinical Pharmacologist
Austin Hospital and
Senior Associate in Medicine
University of Melbourne
Heidelberg, Victoria, Australia

A. van der Dries
Reanimation and Intensive Care
Sint Radboud Hospital
Catholic University of Nijmegen
Nijmegen, The Netherlands

E. van der Kleijn, Ph.D.
Department of Clinical Pharmacy
Sint Radboud Hospital
Catholic University of Nijmegen
Nijmegen, The Netherlands

H.-H. von Albert
Bezirkskrankenhous Günzburg
Fachkrankenhaus für Psychiatrie, Neurologie,
*   und Neurochirurgie*
Akademisches Krankenhaus für die Universität
*   Ulm*
8870 Günzburg, Federal Republic of Germany

T. B. Vree
Department of Pharmacy
Sint Radboud Hospital
Catholic University of Nijmegen
Nijmegen, The Netherlands

Gwendolyn H. Waddell, R. N., BSN,
MSN
Assistant Professor
Duke University School of Nursing
Durham, North Carolina 27710

J. E. Walker, MS, M.D.
Associate Professor
Department of Neurology
University of Texas Health Science Center, and
Chief of Neurology Service
Veterans Administration Medical Center
Dallas, Texas 75235

Arthur A. Ward, Jr., M.D.
Professor and Chairman
Department of Neurological Surgery
University of Washington School of Medicine
Seattle, Washington 98195

Claude G. Wasterlain, M.D.
Professor and Vice Chairman
Department of Neurology
University of California (Los Angeles) School of
*   Medicine, and*
Chief of Neurology Service
Veterans Administration Medical Center
Sepulveda, California 91343

B. J. Wilder, M.D.
Professor and Chief
Neurology Service
Veterans Administration Medical Center, and
Department of Neurology
University of Florida College of Medicine
Gainsville, Florida 32602

Dixon M. Woodbury, Ph.D.
Professor
Division of Neuropharmacology and
*   Epileptology*
University of Utah College of Medicine
Salt Lake City, Utah 84132

Prologue

The earliest reference I have found to status epilepticus, or what can by inference be taken to refer to status epilepticus, dates to the first century. According to that reference, when an epileptic attack extended into the second day, a fatal outcome was to be expected. Depending on the source, this observation has been attributed to a Roman physician, Caelius Aurielianus (5), or to the Greek, Soranus of Ephesus, personal physician to the emperors Trajan and Hadrian (1). Regardless of the source, it suggests that for 2,000 years, we have known that prolonged convulsive states can occur and that they can be serious. Nevertheless, subsequent reports were few and far between, until the 1820s, when a French physician, Calmiel, first clearly articulated the concept of status epilepticus, or *état de mal* as being separate or distinct from individual attacks (5). Since then, more numerous reports of status epilepticus have appeared, and by the 1950s, the concept was extended to include status epilepticus involving other than convulsive seizures. Noting that the increasing attention was roughly coeval with the use of antiepileptic drugs, Hunter (2) in 1959 speculated that the drugs might in some way be responsible for the increased incidence of status epilepticus. Some support for this assumption, other than the well-known risk after sudden withdrawal of drugs, comes from the fact that some of the earliest reported cases of petit mal status were attributed to the use of phenytoin (6). More recently, the apparent paradoxical effects of benzodiazepines both to produce and to control episodes of status epilepticus have been reported (4).

Whether or not the condition is in fact more common now than 100 years ago, and whether or not the drugs cause the condition, it would be difficult to speak of an information explosion in regard to status epilepticus. Virtually every textbook on clinical neurology mentions status epilepticus, but that is about all; such discussions occupy less than one-tenth of one percent of the pages—at least, this is the case for the dozen English language texts I surveyed. The epilepsy indexes (3) recently published by the National Institute of Neurological and Communicative Disorders and Stroke claimed to contain citations to most of the scientific literature on epilepsy as of 1978. Yet only 215 of the total 35,000 citations were indexed as either primary or secondary references to status epilepticus. This volume, then, is a timely and much needed effort to correct this deficiency.

However, in addition to the traditional function of presenting information, this volume also attempts to develop a state of the art about the management of status epilepticus. This takes the form of the summary.

A fundamental problem is the definition of status epilepticus: We will reach consensus on other problems such as incidence and preferred treatment only when we agree on what status epilepticus is. At first thought, this should not be a major problem for the clinician, because the dramatic nature of continuous convulsions should present no problem in recognition. However, it is one thing to recognize when an individual patient is in status epilepticus or close to it, so that something urgent can be done, but it is another matter when we attempt to compare our findings and results with those of other clinicians. For this latter purpose, we must agree upon how long a convulsion lasts and how many attacks occur at what intervals for categorization as status epilepticus.

In status epilepticus, consciousness is not regained between successive attacks as it is with serial seizures. But is there, in fact, any evidence that different pathophysiological mechanisms are operating or that the risks to patients are fundamentally different in these two conditions? If the answer is no, as I suspect it is, then this definition makes a distinction that is of no theoretical or practical value. Even if we could find a rationale for agreement on the role played by the interictal loss of consciousness, it would not be of much help in those situations in which consciousness is not lost, either ictally or interictally—for example, with frequently repeated partial seizures or in petit mal or spike-wave stupor. In our own experience, such cases constitute a significant portion of the total. Can we abstract from the different clinical types of status epilepticus a common principle that will permit a single unifying definition, or, for practical purposes, will we need a series of definitions?

Ideally, our definitions of status epilepticus should be substantive, based on an understanding of the pathophysiological mechanisms involved, but at the same time, relevant to the practical needs of the clinical situation. However, the gaps in our current knowledge are likely to be such that we cannot frame a "unified-field" definition. Thus, we may need two sets of definitions: Those for the clinic probably will be descriptive, whereas those for the laboratory should be operational. I suggest that whatever the definitions, they be compatible with the International Classifications of the Epilepsies and Epileptic Seizures. Although these classifications are arbitrary, they have nevertheless been helpful in efforts to standardize data collection and reporting and thus have facilitated the exchange of information and acquisition of knowledge. The definitions of status epilepticus also will be arbitrary, but they can serve the same important purposes equally well.

There are important issues other than that of definition. With regard to mechanisms, status epilepticus is often considered to be essentially like individual seizures, only much more so. The mechanisms that produce single attacks are presumed to produce status epilepticus, except perhaps that the initiating stimulus, whatever it is, is more intense or prolonged. Conversely, the inhibitory process that stops individual attacks, whatever it is, may be lost. Treatment of status epilepticus relies on the same drugs that are used to prevent individual attacks, with the rationale that if moderate doses control a moderate expression of the epileptic process, then massive doses will control a massive expression of that same process. That they sometimes do work is no more confirmation than the response to bromides can be considered a confirmation of the old sexual venery theory of the cause of epilepsy.

Does status epilepticus in fact occur because of unique biochemical or pathophysiological mechanisms not present in individual attacks? Are the mechanisms different either in the different types of status epilepticus or in identical types of status resulting from different causes? Do the antiepileptic drugs in fact cause many cases of status epilepticus? To what degree do the mechanisms of status epilepticus in experimental models differ because of species differences or because of different methods of inducing the attacks? What drugs are most effective in the various experimental models and clinical situations? What should be done to treat status epilepticus other than administering antiepileptic drugs?

This last question raises the issue of the consequences of status epilepticus. There is evidence that prolonged seizure activity, even in the absence of secondary systemic metabolic abnormalities, results in increased metabolic demands and loss of normal regulatory processes so that the brain appears to consume its own substance. The clinical implications of this finding need to be clarified so that we can try to prevent or at least control the brain's autophagous behavior in status epilepticus. We will need to know, of course, the critical variables that require monitoring in order to measure this process and its response to any treatment.

The choice of drugs will continue to be determined largely by a pharmaceutical rather than by a pharmacodynamic principle. That is, drugs are used more for their solubility (hence, availability for parenteral administration) than for their mechanisms of action. Nevertheless, they are the only treatment we have, and we must continue to use them. Unfortunately, current drug use can only be described as chaotic. Management of the patient with status epilepticus is guided more by the opinion or experience of the clinician than by any rationale based on pharmacological principles or even controlled clinical trials. Nevertheless, some such principles and trials do exist, and are summarized in this volume. It is important that we consider the findings, combine them with the rest of our knowledge, and then use the results as guidelines in the treatment of status epilepticus.

Presented here are but a few of the important questions about status epilepticus. It is the responsibility of the contributors to this volume to identify further questions and to devise general strategies for seeking answers to them.

The collation and synthesis of current knowledge on this subject constitute a truly important effort, because the well-being, even the lives, of future victims of status epilepticus will depend in great degree on the information presented here.

Harold E. Booker
Veterans Administration Central Office
Washington, D.C.

REFERENCES

1. Adams, G. F. (1974): *Cerebrovascular Disability and the Aging Brain.* Churchill-Livingstone, London.
2. Hunter, R. A. (1959/60): Status epilepticus: History, incidence, and problems. *Epilepsia*, 1:162–188.
3. Penry, J. K. (editor) (1978): *Indexes to the Epilepsy Accessions of the Epilepsy Information System*, Vols. *1–3.* D. H. E. W. Publication No. (N.I.H.) 78–1819. U.S. Department of Health, Education, and Welfare, Bethesda, Md.
4. Tassinari, C. A., Dravet, C., Roger, J., Cano, J. P., and Gastaut, H. (1972): Tonic status epilepticus precipitated by intravenous benzodiazepine in five patients with Lennox-Gastaut syndrome. *Epilepsia*, 13:421–435.
5. Temkin, O. (1971): *The Falling Sickness*, ed. 2. The Johns Hopkins Press, Baltimore.
6. Tucker, M., and Forster, F. M. (1950): Petit mal epilepsy occurring in status. *Arch. Neurol. Psychiatry*, 64:823–827.

Advances in Neurology, Vol. 34: Status Epilepticus, edited by A.V. Delgado-Escueta, C.G. Wasterlain, D.M. Treiman, and R.J. Porter. Raven Press, New York © 1983.

1

Status Epilepticus: Frequency, Etiology, and Neurological Sequelae

W. Allen Hauser

"It seems very pretty," she said when she had finished it; "but it's *rather* hard to understand!" (You see she didn't like to confess, even to herself, that she couldn't make it out at all.) "Somehow it seems to fill my head with ideas—only I don't exactly know what they are! However, *somebody* killed *something*; that's clear, at any rate."

(Through the Looking Glass,
—Lewis Carroll)

Information regarding the frequency of status epilepticus, its precipitating and concurrent events, and the prognosis for affected patients is limited to data from case reports and clinical series. Patients are usually identified by searching for a history of status epilepticus in outpatient records of patients with chronic epilepsy, or by reviewing records of hospital admissions for epilepsy. Less frequently, patients are identified at the time of admission for status epilepticus. Most reports have dealt with groups selected by age of occurrence and/or by clinical characteristics associated with the status episode. Thus, there are studies limited to status epilepticus in neonates, children, or adults and studies of status epilepticus in association with febrile illness, head trauma, or brain tumors. Few studies allow comparison of the occurrence of status epilepticus across all age groups and etiologies, and in none is it possible to define a population at risk for which incidence rates may be determined.

Obvious outcome biases will be associated with some of the foregoing methodologies. Evaluation of status epilepticus based on its occurrence in a clinic population of epileptic patients selects for an individual who not only has experienced chronic and recurring seizures but also has survived an episode of status epilepticus. Identification of status epilepticus by review of patients hospitalized with a diagnosis of epilepsy frequently will exclude those with status epilepticus associated with acute systemic or acute neurological insults. In this situation, status epilepticus or epilepsy will seldom be a recorded diagnosis; rather, the diagnosis will be that of the underlying medical or neurological illness.

The definition of status epilepticus has been inconsistent among the published studies. The World Health Organization *Dictionary of Epilepsy* (25) defines status epilepticus as "a condition characterized by an epileptic seizure that is sufficiently prolonged or repeated at sufficiently brief intervals so as to produce an unvarying and enduring epileptic condition." Unfortunately, "unvarying and enduring" has yet to be defined, leaving most authors to formulate their own definitions. "Prolonged motor seizure activity" (57), uncontrolled seizure activity (62), and acute repetitious seizures (70) have all been used to define status after the foregoing definition has been cited.

The absolute duration of continuing seizure activity has been the most common criteria for a diagnosis of status epilepticus, but that duration has varied considerably. On the one hand, patients with seizures as brief as 10 min in duration have been considered to have status epilepticus; on the other hand, Clark and Prout (15,16) considered status to be the maximum development of epilepsy (8–10 hr). Most frequently, status epilepticus has been defined as any seizure lasting 30 min or more (13,14,30,59) or 1 hr or more (1,12). Some authors have included patients who do not regain consciousness between repeated and sequential convulsions, patients who have sequential seizures (34,59,61), and patients who are unable to follow commands after regaining consciousness (59). It is not implicit that these latter patients will meet minimum temporal criteria for status epilepticus (30 or 60 min).

RELATIVE FREQUENCY OF STATUS EPILEPTICUS

No incidence rates for status epilepticus exist; only reports of the relative frequency of status epilepticus among epileptic patients admitted to the hospital, epileptic patients treated in the outpatient clinic, or some combination thereof are available. The proportion of patients with epilepsy who have experienced status epilepticus at some time ranges from 1.3% to 16% (Table 1). Most studies of adults have reported status epilepticus as a first seizure episode to be rare, but a seizure more than 1 hr in duration occurred as the initial seizure in 70% of the cases of status epilepticus reported by Aicardi and Chevrie (1). Conversely, among 1,047 newly diagnosed patients with epilepsy in Minneapolis, 132 (12.6%) had seizures more than 30 min in duration as their initial episodes (30).

Age

It is difficult to find information regarding the age-specific occurrence of status epilepticus, but its relative frequency appears to be greatest in younger age groups. Aicardi and Chevrie (1) reported that 16% of children with the diagnosis of epilepsy prior to age 15 years had experienced status epilepticus at some time, and in this series a higher proportion of patients with epilepsy ex-

perienced status epilepticus in the first 2 years of life than in subsequent years. In Minneapolis, 24% of all children with a first nonfebrile seizure prior to age 10 years presented with status epilepticus, a higher rate than in any other age group (31).

Sex

Aicardi and Chevrie (1) reported a slight excess of males among 239 children with status epilepticus. In this series males outnumbered females among symptomatic seizure cases, but a female excess was noted among idiopathic cases. In Minneapolis, the percentages of patients with first seizures in whom status epilepticus had occurred were similar for males (13%) and females (12%) (30).

Seizure Type

Classification of status epilepticus by seizure type, based on the current international classification of seizures (24), or a modification thereof, has been provided in several studies (Table 2). Prolonged confusional states (nonconvulsive status) associated with either generalized spike-wave EEG patterns (petit mal status) or focal temporal ictal activity (complex partial status), if included, have usually been separately classified, and in none of the large studies of patients with status epilepticus has epilepsia partialis continua (Kojevnikov epilepsy) been discussed as a specific entity.

Distribution by seizure type depends to some extent on the age group studied. In studies including adults (30) or limited to adults (3,13), partial seizures (usually with secondary generalization) have been the prominent seizure type. In children, generalized-onset seizures have represented the predominant seizure type (1). It is unclear to what extent prolonged generalized febrile convulsions account for this excess.

Seizures lasting more than 30 min occur in slightly over 5% of patients experiencing febrile convulsions (29,45,46). Because between 2.5% and 5% of children in the United States are known to experience febrile convulsions, one may estimate the population frequency of status epilepticus due to this one cause to be between 125 and 250 per 100,000 children (31). Roughly 30% of Aicardi's cases of status epilepticus were attributed to febrile convulsions (1). If his series is representative of the relative distribution of status epilepticus as it occurs in the general childhood population, between 4 and 8 of every 1,000 children may be

TABLE 1. *Relative proportions of status epilepticus in selected clinical series*

Reference	N	%	Source
Rowan and Scott (59)	50	0.02	Total hospital admissions, all ages
Hunter (33)	30	1.3	Status in adult epileptic admissions to general hospital, London
Bridge (10)	50	2.2	Outpatients—children with absence seizures only
Celesia (13)	60	2.6	Adults; hospital admissions for epilepsy
Edoo (19)	12	2.8	Referral to EEG lab with diagnosis of epilepsy
Edoo (19)	24	3.3	Admissions to tertiary-care facility for epilepsy
Oxbury and Whitty (54)	86	3.4	All ages; hospital admissions for epilepsy
Janz and Kautz (35)	95	3.7	Status history among adult clinic seizure patients, Heidelberg
Turner (68)	15	5	Outpatients with history of status
Nelson and Ellenberg (45,46)	98	5.4[a]	Febrile convulsions—collaborative perinatal project
Hauser and Kurland (29)	28	5.7[a]	Febrile convulsions—population of Rochester, Minnesota
Oxbury and Whitty (54)	86	6.6	Adults; hospital admissions for epilepsy
Heintel (32)	41	7.6	Status in epileptic admissions to a general hospital
Lennox (37)	124	8	Pediatric clinic seizure patients with a history of status
Chevrie and Aicardi (14)	40	9.1	Status or history of status in inpatients or outpatients with history of seizures in the first year of life
Hauser (30)	132	12.3	Newly diagnosed seizure patients of any age seen in hospital or clinic
Aicardi and Chevrie (1)	239	16	Status or history of status in inpatients with history of seizures under age 15

[a]Proportion of febrile status epilepticus in all patients with febrile seizures.

TABLE 2. *Classification of status epilepticus by seizure type*

			Partial			
Reference	Generalized (%)	Uni-lateral (%)	Motor (%)	Secondary generalized (%)	Other (%)	Non-convulsive (%)
Aminoff and Simon (3)	38			62		
Celesia (13)	27		20	28		25
Hauser (30)	23		72			5
Aicardi and Chevrie (1)	51	39		5	5	
Forster et al. (21)	33		33			33

expected to experience status epilepticus prior to age 15.

ETIOLOGY OF STATUS EPILEPTICUS

Status epilepticus has generally been categorized as either idiopathic (usually status epilepticus in patients with idiopathic epilepsy) or symptomatic. Criteria for inclusion (or exclusion) as an idiopathic case have seldom been defined. Further, authors seldom clearly distinguish between status epilepticus associated with an acute neurological or metabolic insult and status epilepticus occurring in patients with a history of neurological insult produced by a static or slowly progressive neurological deficit. Because the outcomes may be

very different in these two subgroups, it is important to make a distinction between acute and chronic precipitants. Table 3 shows the relative proportions of patients with status epilepticus associated with symptomatic epilepsy from acute CNS insults or systemic disturbances and chronic but static CNS lesions (e.g., stroke, prior encephalitis or anoxic insult) and idiopathic epilepsy, as reported in several clinical series. Idiopathic cases accounted for no more than one-third of status epilepticus cases in most of the clinical series reviewed, and the majority of cases in most series were attributed to symptomatic insults. The only discrepancies occurred in the small series of Edoo (only 12 cases) (20) and the study of neonatal

TABLE 3. *Etiology of status epilepticus*

| | | Symptomatic | | |
| | | Chronic neurological state (%) | Acute systemic or neurological insult (%) | Idiopathic (%) |
Reference	N			
Janz and Kautz (35)	95	55	11	34
Oxbury and Whitty (54)	86	52	12	36
Whitty and Taylor (71)	25	61	22	17
Rowan and Scott (59)	42	56	25	29
Hunter (33)	30	73	0	27
Celesia et al. (12)	60	53	9	38
Aicardi and Chevrie (1)[a]	172	37	29	34
Aminoff and Simon (3)	51	29	45	26
Hauser (30)[a,b]	125	31	35	34
Dreyfus-Brisac and Monod (17)[c]	57	10		90
Edoo (19)	12	6	44	50

[a]Excludes febrile seizures.
[b]First-seizure patients.
[c]Neonatal status.

seizures reported by Dreyfus-Brisac and Monod (17). In the neonatal seizure group, the status epilepticus may have a totally different pathophysiological basis, explaining the apparent excess of idiopathic cases.

Among patients with epilepsy, status epilepticus tends to occur most frequently in those with history of neurological insult prior to the onset of seizures (symptomatic epilepsy) (34,37). In the series of Janz and Kautz (35), status epilepticus occurred in 9% of patients with symptomatic epilepsy, but in only 1.6% of patients with idiopathic epilepsy. In the Minneapolis series of first seizures, 16% of patients with a prior history of CNS insults presented with status epilepticus, compared with 9% of patients with newly identified idiopathic seizures (30).

Specific causes of seizures in status epilepticus patients are outlined in Table 4. The distribution of antecedent illness varies greatly depending on the age group studied. In series limited to children, febrile seizures and CNS infections accounted for the majority of cases of symptomatic status epilepticus. In series including or limited to adults, head trauma, cerebrovascular disease, and CNS neoplasms accounted for the majority of symptomatic status epilepticus.

Janz and Kautz (35) examined the frequency of status epilepticus in patients within specific categories of diseases. In their series, 16% of patients with epilepsy attributed to brain tumors experi-

enced status epilepticus at some time during the course of illness (over half as the first seizure), and status epilepticus occurred at some time in 11% of all patients with posttraumatic epilepsy. In Minneapolis, 40% of patients with a first seizure attributable to CNS infections experienced status epilepticus. The first seizure met status epilepticus criteria in 20%, 16%, and 14% of those cases associated with CNS trauma, neoplasms, and cerebrovascular episodes, respectively.

A propensity for status epilepticus to occur in association with frontal lobe lesions has been observed (29,34,71). In one series, frontal lesions were identified in 74% of patients with status epilepticus associated with CNS neoplasms and 94% of patients with status epilepticus associated with CNS trauma (34). A similar propensity for frontal lesions to be identified at autopsy of patients diagnosed as having status epilepticus was cited by Janz (34). This observation was not confirmed in the autopsied cases reported by Rowan and Scott (59).

It has been suggested that status epilepticus seldom occurs as the initial manifestation of idiopathic epilepsy; rather, it is primarily a concomitant of a chronic epileptic state that in some way establishes a milieu in which status epilepticus can occur (33,34,53). Thus, when status epilepticus occurs in patients with a diagnosis of idiopathic epilepsy, the mean interval between onset of epilepsy and the first episode of status epilepticus is

TABLE 4. *Suspected causes of brain pathology in patients with status epilepticus*

Cause	Celesia (13) N = 60	Rowan and Scott (59) N = 42	Janz and Kautz (35) N = 95	Hauser (30) N = 132	Aicardi and Chevrie (1) N = 239	Oxbury and Whitty (54) N = 86
Idiopathic	38%	11 (29%)	32 (34%)	42 (32%)	59 (25%)	32 (36%)
Craniocerebral trauma	12%	11 (26%)	23 (24%)	23 (17%)	2 (1%)	7 (9%)
Neoplasm	5%	—	24 (25%)	4 (3%)	0	19 (22%)
Cerebrovascular disease	15%	3 (7%)	4 (4%)	17 (13%)	0	13 (15%)
Other	25%	5 (12%)	7 (7%)	20 (15%)	(26%)	2 (2%)
CNS infection	5%	4 (10%)	3 (8%)	19 (15%)	29 (12%)	9 (10%)
Febrile	—	2 (5%)	—	7 (5%)	67 (28%)	—
Congenital abnormalities and birth defects	—	7 (17%)	3 (3%)	—	20 (8%)	4 (5%)

12 years (33,36). Further, the true etiology in "idiopathic" status cases must also be questioned. Although Oxbury and Whitty (53) initially categorized 9 of their patients with status epilepticus as a first seizure as having "idiopathic epilepsy," brain tumors were identified in 7 of these patients within 2 to 7 years after the status episode. Neither of these tenets holds true if patients with first seizures rather than status epilepticus are studied. In the Minneapolis study (30), convulsions lasting longer than 30 min occurred in 8% of all patients with a first seizure that was considered idiopathic, and in none of these patients (followed for a mean of 2 years) have brain tumors been identified.

INDUCERS OF STATUS EPILEPTICUS

A distinction must be made between an acute disease process that may cause status epilepticus and factors that may trigger status epilepticus in epileptic patients. In patients with preexisting epilepsy, status epilepticus has been attributed to withdrawal of anticonvulsant medication, alcohol abuse, sleep deprivation, or intercurrent infection. Some of these same factors (e.g., alcohol withdrawal) considered to be "etiologic" in an individual without a history of epilepsy are considered to be triggering factors in a patient with a history of epilepsy. Discontinuation of anticonvulsant medication frequently has been the sole factor associated with status epilepticus (3,33,59). The intervals between medication withdrawal or reduction and status epilepticus have seldom been designated. When this information has been provided, intervals frequently have been sufficiently long to exclude any known pharmacological effect related to acute reduction of the anticonvulsant concentration in the blood. Tonic status epilepticus has been induced in some patients by intravenous administration of diazepam (58,65).

PROGNOSIS

Patients with status epilepticus may die because of their seizures per se, but more often they die of the acute illness (e.g., meningitis or stroke) that has precipitated the status epilepticus. Mortality data, as reported from several of the clinical series of status epilepticus, are summarized in Table 5. Over the past century, there has been a general reduction in acute mortality. Early deaths in recent studies have occurred almost exclusively in symptomatic cases and have generally been attributed to the precipitating symptomatic illness. Deaths have seldom been reported among patients with idiopathic epilepsy who have status epilepticus. Currently, death attributable to status epilepticus alone is rare. When such deaths do occur they are generally associated with respiratory or cardiac arrest and at times are associated with the intravenous use of anticonvulsant agents. Less obvious causes of seizure-related deaths have been reported; fatalities have been attributed to renal failure secondary to myoglobinuria (64). Patients who have experienced status epilepticus may also be at increased risk of death subsequent to the status epilepticus, but this is usually due to a preexisting condition responsible for the status epilepticus. The contribution of a prolonged seizure to late mortality is unclear.

TIME TRENDS

Hunter (33) contended that status epilepticus was virtually unknown prior to the use of anticonvulsant medication for epilepsy, basing this theory on

TABLE 5. *Mortality among patients with status epilepticus*

Reference	Year	N	Acute mortality (%)			Late mortality (%)
			Seizure	Non-seizure	Total	
Brown (11)	1873				32	
Binswanger (6)	1886				50	
Lorenz (41)	1890				45	
Gowers (27)	1901				18	
Clark and Prout (16)	1904				33	
Turner (68)	1907	15			20	
Hunter (33)	1959				23	
Lennox (37)	1960	127			3	
Janz and Kautz (35)	1963	68			7	
Dreyfus-Brisac and Monod (17)	1964	57				53
Brett (9)	1966					18
Aicardi and Chevrie (1)	1970	237			4	7
Rowan and Scott (59)	1970	42	25	17	23	
Oxbury and Whitty (53)	1971	86	7	7	8	35
Heintel (32)	1972	83	1	24	25	
Celesia (13)	1976	60	7		7	18
Bladin et al. (7)	1977	10				30
Aminoff and Simon (3)	1980	98	2	14	16	
Hauser (30)	1980	132				6

the paucity of reports of prolonged convulsions prior to the introduction of bromides in the nineteenth century. Lennox (37), however, suggested that status epilepticus occurred less frequently in 1960 than earlier in this century. Although there is no proof that the actual incidence of status epilepticus is changing, it does appear that in England the mortality attributable to epilepsy fell dramatically between 1931 and 1956. Although coding practices could account for a portion of this reduction, it seems likely that a true decrease in mortality occurred over this period. More than 25% of these deaths were reported among patients in mental hospitals, and status epilepticus was most frequently indexed as a cause of death among these patients. Thus, by inference, mortality due to status epilepticus may also be decreasing.

In England, status epilepticus was separately indexed as a cause of death from 1949, and Hunter (33) determined annual death rates attributable to status epilepticus from 1949 through 1956. Although there was a trend toward lower rates, the change is not convincing. It is likely that this 7-year window is insufficient to demonstrate a change in the death rate, even if such has occurred, and a reduction over this period would be surprising, because no obvious therapeutic breakthrough occurred during that period.

NEUROLOGICAL SEQUELAE OF STATUS EPILEPTICUS

The relative contribution of a prolonged seizure per se to subsequent neurological abnormalities is difficult to evaluate. In most clinical series, adverse outcomes following status epilepticus have frequently been confounded by history of prior neurological insult, preexisting neurological deficit of uncertain cause, and/or the precipitation of status epilepticus by an entity that itself may be associated with subsequent poor neurological outcome. Adverse outcomes discussed by most authors, aside from mortality, include (a) mental retardation (children) or intellectual deterioration (adults), (b) permanent neurological residual, and (c) continuing recurrent seizures.

Status epilepticus alone has been implicated in the production of brain damage in several neuropathological studies (18,44,48–50,63). Also, there have been individual case reports of cerebral atrophy following status epilepticus, and in two instances serial documentation of cerebral atrophy following status epilepticus was provided. Aicardi and Baraton (2) reported progressive ventricular enlargement in 13 of 15 patients in whom serial pneumoencephalography was performed following status epilepticus, and in the San Francisco General Hospital series 2 patients showed increasing cerebral atrophy on serial CT scanning (3).

Most studies have reported a positive association between adverse outcome and duration of status epilepticus. The proportion of cases with adverse outcomes of all types tends to increase with increasing duration of status epilepticus. An adverse outcome is more likely when a preexisting neurological lesion is identified (54,59). Females experiencing status epilepticus are said to have a higher frequency of adverse outcomes than males. Also, those with a family history of epilepsy are said to have a lower frequency of adverse outcomes (1).

It has been suggested that status epilepticus occurring at an early age has a higher association with long-term neurological sequelae than status epilepticus occurring in older age groups, but this age effect is not universally accepted. Aicardi and Chevrie (1) stated that "prolonged convulsions seem more devastating in young babies. Whether this is due to a great susceptibility of the developing brain or a greater severity and longer duration of convulsions is uncertain." However, Grand (28) stated that "children are more likely to respond to minor brain injury with status epilepticus, with less severe prognosis than in adults."

Few reports have dealt with outcomes of status epilepticus across all ages and by diverse causes. Further, differences in methods of case selection and definitions make direct comparisons between studies difficult. To obtain a comprehensive picture of the frequency of sequelae, one must consider the results from several studies dealing with disparate patient groups.

Reports on status epilepticus, particularly those involving children, tend to originate from specialty hospitals and referral centers; thus the effect of referral bias must also be considered in evaluating outcomes reported from such centers. Many reports on status epilepticus are confounded by the inclusion of both patients with a past history of status epilepticus identified at the time of evaluation for seizures, mental retardation, or other neurological difficulty and patients identified at the time of their status epilepticus and followed prospectively. This will clearly increase the apparent frequency of these complications.

Status Epilepticus in the First Year of Life

Chevrie and Aicardi (14) reported long-term outcomes for 313 of 437 patients with seizures starting in the first year of life. Thirty-five of these patients had status epilepticus. Cases were divided into two groups: cryptogenic (no identified prior neurological insult or abnormality) and symptomatic (prior neurological abnormality, mental retardation, and/or demonstrable brain abnormality). Among the 140 cryptogenic cases of epilepsy, 15 patients (11%) experienced status epilepticus. Although subsequent neurological abnormalities and severe mental retardation occurred in 40% and 27%, respectively, the proportion experiencing adverse outcomes was similar to that among the cryptogenic patients who had not experienced status epilepticus. Even after patients with infantile spasms (a group known to be at high risk for mental retardation and neurological abnormalities) were excluded from the non-status-epilepticus group, the proportions of patients noted to have adverse outcomes were similar in the status epilepticus group and the non-status-epilepticus group.

Symptomatic status epilepticus was associated with higher proportions of subsequent neurological abnormality (50%) and mental retardation (75%), but the proportions were again similar to those noted among patients with symptomatic epilepsy without status epilepticus. Because the outcome measures (mental retardation, neurological deficit) were prerequisites for inclusion in the symptomatic group in some instances, the exact meaning of these very high percentages of adverse outcomes in the symptomatic group is unclear.

Mental retardation occurred more frequently if the status epilepticus episode occurred prior to age 6 months, but the frequency of neurological abnormalities appeared to be independent of age. A history of prenatal or perinatal abnormality prior to status epilepticus was associated with increased frequency of mental retardation or neurological abnormalities. A family history of epilepsy or febrile seizures was associated with decreased frequency of adverse neurological outcomes.

Status Epilepticus in Older Children

Aicardi and Chevrie (1) followed children in whom status epilepticus occurred before the 15th birthday and reported the frequency of untoward sequelae. Among 239 patients, 63 (26%) had concurrent systemic or CNS insults, 67 (28%) had febrile seizures, 50 (21%) had chronic encephalopathy, and 59 (25%) had no concurrent illness or prior neurological abnormality. Unfortunately, only 142 of these patients (59%) were seen at the time status epilepticus occurred. The other 97 (41%) were identified subsequent to the first status episode "for investigation of sequelae, residual epilepsy or because of recurrent status." Many of these patients had experienced recurrent seizures prior to the episode of status epilepticus.

Among all status epilepticus patients, 73% have experienced subsequent seizures. However, among those patients presenting with status epilepticus, only 36% have had subsequent seizures. Abnormal neurological findings after the status episode were noted in 88 patients (37%). Among this number, 41 patients (15%) had abnormalities that were identified prior to the status episode. Mental retardation occurred in 114 (48%), but 36 (15%) were known to have had an abnormal mental status prior to the status episode.

Febrile Status Epilepticus

Patients with febrile seizures are known to be at increased risk for subsequent epilepsy. This risk is higher among children experiencing more prolonged convulsions (45). The risk for recurrent afebrile seizures among patients experiencing febrile status (convulsions lasting longer 30 min) in the absence of preexisting neurological disease is 8% by age 20 (5). This compares with a 1% risk for recurrent seizures by that age in the general population and a 3% risk for recurrent seizures for those with brief "simple" febrile convulsions (5,31).

Lindsay, Ounsted, and associates (38–40,52) have evaluated long-term outcomes in a group of 100 children with "temporal lobe epilepsy." As shown in Table 6, three subgroups were studied: those with a history of status epilepticus (predominantly febrile) prior to the diagnosis of temporal lobe epilepsy, those with a history of neurological dysfunction, and those with neither status epilepticus nor neurological abnormality at the time of onset of seizures (idiopathic cases). Given the mean age at onset of febrile seizures (18 months), it is not surprising that patients with status epilepticus in this series were significantly younger at the time of the first seizure (16 months) than those with either prior CNS insults (36 months) or idiopathic epilepsy (58 months). The (febrile) status epilepticus group also had an earlier age of onset for temporal lobe epilepsy than the other two groups.

TABLE 6. *Outcome for 100 children with temporal lobe epilepsy*

	Prior status $N = 32$	Prior insult $N = 35$	Idiopathic $N = 33$
Mean age at first seizure (months)	16	36	58
Mean age at temporal lobe seizure (months)	50	67	90
Mean IQ, performance	80	82	105
Mean IQ, verbal	78	76	105
Hyperkinesis (%)	28	40	9
Seizure-free at follow-up (%)	31	14	55
Independent with seizures at follow-up (%)	25	31	40
Dependent or institutionalized at follow-up (%)	38	46	6

From Lindsay et al. (38–40).

IQ test results were significantly lower and the frequency of hyperkinesis was greater in the status epilepticus group than in the idiopathic cases. In both of these aspects, the status epilepticus patients were similar to those with prior neurological insults. In an evaluation of functional outcome, status epilepticus patients were intermediate between the idiopathic patients and the neurological insult patients in regard to the proportion capable of living independently and the proportion who were seizure-free at follow-up. Psychiatric and other social outcomes were evaluated, but data on status epilepticus patients were not provided separately.

In 54% of status epilepticus cases, a first-degree relative also had seizures. Status epilepticus patients with a positive family history were more likely to have well-controlled seizures or to have achieved total seizure remission than status epilepticus patients without a family history of seizures.

As in Aicardi's study, patients with early onset of seizures were more likely to demonstrate problems at follow-up than those with late onset, but the frequency of adverse outcome among patients with status epilepticus at an early age was no greater than that for seizure patients with onset at a similar age.

Status Epilepticus in Adults

Much less information regarding neurological sequelae following status epilepticus is available for adults. Studies of adults have included few cases of status epilepticus as an initial event. Thus, for adults, interpretation of the causal sequence of neurological difficulty after an episode of status epilepticus is even more frequently confounded by preexisting epilepsy and the conditions responsible for epilepsy than in studies of children. In only two adult series have outcomes other than mortality been evaluated. Among 47 patients followed after status epilepticus by Oxbury and Whitty (54), 5 patients showed evidence of subsequent neurological deterioration. Encephalitis was the cause of status epilepticus in 3 of these patients, whereas in the other 2 patients (both of whom had suffered from "idiopathic" seizures for several years prior to the status episode) there was evidence of progressive neurological deterioration preceding the occurrence of status epilepticus. Aminoff and Simon (3) reported intellectual impairment of neurological dysfunction in 11 of 84 survivors of episodes of status epilepticus at San Francisco General Hospital. In 4 of these patients the deterioration could be attributed to the underlying cause of the status epilepticus; in 7 patients, status epilepticus itself was the only factor identified.

NONCONVULSIVE STATUS EPILEPTICUS

A number of case reports of patients with "nonconvulsive status" have reached the medical literature over the past 35 years. This term includes patients with "absence status" (4,8,9,22,23,44, 47,51,58,60,66,67) and patients with "complex partial" status (20,21,42,43,55,69).

Absence status (petit mal status, prolonged petit mal automatism, spike-wave stupor, epilepsia minor continua) is manifest clinically by a prolonged confusional state frequently associated with myoclonic jerks (4). Usually these patients have a history of generalized seizures. Interictally, patients demonstrate spike-wave EEG patterns, but during the absence status episode the EEG patterns may include continuous or intermittent generalized spikes and waves or a generalized rhythmic slowing. Multifocal spikes have also been described (9).

Absence status may occur at any age, but it is said to be rare before age 10. This phenomenon occurs in 3% of all absence patients, although over 10% of adults who continue to suffer from absence seizures are said to have absence status at some time (4,26). The absence status episodes frequently are terminated by generalized tonic-clonic seizures.

Another form of nonconvulsive status has been termed partial complex status (psychomotor status or temporal lobe status). Partial complex status may occur in association with a preexisting convulsive disorder (presumably in patients with partial complex seizures) or as the sole manifestation of an epileptic condition (20). Electroencephalographically, the ictal patterns consist of continuous epileptiform activity, at times localized to one temporal area but frequently shifting over from one hemisphere to the other or involving the front temporal areas bilaterally. Partial complex status epilepticus has been less frequently reported than absence status.

Among 60 adult patients with status epilepticus reported by Celesia (13), 15 (25%) experienced nonconvulsive status. Petit mal (absence) status epilepticus was diagnosed in 13 of these cases, and psychomotor status (complex partial) was diagnosed in 2 cases. In a German study of 100 patients with status epilepticus, 35 (35%) had nonconvulsive status (33 petit mal, 2 psychomotor) (21). If this proportion of patients with nonconvulsive status among these series is representative, many patients with nonconvulsive status go unidentified. In the study of first seizures in Minneapolis (30), 6 of the 125 patients having status epilepticus as a first seizure event experienced nonconvulsive status.

Seldom has long-term outcome for patients with nonconvulsive status been evaluated. Most large studies of status epilepticus (particularly among adults) have dealt only with patients with generalized convulsive episodes. Although prolonged postictal deficits have been documented in some cases, no evidence of permanent intellectual deterioration has yet been reported.

Brett (9) reported 22 cases of "minor epileptic status" involving children, differentiating these cases from "petit mal status" by the presence of myoclonus and less frequently occurring spike-wave patterns on EEG. These status episodes lasted from days to months. Seizures preceded the onset of these status episodes in 68%. At long-term follow-up, 4 of these patients had died (1 patient in generalized status). Only 6 patients (27%) remained intellectually normal, and degenerative neurological syndromes were identified at follow-up in 14%. The causal sequence of deterioration in the remainder was not clear.

Gall and associates (23) reported frontal lobe abnormalities in 7 adults with absence status who had CT scans. In 1 patient a lucency was noted, and in 6 patients atrophy or asymmetric ventricles were noted. Four of these patients were over age 60, and in the absence of a control (nonseizure) population, the interpretation of such ventricular enlargement remains unclear.

Case reports of electrical status epilepticus are rare, and these patients usually are identified during the course of an evaluation for epilepsy. Even less frequently identified are patients with continuous ictal EEG abnormalities during sleep. The prognosis for such patients is uncertain. Patry and associates (56) reported 6 cases of electrical status occurring during sleep; all these patients were mentally retarded, and 5 had epilepsy.

SUMMARY

Status epilepticus is associated with high mortality and is a predictor of poor neurological outcome; yet the contribution of prolonged seizures to mortality and the causal sequence for neurological damage remain unclear. Many cases of status epilepticus are precipitated by illnesses that themselves are associated with increased mortality and morbidity. In studies of children, status epilepticus appears to be no better a predictor of an adverse outcome than is any seizure disorder starting at a similar age. Status epilepticus is a conditon in which fast and definitive medical intervention is warranted. Random assignment to treatment groups is difficult. Evaluation of the effect of duration of seizures is also difficult, because those patients responding promptly to treatment may be quite a different population than those not responding.

The study of cases of "nonconvulsive" status may provide information regarding the effect of these continuing ictal brain discharges, which can be evaluated without the confounding effects of concomitant metabolic (e.g., anoxic, pH, electrolyte) disturbances that accompany most cases of generalized status epilepticus.

It is possible that appropriately designed prospective studies of status epilepticus and/or case-control studies will assist in evaluating the contribution of a prolonged seizure per se over and above that associated with preexisting or concurrent illness.

ACKNOWLEDGMENTS

This research was supported in part by the Comprehensive Epilepsy Program, University of Minnesota grant 1-PO5-NS-16308-01 from the National Institute of Neurological and Communicative Disorders and Stroke.

The assistance of Connie M. Eves in manuscript preparation and typing is appreciated.

REFERENCES

1. Aicardi, J., and Chevrie, J. J. (1970): Convulsive status epilepticus in infants and children: A study of 239 cases. *Epilepsia*, 11:187–197.
2. Aicardi, J., and Baraton, J. (1971): A pneumoencephalographic demonstration of brain atrophy following status epilepticus. *Dev. Med. Child Neurol.*, 13:660–667.
3. Aminoff, M. J., and Simon, R. P. (1980): Status epilepticus: Causes, clinical features and consequences in 98 patients. *Am. J. Med.*, 69:657–666.
4. Andermann, F., and Robb, J. P. (1972): Absence status: A reappraisal following review of thirty-eight patients. *Epilepsia*, 13:177–187.
5. Annegers, J. E., Hauser, W. A., Elveback, L. R., and Kurland, L. T. (1979): The risk of epilepsy following febrile convulsions. *Neurology (Minneap.)*, 29:297–303.
6. Binswanger, O. (1886): *Eulenberg's Realencyclopadie, Vol. 6*; cited in Turner, W. A. (1907): *Epilepsy.* Macmillan, London.
7. Bladin, P. F., Vajda, F. J., and Symington, G. R. (1977): Therapeutic problems related to tonic status epilepticus. Proceedings of the Australian Association of Neurologists. *Clinical and Experimental Neurology*, 14:203–207.
8. Bower, B. D. (1972): Minor epileptic status. *Dev. Med. Child Neurol.*, 14:80–81.
9. Brett, E. M. (1966): Minor epileptic status. *J. Neurol. Sci.*, 3:52–75.
10. Bridge, E. M. (1949): *Epilepsy and Convulsive Disorders in Children.* McGraw-Hill, New York.
11. Browne, J. C. (1873): Notes on epilepsy and its pathological consequences. *J. Ment. Sci.*, 19:19–46; cited in Clark, L. P., and Prout, T. P. (1904): *Am. J. Insan.*, 61:81–108.
12. Celesia, G. G., Messert, B., and Murphy, M. J. (1972): Status epilepticus of late adult onset. *Neurology (Minneap.)*, 22:1047–1055.
13. Celesia, G. G. (1976): Modern concepts of status epilepticus. *J.A.M.A.*, 235:1571–1574.
14. Chevrie, J. J., and Aicardi, J. (1978): Convulsive disorders in the first year of life: Neurological and mental outcome and mortality. *Epilepsia*, 19:67–74.
15. Clark, L. P., and Prout, T. P. (1903): Status epilepticus: A clinical and pathological study in epilepsy. *Am. J. Insan.*, 60:291–306.
16. Clark, L. P., and Prout, T. P. (1904): Status epilepticus: A clinical and pathological study in epilepsy. *Am. J. Insan.*, 61:81–108.
17. Dreyfus-Brisac, C., and Monod, N. (1964): Electroclinical studies of status epilepticus and convulsions

in the newborn. In: *Neurological and Electroencephalographical Studies in Infancy*, edited by P. Kellaway and I. Petersen, pp. 250–271. Grune & Stratton, New York.

18. Earle, K. M., Baldwin, M., and Penfield, W. (1953): Incisural sclerosis and temporal lobe seizures produced by hippocampal herniation at birth. *Arch. Neurol. Psychiatr.*, 69:27–42.

19. Edoo, B. B. (1970): Clinico-electroencephalographic features of status epilepticus in Accra. *Ghana Med. J.*, 9:70–79.

20. Engel, J., Ludwig, B. I., and Fetell, M. (1978): Prolonged partial complex status epilepticus: EEG and behavioral observations. *Neurology (Minneap.)*, 28:863–869.

21. Forster, C., Ross, A., and Kugler, J. (1969): Psychomotor status epilepticus. *Electroencephalogr. Clin. Neurophysiol.*, 27:211.

22. Friedlander, W. J., and Feinstein, G. H. (1956): Petit mal status, epilepsia minoris continua. *Neurology (Minneap.)*, 6:357–362.

23. Gall, M., Scollo-Lavizzari, G., and Becker, H. (1978): Absence status in the adult. *Eur. Neurol.*, 17:121–128.

24. Gastaut, H. (1970): Clinical and electroencephalographical classification of epileptic seizures. *Epilepsia*, 11:102–113.

25. Gastaut, H. (editor) (1973): *Dictionary of Epilepsy, Part I: Definitions*. World Health Organization, Geneva.

26. Gibbs, F. A., and Gibbs, E. L. (1952): *Atlas of Electroencephalography, Vol. 2: Epilepsy*, p. 55. Addison Wesley, Cambridge, Mass.

27. Gowers, W. R. G. (1901): *Epilepsy and Other Chronic Convulsive Diseases*, ed. 2. Churchill, London.

28. Grand, W. (1974): The significance of post-traumatic status epilepticus in childhood. *J. Neurol. Neurosurg. Psychiatry*, 37:178–180.

29. Hauser, W. A., and Kurland, L. T. (1975): The epidemiology of epilepsy in Rochester, Minnesota, 1935 through 1967. *Epilepsia*, 16:1–66.

30. Hauser, W. A. (1980): Epidemiology, morbidity and mortality of status epilepticus. Presented at the International Symposium on Status Epilepticus, Santa Monica, California.

31. Hauser, W. A. (1981): The natural history of febrile seizures. In: *Febrile Seizures*, edited by K. B. Nelson and J. H. Ellenberg, pp. 5–17. Raven Press, New York.

32. Heintel, H. (1972): *Status Epilepticus, Etiology, Clinical Aspects and Lethality*, pp. 1–116. Gustav Kischer Verlag, Stuttgart.

33. Hunter, R. A. (1959/60): Status epilepticus: History, incidence and problems. *Epilepsia*, 1:162–188.

34. Janz, D. (1964): Status epilepticus and frontal lobe lesions. *J. Neurol. Sci.*, 1:44–457.

35. Janz, D., and Kautz, G. (1963): The aetiology and treatment of status epilepticus. *Dtsch. Med. Wochenschr.*, 88:2189.

36. Janz, D. (1961): Conditions and causes of status epilepticus. *Epilepsia*, 2:170–177.

37. Lennox, W. G. (1960): *Epilepsy and Related Disorders, Vol. 1*. Little, Brown, Boston.

38. Lindsay, J., Ounsted, C., and Richards, P. (1979): Long-term outcome in children with temporal lobe seizures. I. Social outcome and childhood factors. *Dev. Med. Child Neurol.*, 21:285–298.

39. Lindsay, I., Ounsted, C., and Richards, P. (1979): Long-term outcome in children with temporal lobe seizures. II. Marriage, parenthood, and sexual indifference. *Dev. Med. Child Neurol.*, 21:433–440.

40. Lindsay, J., Ounsted, C., and Richards, P. (1979): Long-term outcome in children with temporal lobe seizures. III. Psychiatric aspects in childhood and adult life. *Dev. Med. Child Neurol.*, 21:630–636.

41. Lorenz (1890): Diss. Inaug., Kiel; cited in Turner, W. A. (1907): *Epilepsy*, Macmillan, London.

42. Markand, O. M., Wheeler, G. L., and Pollack, S. L. (1978): Complex partial status epilepticus (psychomotor status). *Neurology (Minneap.)*, 28:189–196.

43. Mayeux, R., and Leuders, H. (1978): Complex partial status epilepticus: Case report and proposal for diagnostic criteria. *Neurology (Minneap.)*, 28:957–961.

44. Meyer, A., Beck, E., and Shepherd, M. (1955): Unusually severe lesions in the brain following status epilepticus. *J. Neurol. Neurosurg. Psychiatry*, 18:24–33.

45. Nelson, K. B., and Ellenberg, J. H. (1976): Predictors of epilepsy in children who have experienced febrile seizures. *N. Engl. J. Med.*, 295:1030–1033.

46. Nelson, K. B., and Ellenberg, J. H. (1978): Prognosis in children with febrile seizures. *Pediatrics*, 61:720–727.

47. Niedermeyer, E., Fineyre, F., Riley, T., and Uematsu, S. (1979): Absence status (petit mal status) with focal characteristics. *Arch. Neurol.*, 36:417–421.

48. Noel, P., Cornil, A., Chailly, P., and Flament-Durand, J. (1977): Mesial temporal haemorrhage, consequence of status epilepticus. *J. Neurol. Neurosurg. Psychiatry*, 40:932–935.

49. Norman, R. M. (1964): The neuropathology of status epilepticus. *Medicine and Law*, 4:660–667.

50. Norman, R. M. (1962): Neuropathological findings in acute hemiplegia in childhood. With special reference to epilepsy as a pathogenic factor. *Little Clubs Clin. Dev. Med.*, 6:37–48.

51. Novak, J., Corke, P., and Fairley, N. (1971): "Petit mal status" in adults. *Dis. Nerv. Syst.*, 32:245–248.

52. Ounsted, C., Lindsay, J., and Norman, R. (1966): *Biological Factors in Temporal Lobe Epilepsy*. Lanenham Press, Lavenham, Suffolk, England.

53. Oxbury, J. M., and Whitty, C. W. M. (1971): The syndrome of isolated epileptic status. *J. Neurol. Neurosurg. Psychiatry*, 34:182–184.

54. Oxbury, J. M., and Whitty, C. W. M. (1971): Causes and consequences of status epilepticus in adults: A study of 86 cases. *Brain*, 94:733–744.

55. Pasquet, E. G., de Gaudin, E. S., Bianchi, A., and De Mendilaharsu, S. A. (1976): Prolonged and monosymptomatic dysphasic status epilepticus. *Neurology (Minneap.)*, 26:244–247.

56. Patry, G., Lyagoubi, S., and Tassinari, A. (1971): Subclinical "electrical status epilepticus" induced by sleep in children. *Arch. Neurol.*, 24:242–252.

57. Prensky, A. L., Raff, M. C., Moore, M. J., and Schwab, R. S. (1964): Intravenous diazepam in the treatment

of prolonged seizure activity. *N. Engl. J. Med.*, 276:779–784.

58. Prior, P. M., MacLaine, M., Scott, D. F., and Laurence M. (1972): Tonic status epilepticus precipitated by intravenous diazepam in a child with petit mal status. *Epilepsia*, 13:467–472.
59. Rowan, A. J., and Scott, D. F. (1970): Major status epilepticus: A series of 42 patients. *Acta Neurol. Scand.*, 46:573–584.
60. Sapier, J. R., and Lossing, J. H. (1974): Prolonged trance-like stupor in epilepsy. *Arch. Intern. Med.*, 134:1079–1082.
61. Sawyer, G. T., Webster, D. D., and Schutz, J. (1968): Treatment of uncontrolled seizure activity with diazepam. *J.A.M.A.*, 203:913–918.
62. Scott, J. S., and Masland, R. L. (1952): Occurrence of "continuous symptoms" in epilepsy patients. *Neurology*, 2:297–301.
63. Scholz, W. (1951): *Die Krampfschadigungen des Gehirns*. Springer-Verlag, Berlin.
64. Singhal, P. C., Chugh, K. S., and Gulati, D. R. (1978): Myoglobinuria and renal failure after status epilepticus. *Neurology (Minneap.)*, 28:200–201.
65. Tassinari, C. A., Dravet, C., Roger, J., Cano, J. P., and Gastaut, H. (1972): Tonic status epilepticus precipitated by intravenous benzodiazepine to five patients with the Lennox-Gastaut syndrome. *Epilepsia*, 13:421–435.
66. Thompson, S. W., and Greenhouse, A. H. (1968): Petit mal status in adults. *Ann. Intern. Med.*, 68:1271–1279.
67. Tucker, W. M., and Forster, F. M. (1950): Petit mal epilepsy occurring in status. *Arch. Neurol. Psychiatry*, 64:823–827.
68. Turner, W. A. (1907): *Epilepsy*, pp. 101–105. Macmillan, London.
69. Vernea, J. J. (1974): Partial status epilepticus with speech arrest. *Proc. Aust. Assoc. Neurol.*, 11:224–228.
70. Wallis, W., Kutt, H., and McDowell, F. (1968): Intravenous diphenylhydantoin in treatment of acute repetitive seizures. *Neurology (Minneap.)*, 18:513–525.
71. Whitty, C. W. M., and Taylor, M. (1949): Treatment of status epilepticus. *Lancet*, 2:591–594.

Advances in Neurology, Vol. 34: Status Epilepticus, edited by A.V. Delgado-Escueta, C.G. Wasterlain, D.M. Treiman, and R.J. Porter. Raven Press, New York © 1983.

2

Classification of Status Epilepticus

Henri Gastaut

> As long as one uses only symptoms for the basis of a classification, it will vary like our spirits, for each person will construct a framework according to the way in which he sees these same symptoms.
>
> Bichat, 1802

The current classification of status epilepticus was elaborated in Marseilles, France, in October 1962 during the tenth European conference on epileptology and clinical neurophysiology. This conference was appropriately devoted to the study of "serial seizures and status epilepticus." Until 1962, no attempt had been made to achieve a classification of status epilepticus for the simple reason that subsequent to studies by Calmeil (13) and Bourneville (9) in the nineteenth century the term was used to designate a single indivisible entity characterized by rapidly recurrent grand mal seizures accompanied by coma, hyperthermia, and grave neurovegetative disturbances that could rapidly lead to a fatal outcome.

Such a restrictive conception of status epilepticus was still held by Penfield and Jasper (69) in 1954, and even more curiously, by Lennox (53) in 1960. Indeed, the latter author limited an entire chapter of his treatise on epilepsy to the status epilepticus described by Calmeil and Bourneville, whereas a paragraph in the chapter devoted to petit mal epilepsy dealt with "petit mal status" identified by the author 15 years earlier. Several authors prior to Lennox had already begun to use the term "status" to designate serially repeated seizures not involving grand mal. Such descriptions included

"status myoclonicus" in 1903 (16), "status hemiepilepticus idiopathicus" in 1904 (59), "Jacksonian status epilepticus" in 1923 (72), and "temporal lobe status" in 1956 (39). But despite the terminology used, none of the authors in question considered the entity they described as meriting stricto-sensu the designation status epilepticus similar to that described by Calmeil and Bourneville.

During the 1962 conference in Marseilles, 103 participants presented 237 EEG clinical cases of abnormally prolonged or serially repeated seizures, most of which did not correspond to the definition of status epilepticus accepted at that time. Accordingly, it was decided to change the historical definition of the term to an etymological one in keeping with the Latin meaning of *status*, i.e., "a manner of being fixed and durable." The conference thus proposed to define status epilepticus as "a condition characterized by an epileptic seizure which is so frequently repeated or so prolonged as to create a fixed and lasting epileptic condition." Implicit in this definition was the existence of as many types of status epilepticus as there are types of epileptic seizures. However, because an international classification of epileptic seizures (also in preparation at that time) was to be presented 2 years later at the thirteenth conference at Marseilles, it was decided to await that conference for simultaneous presentation of the classification of status epilepticus. Accordingly, the latter was first published in 1967 by Gastaut (24) in the proceedings of the 1962 Marseilles conference (37) before being officially adopted in 1970 by the International League against Epilepsy in an appendix to the international classification of epileptic seizures (25). The classification of status epilepticus was subsequently included in the World Health Organization's *Dictionary of Epilepsy* (26) in 1973. Following those milestones, in 1974 and 1975 the classification was incorporated in the chapters devoted to status epilepticus in the *Handbook of Clinical Neurology* (76) and the *Handbook of Electroencephalography and Clinical Neurophysiology* (41). Finally, this classification is commonly used throughout the world, with the exception of a few details to be discussed later.

Theoretically, the classification identifies as many types of status epilepticus as there are types of seizures described in the international classification of epileptic seizures and groups together all these types of status epilepticus in the same three categories that group together epileptic seizures. For this reason, the discussion to follow deals successively with generalized, partial, and unilateral status epilepticus.

GENERALIZED STATUS EPILEPTICUS

Generalized status epilepticus can be divided into two categories according to whether or not the condition is accompanied by bilateral convulsions.

Convulsive Generalized Status Epilepticus

Tonic-Clonic Status Epilepticus (Grand Mal Status Epilepticus)

This name refers to the historical status epilepticus as first described by Calmeil in 1824 (13), i.e., "there is a succession of up to as many as forty or sixty uninterrupted epileptic attacks. The danger is urgent; many patients die. This is what the patients amongst themselves call 'état de mal.'"

Tonic-clonic status epilepticus is almost exclusively observed in adults, especially men, and it is characterized by one of the following two kinds of tonic-clonic seizures: (a) seizures that are generalized from the onset occurring in patients known to have primary generalized epilepsy (Figs. 1A and

B); (b) more frequently, tonic-clonic seizures that are secondarily generalized, after an initially partial onset (Fig. 2A). With the second type, half of the patients are known to have partial epilepsy, whereas the other half are not known epileptics, although they do present potentially epileptogenic brain lesions (most often in the frontal region) that are responsible for the initial status epilepticus (isolated or lone status epilepticus). EEG recordings obtained during status epilepticus are obviously of prime importance for differentiating between seizures with a partial onset and those with a generalized onset.

Grand mal status, be it with generalized or secondarily generalized onset, is often triggered by conditions that lead to a lowering of the convulsant threshold (e.g., metabolic or ionic disturbances secondary to liver or kidney failure, serious infection, etc.; toxic disturbances, including therapeutic accidents; untimely withdrawal of anticonvulsant therapy).

Tonic-clonic status epilepticus generally lasts about 48 hr, with four to five seizures per hour. The duration and magnitude of the seizures, especially in the tonic phase, tend to diminish as the status epilepticus progresses. In some patients the seizures become subclinical; only being detected on the EEG, which shows signs of marked brain suffering between the ictal discharges.

Despite recent therapeutic progress, the death rate remains high, especially in cases of secondarily generalized status epilepticus (Fig. 2B), varying from 6% to 20% of cases, according to various authors.

Tonic Status Epilepticus

Tonic status epilepticus was identified only after Gastaut et al. (36) described tonic seizures in 1962; its first description, reported by the same authors, dates back only about 15 years (40). Tonic status epilepticus is relatively frequent; according to Ohtahara et al. (64) approximately half their cases of status epilepticus in children are of this type.

From practically every viewpoint, tonic status epilepticus can be contrasted with the tonic-clonic status epilepticus of adults: (a) Tonic status epilepticus is found only in children or adolescents with secondary generalized epilepsy, generally belonging to the Lennox syndrome; (b) the duration of tonic status epilepticus is much longer (days or even weeks); (c) tonic status epilepticus features seizures that are more numerous (about 10 per

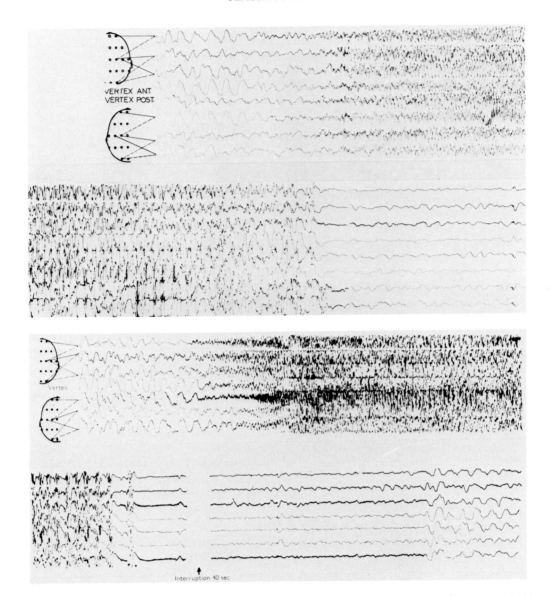

VERTEX ANT.
VERTEX POST.

Vertex

Interruption 40 sec

FIG. 1. Tonic-clonic or "grand mal" status epilepticus with seizures generalized from the onset in a 5-year-old girl with primary generalized epilepsy. The two seizures, recorded at an interval of 25 min, should be considered bilateral and synchronous from the onset even though the epileptic recruiting rhythm begins a few seconds earlier in one hemisphere (left hemisphere in Fig. 1A, right hemisphere in Fig. 1B), a common finding in primary generalized seizures. During the period between seizures, basic EEG activity is markedly abnormal, displaying nonreactive delta rhythm, in accordance with the clinical signs of deep coma. Full regression without sequelae occurred on the third day of status epilepticus.

hour) but much less pronounced than those of grand mal status epilepticus (indeed, seizure intensity is sometimes so low that the seizures are clinically almost imperceptible, thus requiring EEG identification of their accompanying generalized electrodecremental event or burst of recruiting epileptic rhythm) (Fig. 3); (d) finally, the outcome is less severe, because coma and total electrical disorganization between seizures occur in only 50% of cases, and the mortality is currently less than 3%.

Clonic Status Epilepticus

Clonic status epilepticus is seen only in infants and very young children (90% of cases occur be-

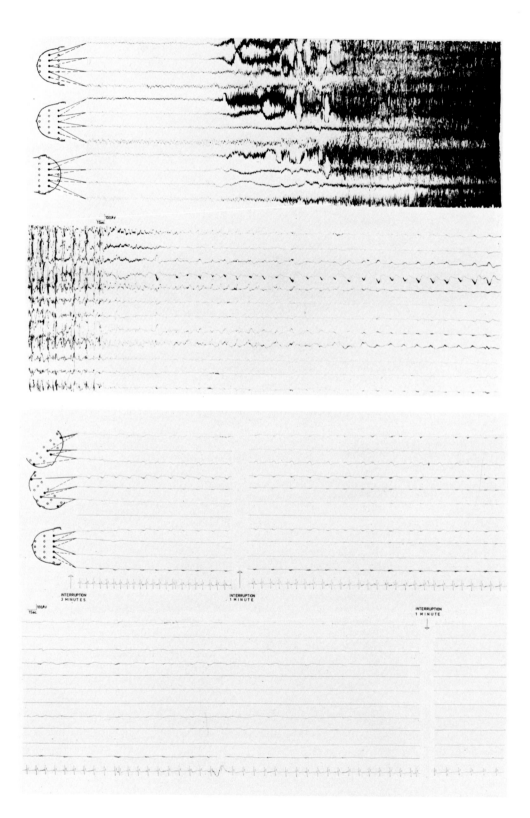

fore 5 years of age). In 25% of patients, clonic status epilepticus is the inaugural symptom of an acute brain lesion (meningoencephalitis, dehydration or metabolic disturbances, etc.); in another 25%, clonic status epilepticus is a consequence of chronic encephalopathy (with or without prior epilepsy); the remaining 50% of cases occur in apparently normal patients. In the latter group, the status epilepticus is termed "cryptogenic," and in about two-thirds of such cases it occurs during hyperthermia, thus resembling a hyperthermic convulsion, but of long duration. It should be noted that the name status epilepticus is used in children to designate a seizure lasting more than 1 hr (2) or even 30 min (17).

Clonic status epilepticus is remarkably frequent, representing more than 50% of generalized convulsive status epilepticus cases in children, according to Aicardi and Chevrie (2) and more than 80% of such cases reported by Congdon and Forsythe (17). It is thus rather curious that a precise EEG clinical description of clonic status epilepticus has not been reported. In our experience, clonic status epilepticus displays the following features: Clinically, the jerks are of low amplitude, bilateral but often asymmetrical and asynchronous, and recurring arrhythmically; the EEG reveals a discharge of high-amplitude bilateral and synchronous delta waves, mixed with bursts of spikes or epileptic recruiting rhythm, thus forming with them some arrhythmic spike-wave patterns (Fig. 4).

The prognosis in clonic status epilepticus depends on the cause. The prognosis is especially severe when status epilepticus is secondary to an acute brain lesion, but it is relatively benign in cryptogenic cases, which are easily arrested by parenteral administration of diazepam or clonazepam.

Myoclonic Status Epilepticus

It is unfortunate that this term is used to designate two myoclonic syndromes whose causes, symptoms, and prognoses are so distinct that their differentiation is absolutely necessary. Such distinction is all the more important because only one of the two syndromes merits inclusion in the domain of status epilepticus.

Myoclonic status epilepticus (stricto-sensu) occurring in patients with generalized epilepsy. Two subgroups can be described, according to whether the generalized epilepsy is of the primary or secondary type.

1. Myoclonic status epilepticus in primary generalized epilepsy is to our knowledge an exceptional finding, because aside from four cases presented by Mertens and ourselves at the 1962 Marseilles conference (74), only cases termed "impulsive petit mal status" reported by Janz (49), Gruneberg and Helmchen (45), and Schneemann et al. (77) and those designated "myoclonic status with multiple spike-wave" published by Ohtahara et al. (64) have been published. This type of status epilepticus, peculiar to children and adolescents, features massive bilateral myoclonias repeated at irregular intervals and often grouped in salvos, and the EEG shows the classic multiple spike-wave (Fig. 5). Consciousness is remarkably intact, the duration of status epilepticus is short (a few hours to 1 day), and the prognosis is excellent.

2. Myoclonic status epilepticus in secondary generalized epilepsy in children is far more frequent, but quite different and less typical, as shown by the following: (a) myoclonias consistently bilateral but often asymmetrical, asynchronous, and of smaller amplitude; (b) clouding of consciousness that dominates the clinical picture; (c) EEG no longer featuring typically multiple spike-waves, but rather arrhythmically repeated spike-waves interspersed with high-amplitude delta rhythm mixed with bursts of theta waves and epileptic recruiting rhythm. As will be discussed later, several authors, including Storm Van Leeuwen (82) and ourselves, consider that such status epilepticus is in fact absence status camouflaged by myoclonus rather than

FIG. 2. Tonic-clonic or "grand mal" status epilepticus with secondarily generalized seizures after a right-sided versive onset (two to three seizures per hour) in a 55-year-old man. The patient had no history of epilepsy, whereas a grave head trauma had occurred. The tonic-clonic seizure recorded in Fig. 2A begins with a left temporal discharge of spikes accompanied by deviation of the head and eyes to the right followed by right hemiclonus (note the pronounced muscular artifacts recorded by the right EEG electrodes); secondarily generalization then occurs (muscular artifacts are bilateral). The patient died (Fig. 2B) a few minutes after this seizure. Note the definitive electrical silence while the heart continues to beat.

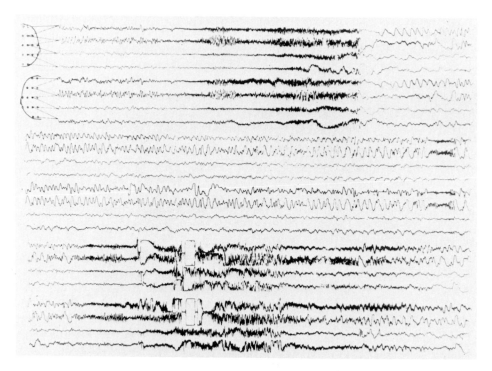

FIG. 3. Tonic status epilepticus, 48 hr after the onset (about 40 seizures per hour), in a 15-year-old boy with Lennox-Gastaut syndrome. Two tonic seizures, lasting 20 and 40 sec, respectively, were recorded during a 3-min period. Note the interictal signs of brain suffering (bilateral frontal delta rhythm) in accordance with the clinical signs of light coma. The second segment shows a brief burst of recruiting rhythm corresponding to infraclinical tonic seizure. Status epilepticus continued for 3 days, the seizures occurring with the same frequency but with a progressively lower intensity, finally becoming entirely infraclinical. Full regression occurred on the fifth day.

true myoclonic status. In this respect, Ohtahara et al. (64) described a paradoxical situation when they placed such myoclonic status epilepticus in the category of nonconvulsive status epilepticus in childhood, next to absence status.

So-called myoclonic status epilepticus during acute or subacute brain disorders in nonepileptics. In contrast with the two preceding subtypes of status epilepticus, this variety of status epilepticus involves myoclonic manifestations, generally occurring in adults, and they are always secondary to acute or subacute encephalopathy whose origin is metabolic (liver or kidney failure and especially anoxia), toxic (especially methylbromide and chloralosis intoxication), viral (Creutzfeldt-Jakob disease), or degenerative (Ramsay Hunt syndrome, neurolipidosis, and especially Unverricht-Lundborg syndrome). In such cases the EEG signs are those of the underlying disorder, e.g., periodic spikes in neurolipidosis (Fig. 6), anoxic encephalopathy or rolandic spikes evoked by jerks in cases

of methylbromide intoxication or Lance-Adams syndrome. The outcome is always very severe, if not fatal.

It is our opinion that this type of myoclonic syndrome should not be regarded as status epilepticus in the strict sense of the term. For example, it would seem more appropriate to refer to the late myoclonic phase of neurolipidosis rather than myoclonic status epilepticus in the course of neurolipidosis.

Nonconvulsive Generalized Status Epilepticus

Absence Status

This type of status epilepticus, characterized by clouding of consciousness, was identified by Lennox (52) in 1945. Because the condition is accompanied by discharges of spike-waves, as encountered by Lennox 10 years earlier in cases of petit mal absence, he proposed the term "petit mal status."

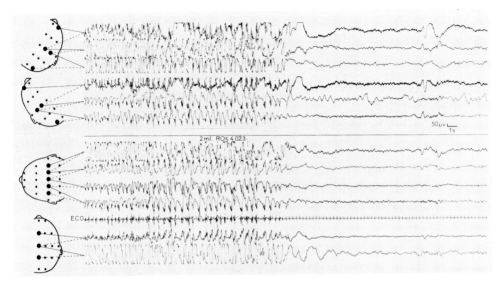

FIG. 4. The end of a clonic status epilepticus occurring without interruption for 2 hr after delivery in a 30-year-old woman. As a young child the patient presented long-lasting febrile convulsions of the same type. Status epilepticus was arrested 40 sec after intravenous injection of clonazepam. Note the clonus recorded as muscular artifacts on the electrocardiogram.

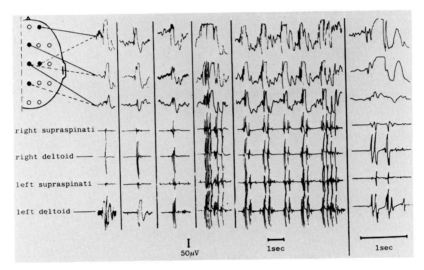

FIG. 5. True myoclonic status epilepticus, 48 hr after the onset, due to sudden withdrawal of medication in a 15-year-old boy with primary generalized epilepsy. The EEG of the central brain regions and EMG of the left and right supraspinous and deltoid muscles show the relationship between each cortical spike of the bilateral polyspike-waves and the corresponding muscle potential. The patient's state of consciousness was perfectly normal, as shown by the results of different psychological tests (Bender, W.I.S.C., taping, etc.) that were identical to those obtained prior to status epilepticus.

The same terminology was employed without reservation during the decade following the original description of petit mal status (12,43,51,57, 78,84,87). However, numerous subsequent observations have clearly shown that such status epilepticus (a) is only exceptionally composed of typical petit mal absence with spike-waves at 3 Hz repeated at short time intervals or prolonged without interruption, (b) is only exceptionally seen in patients presenting primary generalized epilepsy with

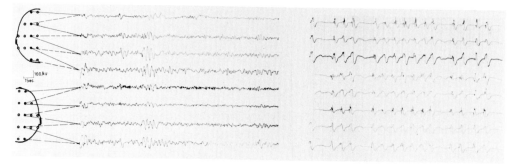

FIG. 6. So-called myoclonic status epilepticus, 12 hr after the onset and 35 min before death, in a 5-year-old child with Batten's disease. The history of Batten's disease dated back 2 years (tracing on the left) and had led to overall dementia. Status epilepticus, with massive bilateral myoclonus in flexion recurring about once every second (tracing on the right), began only 12 hr prior to death in this patient. Accordingly, it is preferable to refer to this case as the terminal myoclonic phase of neurolipidosis rather than true myoclonic status epilepticus.

typical petit mal absences, (c) is also observed in patients with primary generalized epilepsy without petit mal absences (or a long time after disappearance of such absences), (d) is especially frequent in cases of secondary generalized epilepsy with minor seizures different from petit mal, and (e) in the latter case is accompanied by spikewaves different from those of typical petit mal, often recurring with a frequency less than 3 Hz or arrhythmically dispersed over slow dysrhythmia mixed with spikes. Subsequent to these observations it became apparent that the term "petit mal status" was too restrictive, thus leading to other proposed terms, such as "epileptic twilight states with spikes and waves" (93), "epilepsia minoris continua" (22), "minor epileptic status" (11), "spike-wave stupor" (62), and "absence status" (25,55). The latter term, absence status, was finally retained by the Terminology Committee of the International League against Epilepsy in its classification of seizures published in 1970 (25). This term was also adopted by the experts of the W. H. O. in their *Dictionary of Epilepsy* published in 1973 (26). The term absence status is largely used around the world (3,14,23, 56,61,64,65,86), but the older term petit mal status also persists (4,7,44,47,54,63,70,71,79,81–83,90). Other terms, including "epileptic twilight state" (6), "spike-wave stupor" (58), and "minor epileptic status" (10,48,64) are only exceptionally employed.

Thus, there are problems of both terminology and nosography, because certain authors (5,56, 64,65) accept the existence of several types of

nonconvulsive generalized status epilepticus and employ several of the previously mentioned terms to designate these different types of status epilepticus. According to certain authors, the following two major types of such status epilepticus can then be distinguished:

1. "Petit mal status" or "typical absence status" or "spike-wave stupor" would occur in children or adolescents presenting primary generalized epilepsy with petit mal absences. Such status epilepticus (with an excellent prognosis) would feature pure mental confusion, with rhythmic discharge of spike-waves at 3Hz. Based on the work of Andermann and Robb (3) and on two studies by Hosokawa (cited by the authors), Ohtahara et al. (64) proposed that the term petit mal status be reserved for cases where the discharges of spike-waves at 3 Hz are repeated in closely spaced bursts corresponding to a series of petit mal absences (Fig. 7), whereas the term spike-wave stupor would be exclusive to cases where the 3-Hz spike-wave discharge is uninterrupted (Fig. 8), corresponding to a prolonged petit mal absence.

2. "Minor status epilepticus" or "atypical absence status" would occur in infants and young children presenting secondary generalized epilepsy (mainly Lennox syndrome). Such status epilepticus, with a somber prognosis, would feature more marked mental confusion, sometimes associated with myoclonus and tonic or atonic seizures, as well as rhythmically recurrent spike-waves at frequencies less than 3 Hz (2 or even 1 Hz) or arrhythmic spike-waves or, even more frequently, diffuse slow (theta or delta) high-amplitude background

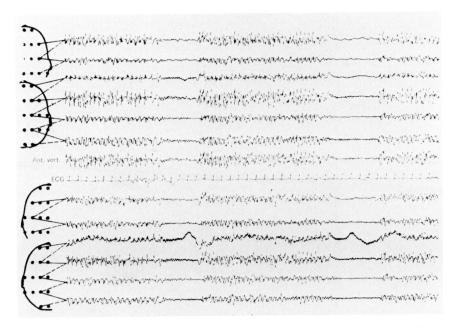

FIG. 7. Absence status epilepticus of 5 hr duration in a 44-year-old menopausal woman. The patient's history revealed the occurrence of petit mal absences at puberty and a few grand mal menstrual seizures at 30 years of age. The EEG shows spike-wave complexes, with rhythmic recurrence three times per second, grouped in bursts lasting about 10 sec. Normal background activity lasting 3 to 5 sec occurs between the bursts. This case can thus be referred to as typical absence status or even petit mal status epilepticus.

activity with superimposed bursts of fast activity (10-Hz recruiting rhythm) and occasional bursts of spike-wave complexes (Fig. 9).

Ohtahara et al. (64) went even further, because paradoxically they placed the following in the domain of nonconvulsive status epilepticus in childhood: (a) tonic status epilepticus, arguing that it occurs in children with Lennox syndrome and is accompanied by slow spike-waves between the tonic seizures; (b) myoclonic status epilepticus, because it occurs in children or adolescents with primary generalized epilepsy and is accompanied by multiple spike-waves; (c) subclinical electrical status epilepticus induced by sleep, as described by Patry et al. (68), although this entity is not status epilepticus in the clinical sense of the term.

I am not in favor of distinguishing the two varieties of nonconvulsive generalized status epilepticus. However, if such a distinction must be made, and in order to simplify the terminology, then it would seem appropriate to employ the terms typical absence status and atypical absence status, both of which retain the common designation of absence status. This latter point is all the more

significant because with respect to semiology, etiology, and prognosis the distinction between typical and atypical absence status is debatable, whereas both subtypes of status epilepticus respond identically to the same treatment.

From the standpoint of semiology, neither the form of the spike-waves nor their frequency and rhythmicity allow easy distinction between typical and atypical absence status; e.g., rhythmic slow spike-waves or arrhythmic spike-waves mixed with delta activity can be observed in absence status of both primary and secondary generalized epilepsy.

Etiological significance is all the more a relative phenomenon, because atypical absence status (the most frequent) is far from being peculiar to secondary generalized epilepsy and Lennox syndrome; i.e., atypical absence status can be observed in the purest cases of primary generalized epilepsy and even in healthy nonepileptic women at menopause.

With these considerations in mind, it can be said that the prognosis is not related to the semiological type of absence status, but rather to the underlying pathological process in such patients. For example,

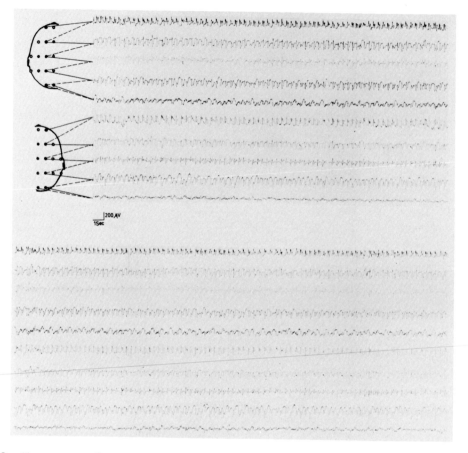

FIG. 8. Absence status epilepticus 36 hr after the onset in a 16-year-old boy presenting petit mal absences since the age of 4 years. The spike-waves recur rhythmically three times per second without interruption (3 hr interruption between the upper and lower tracings). This case can thus be referred to as typical absence status or petit mal status as well as spike-wave stupor.

atypical absence status involves a poor prognosis in a child with Lennox syndrome, whereas the prognosis is good for a healthy 50-year-old woman who first presented primary generalized epilepsy in adolescence. This view is obviously in direct opposition to that held by Doose and Völzke (21,89). According to those authors, atypical absence status occurring in children with cryptogenic Lennox syndrome (also called centrencephalic myoclonic-astatic petit mal) would be directly responsible for progressive mental retardation, which those authors qualify as dementia.

Finally, with respect to treatment, all types of absence status, regardless of clinical and EEG signs, regress in the same manner a few seconds or minutes after parenteral administration of diazepam or clonazepam.

Atonic and Akinetic Status Epilepticus

This type of status epilepticus is peculiar to very young children and generally arises during hyperthermia, thus resembling a long-lasting atonic or akinetic febrile convulsion. In such cases the infant remains immobile (without or with tonus), the eyes often are revulsed, and consciousness is totally absent. It is not rare to observe a few minor clonias from time to time. The EEG features a bilateral and synchronous discharge of slow waves from which stand out a few spikes, thus forming some spike-wave patterns (Fig. 10). The outcome often is remarkably benign.

PARTIAL STATUS EPILEPTICUS

The term partial status epilepticus should be strictly limited to those cases of status epilepticus

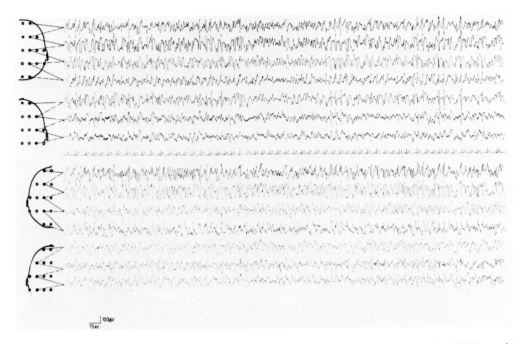

FIG. 9. Absence status of 8 days' duration in a 9-year-old boy with Lennox-Gastaut syndrome. The EEG shows slow theta and delta dysrhythmia with superimposed fast or slow spike-waves. This case should be referred to as atypical absence status epilepticus.

featuring partial seizures repeated over short intervals *without secondary generalization*. This point merits emphasis, because status epilepticus constituted by the repetition of secondarily generalized partial seizures belongs to the group of tonic-clonic status epilepticus due to: (a) the predominance of the generalized convulsive symptoms (which thus relegates the partial onset of each seizure to a position of secondary importance); (b) especially the importance of interictal disturbances of consciousness and neurovegetative regulation; and (c) the severity of the prognosis.

Like all types of status epilepticus, partial status epilepticus can occur in known epileptics and non-epileptics, representing in the latter group the initial epileptic manifestation of a latent or overt brain lesion. Partial status epilepticus is divided into two categories based on whether the symptoms are elementary or complex.

Elementary Partial Status Epilepticus

Theoretically, there are as many types of elementary partial status epilepticus as there are types of partial epileptic seizures displaying elementary symptoms. However, from the practical standpoint, two types are encountered with sufficient

frequency as to require clear distinction: (a) somatomotor status epilepticus, which, according to Passouant et al. (67), accounts for two-thirds of all cases of partial status epilepticus occurring in known epileptics; (b) dysphasic status epilepticus, which is far less frequent but has been well studied.

Somatomotor Status Epilepticus

Unfortunately, the term somatomotor status epilepticus is used to describe two convulsive syndromes whose causes, symptoms, and prognoses are so different as to warrant their differentiation. Strictly speaking, only one of these two syndromes merits the designation somatomotor status epilepticus.

Somatomotor status epilepticus (stricto-sensu) occurring during the course of or at the onset of somatomotor partial epilepsy. This type of status epilepticus is characterized by the more or less frequent repetition (several dozen to hundreds per day) of typical clinical and EEG somatomotor seizures (Fig. 11). Seizures with or without Jacksonian march, with more or less pronounced ictal EEG discharges in the rolandic region, and with well-preserved consciousness and neurovegetative regulation both during and between the seizures. One

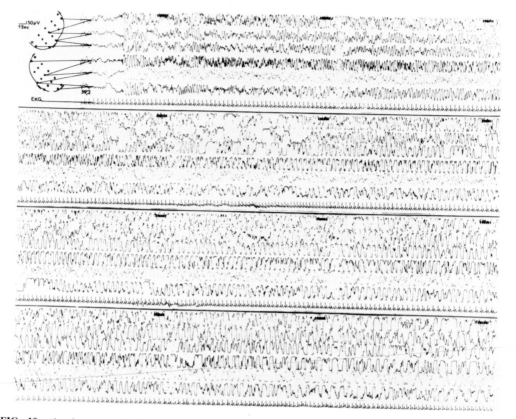

FIG. 10. Atonic status epilepticus lasting 45 min, experimentally induced by raising the body temperature to 39°C in a child presenting naturally occurring febrile seizures of the same type. The figure shows the onset and first 4 min of status, featuring epileptic recruiting rhythm progressively hidden by delta activity, thus presenting the aspect of spike-waves. Entirely devoid of muscle tonus, the child is immobile and unconscious with the eyes deviated upward. Tonus briefly recurs from time to time, leading to short periods of body stiffness.

particular subtype is represented by the persistence of localized segmental myoclonus between the somatomotor seizures and is referred to as epilepsia partialis continua or Kojevnikov's syndrome.

About half the cases of such somatomotor status epilepticus occur in patients with known epilepsy, whereas the other half of the cases arise in nonepileptics. In the latter group, the patients are elderly, and according to Gastaut et al. (29) the inaugural episode of status epilepticus commonly reflects the existence of metastatic embolus or asymptomatic sylvian ischemia.

Most cases of such somatomotor status epilepticus yield to medical therapy, although rare cases may undergo progressive transformation to grand mal by secondary generalization of the seizures.

*So-called somatomotor status epilepticus accompanying severe brain lesions in nonepilep-*tics. The clinical picture is completely different from that of the preceding type; i.e., repeated somatomotor seizures are not observed. On the contrary, this syndrome features periodic repetition of localized myoclonus not at all resembling that of Kojevnikov's syndrome. Such myoclonus, which generally involves the proximal part of a limb or one side of the trunk or flank, is periodically repeated about once per second and is accompanied by periodic lateralized epileptiform discharges in the contralateral hemisphere (Fig. 12). This particular syndrome, observed almost exclusively in older patients, is related to the presence of either interterritorial cerebral infarction or, less frequently, metastatic tumor or brain contusion (15,31,60). It is our opinion that this myoclonic syndrome should not be considered as true status epilepticus. For example, it would seem more ap-

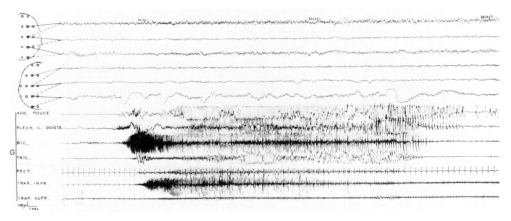

FIG. 11. True somatomotor status epilepticus, of several hours duration, in a 15-year-old boy with Jacksonian epilepsy of the left upper limb. Over 100 seizures were recorded over several hours. The tenth seizure is shown in the figure. Note that the ictal discharge in the right Rolandic region is clearly visible and that the convulsions are progressively extending on the left side from the adducens of the thumb to the common flexor of the fingers, triceps, biceps, pectoralis, and trapezius (Jacksonian march). Abbreviations: Add. Pouce = adductor pollicis; Flech. C. Doigts = common flexor of the finger; Bic. = biceps; Tric. = triceps; Pect. = pectoralis; Trap. infr. = trapezius inferior; Trap. supr. = trapezius superior; G = left.

propriate to speak of the initial myoclonic phase of interterritorial infarction (i.e., infarction in the boundary zone separating the three areas of cortical arterial supply) rather than somatomotor status epilepticus or epilepsia partialis continua in the course of interterritorial infarction.

Dysphasic or Aphasic Status Epilepticus

Although it is much less frequent than somatomotor status epilepticus, dysphasic or aphasic status epilepticus is a well-documented syndrome; four reports of language evaluation during EEG recording of serially repeated seizures have been published (8,19,27,46,85).

Such status epilepticus is characterized by an episode of aphasia, sometimes associated with alexia and agraphia, lasting several hours or days. The following two subtypes have been identified: (a) language is disturbed only during seizures, thus allowing the patient normal oral expression between seizures; (b) language disturbances persist during the interictal period. In the latter case, the episode of aphasia is obvious and thus does not get overlooked by the observer, whereas in the former subtype the disturbance may be missed, because aphasia lasts only 10 to 20 sec, being repeated every 2 or 3 min. Accordingly, dysphasic status may possibly be more frequent than is currently believed.

Other Types of Elementary Partial Status Epilepticus

Such cases are remarkably rare. Only 9 cases confirmed by EEG recordings during status epilepticus have been encountered in our experience.

Adversive status epilepticus. Briefly reported by a few authors (14,73), this type of status epilepticus is certainly exceptional if one is cautious to exclude both secondarily generalized tonic-clonic status epilepticus with seizures commencing with adversion and tonic status epilepticus with predominantly unilateral seizures accompanied by conjugate deviation of the head and eyes. We have encountered only 5 such cases confirmed by EEG showing ictal discharges (precentral in 3 cases, preoccipital in 2 cases).

One may include in this group serially repeated oculo-clonic seizures with contralateral occipital discharges, of which the first cases were reported in 1953 (35).

Somatosensory status epilepticus. This type of status epilepticus is also exceptional if caution is used to distinguish somatosensory status epilepticus from the relatively commonplace episodes of continuous unilateral dysesthesia. The latter, even when detected in patients with somatomotor or somatosensitive partial epilepsy, does not necessarily represent status epilepticus. Indeed, much time has passed since Scott and Masland (80) first

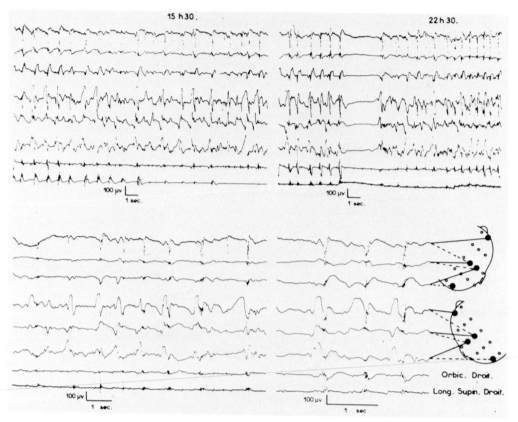

FIG. 12. So-called somatomotor status epilepticus accompanying interterritorial infarction of the left hemisphere in a 66-year-old man. The EEG shows the characteristic periodic lateralized epileptiform discharges recurring about once every second on the left hemisphere and regularly accompanied by contraction of the right hemiface and proximal upper limb (recorded on the orbicularis and long supinator muscles). These phenomena are recorded at two different speeds, as shown in the upper and lower tracings. The patient died 48 hr after the onset of status. Autopsy examination confirmed the diagnosis, showing infarction of the region bordering the territories of the middle and posterior cerebral arteries of the left hemisphere. Transient myoclonus of this type may or may not be considered as status epilepticus. However, this type of myoclonus must be distinguished from Kojevnikov's epilepsia partialis continua, which always results from a very localized lesion of the prerolandic circumvolution and not from a diffuse parieto-temporo-occipital lesion. Abbreviations: Orbic. Droit. = right orbicularis; Long. Supin. Droit. = right long supinator.

described the "continuous symptoms" or "continuous aura" that only reflect the interictal recurrence of the irritative properties of an epileptogenic focus. In patients presenting somatomotor epilepsy with a somatosensitive component, we have seen only 1 case of somatosensitive seizures recurring as status epilepticus with ictal EEG discharges in the region of Rolando, and many cases of continuous hemidysesthesia without EEG signs other than eventual interictal paroxysms.

Elementary visual status epilepticus. This type of status epilepticus is also exceptional if: (a) elementary visual seizures are defined as those both originating in the occipital region and accompanied by scintillating phosphenes and not visual illusions

or hallucinations and; (b) one does not include in the domain of status epilepticus continuous phosphenes (in one or both visual fields) that correspond to an "epileptic continuous symptom" as defined by Scott and Masland (80). In patients presenting occipital epilepsy, we have encountered only 2 cases of repeated elementary visual seizures in the form of status epilepticus with ictal EEG discharges in the contralateral occipital region. On the other hand, 5 cases of continuous phosphenes were observed without EEG signs other than interictal paroxysms over the contralateral occipital pole.

Autonomic status epilepticus. Although convincing evidence is scarce, the existence of repeated or prolonged epileptic seizures has often been considered at the origin of recurrent episodes of abdominal pain, vomiting, headache, etc. It is obvious that this "borderland of epilepsy" has been abusively extended. Nevertheless, abdominal status epilepticus certainly exists, because on one occasion (33) we were able to induce such a status in a patient with abdominal epilepsy and produce an EEG tracing of several hours' duration.

Complex Partial Status Epilepticus

Since the first description of complex partial status epilepticus was reported by Gastaut et al. (39) in 1956, about 50 such cases have been published and reviewed by Wolf (92), Gastaut (28), and Karbowski (50). These cases all involved seizures with complex temporal symptoms and were referred to as "temporal lobe status epilepticus," "psychomotor status epilepticus", "status psychomotoricus," or, more recently, "complex partial status epilepticus." Unfortunately, only one-third of these cases were accompanied by EEG proof that status epilepticus was indeed present, rather than a psychotic state of short duration, which, according to most authors after the initial work of Dongier (20), is fairly often observed in patients with temporal lobe epilepsy.

Although it is seen mainly in adults, temporal lobe status epilepticus can be encountered in patients of all ages. The duration of status epilepticus ranges from a few hours to days or even weeks. According to Gastaut and Tassinari (41), two subtypes exist: (a) shortly spaced temporal seizures displaying classic psychomotor, psychosensorial, or psychoaffective symptoms; (b) status featuring a continuous, long-lasting episode of mental confusion with or without automatic behavior and psychosensorial or psychoaffective phenomena. Obviously, when EEG confirmation is lacking, the latter subtype may be mistakenly diagnosed instead of the interictal psychotic episodes, which are entirely different from true status epilepticus. Nevertheless, even in the absence of ictal EEG discharges, episodic behavior considered as psychotic and interictal may possibly reflect successive seizures involving deep-lying structures accessible only to stereo-EEG. This seems to be the case in the remarkable study reported by Wieser (91), who correlated the different components of highly fluctuating psychosensorial symptoms (visual or auditory hallucinations, clouding of consciousness, visceral sensations, etc.) with deep-lying temporal discharges recorded by stereo-EEG (lingual gyrus, gyrus of Heschl, hippocampus, amygdala, etc.), whereas ictal discharges were not found on conventional EEG tracings.

Five cases of complex partial status epilepticus of extratemporal origin have been reported to date (18,35,66). All such cases involved visual hallucinatory status epilepticus whose occipital origin was confirmed by the site of ictal EEG discharges and, in three cases, by the association of "epileptic nystagmus" and visual hallucinations (35,66).

UNILATERAL STATUS EPILEPTICUS

Already known to very early authors, notably Voisin (88), who published a remarkable clinical description in his treatise on epilepsy in 1897, unilateral status epilepticus was identified along with its complications by a group of workers in Marseilles based on EEG-clinical (42,75), anatomical (34), and CT evidence (32).

Unilateral status epilepticus is encountered only in infants and very young children (75% of patients are less than 3 years old). In about half these patients unilateral status epilepticus is the initial symptom of an acute brain lesion (arterial and especially venous thrombosis, subdural hematoma, brain contusion, etc.) or a complication of chronic encephalopathy (with or without prior epilepsy). In the remaining half of these cases, unilateral status epilepticus arises in apparently normal subjects and is referred to as cryptogenic. Among this latter group, two-thirds of cases occur in the course of hyperthermia and thus present as long-lasting (more than 30 or 60 min) unilateral hyperthermic convulsions. The unilateral nature of the seizure can be accounted for by (a) an initially focal discharge that generalizes to an entire hemisphere or, conversely, (b) localization on one hemisphere (due to immaturity of the commissural fibers) of an initially generalized discharge.

Unilateral status epilepticus is remarkably frequent, representing at least 40% of convulsive status epilepticus cases in children (2). The seizures, practically always of the hemiclonic type, as described by Gastaut et al. (30,36), last several hours or even days. Thus, unilateral status epilepticus presents the same features as generalized clonic status epilepticus, discussed previously, but is localized to one side of the body, with EEG discharges occurring in the contralateral hemisphere. The clonic seizures involve the entire right or left body half, but their frequency and amplitude sometimes vary from one segment to another; further-more, clonus may stop in one segment but continue in another and, in some cases, even change over to the other side of the body (alternate seizures) or become bilateral during a certain period of time. When status is sufficiently long-lasting, conscious-ness undergoes progressive deterioration, leading to coma and respiratory disturbance. At the end of status, hemiplegia is consistently present and is a function of the duration of the hemiconvulsive episode, either transitory or permanent. Unilateral status epilepticus is accompanied by a discharge of generalized slow waves that display a much higher amplitude on the contralateral hemisphere, in which the slow waves are associated with a predominantly posterior epileptic recruiting rhythm, thus forming with it a more or less typical aspect of spike-waves. After status has ended, slow waves persist on the posterior part of the involved hem-isphere, later yielding to either a normal basic rhythm in cases with favorable outcome or a depressed basic rhythm when sequelae persist (Fig. 13).

Although death is rare in the course of unilateral status epilepticus (about 5% of cases), sequelae are frequent, i.e., definitive hemiplegia in one-third of cases, half of which are complicated by partial epilepsy (commonly of the temporal lobe

variety). Such cases represent the HH syndrome (hemiconvulsions-hemiplegia) or the HHE syn-drome (hemiconvulsions-hemiplegia-epilepsy) (Fig. 14), as described by Gastaut et al. (32,34,42,75), later confirmed by Aicardi et al. (1), and recog-nized by the WHO in its *Dictionary of Epilepsy* (26) and by the American Heart Association in its report of the Joint Committee for Stroke Facilities (Stroke in Children, Part I, 1973). Fortunately, the discovery of injectable anticonvulsant benzodiaze-pines (diazepam, clonazepam), coupled with the good working knowledge of pediatricians, for whom any hemiclonic seizure lasting more than 10 min is an emergency, has led to a marked reduction in the frequency and sequelae of unilateral status epi-lepticus over the past decade (Fig. 14). With this fact in mind, the intention of the Terminology Committee of the International League against Epi-lepsy to remove the term unilateral seizure and thus unilateral status epilepticus from the inter-national classification of epileptic seizures should be deplored.

ERRATIC STATUS EPILEPTICUS

This type of status epilepticus, usually discussed along with unilateral status epilepticus, should log-ically be considered separately because of certain

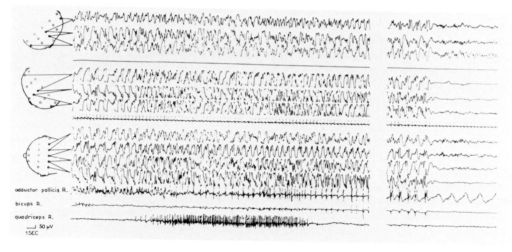

FIG. 13. Right hemiclonic status epilepticus, 2 hr after the onset, in an 8-month-old infant. The patient's history revealed the occurrence of a few short-lasting left and right hemiclonic seizures. The EEG recording on the left, taken in the midst of status, features bilateral and synchronous high-amplitude delta activity associated with epileptic recruiting rhythm, thus taking on the aspect of rudimentary spike-waves; delta waves and especially the recruiting rhythm predominate on the left hemisphere, whereas the clonus is only recorded on the muscles of the right half of the body, the frequency and amplitude of muscle clonus differing on the upper limb (adducens of the thumb, biceps) and lower limb (quadriceps). The tracing on the right shows the end of status, with subsequent total electrical depression on the left hemisphere corresponding to postictal right hemiplegia.

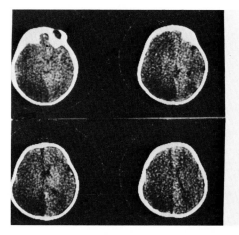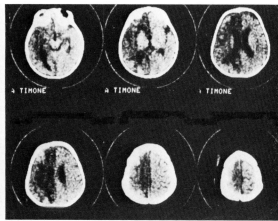

FIG. 14. Computed tomography shows the tragic outcome of right hemiclonic status epilepticus due to hyperthermia in a 1-year-old infant. The CT scans shown on the left were made only 1 day after the end of status epilepticus. Note the presence of left hemispheric edema resulting from the epileptic discharge of this hemisphere during 18 hr. The edema is evidenced as a diffuse hypodensity predominating in the posterior region of the enlarged left hemisphere, with compression of the right hemisphere (space-occupying effect). The CT scans on the right, obtained 50 days after the end of status epilepticus, show marked cortical/subcortical atrophy of the left hemisphere subsequent to edema. Note the presence of less pronounced right hemispheric atrophy. This case illustrates the development of HH syndrome over a 2-month period, with rapid progression to HHE syndrome in a patient with hemiclonic status epilepticus that was arrested too late.

particular characteristics. Erratic status epilepticus is exclusive to neonates and features the repetition of short-spaced erratic seizures. Clinically, the seizures display more or less rhythmically repeated low-amplitude convulsions involving a restricted part of the body (e.g., hemiface, or only the palpebral commissure, chin, or tongue), and thus they often go unnoticed. The EEG reveals localized discharges often changing from one part of a hemisphere to another part of the same or opposite hemisphere, without a strict correspondence to the site of the convulsions.

The outcome is unfavorable in most cases, especially when status epilepticus occurs soon after birth. In this respect, erratic status epilepticus occurring during the first 3 days of life (consistently secondary to a severe prenatal or neonatal lesion) leads to death or serious encephalopathic sequelae in half of the cases, or even in all cases when status epilepticus occurs within hours of birth. Conversely, erratic status epilepticus that arises after the fourth postpartum day (often secondary to a metabolic disturbance) has a more favorable prognosis.

CONCLUSION

The current classification of status epilepticus presents the advantage and disadvantage of being based exclusively on symptoms. The obvious disadvantage is that such a classification is unstable and is interpreted differently according to one's perception of the symptoms. The advantage is that it precisely corresponds to the current semiological classification of epileptic seizures, a feature that is of particular usefulness to epileptologists, i.e., those who are specialists in the diagnosis and treatment of all forms of epilepsy occurring at all ages. However, aside from this small group of specialists, the present classification may be problematic for pediatricians, who are not familiar with epilepsy in adults, and for neurologists, who are unfamiliar with childhood epilepsy. Accordingly, it would appear useful, as a tentative conclusion, to present briefly the semiological forms of status epilepticus as functions of the affected age groups and prognoses.

Status Epilepticus in Neonates (First Month of Life)

Erratic status epilepticus is by far the most frequent type. The prognosis is always very poor, especially when status epilepticus occurs close to birth.

Myoclonic status epilepticus is exceptionally observed. The features are repeated massive bilateral arrhythmic myoclonias with EEG signs of "burst suppression." This type of status epilepticus is commonly related to hyperglycinemia. The outcome is fatal.

Status Epilepticus in Infants and Young Children

During the first 6 years of life the different types of status epilepticus are as peculiar as their component seizures. The following can be identified:

Clonic status epilepticus and *hemiclonic status epilepticus* are by far the most frequent. The prognoses are entirely different according to whether status epilepticus occurs in a child with an acute brain lesion or chronic encephalopathy or a normal subject during the course of hyperthermia. In the latter case, where the prognosis is much better, it should be emphasized that prolonged clonic and chiefly hemiclonic febrile status can leave very severe sequelae if not quickly arrested by parenteral administration of a benzodiazepine.

Atonic and akinetic status epilepticus is exceptional and is consistently benign. Spontaneous arrest of status epilepticus occurs within a few hours.

Absence status epilepticus has a benign short-term prognosis because status epilepticus yields to parenteral benzodiazepine after a few seconds or minutes. The long-term prognosis is not worse, even when absence status epilepticus is observed in secondary generalized epilepsy associated with progressive mental retardation, because the latter finding is not directly related to the presence or the degree of absence status.

Tonic status epilepticus has a more reserved prognosis than absence status epilepticus because it does not necessarily respond to treatment and, in exceptional cases, can lead to death.

Status Epilepticus in Older Children and Adolescents

Throughout these years of transition, status epilepticus progresses from the typical childhood forms to those of the adult. Accordingly, in this age range, the following are seen:

Absence status epilepticus and tonic status epilepticus are still encountered.

Clonic and hemiclonic status epilepticus and atonic and akinetic status epilepticus are no longer observed.

Myoclonic status epilepticus of primary generalized epilepsy begins to appear in this age group.

Grand mal status epilepticus (especially with seizures generalized from the onset in patients with known generalized epilepsy) and *partial status epilepticus* become progressively more frequent.

Status Epilepticus in Adults and the Elderly

After adolescence, status epilepticus is practically limited to the following types:

Grand mal status epilepticus (especially with secondarily generalized seizures occurring in nonepileptics) and *partial status epilepticus* (especially somatomotor status epilepticus in epileptics as well as so-called somatomotor status epilepticus in nonepileptics).

Absence status epilepticus may be encountered, almost exclusively at menopause in women who often have a personal or family history of primary generalized epilepsy.

A physiopathogenic classification distinguishing status epilepticus with short-spaced epileptic seizures from that composed of a single prolonged seizure (eventually and accessorily fragmented) would also be useful from the therapeutic standpoint. Indeed, only the latter group (clonic, hemiclonic, atonic, akinetic, and absence status epilepticus) almost regularly and systematically yields to parenteral administration of benzodiazepine.

However, it would be regrettable to simultaneously adopt several modes of classification for the same series of entities. It is for this reason that we propose to retain the current semiological classification of status epilepticus, supplementing it with etiopathogenic, prognostic, and therapeutic considerations necessary for a clear understanding.

REFERENCES

1. Aicardi, J., Amsili, J., and Chevrie, J. (1969): Acute hemiplegia in infancy and childhood. *Dev. Med. Child Neurol.*, 11:162–173.
2. Aicardi, J., and Chevrie, J. (1970): Convulsive status epilepticus in infants and children. *Epilepsia*, 11:187–197.
3. Andermann, F., and Robb, J. (1972): Absence status, a review of 38 patients. *Epilepsia*, 13:177–187.
4. Assael, M. (1972): Petit mal status without impairment of consciousness. *Dis. Nerv. Syst.*, 33:526–528.
5. Bauer, G. (1976): Psychic changes with continuous epileptic discharges. *Electroencephalogr. Clin. Neurophysiol.*, 41:188.
6. Belafsky, M., Carwile, S., Miller, P., and Escueta, A. (1976): Prolonged twilight states. *Neurology (Minneap.)*, 26:366.

7. Böhm, M. (1969): Status epilepticus petit mal: An adult case. *Electroencephalogr. Clin. Neurophysiol.*, 26:229.

8. Boudouresques, J., Roger, J., and Gastaut, H. (1962): Crises aphasiques subintrantes chez un épileptique temporal. *Rev. Neurol. (Paris)*, 106:381–393.

9. Bourneville, D. (1876): *Recherches cliniques et thérapeutiques sur l'épilepsie et l'hystérie*. Delahaye et Lecrosnier, Paris.

10. Bower, B. (1972): Minor epileptic status. *Dev. Med. Child Neurol.*, 14:80–81.

11. Brett, E. (1966): Minor epileptic status. *J. Neurol. Sci.*, 3:52–75.

12. Bridge, E. (1949): *Epilepsy and Convulsive Disorders in Children*. McGraw-Hill, New York, p. 670.

13. Calmeil, L. (1824): *De l'Epilepsie*. thèse, Paris.

14. Celesia, G., Messert, B., and Murphy, J. (1972): Status epilepticus of late adult onset. *Neurology (Minneap.)*, 22:1047–1055.

15. Chatrian, G., Shaw, C., and Leffman, H. (1964): The significance of periodic lateralized epileptiform discharges. *Electroencephalogr. Clin. Neurophysiol.*, 17:177–193.

16. Clark, L., and Prout, T. (1903–4): Status epilepticus: A clinical and pathological study in epilepsy. *Am. J. Insan.*, 60:291–306, 645–675; 61:81–108.

17. Congdon, P., and Forsythe, W. (1980): Intravenous clonazepam in treatment of status epilepticus in children. *Epilepsia*, 21:97–102.

18. Corin, S. (1973): Visual status epilepticus. *Neurology, (Minneap.)*, 23:434.

19. De Pasquet, E., Gaudin, E., Bianchi, A., and De Mendilaharsu, S. (1976): Prolonged and monosymptomatic dysphasic status epilepticus. *Neurology (Minneap.)*, 26:244–247.

20. Dongier, S. (1959–60): Statistical study of clinical and EEG manifestations of 536 psychotic episodes occurring in 516 epileptics between clinical seizures. *Epilepsia*, 1:117–142.

21. Doose, H., and Völzke, E. (1979): Petit mal status in early childhood. *Neuropediatrie*, 10:10–14.

22. Friedlander, W., and Feinstein, G. (1956): Petit mal status; epilepsia minoris continua. *Neurology (Minneap.)*, 6:357–362.

23. Gall, M., Scollo-Lavizzari, G. and Becker, H. (1978): Absence status in the adult. *Eur. Neurol.*, 17:121–128.

24. Gastaut, H. (1967): À propos d'une classification symptômatologique des états de mal épileptiques. In: *Les états de mal épileptiques*, edited by H. Gastaut, J. Roger, and H. Lob, pp. 1–8. Masson, Paris.

25. Gastaut, H. (1970): Clinical and electroencephalographic classification of epileptic seizures. *Epilepsia*, 11:102–113.

26. Gastaut, H. (1973): *Dictionary of Epilepsy*. World Health Organization, Geneva.

27. Gestaut, H. (1979): Aphasia. The sole manifestation of focal status epilepticus. *Neurology (Minneap.)*, 29:1638 (letter).

28. Gastaut, H. (1980): *L'epilepsie temporale*. La Concours Médical, Paris.

29. Gastaut, H., Boudouresques, G., Gastaut, J. L., and Michel, B. (1977): Jacksonian epileptic seizures as inaugural manifestations of sylvian infarctus. In: *Computerized Axial Tomography in Clinical Practice*, edited by G. Boulay and I. F. Moseley, pp. 237–245. Springer-Verlag, New York.

30. Gastaut, H., Broughton, R., Tassinari, C., and Roger, J. (1974): Unilateral epileptic seizures. In: *Handbook of Clinical Neurology, Vol. 15*, edited by P. J. Vinken and G. W. Bruyn, pp. 235–245. American Elsevier, New York.

31. Gastaut, H., and Naquet, R. (1966): Étude électroencephalographique de l'insuffisance circulatoire cérébrale chronique. In: *Symposium International sur le circulation cérébrale*, pp. 163–191. Editions Sandoz, Paris.

32. Gastaut, H., Pinsard, N., Gastaut, J. L., Regis, H., and Michel, B. (1979): Acute hemiplegia in children. In: *Advances in Neurology, Vol. 25*, edited by M. Goldstein et al., pp. 329–337. Raven Press, New York.

33. Gastaut, H., and Poirier, F. (1964): Experimental induction of abdominal seizures. *Epilepsia*, 5:256–270.

34. Gastaut, H., Poirier, F., Payan, H., Salamon, G., Toga, M., and Vigouroux, M. (1959): H. H. E. syndrome: Hemiconvulsion-hemiplegia-epilepsy. *Epilepsia*, 1:418–447.

35. Gastaut, H., and Roger, A. (1954): Les formes inhabituelles de l'épilepsie: le nystagmus épileptique. *Rev. Neurol. (Paris)*, 90:130–132.

36. Gastaut, H., Roger, J., Faidherbes, J., Ouahchi, S., and Franck, G. (1962): Nonjacksonian hemiconvulsive seizures and one-sided generalized epilepsy. *Epilepsia*, 3:56–68.

37. Gastaut, H., Roger, J., and Lob, H. (1967): *Les états de mal épileptiques*. Masson, Paris.

38. Gastaut, H., Roger, J., Ouahchi, S., Timsit, M., and Broughton, R. (1963): An electro-clinical study of generalized epileptic seizures of tonic expression. *Epilepsia*, 4:15–44.

39. Gastaut, H., Roger, J., and Roger, A. (1956): Sur la signification de certaines fugues épileptiques: état de mal temporal. *Rev. Neurol. (Paris)*, 94:298–301.

40. Gastaut, H., Roger, J., and Poire, R. (1967): Les états de mal généralisés toniques. In: *Les états de mal épileptiques*, edited by H. Gastaut, J. Roger, and H. Lob, pp. 44–76. Masson, Paris.

41. Gastaut, H., and Tassinari, C. (1975): Status epilepticus. In: *Handbook of Electroencephalography and Clinical Neurophysiology, Vol. 13A*, edited by H. Gastaut, pp. 39–45. Elsevier, Amsterdam.

42. Gastaut, H., Vigouroux, M., Trevisan, C., and Regis, H. (1957): Le syndrome hémiconvulsions-hémiplégie-epilepsie (syndrome H. H. E.). *Rev. Neurol. (Paris)*, 97:37–52.

43. Gibbs, F., and Gibbs, E. (1952): *Atlas of Electroencephalography, Vol. 2*, Addison-Wesley, Cambridge, Mass.

44. Groh, C., and Rosenmayer, F. (1974): Isolierter petit mal Status. *Dtsch. Med. Wochenschr.*, 99:379–385.

45. Gruneberg, F., and Helmchen, H. (1969): Impulsiv—petit mal—Status und paranoide Psychose. *Nervenarzt.*, 40:381–385.

46. Hamilton, N., and Matthews, T. (1979): Aphasia, the sole manifestation of focal status epilepticus. *Neurology (Minneap.)*, 29:745–748.

47. Hess, R., Scollo-Lavizzari, G., and Wyss, F. (1971): Borderline cases of petit mal status. *Eur. Neurol.*, 5:137.

48. Jamison, D. (1973): Minor epileptic status with contractures. *Proc. R. Soc. Med.*, 66:1068–1069.

49. Janz, D. (1963): *Die Epilepsien, Spezielle Pathologie und Therapie*. Georg Thieme Verlag, Stuttgart.

50. Karbowski, K. (1980): *Status psychomotoricus*. Hans Huber, Berne.

51. Kellaway, P., and Chao, D. (1955): Prolonged status epilepticus in petit mal. *Electroencephalogr. Clin. Neurophysiol.*, 7:145.

52. Lennox, W. (1945): The petit mal epilepsies—their treatment with tridione. *J. A. M. A.*, 129:1069–1073.

53. Lennox, W. (1960): *Epilepsy and Related Disorders*, Little-Brown, Boston.

54. Lipman, I., Isaacs, E., and Suter, C. (1971): Petit mal status epilepticus. *Electroencephalogr. Clin. Neurophysiol.*, 30:159–165.

55. Lob, H., Roger, J., Soulayrol, R., Regis, H., and Gastaut, H. (1967): Les états de mal généralisés à expression confusionnelle (états de petit mal ou états d'absence). In: *Les états de mal épileptiques*, edited by H. Gastaut, J. Roger, and H. Lob, pp. 91–128. Masson, Paris.

56. Lugaresi, E., Pazzaglia, P., and Tassinari, C. (1971): Differentiation of "absence status" and "temporal lobe status". *Epilepsia*, 12:77–87.

57. Mann, L. (1954): Status epilepticus occurring in petit mal. *Bull. Los Angeles Neurol Soc.*, 19:96–104.

58. Moe, P. (1971): Spike-wave stupor. *Am. Dis. Child.*, 121:307.

59. Muller, J. (1904): Status hemi-epilepticus idiopathicus. *Dtsch. Zeitsch. Nerven.*, 28:31.

60. Naquet, R., Franck, G., and Vigouroux, R. (1915): Décharge paroxystiques du carrefour pariéto-temporo-occipital. *Zentralbl. Neurochir.*, 4/5:153–180.

61. Niedermeyer, E., Fineyre, F., Riley, T., and Uematsu, S. (1979): Absence status (petit mal status) with focal characteristics. *Arch. Neurol.*, 36:417–421.

62. Niedermeyer, E., and Khalifeh, R. (1965): Petit mal status (spike-wave stupor). *Epilepsia*, 6:250–262.

63. Novak, J., Corke, S., and Fairley, R. (1971): Petit mal status in adults. *Dis. Nerv. Syst.*, 32:245–248.

64. Ohtahara, S., Oka, E., Yamatogi, Y., Ohtsuka, Y., Ishida, T., Ichiba, N., Ishida, S., and Miyake, S. (1979): Non-convulsive status epilepticus in childhood. *Folia Psychiatr. Neurol. Jpn.* 33:345–351.

65. Oller-Daurella, L. (1974): Les états confusionnels (états d'absence). *Acta Neurol. Belg.*, 74:265–275.

66. Palem, R., Force, L., and Esvan, J. (1980): Hallucinations critiques épileptiques à propos d'un état de mal oculo-clonique. *Ann. Med. Psychol. (Paris)*, 2:161–190.

67. Passouant, P., Cadilhac, J., Ribstein, M., Delange, M., and Castan, Ph. (1967): Les états de mal partiels. In: *Les états de mal épileptiques*, edited by H. Gastaut, J. Roger, and H. Lob, pp. 152–181. Masson, Paris.

68. Patry, G., Lyagoubi, S., and Tassinari, C. (1971): Subclinical electrical status epilepticus induced by sleep in children. *Arch. Neurol.*, 24:242–252.

69. Penfield, W., and Jasper, H. (1954): *Epilepsy and the Functional Anatomy of the Human Brain*. Little-Brown, Boston.

70. Pruell, G. (1969): The petit mal status of Lennox. *Munch. Med. Wschr.*, 193:269.

71. Rambaud, G. (1970): *Status petit mal*. Thèse, Lyon.

72. Roger, H., and Pourtal, L. (1923): État de mal Jacksonien traumatique tardif par kyste traumatique cérébral de la région frontale. *Marseille Médical*, 1922, pp. 203–218; analysé *Rev. Neurol.*, *(Paris)*, 2:150.

73. Roger, J., Dravet, C., Bureau, M., Dalla Bernardina, B., Mesdjian, E., and Tassinari, C. A. (1978): États de mal partiels chez l'enfant et l'adolescent. In: *Progressi in epileptologia*, edited by F. Angeleri and R. Canger, pp. 195–201. Tipographia di Milano, Milano.

74. Roger, J., Lob, H., Regis, H., and Gastaut, H. (1967): Les états de mal généralisés myocloniques. In: *Les états de mal épileptiques*, edited by H. Gastaut, J. Roger, and H. Lob, pp. 77–84. Masson, Paris.

75. Roger, J., Lob, H., Regis, H., and Gastaut, H. (1967): Les états de mal hémicloniques. In: *Les États de Mal Epileptiques*, edited by H. Gastaut, J. Roger, and H. Lob, pp. 140–151. Masson, Paris.

76. Roger, J., Lob, H., and Tassinari, C. (1974): Status epilepticus. In: *Handbook of Clinical Neurology, Vol. 15*, edited by P. J. Vinken and G. W. Bruyn, pp. 145–188. American Elsevier, New York.

77. Schneemann, N., Brune, F., and Busch, H. (1969): Impulsiv petit mal und Dammerzustand. *Schweiz. Arch. Neurol. Neurochir. Psychiatr.*, 105:281–292.

78. Schwab, R. (1953): A case of status epilepticus in petit mal. *Electroencephalogr. Clin. Neurophysiol.*, 5:441–442.

79. Schwartz, M. S., and Scott, D. F. (1971): Isolated petit mal status presenting de novo in middle age. *Lancet*, 2:1399–1401.

80. Scott, J. S., and Masland, R. L. (1953): Occurrence of "continuous symptoms" in epilepsy patients. *Neurology (Minneap.)*, 3:297–301.

81. Shev, E. (1968): Adult petit mal with special reference to petit mal status. *Electroencephalogr. Clin. Neurophysiol.*, 24:396.

82. Storm Van Leeuwen, W., Jennekens, F., and Elink Sterk, C. (1969): A case of petit mal status with myoclonus. *Epilepsia*, 10:407–414.

83. Thompson, S. W., and Greenhouse, A. H. (1968): Petit mal status in adults. *Ann. Intern. Med.*, 68:1271–1279.

84. Tucker, W., and Forster, F. (1950): Petit mal epilepsy occurring in status. *Arch. Neurol. Psychiatry (Chicago)*, 64:823–827.

85. Vernea, J. (1974): Partial status epilepticus with speech arrest. *Proc. Aust. Assoc. Neurol.*, 11:223–228.

86. Visser, S. (1970): Absence-status. *Ned. Tijdschr. Geneeskd.*, 114:1437–1440.

87. Vizioli, R., and Magliocco, E. (1953): A case of prolonged petit mal seizures. *Electroencephalogr. Clin. Neurophysiol.*, 5:439–440.

88. Voisin, J. (1897): *L'épilepsie*. Félix Alcan, Paris.

89. Völzke, E., and Doose, R. H. (1979): Petit mal status and dementia. *Epilepsia*, 20:183.

90. Weissberg, J. (1975): A case of petit mal status. *Am. J. Psychiatry*, 132:1200–1221.

91. Wieser, H. (1980): Temporal lobe or psychomotor status epilepticus. *Electroencephalogr. Clin. Neurophysiol.*, 48:558–572.

92. Wolf, P. (1970): Zur Klinik und Psychopathologie des Status psychomotoricus. *Nervenarzt*, 41:603–610.

93. Zappoli, R. (1955): Prolonged epileptic twilight state with almost continuous "wave-spikes." *Electroencephalogr. Clin. Neurophysiol.*, 3:421–423.

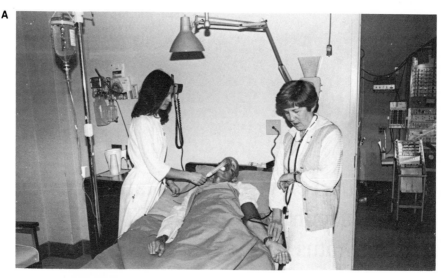

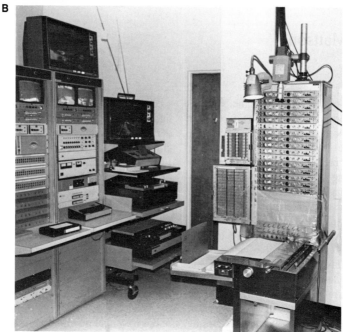

FIG. 1. **A:** A patient room in the Seizure Unit, equipped with suction and oxygen. A wall-mounted camera (not seen) with remote-control zoom lens and automatic iris monitors the patient's activity. EEG signals are transmitted by hard wire or telemetry to the adjoining monitoring room. **B:** The monitoring room, housing polygraphs, videotape recorders, and monitors displaying split-screen clinical/EEG activity on line or in replay.

rienced nurses able to provide necessary critical care.

As soon as a patient arrives at the Seizure Unit, and while other immediate needs are being met, collodion-fixed electrodes are applied to the scalp and chest. Recording of clinical and electrographic events is begun as soon as possible. The videotape recording of seizures may be viewed by one member of the team while others are treating the patient. Interictally, or when time allows, the events are critically reviewed by replaying the videotape recording.

OBSERVATIONS

During the past 10 years, approximately 2,000 different patients have been admitted to our In-patient Seizure Unit. An intensive review of the reasons for admission for 388 patients in a 3-year period indicated that 88 (23%) were admitted for acute seizures, serial seizures, or status epilepticus (6). An exact number is not available, but well over 200 patients with serial seizures or convulsive status epilepticus have been managed during this decade. Many patients with convulsive status epilepticus were not initially managed in the Seizure Unit but were treated in the emergency room and transferred to the medical or neurological intensive care units if intubation and respiratory support were required. The patients seen and managed for serial seizures or status epilepticus in the Seizure Unit came directly from the emergency room or were transferred from other medical and surgical units within the hospital. Some patients developed serial seizures while in the Seizure Unit as a consequence of purposeful medication withdrawal for patients for whom the diagnosis of epilepsy needed to be established or for those with intractable seizures in whom the onset of attacks was being localized in preparation for surgical treatment (14).

APPLICATION AND VALUE OF INTENSIVE MONITORING

Intensive CCTV/EEG monitoring has proved to be especially helpful in several ways, each of which will be discussed separately.

Monitoring and Videotape Recording of the Patient's Condition

The occurrence of status epilepticus or serial seizures calls for immediate support of the patient's vital functions. During and between seizures, nurses and physicians are of necessity occupied with such tasks as protecting the patient from falling, injuring himself, and biting his tongue. Several people may be required to turn the patient to allow drainage of saliva to maintain a good airway. One nurse may be preparing an antiepileptic drug for administration, and another may be drawing blood for diagnostic tests. In such a setting there is little opportunity for careful observation of the onset of the attack and other, sometimes subtle, but important, characteristics of the attack. Even changes in respiration, pulse rate, and blood pressure may be difficult to document until the seizure is controlled.

Videotape recording of the clinical events, with simultaneous recording of the EEG, pulse, and respiration will document details of the attack for later review. The recording of rapid and/or irregular pulse and slow respiration may alert the staff to the need for respiratory support, with or without intubation. The EEG may disclose otherwise clinically unrecognized or subclinical seizure activity, indicating a need for more or different antiepileptic drug therapy. Such recording of electrical seizure activity and vital functions serves as a guide to the physician in determining the rate and quantity of drugs to be infused until reports of antiepileptic drug concentrations become available.

Case 1. A 40-year-old man was admitted to the Seizure Unit with repeated tonic-clonic seizures and incomplete recovery of consciousness between attacks. Intravenous phenytoin markedly decreased the frequency and severity of the convulsive attacks, but he remained only partly responsive interictally. His level of confusion varied during the hours between obvious seizures. Intensive monitoring revealed marked generalized EEG slowing, with periodic partial seizures characterized by semirhythmic, 6-Hz sharp waves arising from the right temporal parietal area. The episodes of maximal confusion corresponded to the presence of the EEG seizure activity, indicating that the patient was continuing to have multiple partial seizures not readily recognizable by motor activity. Intravenous phenobarbital was added to the phenytoin, resulting in marked decreases in both frequency and severity of attacks. Periodic lateralized epileptiform discharges (PLED) continued from the right hemisphere. Because the patient's respirations were quite shallow and high plasma concentrations of antiepileptic drugs had already been obtained, additional drugs were not administered. The subsequent results of cerebrospinal fluid analysis disclosed evidence of meningitis. The patient slowly improved over subsequent days, although the EEG did not clear of PLED activity until the fifth day.

Intensive monitoring of this patient indicated diffuse as well as focal disturbance of function, confirmed by subsequent cerebrospinal fluid evidence of meningitis. It also disclosed that confusional episodes between convulsive attacks were associated with electrographic seizures, and this led to more vigorous treatment and better control.

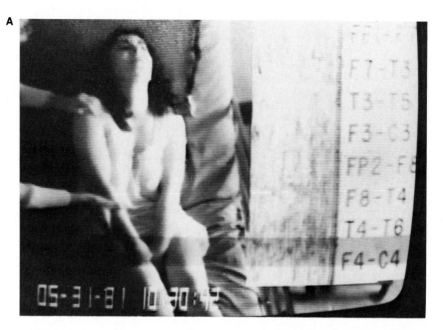

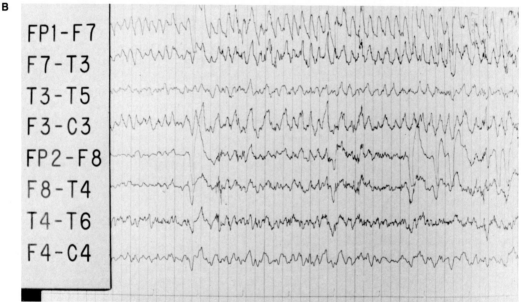

FIG. 2.   A: A tonic-clonic seizure without clinically obvious focal onset. **B:** The paper printout of the EEG recorded at the onset of the seizure and displayed simultaneously on split-screen TV showed that the attack was of secondary generalized type, with a left temporal focal onset.

Intensive monitoring allowed surveillance of the electrical seizure activity, and polygraphic recording documented some mild compromise in respi-rations after drug therapy; so treatment was not pursued to the point of needing intubation and respiratory support.

Seizure Type

The recording of clinical and EEG activity aids in the classification of the seizure type. Convulsive seizures may be characterized as tonic-clonic, tonic, clonic, or massive myoclonic. They also can be identified as primary generalized, secondary generalized, or multifocal in onset. The definition or classification of the seizure type (see Chapter 2) is of great importance in providing insight as to the underlying cause and the selection of optimal treatment. Clinical or EEG detection of the focal onset of a seizure suggests the area of the brain from which the attack originates and indicates the probability of a lesion in the area. In seizures of unknown cause, such localized findings focus a diagnostic search for an underlying structural abnormality such as tumor, abscess, or vascular lesion. Phenytoin is a drug of choice in such instances. On the other hand, a generalized onset, especially when associated interictally with generalized spike-wave discharges, makes a diagnosis of primary generalized epilepsy or withdrawal seizures more likely, and extensive neurodiagnostic studies often will not be required. Treatment with a benzodiazepine or phenobarbital may be more effective than phenytoin in such cases.

Case 2. A 24-year-old woman had repeated episodes of blank staring, with some minimal automatisms, followed by tonic-clonic seizures. As part of an evaluation prior to possible surgical therapy, some antiepileptic drugs were withdrawn, and that precipitated typical seizures occurring serially. The attacks were characterized by loss of awareness, progressing to tonic-clonic activity (Fig. 2). The seizures began with arrest of clinical activity associated with buildup of rhythmic 5- to 6-Hz theta in the left temporal area. Subsequent generalized spread was seen at the time of loss of consciousness and tonic-clonic movements. The seizures were clearly identified as being of the secondary generalized tonic-clonic type, arising from a left temporal focus. Intravenous phenytoin promptly controlled the attacks.

This patient's tonic-clonic attacks were shown on the EEG to have a focal onset, indicating the probable source of the seizures and a classification of secondary generalized type. Such findings often indicate underlying structural disease and may require further diagnostic evaluation. This is especially important in patients with new onset of seizures of unknown cause.

Case 3. An 18-year-old woman was admitted to the Seizure Unit, having had four seizures within the preceding 2 hr, with only partial recovery of consciousness between attacks. Her history showed that she had had recurrent seizures for the past 5 years. A prior diagnostic evaluation had shown no abnormalities. Shortly after admission, while intensive monitoring was being carried out, the patient was noted to be only partly in contact on attempted conversation with the medical staff. During this time, very frequent polyspike-and-wave bursts were observed in generalized distribution and were greatly increased during photic stimulation. Despite a phenytoin concentration of 18 μg/ml, the patient progressed to another tonic-clonic seizure. Intravenous phenobarbital was administered, and the patient had no further attacks. Subsequent questioning revealed that the patient had been taking pentobarbital for sleep and using alcohol excessively until 24 hr before admission.

The finding of generalized spike-wave activity and subclinical absence status made it apparent that the patient had primary generalized seizures. On this basis it was concluded that extensive neurodiagnostic studies, such as CT scans, lumbar puncture, and angiography, were not needed. The presence of a photoconvulsive response probably was related to the diagnosis of primary generalized epilepsy, but it may have been enhanced by barbiturate and/or alcohol withdrawal. In other patients with unexplained repeated seizures, photic sensitivity may be an important clue to a withdrawal response to alcohol or sedative drugs, thus helping in the diagnosis and allowing selection of cross-tolerant drugs such as benzodiazepines, barbiturates, or paraldehyde for treatment rather than phenytoin. Indeed, in this patient, the occurrence of repeated convulsive tonic-clonic attacks, despite high therapeutic concentrations of phenytoin, led to a shift in treatment to phenobarbital, with prompt termination of attacks. Subsequently, this patient was effectively treated with phenobarbital and sharp limitation of alcohol use.

Case 4. A 26-year-old white male with a 2-year history of seizures was admitted to the Seizure Unit because of repeated seizures. Jerking convulsive activity had been noted by the family for several hours, culminating in an attack in which he fell from bed and suffered multiple superficial injuries. Intensive CCTV/EEG monitoring revealed almost continuous myoclonic seizures, with associated generalized polyspike-and-wave discharges occur-

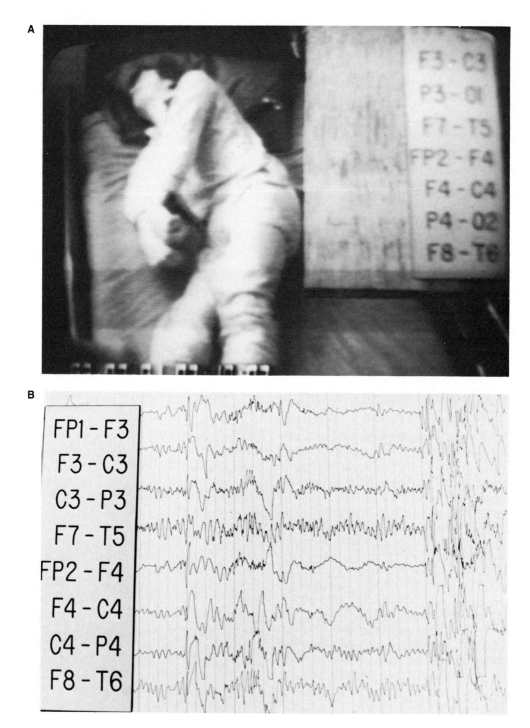

FIG. 3. A: Tonic-clonic seizures after myoclonic status epilepticus. **B:** Interictally the EEG shows polyspike-and-wave discharges, supporting a diagnosis of primary generalized epilepsy.

ring every 5 to 10 sec (Fig. 3). These culminated in another clonic-tonic-clonic seizure, despite a high therapeutic concentration of phenytoin. After parenteral diazepam was given, valproic acid therapy was initiated, and the patient has had no further seizures. Phenytoin was discontinued subsequently without any recurrence of attacks.

Intensive monitoring of the patient's repeated attacks revealed primary generalized seizures of myoclonic and tonic-clonic type. The attacks typically occurred during the night and on awaking. Intensive monitoring throughout the night made it evident that the patient was having myoclonic status epilepticus. Shifting from treatment with phenytoin to valproic acid resulted in complete control of the attacks.

Diagnosis of Epilepsy

Most patients with convulsive status epilepticus have seizures of obvious epileptic type, with tongue biting, incontinence, cyanosis, and associated motor activity. It is not infrequent that some patients also may have attacks for which a specific diagnosis of epilepsy is unclear or uncertain. Seizures may become modified and atypical after acute antiepileptic drug therapy. A question may arise as to the nature of the continuing episodes. In our previous analysis of intractable seizures, we found that 20% of patients referred to the Seizure Unit were having attacks of nonepileptic type, even though most also had well-established diagnoses of epilepsy (6). These alternative diagnoses included movement disorders, at times secondary to toxic effects of antiepileptic drug, hypoxia, or ischemic episodes and, most often, "hysterical" seizures or pseudoseizures. The latter constituted one of the most frequent nonepileptic diagnoses in patients with uncontrolled, recurrent attacks. Fifteen percent of patients admitted to the unit proved to be having pseudoseizures. Rodin et al. (12) have observed a similar surprisingly high frequency of patients with pseudoseizure status epilepticus.

Case 5. A 16-year-old boy with well-documented absence and tonic-clonic seizures was admitted to the Seizure Unit for apparent repeated convulsive attacks. Episodes of absence status culminating in multiple tonic-clonic attacks had occasionally required hospitalization previously. On this occasion, his mother found him lying on the kitchen floor in a pool of vomitus, poorly responsive, and cyanotic. On admission, it was observed that the patient had frequent tonic activity, with

no recovery of consciousness between attacks. Surprisingly, the monitoring revealed that no electrographic seizure activity accompanied his tonic episodes. The recording was characterized by low-voltage slow waves, with loss of normal background frequencies. The patient's clinical status worsened, and he was transferred to the intensive care unit for respiratory support. Plasma phenytoin concentration was 18 μg/ml, and plasma phenobarbital concentration was 60 μg/ml. The atypical findings on intensive EEG monitoring, as well as the high therapeutic concentrations of the drugs, led us to assume drug overdose, with possible aspiration and secondary hypoxia. Care was directed toward support of vital functions, and the patient gradually made a full recovery. Subsequently, he confessed to having made a suicide attempt by taking an overdose of phenobarbital.

The intensive monitoring of an apparently severe, complicated tonic status epilepticus without EEG seizure discharge led us to suspect hypoxic tonic posturing, rather than seizure activity. Without this supplementary information, the seizurelike episodes probably would have been treated with increasingly vigorous administration of antiepileptic drugs, further aggravating the respiratory problem. Intensive monitoring led to a correct diagnosis, followed by support of vital functions, withholding of further antiepileptic drugs, and subsequent recovery.

Case 6. A 30-year-old woman was transferred to the Seizure Unit from another hospital with a history of multiple recurrent attacks unresponsive to parenteral administration of therapeutic doses of phenytoin, phenobarbital, and diazepam. Interictal EEGs previously had shown temporal sharp wave activity. The patient had a lengthy psychiatric history, and the thrashing character of the attacks appeared to the referring neurologist to be atypical of epilepsy. Intensive CCTV/EEG monitoring of the patient revealed repeated attacks of stiffening and thrashing movements of all extremities. During periods of quiet between the motor activity, the patient was totally unresponsive and limp. The simultaneous EEG recording showed movement artifact during the motor component. When movement artifact did not obscure the EEG, a well-organized alpha background was present, although the patient was seemingly comatose and unresponsive (Fig. 4). A diagnosis of pseudoseizure status epilepticus was made, and further administration of antiepileptic drugs was withheld.

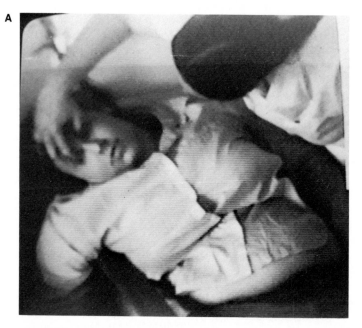

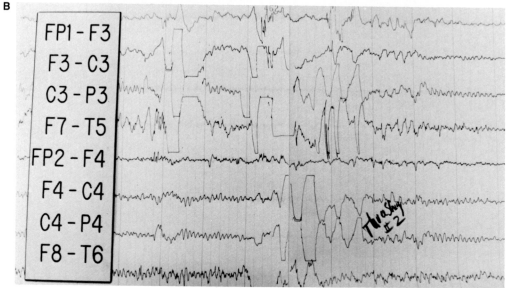

FIG. 4. A: Thrashing convulsive movements were intermixed with unresponsive periods. **B:** Simultaneously recorded EEG revealed normal alpha activity disrupted only by movement artifact, supporting the clinical suspicion of pseudoseizures.

The patient was treated psychiatrically, and the attacks terminated.

The simultaneous recording of muscle artifact on the EEG and normal or nonictal patterns except during movement greatly assisted in characterizing the convulsive attacks as nonepileptic. Although complex partial seizures or simple partial seizures may occur in the presence of a normal scalp-recorded EEG, a typical convulsive tonic-clonic seizure should alter the recording in some way. Videotape recording of the attacks allows careful attention to details of the clinical events; it can be particularly useful in patients in whom the distinction between hysterical seizures and epileptic seizures is most difficult (1). Even though attacks are videotaped, supplementary examination by medical personnel during and between attacks may give useful diagnostic clues. For example, findings of semipurposeful activity, resistance to eye opening, or even termination of an attack on direct command give important support for the diagnosis of hysteria. Conversely, the EEG during recurrent, apparently hysterical, attacks with considerable thrashing may reveal frank epileptiform changes even though the interictal recording is normal and nonspecific. Other useful diagnostic clues during or immediately after the attack include tonic activity of one extremity, lip smacking, automatisms, and dilated unresponsive pupils. All suggest that apparently nonepileptic series of attacks are true severe complex partial seizures, which require appropriate antiepileptic drug therapy (3). Such findings may be evident only on repeated videotape review.

Case 7. A 14-year-old boy with Lennox-Gastaut syndrome and poorly controlled seizures was transferred to the Seizure Unit from another hospital because of continued tonic attacks, despite administration of diazepam, carbamazepine, and phenytoin. At the time of admission, the patient was poorly responsive, and the EEG revealed diffuse slowing, with an occasional slow spike-wave complex similar to patterns previously seen on interictal recordings. Approximately every 3 to 4 hr, and coming 1 to 2 hr after administration of his regular doses of antiepileptic drugs, the patient began to exhibit semicontinuous extensor posturing of the arms and legs, which persisted for approximately 60 to 90 min. The EEG did not show any seizure activity. The predose plasma carbamazepine concentration was 7 μg/ml, but it rose to 14 μg/ml during this motor activity. Carbamazepine had been given prior to admission in doses of 700 mg twice daily. The dosage was altered to 300 mg four times daily, and the episodes disappeared. To clarify the situation, carbamazepine was again administered in twice-daily doses, and the dystonic activity recurred. Following adjustment of the dosage schedule, the patient returned to his usual condition.

The patient's apparently uncontrolled status epilepticus proved on intensive monitoring to be a drug-induced dystonic reaction similar to his tonic seizures, and it was corrected by rescheduling the dosage of carbamazepine to avoid peak concentrations.

CONCLUSIONS

These case reports illustrate the considerable value of CCTV/EEG monitoring in the diagnosis and management of convulsive status epilepticus. Despite the advantages of intensive monitoring, several factors may limit the utilization of this procedure. Foremost is the lack of fully staffed and equipped epilepsy units in most hospitals, even in major medical centers. This can be expected to change in coming years. Even where such a unit is available, some patients with severe convulsive status epilepticus requiring intubation will need to be managed in a medical or neurological intensive care unit designed to maintain vital functions. Some hospitals not having an epilepsy unit might establish a bed for CCTV/polygraphic monitoring within the intensive care unit for a relatively modest cost. This could provide surveillance and diagnostic information not only for patients with acute seizures but also for those with other acute neurological disorders. In the absence of CCTV/EEG facilities, a portable EEG brought to the emergency room or intensive care unit can provide some of the benefits of intensive monitoring and videotape recording.

CCTV/EEG monitoring supplements but does not replace clinical patient evaluation. A passive recording device, it cannot test the patient ictally or interictally for disturbances such as dysphasia, weakness, incontinence, or subtle pupillary changes (3). Ultimately, the findings on CCTV/EEG are of most value when interpreted in concert with other clinical and laboratory findings.

REFERENCES

1. Desai, B. T., Porter, R. J., and Penry, J. K. (1982): Psychogenic seizures. A study of 42 attacks in six patients with intensive monitoring. *Arch. Neurol.* 39:202–209.
2. Escueta, A. V., Kunze, U., Waddell, G., Boxley, J., and Nadel, A. (1977): Lapse of consciousness and automatisms in temporal lobe epilepsy: A videotape analysis. *Neurology (Minneap.),* 27:144–155.
3. Fay, M. L., and Mattson, R. H. (1980): Clinical testing during intensive monitoring of ictal events. In: *Advances in Epileptology: The Xth Epilepsy International Symposium,* edited by J. A. Wada and J. K. Penry, pp. 65–68. Raven Press, New York.
4. Holmes, G. L., McKeever, M., and Russman, B. S. (1981): Long term monitoring of seizure patients. *Conn. Med.,* 45:358–362.
5. Ives, J. R., and Gloor, P. (1978): A long term timelapse video system to document the patient's spon-

taneous clinical seizure synchronized with the EEG. *Electroencephalogr. Clin. Neurophysiol.*, 45:412–416.

6. Mattson, R. H. (1980): Value of intensive monitoring. In: *Advances in Epileptology: The Xth Epilepsy International Symposium*, edited by J. A. Wada and J. K. Penry, pp. 43–51. Raven Press, New York.

7. Penry, J. K., and Porter, R. J. (1977): Intensive monitoring of patients with intractable seizures. In: *Epilepsy, The Eighth International Symposium*, edited by J. K. Penry, pp. 95–101. Raven Press, New York.

8. Penry, J. K., Porter, R. J., and Dreifuss, F. E. (1975): Simultaneous recording of absence seizures with videotape and electroencephalography. *Brain*, 98:427–440.

9. Porter, R. J. (1980): Methodology of continuous monitoring with videotape recording and electroencephalography. In: *Advances in Epileptology: The Xth Epilepsy International Symposium*, edited by J. A. Wada and J. K. Penry, pp. 35–42. Raven Press, New York.

10. Porter, R. J., Penry, J. K., and Lacy, J. R. (1977): Diagnostic and therapeutic reevaluation of patients with intractable epilepsy. *Neurology (Minneap.)*, 27:1006–1011.

11. Porter, R. J., Penry, J. K., and Wolf, A. A. (1976): Simultaneous documentation of clinical and electroencephalographic manifestations of epileptic seizures. In: *Quantitative Analytic Studies in Epilepsy*, edited by P. Kellaway and I. Petersén, pp. 253–268. Raven Press, New York.

12. Rodin, E., Chayasirisobohon, A., and Deremo, J. (1981): EEG recordings of psychogenic seizures and diagnosis of pseudo status epilepticus. *Electroencephalogr. Clin. Neurophysiol.*, 51:73P.

13. So, E. L., and Penry, J. K. (1981): Epilepsy in adults. *Ann. Neurol.*, 9:3–16.

14. Williamson, P. D., Spencer, D. D., Spencer, S. S., and Mattson, R. H. (1980): Presurgical intensive monitoring using depth electroencephalography in temporal lobe epilepsy. In: *Advances in Epileptology: The Xth Epilepsy International Symposium*, edited by J. A. Wada and J. K. Penry, pp. 73–81. Raven Press, New York.

Advances in Neurology, Vol. 34: Status Epilepticus, edited by A.V. Delgado-Escueta, C.G. Wasterlain, D.M. Treiman, and R.J. Porter. Raven Press, New York © 1983.

4

Etiology of Convulsive Status Epilepticus

Dieter Janz

This chapter will treat the etiology, cerebral topology, and immediate precipitating factors associated with convulsive status epilepticus in juveniles and adults. The discussion will be confined to the status epilepticus of generalized tonic-clonic seizures (hereafter referred to as grand mal status), irrespective of whether or not the seizures were preceded by focal symptoms, and it will omit the forms of status epilepticus with only clonic or only tonic seizures, which according to Gastaut (7) also belong to convulsive status epilepticus.

ETIOLOGY

The development of conceptions on the etiology of grand mal status is fittingly illustrated by the contrast between Gowers's (8) remark in 1899, "Nothing is known of its immediate cause," and mine (17) in 1969, "A status epilepticus [meaning grand mal status] is presumably always the expression of organic brain damage." My statement, which naturally had only hypothetical character, was based on three generally accepted observations: (a) The etiology of grand mal status is more often known than unknown. (b) Grand mal status is rarely, if ever, the first manifestation of idiopathic epilepsy. (c) Grand mal status in the course of idiopathic epilepsy is not an inevitable symptom but a complication that commonly supposes a disease of long standing.

In all published reports on the etiology of grand mal status, the cases with known causes outnumber those with unknown causes. The ratio is on the average about ¾ to ¼ (Table 1). Grand mal status among patients with epileptic seizures of known and unknown origin is about five to six times more frequent in patients with seizures of defined cause than in patients with seizures of undefinable cause (9,16). Our data show that the preponderance of symptomatic status episodes results mainly from a higher proportion of seizures caused by brain tumors and traumatic brain damage and less from other causes. Grand mal status occurred in only 1.6% of the cases of cryptogenic epilepsy, but it occurred in 15.8% of patients with tumor-related epilepsy and in 10.7% of those with traumatic epilepsy, as against 5.4% of patients with epilepsy of other known causes (Table 2).

TABLE 1. *Etiology of grand mal status*

References	Cause		
	Known (N)	Unknown (N)	Total (N)
Whitty and Taylor (39)	22	3	25
Hunter (13)	22	8	30
Janz (16)	95	43	138
Oxbury and Whitty (27)	64	32	96
Heintel (9)	67	16	83
Meier (25)	46	19	65
Littann-Masuhr (23)	52	20	72
Total	368	141	509
%	72	28	100

TABLE 2. *Incidence and etiology of status epilepticus*

Epilepsy	Total	With status	Percentage
Cryptogenic	1,885	30	1.6
Symptomatic	703	65	9.0
Tumors	152	24	15.8
Trauma	215	23	10.7
Other types	336	18	5.4
	2,588	95	3.76

From Janz (16).

The figure in Heintel's excellent monograph (9) shows basically the same situation (Fig. 1). In comparison with the cases of epilepsy without grand mal status, the causes in cases of grand mal status were much more often known than unknown. Again, a relatively greater proportion of tumors and brain trauma, and also infectious brain diseases, was evidently responsible for the status.

Among the specific causes of grand mal status in patients with neurological disorders, brain trauma and brain tumors come first, with about 20% each, followed by cerebral vascular diseases, encepha-

litis, perinatal brain damage, and other causes (Table 3). Heintel (9) has demonstrated that tumors, trauma, and inflammatory brain processes have a statistically significant association with grand mal status, whereas vascular processes and perinatal damage do not. Among the brain tumors, the tendency toward or against status varies from type to type. Astrocytomas have a significant disposition to grand mal status, whereas meningiomas lead to status less often than would be expected with an average distribution (9).

Among the types of traumatic brain damage, open brain injuries are associated with status epilepticus three times more often than closed contusions. Of 192 patients with traumatic epilepsy without status, 81 had open brain damage, and of 23 brain-injured patients with status, 16 had open brain injuries ($p < 0.05$) (14). Grand mal status often occurs in the acute phase after a severe head injury, as was shown in 10 of the 14 traumatic cases of Oxbury and Whitty (28) and in 6 of the 14 traumatic cases in a prospective series recently studied systematically over a period of 2 years in

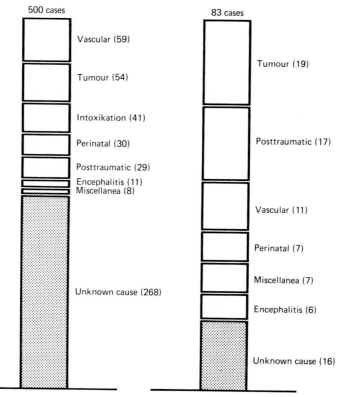

FIG. 1. Causes of epilepsy without status epilepticus *(left)* and of epilepsy with status epilepticus *(right)*. (From Heintel, ref. 9, with permission.)

TABLE 3. *Causes of grand mal status*

References	Tumor (N)	Trauma (N)	Encephalitis (N)	Vascular (N)	Perinatal (N)	Miscellaneous (N)	Total (N)
Whitty and Taylor (39)	4	13	3	—	1	1	25
Hunter (13)	4	—	4	—	3	11	30
Janz (16)	35	30	9	9	5	7	138
Oxbury and Whitty (27)	19	14	9	13	4	5	96
Heintel (9)	19	17	6	11	7	7	83
Meier (25)	12	17	3	9	—	5	65
Littann-Masuhr (23)	8	14	6	6	11	7	72
Total	101	105	40	48	31	43	509
%	20	21	8	9	6	8	100

Berlin (23). Among these patients with early post-traumatic grand mal status, 4 were alcoholics who had suffered cerebral contusion, and in 1 patient a subdural hematoma had occurred as a result of a fall either during intoxication or during an epileptic withdrawal seizure.

According to Heintel (9), inflammatory and infectious brain diseases predispose to grand mal status. The assumption has been verified at the 5% level. In his small standard work, he listed all reported cases and forms of viral, allergic, bacterial, and cysticercal encephalitis in which grand mal status had occurred.

The incidence of grand mal status in cerebrovascular diseases and perinatal brain damage is not significantly greater than would be expected by chance, as Heintel (9) was able to show statistically in comparison with cases of vascular and perinatal epilepsy not accompanied by convulsive status epilepticus of the grand mal type. He pointed out that status epilepticus as a symptom of an infarction, hemorrhage, or venous and sinus thrombosis has a less favorable prognosis than status that occurs in the course of a chronic vascular disorder such as cerebral arteriosclerosis.

The enumeration of all the other reported causes of grand mal status fills a long list that covers six pages of Heintel's monograph (9): drugs and chemicals; metabolic disorders; degenerative, heredodegenerative, demyelinating, and storage diseases; states of cerebral anoxia; intracranial and intraspinal operations; alcoholism; such processes as cerebral edema after strangulation or insolation.

In contrast to the numerous causes that lead to grand mal status via a definable metabolic disorder or morphological brain damage is the fact that grand mal status in epilepsy of unknown origin is relatively rare and (as many investigators have em-

phasized) never marks the beginning of idiopathic epilepsy (2,9,10,13,21,27,28,32). It seems reasonable, therefore, to assume that status epilepticus in the course of idiopathic epilepsy cannot be a natural and inevitable event but only occurs under particular conditions. Apart from the immediate precipitating factors (to which we shall return later), one obvious condition of grand mal status in cryptogenic epilepsy is a disease of long standing. The average duration of epilepsy in the patients of Janz was 13 years (14), and in the patients of Heintel (9) it was 15.5 years. Oxbury and Whitty (28) distinguished two groups, one with progressive deteriorating epilepsy with focal abnormalities in the temporal lobes in which the first status occurred on average after 6 years of illness, the other with epilepsy without signs of progressive deterioration and with generalized abnormalities in the EEG in which the first grand mal status occurred after an average of 18 years. Because in the course of long-standing epilepsy the chance of secondary epileptogenic brain damage increases, it seems reasonable to assume that status even in idiopathic epilepsies is a symptom of a functional disturbance caused by altered morphology, in other words, that the idiopathic epilepsy has with the passage of time and in consequence of its own attacks become a symptomatic epilepsy. If this is accepted, all grand mal status can be considered as a manifestation of symptomatic epilepsy (15,16).

TIME OF MANIFESTATION IN THE COURSE OF ILLNESS

For the etiological diagnosis, it is important to know at what point in the course of illness the first grand mal status occurs. We suggested using the term "initial" for cases presenting with status as the first manifestation of epilepsy, "isolated" for cases presenting with status as the only manifestation of epilepsy, and "intercurrent" for cases with status occurring in the course of already established epilepsy (14). Heintel (9) supplemented this by suggesting the term "iterated" for cases of epilepsy presenting with several episodes of status as the only manifestation. Table 4, in which the results of Janz (16) and Heintel (9) are combined, shows that, apart from epilepsy of unknown origin, intercurrent status is found most frequently in residual epilepsy as a result of perinatal damage and in traumatic epilepsy. Isolated status occurs relatively often in encephalitis, vascular processes, and brain tumors, but also after head injuries. Brain tumors and traumatic brain damage are also the domain of courses with iterated status. Initial status as the first manifestation of epilepsy is found relatively frequently in tumors and vascular processes and is relatively uncommon in encephalitis and perinatal brain damage. The placement of 6 patients in the group of initial status in cryptogenic epilepsy is questionable. The EEGs in 2 men (24 and 29 years old) revealed with regular symmetrical spike-wave activity that at least the subclinical discharges were of long standing. In the remaining 4 patients the status episode had occurred so long ago that the circumstances could not be exactly elucidated.

SITES OF CEREBRAL DAMAGE

In many cases, grand mal status appears to be a symptom of acute or chronic diffuse brain damage. However, when it is based on circumscribed brain damage it is mostly a case of a unilateral lesion of the frontal lobes (2,4,5,9,14,15,25,27–

TABLE 4. *Causes and relationship of grand mal status to the overall course of epilepsy*

Grand mal status	Isolated (N)	Initial (N)	Intercurrent (N)	Total (N)
Tumor	20	11	23	54
Trauma	13	3	31	47
Encephalitis	11	1	3	15
Vascular	10	4	6	20
Perinatal	1	1	10	12
Miscellaneous	9	1	4	14
Cryptogenic	2	6	51	59
Total	66	27	128	221
%	30	12	58	100

Data from Janz (16) and Heintel (9).

29,37–39). This observation can be of considerable diagnostic value in determining the location and nature of brain tumors. Of our 123 patients who had tumors associated with epileptic seizures, 27 had one or more attacks of grand mal status. In 20 of these patients the tumors were situated in the frontal lobes (Table 5). Heintel (9), who gave an analogous synoptic presentation of the nature and location of 58 cases of tumor-related epilepsy, came to the same result, because 13 of 18 cases of grand mal status were found to be caused by tumors of the frontal lobe, and 3 cases were associated with tumors of the central region (Fig. 2). It is, in particular, the frontally situated astrocytomas that are associated with status, in contrast to the frontally situated glioblastoma multiforme, which is rarely the cause of grand mal status. Oxbury and Whitty (27,28) suggested that status is especially associated with frontal tumors only in those cases where it is the first (initial or isolated) manifestation of neurological disease.

Epileptic seizures following head trauma further underline the localizing significance of grand mal status, particularly those following open head injuries. Of 215 patients with traumatic epilepsy, 23 (10.7%) had one or more episodes of status (Table 2). Open head injuries lead to status three times more often (16.5%) than closed injuries (5.9%) (14,16). Table 6 shows the incidence of status in 97 cases of open injury and correlates it to the site of the lesions. Here the association of grand mal status with frontal lobe damage is even more marked than in cases of tumor-related epilepsy, for 15 of the 16 traumatic status episodes developed in relation to damage to the frontal lobes (Fig. 3). The sites of the traumatic lesions in 8 cases of convulsive status epilepticus reported by Heintel (9) concerned the frontal or central regions of the brain in 6 cases and the parietal lobes in 2 cases. The only cases of grand mal status after surgical intracranial procedures reported by Oxbury and Whitty (28) concern surgical frontal lobe damage.

During my stay at the National Hospital, Queen Square, in London, I was able to study the case histories of 20 patients suffering from postleukotomy epilepsy. Almost half of these patients had had one or more episodes of status epilepticus, and in several the recurrent episodes of status, the iterated cases of status epilepticus of Heintel (9), were the only epileptic manifestations (16). The incidence of grand mal status in cases of postleukotomy epilepsy has been reported to be 23% (6).

TABLE 5. *Locations and types of tumors in 123 patients with tumor-related epilepsy*

Type of tumor	Frontal	Parietal	Temporal	Occipital	
With status epilepticus					
Astrocytoma	10	—	—	—	
Oligodendroglioma	3	—	1	—	
Glioblastoma multiforme	—	3	2	1	
Meningioma	1	—	—	—	
Other	6	—	—	—	
Total	20	3	3	1	27
Without status epilepticus					
Astrocytoma	4	10	5	—	
Oligodendroglioma	8	5	5	1	
Glioblastoma multiforme	5	8	2	—	
Meningioma	4	19	3	2	
Other	2	7	5	1	
Total	23	49	20	4	96
Total of tumors	43	52	23	5	123

From Janz (16).

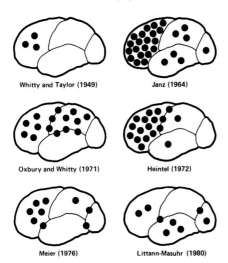

Whitty and Taylor (1949) Janz (1964)

Oxbury and Whitty (1971) Heintel (1972)

Meier (1976) Littann-Masuhr (1980)

FIG. 2. Locations of brain tumors in cases of grand mal status.

In 10 patients, status was the only, or almost the only, manifestation of a traumatic frontal lobe epilepsy, as it may be called.

Peters (30), in a postmortem study involving 13 patients with open head injuries who died in grand mal status, found that 8 of these patients had lesions deep in the white matter of the frontal lobes. Peiffer (29) examined the brains of 97 patients with symptomatic epilepsy who had had episodes of status epilepticus. He found that 77 of these, or 87%, had frontal lobe damage.

PRECIPITATING FACTORS

A distinction must be made between the underlying causes of convulsive status epilepticus and the immediate precipitating factors. The latter are, according to Heintel (9), factors that in manifest epilepsy, irrespective of cause, elicit a status epilepticus that probably would not have occurred without these factors. According to the authors who have reported on this (2,3,9,13,15,20,25,33), in one-third to two-thirds of the cases of grand mal status, directly preceding circumstances can be identified that probably were relevant to its elicitation. The circumstances found most frequently are errors in medication and intercurrent infections. Errors in medication account for about half the cases with known precipitating factors and always involve a reduction below the effective dosage either through a change in drug or relative or absolute drug withdrawal. The fault can result from incorrect prescription by the physician or from omission on the part of the patient, and it often occurs in combination with events that, as in the case of intercurrent infection or alcohol excess, can themselves be precipitating factors. The feature common to these processes appears to be that there is a sudden and considerable drop in a given dosage, especially because elicitation of status epilepticus has never been reported in a case of a carefully planned step-by-step reduction in dosage (11,18,19,26). The observation of a connection between errors in medication and elicitation of grand

TABLE 6. *Incidence of status epilepticus and sites of lesions in 97 cases of open head injury*

	Frontal	Parietal	Temporal	Occipital	
Epilepsies with status	15 (94%)	1 (6%)	—	—	16 (100%)
Epilepsies without status	11 (13.5%)	49 (60%)	12 (15%)	9 (11%)	81 (100%)
Total	26 (27%)	50 (51%)	12 (12%)	9 (9%)	97 (100%)

From Janz (16).

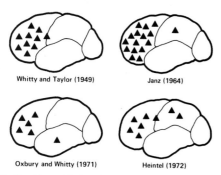

Whitty and Taylor (1949)   Janz (1964)

Oxbury and Whitty (1971)   Heintel (1972)

FIG. 3. Sites of lesions in cases of open head injury and grand mal status.

mal status substantiates the hypothesis of Hunter (13) that the increasing incidence of status epilepticus since the nineteenth century coincides with the introduction of treatment with antiepileptic drugs.

Infections accounted for about 25% of the known precipitating factors and were mainly infections of the respiratory tract. Hunter (13) suspected that infections acted by means of "internal withdrawal" of antiepileptic drugs. Although this hypothesis was voiced 20 years ago, and although the mutual effects of temperature and drug actions were described even earlier as a formidable problem (31), the pharmacokinetics of antiepileptic drugs during fever have, to my knowledge, not hitherto been analyzed. Hunter's (13) hypothesis is still interesting, even though it does not apply to all observations, as there are a number of cases known in which grand mal status occurred during an infection without drugs being taken (9,15). In particular, in cases of posttraumatic epilepsy after open brain injuries, there has been a grand mal status with acute exacerbations of chronic inflammations in the neighborhood of brain scars, sometimes in connection with a general infection.

Alcohol, by either intoxication or withdrawal, and sleep withdrawal are reported relatively seldom as precipitating factors. Whereas sleep withdrawal generally becomes relevant in combination with one of the other factors given, in chronic alcoholism relative or absolute alcohol withdrawal alone can elicit grand mal status. Among 241 patients with withdrawal seizures, Victor and Brausch (36) found 8 patients with status epilepticus. As an additional factor, and possibly the determining factor for the status, in 2 of 4 cases in our last series (23) we found immediately preceding head trauma without traumatic lesions being shown in the cranial computerized tomograms. Thus the question arises whether and in what manner the pathogenic conditions differ for alcohol withdrawal seizures occurring singly, in series, or in status form.

The other factors reported as occasionally eliciting grand mal status in the case of prior brain damage include physical exertion, excessive fluid intake, pneumoencephalography, carotid angiography, radiation therapy of the brain, high-voltage trauma, insolation (14,15), neuroleptic and psychotropic drugs (1,22), and pregnancy and delivery (12,24,34,35).

CONCLUSION

A pathogenic concept deriving from all the clinical experiences mentioned earlier must be based on the fact that grand mal status can be caused by diffuse brain affections as well as by local brain lesions, particularly those of frontal localization. In trying to find a common denominator, it still seems to be likely that the rather uninhibited recurrence of attacks that characterizes status is somehow linked with a structural or functional interruption of thalamocortical fibers belonging to a nonspecific projection system passing from the reticular formation up to the cortex via the thalamus. Lesions in the white matter of the frontal lobes obviously act through an extensive interruption of this inhibiting system. In patients with diffuse brain damage, incipient brain edema may lead to status when it spreads into the centrum semiovale, inducing functional damage or blocking of thalamocortical connections, because it is known that the white matter is particularly prone to edema. I admit, however, that I am touching on problems that are beyond the fringe of clinical neurology and properly belong to neurophysiology and neuropathology.

REFERENCES

1. Alderton, H. R., and Hoddinot, B. A. (1964): A controlled study of the use of thioridazine in the treatment of hyperactive and aggressive children in a children's psychiatric hospital. *Can. Psychiatr. Assoc. J.*, 9:239–247.
2. Aminoff, M. J., and Simon, R. P. (1980): Status epilepticus. Causes, clinical features and consequences in 98 patients. *Am. J. Med.*, 69:657–666.
3. Anton, L. S., Estrada, R., Rosello, H., and Begueria, R. (1977): Status epilepticus. Estudio de 105 casos durante 1972–1973. *Neurol. Neurocir. Psiquiatr.*, 18(Suppl.):325–337.
4. Celesia, C. G., Messert, B., and Murphy, M. J. (1972): Status epilepticus of late adult onset. *Neurology (Minneap.)*, 22:1047–1055.
5. Corkill, A. G. L. (1966): Indications for surgery in recurrent status epilepticus. *Practitioner*, 197:208–209.
6. Feuillet, C., Poiré, R., Mabille, P., and Degraeve, M. (1963): Séquelles convulsives de la lobotomie préfrontale données cliniques et numériques sur une série homogène de 447 opérés, intérêt en matière d'epilepsie traumatique. *Rev. Neurol. (Paris)*, 109:366–378.
7. Gastaut, H. (1982): Classification of status epilepticus. (Chapter 2, this volume).
8. Gowers, W. R. (1899): Epilepsy. In: *A System of Medicine*, edited by T. C. Allbut. Macmillan, London.
9. Heintel, H. (1972): *Der Status epilepticus, seine Aetiologie, Klinik und Letalität. Eine klinisch-statistische Analyse*. Gustav Fischer, Stuttgart.
10. Heycop ten Ham, M. W. van, Kuijer, A., and Lorentz de Haas, A. M. (1967): Recherches sur la genèse de l'état de mal. In: *Les états de mal épileptiques*, edited by H. Gastaut, J. Roger, and H. Lob. Masson, Paris.
11. Heycop ten Ham, M. W. van (1980): Complete recovery from epilepsy? Discontinuation of antiepileptics after 5 or more seizure free years. *Huisarts N. Wetenschap.*, 23:309–311.
12. Huhmar, E., and Järvinen, P. A. (1961): Relation of epileptic symptoms to pregnancy, delivery and puerperium. *Ann. Chir. Gynaecol.*, 50:49–64.
13. Hunter, R. H. (1959–60): Status epilepticus: History, incidence and problems. *Epilepsia (Amst.)*, 4:162–188.
14. Janz, D. (1960): Status epilepticus und Stirnhirn. *Dtsch. Z. Nervenheilk.*, 180:562–594.
15. Janz, D. (1961): Conditions and causes of status epilepticus. *Epilepsia*, 2:170–177.
16. Janz, D. (1964): Status epilepticus and frontal lobe lesions. *J. Neurol. Sci.*, 1:446–457.
17. Janz, D. (1969): *Die Epilepsien*. Thieme, Stuttgart.
18. Janz, D., and Sommer-Burkhardt, E. -M. (1976): Discontinuance of antiepileptic drugs in patients with epilepsy, who have been seizure free for more than two years. In: *Epileptology*, edited by D. Janz. Thieme, Stuttgart.
19. Juul-Jensen, P. (1968): Frequency of recurrence after discontinuance of anticonvulsant therapy in patients with epileptic seizures. Follow-up after 5 years. *Epilepsia*, 9:11–16.
20. Kás, S., and Országh, J. (1976): Clinical study of status epilepticus. Review of 111 statuses. *Acta Univ. Carol. [Med.] (Praha)*, 22:133–178.
21. Ketz, E., and Meier, H. -R. (1979): Verlauf- und prognosebestimmende Faktoren beim Grand mal-Status. *Akt. Neurol.*, 6:233–239.
22. Liddel, D. W., and Retterstöl, N. A. (1957): The occurrence of epileptic fits in leucotomized patients receiving chlorpromazine therapy. *J. Neurol. Neurosurg. Psychiatry*, 20:105–107.
23. Littann-Masuhr, C. (1981): Grand mal-Status. Klinische und computertomographische Befunde. Unpublished manuscript.
24. McClure, J. H. (1955): Idiopathic epilepsy in pregnancy. *Am. J. Obstet. Gynecol.*, 70:296–301.
25. Meier, H. R. (1976): Der Status epilepticus in einem neurochirurgischen Krankengut, Ursache, auslösende Faktoren, Verlauf und Therapie. Inaugural Dissertation, Zürich.
26. Oller-Daurella, L., Oller, L., and Pamies, R. (1977): Clinical, therapeutic and social status of epileptic patients without seizures for more than 5 years. In: *Epilepsy*, edited by J. K. Penry. Raven Press, New York.
27. Oxbury, J. M., and Whitty, C. W. M. (1971): Causes and consequences of status epilepticus in adults. A study of 86 cases. *Brain*, 94:733–744.
28. Oxbury, J. M., and Whitty, C. W. M. (1971): The syndrome of isolated epileptic status. *J. Neurol. Neurosurg. Psychiatry*, 34:182–184.
29. Peiffer, J. (1963): *Morphologische Aspekte der Epilepsien, pathogenetische, pathologisch-anatomische und klinische Probleme der Epilepsien*. Springer, Berlin.
30. Peters, G. (1962): *Ergebnisse vergleichender anatomisch-pathologischer und klinischer Untersuchungen an Hirngeschädigten*. Thieme, Stuttgart.
31. Richards, R. K., and Taylor, J. D. (1956): Some factors influencing distribution, metabolism and action of barbiturates: A review. *Anesthesiology*, 17:414–458.
32. Roger, J., Lob, H., and Tassinari, C. A. (1974): Status epilepticus. In: *Neurology, Vol. 15, The Epilepsies*, edited by O. Magnus and A. M. Lorentz de Haas. North Holland, Amsterdam.
33. Rowan, A. J., and Scott, D. F. (1970): Major status epilepticus. A series of 42 patients. *Acta Neurol. Scand.*, 46:573–584.
34. Sachs, E. (1910): Status epilepticus und Schwangerschaft. *Mschr. Geburtsh. Gynäk.*, 32:649–672.
35. Schmidt, D. (1982): The effect of pregnancy on the natural course of epilepsy. In: *Epilepsy, Pregnancy and the Child*, edited by D. Janz, L. Bossi, M. Dam, H. Helge, A. Richens, and D. Schmidt, Raven Press, New York.
36. Victor, M., and Brausch, J. (1967): The role of abstinence in the genesis of alcoholic epilepsy. *Epilepsia*, 8:1–20.

37. Whitty, C. W. M. (1956): The diagnosis of epilepsy. *J. Indian Med. Assoc.*, 3:1268–1275.
38. Whitty, C. W. M. (1961): Focal epilepsy and the study of cortical function. *Med. J. Aust.*, 48:1–8.

39. Whitty, C. W. M., and Taylor, M. (1949): Treatment of status epilepticus. *Lancet*, 2:591–594.

Advances in Neurology, Vol. 34: Status Epilepticus, edited by A.V. Delgado-Escueta, C.G. Wasterlain, D.M. Treiman, and R.J. Porter. Raven Press, New York © 1983.

5

Prognosis in Convulsive Status Epilepticus

Gastone G. Celesia

Social, economic, and scientific changes in the last decade have profoundly influenced our daily medical practice. Many patients affected with previously fatal diseases (e.g., renal failure) are now alive under close medical management. In epilepsy, the introduction of new anticonvulsants, general monitoring of plasma drug levels, and utilization of new neuro-imaging techniques have greatly improved our diagnostic skills and therapeutic achievements. Whether or not these complex and multifactorial changes have influenced the causes, prevalence, and outcome of convulsive status epilepticus is unclear. In order to determine the effects of these changes, all cases of convulsive status epilepticus seen at the University of Wisconsin Hospitals/Veterans Administration Hospital Health Center complex between 1970 and 1980 were reviewed.

Convulsive status epilepticus was defined as a seizure characterized by the presence of muscle twitchings or clonic jerks persisting for at least 30 min or a seizure that, as defined by the International League against Epilepsy, "is repeated frequently enough to produce a fixed and enduring epileptic condition" lasting at least 30 min (5). Convulsive status was subdivided into two major categories: partial and generalized (Table 1). The classification outlined in Table 1 differs somewhat from the classification proposed by H. Gastaut in Chapter 2. The simple clinical observation that motor manifestations and particularly muscle jerks are either focal or generalized is at the base of this

TABLE 1. *Classification of convulsive epilepticus*

Partial or focal
  Motor status (Jacksonian status)
  Epilepsia partialis continua
Generalized
  Primary generalized
    Tonic-clonic status (grand mal status)
    Tonic status
    Status myoclonicus
  Partial with secondary generalization
    Partial motor with secondary generalization
    Partial adversive with secondary generalization

classification. Partial or focal status is further subdivided into motor or Jacksonian status and epilepsia partialis continua. Jacksonian status is characterized by recurring rhythmic motor twitches and a Jacksonian march with progressive recruitment of additional muscles, whereas epilepsia partialis continua refers to continuous rhythmic clonic jerks that remain localized to a limb or part of a limb. Generalized status is subdivided into primary generalized and partial status with secondary generalization in accordance with the international classification of epileptic seizures (5).

ETIOLOGY

Status epilepticus was found in 78 patients. There were 28 females and 50 males, ranging in age from 1.4 to 80 years (mean 41.4 years). The duration of status varied from 45 min to 2.5 months (mean 56 hr). The causes were varied. Sixty-one cases

(78%) were symptomatic of various central nervous system diseases (Table 2). Six cases (8%) were related to primary generalized epilepsy; the remaining 11 cases (14%) were of unknown cause. It is of interest that 8 (13%) of the 61 cases of symptomatic status were related to metabolic disturbances, comprising 3 cases of hyperosmolar nonketotic hyperglycemia and 1 case each of the following: renal failure with uremia, hyponatremia, and metabolic acidosis; respiratory alkalosis and electrolyte imbalance; metabolic alkalosis and hypokalemia; water intoxication and hyponatremia; hypoglycemia and hypokalemia.

Status epilepticus was caused by brain tumors in only 7 patients. Three patients had primary brain tumors (glioblastoma multiforme, astrocytoma, meningioma), and the remaining 4 patients had brain metastases.

The relationships between types and causes of status epilepticus are shown in Table 3. Note that

status myoclonicus was always secondary to a symptomatic cause, whereas all other types of status were related to chronic epilepsy or other diseases affecting the central nervous system.

PROGNOSIS AND THERAPY

Mortality varied in relation to the type and cause of status. Only 1 (6%) of the 17 patients with chronic epilepsy died. This patient was a 30-year-old woman in grand mal status who died in coma related to respiratory failure following phenobarbital therapy. Death occurred 20 hr after cessation of status epilepticus and 19 hr after respiratory arrest. Autopsy revealed severe generalized anoxic encephalopathy.

Seventeen (28%) of the 61 patients with symptomatic epilepsy died. Status was the direct cause of death in 6 patients. The remaining 11 patients died from the underlying neurological disease responsible for the status epilepticus; their deaths occurred during the first 10 months following the onset of epileptic status.

A variety of drugs were used to control status, but none was subjected to the rigors of a controlled clinical trial. Therapeutic failures could be classified into four types: patient death in status epilepticus; status gradually changing to frequent uncontrollable recurrent seizures; status ceasing, but patient left comatose and subsequently dying; status ceasing, but patient left with permanent neurological deficit. Failures occurred in 27 (35%) of the patients (Table 4). The causes of failure could be subdivided into two major categories: intract-

TABLE 2. *Causes of symptomatic status (61 cases)*

Cause	No.	Percent
Cerebrovascular	17	28
Head trauma	9	15
Metabolic	8	13
Brain tumor	7	11
Alcohol-related	5	8
CNS degenerative diseases	4	7
Anoxia	3	5
Multifactorial	2	3
Infective	1	2
Miscellaneous (multiple sclerosis, hydrocephalus)	5	8

TABLE 3. *Relationships between causes and types of convulsive status epilepticus*

Cause	No. of cases	Primary generalized (grand mal)	Partial with secondary generalization	Status myoclonicus	Motor Jacksonian	Epilepsia partialis continua
Primary generalized epilepsy	6	6	—	—	—	—
Unknown	11	2	4	—	2	3
Symptomatic	61	13	26	4	11	7
Head trauma	9	3	5	—	1	—
Cerebrovascular	17	1	6	—	7	3
Metabolic	8	2	1	2	1	2
Alcohol-related	5	1	4	—	—	—
Brain tumor	7	1	4	—	1	1
Miscellaneous	5	2	3	—	—	—
CNS degenerative	4	1	1	1	—	1
Anoxia	3	1	—	1	1	—
Multifactorial	2	1	1	—	—	—
Infective	1	—	1	—	—	—

TABLE 4. *Causes of therapeutic failure in convulsive status epilepticus*

Cause	No. of cases
Intractable status (20 cases)	
Acute massive destructive brain lesions	14
Irritative brain lesions, progressing to neuronal destruction	3
Chronic epilepsy with slowly deteriorating course	2
Unknown	1
Unsatisfactory management (7 cases)	
Inadequate anticonvulsant dosage	3
Failure to maintain adequate respiration	2
Wrong route of administration	1
Failure to continue maintenance dosage of anticonvulsants	1

able status (20 cases, or 26%); unsatisfactory medical management (7 cases, or 9%). Good control of status epilepticus was achieved with various anticonvulsants or an effective medical regimen in 51 cases (65%).

COMMENT

Convulsive status epilepticus, either partial or generalized, is most often symptomatic of a central nervous system disease (1–3,7–9,16,18,19,23,25). Table 5 shows a comparison of our present series with previously reported causes of generalized grand mal status. Seventy-one percent of 329 cases were secondary to diseases affecting the central nervous system. The three leading causes of status epilepticus in our series were cerebrovascular disease, head trauma, and metabolic disorders, comprising 56% of all the symptomatic causes of status. These etiological factors are not in agreement with the emphasis placed by previous authors on primary

brain tumors (7–9,16) as the most frequent cause of symptomatic status. In our series, brain tumors represented only 11% of the causes of symptomatic status and were most often metastatic. These changes are a reflection of the increased prevalence of cerebrovascular diseases, trauma, and metabolic encephalopathies in America. Another interesting observation was the occurrence of focal status epilepticus in 4 patients having metabolic and anoxic encephalopathy. Two of these patients had epilepsia partialis continua, one related to hypoglycemia and hypokalemia and the other related to hyperosmolar nonketotic hyperglycemia. Singh et al. (21,22) reported 21 patients in whom the predominant symptom of nonketotic hyperglycemia was epilepsia partialis continua, which occurred during the initial phase of hyponatremia and mild hyperosmolality. These observations suggest that in the search for causative factors, any form of convulsive status requires careful neurological evaluation. Whereas the possibility of an expanding lesion should always be kept in mind, a complete metabolic screening must be carried out in every case. The importance of metabolic disorders, including drug-related abnormalities and anoxia as important causative factors in status epilepticus, has also been noted in two recent surveys in Miami (6) and San Francisco (20).

Convulsive status epilepticus is a medical emergency involving great morbidity and mortality (1,2,4,20). The prognosis varies in relation to the cause of the status. The mortality from status was low (6%) among patients with chronic epilepsy, but it reached 28% in cases of symptomatic status. The low mortality among patients without underlying structural brain disorders probably reflects the improved therapeutic management of status epilepticus, whereas death in cases of symptomatic

TABLE 5. *Comparison of frequencies of symptomatic status in various studies*

Reference	No. of cases	Status in chronic epileptics		Symptomatic status	
		No.	%	No.	%
Whitty and Taylor (25)	25	4	16	21	84
Hunter (7)	30	8	27	22	73
Janz (8)	95	30	32	65	68
Rowan and Scott (19)	42	9	21	33	79
Oxbury and Whitty (16)	86	32	37	54	63
Celesia (present series)	51	12	24	39	76
Totals	329	95	29	234	71

status most often reflects the inexorable destructive nature of the central nervous system disease.

An effort has been made in this series to analyze the causes of treatment failure in an attempt to learn whether or not it is possible to improve our therapeutic successes. Twenty-six percent of the therapeutic failures were related to intractable status epilepticus. The majority of the cases were due to acute massive destructive brain lesions. Wallis et al. (24) and Prensky et al. (17) noted a similar phenomenon. The underlying organic disease causing status cannot be altered by anticonvulsants. Another cause of failure occurred in some cases of epilepsia partialis continua and partial motor status. Focal seizures persisted until they were substituted by a permanent paralysis of the affected part. It is presumed that the epileptic neurons responsible for the status died because of either excessive metabolic demand or progression of the organic disease that triggered their initial firing. There is some evidence that partial motor status, if left unchecked, may lead to irreversible neuronal loss. Knopman et al. (12) reported that epilepsia partialis continua in the right arm and leg of a 48-year-old woman lasted for 4 weeks until the woman died. Diffuse neuronal necrosis was found in the left hemisphere; the right hemisphere and the cerebellum were spared. Oxbury and Whitty (16) were the first to describe another type of intractable status that occurred in 5 of their 86 patients. It took the form of chronic epilepsy with a slowly deteriorating course. These patients had frequent and poorly controlled seizures and developed grand mal status that was difficult to control. They had a slowly deteriorating course, with frequent seizures and impairment of mental functions. Little is known about the initial factors triggering the slow deterioration. Serial grand mal seizures and/or convulsive status may produce irreversible neuronal destruction. Extensive neuronal loss and dense fibrous gliosis of Ammon's horns, neocortex, thalamus, and cerebellum have been reported in such cases (13–15). In our series, these cases represented only 3% of treatment failures. Unsatisfactory medical management caused treatment failure in 7 cases. Some patients were later controlled by a change in therapy, but 3 patients were left with permanent irreversible brain damage, and 1 patient died of respiratory arrest. The reasons for the failure to control status epilepticus were similar to those noted by Janz and Kautz (10) and Khalid and Schulz (11): (a) inadequate anticonvulsant dosage, (b) failure to maintain adequate respiration during administration of anticonvulsants, (c) wrong route of administration, and (d) failure to continue treatment after initial success.

Most of these errors were caused by unawareness of adequate management of convulsive status. These cases can and should be receiving better management. It should be our task as practicing neurologists to instruct our junior colleagues and our emergency room medical personnel about the necessity for aggressive medical therapy for status epilepticus, using the proper anticonvulsants given by the proper route in sufficient dosage, with constant attention to patent and adequate airways.

This educational task should be a continuing one to keep the medical profession aware of new therapeutic approaches and improved management techniques as they develop.

ACKNOWLEDGMENT

This project was supported in part by the Medical Research Section of the Veterans Administration.

REFERENCES

1. Celesia, G. G. (1976): EEG monitoring in status epilepticus. In: *Epileptology*, edited by D. Janz, pp. 328–337. G. Thieme, Stuttgart.
2. Celesia, G. G. (1976): Modern concepts of status epilepticus. *J. A. M. A.*, 12:1571–1574.
3. Celesia, G. G., Messert, B., and Murphy, M. J. (1972): Status epilepticus of late adult onset. *Neurology (Minneap.)*, 22:1047–1055.
4. Conomy, J. P., and McNamara, J. O. (1974): Emergency management of the patient with seizures. Part 2. Generalized status epilepticus. *Postgrad. Med.*, 55:71–74.
5. Gastaut, H. (1969): Clinical and electroencephalographic classification of epileptic seizures. *Epilepsia*, 10(Suppl.):S2–S13.
6. Ginsberg, P. L., Fischer, K. C., and Richey, E. T. (1976): Status epilepticus: Clinical, electrical, and therapeutic considerations in a general hospital population. *Neurology (Minneap.)*, 26:342.
7. Hunter, R. A. (1959): Status epilepticus: History, incidence, and problems. *Epilepsia*, 1:162–188.
8. Janz, D. (1961): Conditions and causes of status epilepticus. *Epilepsia*, 2:170–177.
9. Janz, D. (1964): Status epilepticus and frontal lobe lesions. *J. Neurol. Sci.*, 1:446–457.
10. Janz, D., and Kautz, C. (1963): Atiologie und therapie des status epilepticus. *Dtsch. Med. Wochenschr.*, 88:2189–2194.
11. Khalid, M. S., and Schulz, H. (1976): The treatment and management of emergency status epilepticus. *Epilepsia*, 17:73–76.

12. Knopman, D., Margolis, G., and Reeves, A. G. (1977): Prolonged focal epilepsy and hypoxemia as a cause of focal brain damage: A case study. *Ann. Neurol.*, 1:195–198.

13. Meyer, A., Beck, E., and Shepherd, M. (1955): Unusually severe lesions in the brain following status epilepticus. *J. Neurol. Neurosurg. Psychiatry*, 18:24–33.

14. Norman, R. M. (1964): The neuropathology of status epilepticus. *Med. Sci. Law*, 4:46–51.

15. Norman, R. M., Sandry, S., and Corsellis, J. A. N. (1974): The nature and origin of patho-anatomical change in the epileptic brain. In: *Handbook of Clinical Neurology, Vol. 15, The Epilepsies*, edited by O. Magnus and A. M. Lorentz de Haas, pp. 611–620. North Holland, Amsterdam.

16. Oxbury, J. M., and Whitty, C. W. M. (1971): Causes and consequences of status epilepticus in adults. *Brain*, 94:733–744.

17. Prensky, A. L., Raff, M. C., Moore, M. J., and Schwab, R. S. (1967): IV diazepam in the treatment of prolonged seizure activity. *N. Engl. J. Med.*, 276:779–784.

18. Roger, J., Lob, H., and Tassinari, C. A. (1974): Status epilepticus. In: *Handbook of Clinical Neurology, Vol. 15, The Epilepsies*, edited by O. Magnus and A. M. Lorentz de Haas, pp. 145–188. North Holland, Amsterdam.

19. Rowan, A. J., and Scott, D. F. (1970): Major motor status. *Acta Neurol. Scand.*, 46:573–584.

20. Simon, R. P., and Aminoff, M. J. (1980): Clinical aspects of status epilepticus in an unselected urban population. *Ann. Neurol.*, 8:93.

21. Singh, B. M., Gupta, D. R., and Strobos, R. J. (1973): Nonketotic hyperglycemia and epilepsia partialis continua. *Arch. Neurol.*, 29:287–290.

22. Singh, B. M., and Strobos, R. J. (1980): Epilepsia partialis continua associated with nonketotic hyperglycemia: Clinical and biochemical profile of 21 patients. *Ann. Neurol.*, 8:155–160.

23. Turner, W. A. (1907): *Epilepsy*. Macmillan, London.

24. Wallis, W., Kutt, H., and McDowell, F. (1968): IV DPH in treatment of acute repetitive seizures. *Neurology (Minneap.)*, 18:513–525.

25. Whitty, C. W., and Taylor, M. (1949): Treatment of status epilepticus. *Lancet*, 2:591–594.

Advances in Neurology, Vol. 34: Status Epilepticus, edited by A.V. Delgado-Escueta, C.G. Wasterlain, D.M. Treiman, and R.J. Porter. Raven Press, New York © 1983.

6

Petit Mal Status

Roger J. Porter and J. Kiffin Penry

Status epilepticus is virtually as heterogeneous as epilepsy itself (3). Although only convulsive status is immediately life-threatening, the various types of nonconvulsive status, such as simple partial status (epilepsia partialis continua), complex partial status (psychomotor status), and petit mal status (spike-wave stupor), may be seriously disabling. Of this latter group, petit mal status is the most frequently observed and the most varied in its nature and form. This chapter will consider petit mal status and contrast it with complex partial status, the seizure type with which it may be confused.

TERMINOLOGY

Petit mal status is known by a variety of names, most of which have attempted to describe some of the many phenomena observed (1). The name spike-wave stupor has some distinct advantages: (a) It is nonspecific and therefore relates well to the heterogeneity of the disorder, and (b) it implies a behavioral change without convulsions. Unfortunately, the name is a clinical-EEG hybrid without relationship to modern classifications of epileptic seizures. The name absence status is much more specific. It relates primarily to the carefully delineated clinical description of absence seizures (30), and when the absence seizures occur in a continuing state, it is appropriate to refer to this condition as absence status. The much less specific names nonconvulsive status and minor status fail even to distinguish the continuing petit mal or absence seizure from epilepsia partialis continua or complex partial status. The names epilepsia minoris continua, status pyknolepticus, prolonged epileptic twilight state, and prolonged behavioral disturbances as ictal phenomena all attempt to convey the concept of the continuous state of altered consciousness (and altered behavior) that occurs during an attack. One investigator even suggested "centrencephalic condition of prolonged disturbance of consciousness," abbreviated CCC (15). None of these names is adequately descriptive, and some are even inaccurate.

We have chosen the name petit mal status because it is widely used to describe seizures other than generalized tonic-clonic attacks, simple partial seizures, or complex partial seizures. The name has been used synonymously with absence status by many, but much less specifically by others. It implies a behavioral change and a generalized EEG abnormality, both of which are criteria for the population of patients described here. The name petit mal status will therefore be used in this chapter nonspecifically, whereas the name absence status, considered a subset of the overall petit mal status group, will refer specifically to absence seizures.

CLINICAL CHARACTERISTICS

Clinically, the most apparent feature of petit mal status is the state of altered consciousness and/or behavior that may be highly variable in an individual or among patients. The spectrum of altered consciousness was well summarized by Andermann and Robb (1). They described some petit mal status patients who were "normal" and were "only aware of a lack of efficiency," as well as those who were barely responsive during their attacks. Most patients are dull and confused, and responsiveness in the large majority will be neither normal nor totally lacking, but somewhere in between. Most are lethargic; they speak slowly, with decreased spontaneity, and are variably disoriented. Many will have spontaneous or environmentally induced automatisms and may be able to eat and drink, dress themselves, withdraw from painful stimuli, walk about, and even, in some cases, carry out simple commands.

These patients do not exhibit gross tonic-clonic activity, but they may have occasional myoclonic jerks of the extremities or, more commonly, of the eyelids, much as observed in classic absence seizures (30).

AGE AT ONSET

Petit mal status may begin at any time of life. Its onset may be the first sign of epilepsy, although the overwhelming majority of patients have epilepsy before the first attack of petit mal status. In Fig. 1, the age at onset of petit mal status was compared with the number of years of preexisting epilepsy in 62 patients from various reports (2,5,6,9–13,16–18,21,23–27,32–40). Excluded were cases of petit mal status in which the attacks were not distinct, such as Lennox-Gastaut syndrome. Cases of petit mal status induced by convulsant drugs were also excluded. Epilepsy beginning "in childhood" was considered arbitrarily as beginning at 8 years of age. In only 9 of the 62 patients (15%) was petit mal status the first sign of epilepsy. In many patients, however, decades separated the first occurrence of epilepsy and the first episode of petit mal status.

A distinct subgroup of patients experience petit mal status during the childhood and adolescent years when absence seizures begin. When the absence attacks are frequent, there may be a higher incidence of petit mal status, better named absence status. Any patient with absence seizures who has an unexpected, prolonged attack of altered consciousness should first be evaluated for absence status (a prolongation of the usual attacks) rather than a new and different seizure type such as complex partial seizures, a more unlikely possibility.

Another subgroup of patients with petit mal status is less well defined. They are the elderly who usually have no documented history of seizures but suddenly experience altered responsiveness. Petit mal status in the elderly may be much more

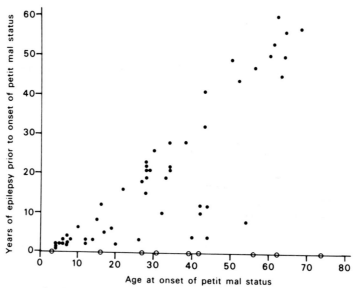

FIG. 1. Age at onset of petit mal status in relation to years of preexisting epilepsy. Onset of petit mal status varied from 3 to 74 years of age in 53 patients with epilepsy for <1 to 63 years *(filled circles).* The first bout of petit mal status occurred at ages 3 to 73 in 9 patients without a history of epilepsy *(open circles).*

resistant to therapy than that seen in the younger population.

BEHAVIORAL ALTERATIONS

The alterations in behavior during petit mal status are known from the general descriptions of relatives, nurses, physicians, and various other observers. Some EEG observations may be made after an attack, and occasionally during an attack, but a second-to-second correlation of behavioral and EEG alterations is not usually accomplished. The limits of general clinical observation have been discussed previously (28). Performance during petit mal status is altered least during the intervals between generalized spike-and-wave bursts, when the EEG may show only slow waves or generalized low-voltage theta activity (28).

In several studies, the performances during spike-and-wave paroxysms of a subgroup of individuals with petit mal status, mostly children with clearly defined absence seizures, were studied in detail (8, 14,29,31). When the scalp-recorded EEG was fully generalized and at highest voltage, performance was maximally impaired. There was no response unless strong and repetitive stimuli disrupted the generalized spike-and-wave discharge. It can be concluded from these studies that behavior is always altered during generalized, continuous spike-and-wave discharge in the EEG, although the spectrum of abnormal behavior may range from only a slight increase in reaction time to deep stupor. The latter is characterized by loss of response to stimuli in all modalities of sensation except withdrawal to painful stimuli.

PRECIPITATING FACTORS

More often than with the other types of epileptic seizures, patients with petit mal status can discern some internal or external factor that triggers the onset of their attacks (Table 1). We have noted sleep deprivation and pneumonia to be precipitants of petit mal status in children whose seizures had been completely controlled on ethosuximide. Other causes include pregnancy (10), renal failure (38), hypocalcemia (39), head trauma (20), and the use of convulsants such as megimide (13) and methohexitone (22).

EEG CHARACTERISTICS

The heterogeneity of patients with petit mal status is reflected in the wide variations in ictal EEGs.

TABLE 1. *Absence status:*
Circumstances of its occurrence

Spontaneous, precipitated by
Hyperventilation
Intermittent photic stimulation
Drug withdrawal
Metrazol activation
Emotion
Tension
Grief
Excitement
Fatigue
Minor trauma
Related to
Menstrual cycle
Sleep-waking cycle

From Andermann and Robb (1).

The classic, more or less continuous, 3/sec spike-and-wave has been described by many observers, and it likely correlates best with the typical absence seizure seen predominantly in childhood and early adolescence. Variations on the 3/sec spike-and-wave include 3 to 4/sec spike-and-wave (6,9–11), 4/sec spike-and-wave (5), 4 to 6/sec spike-and-wave (12), and irregular 3 to 5/sec slow waves with intermingled spikes (35). Other ictal abnormalities bear little relationship to the classic spike-and-wave discharge; they include irregular slow spikes and waves (4), 1/sec bursts of sharp waves and spikes (17), prolonged bursts of spike activity (32), and even generalized, periodic, high-voltage triphasic sharp waves at 2 to 3/sec (34). It is safe to conclude from these data that virtually any generalized continuous or nearly continuous abnormality could be a substrate for this syndrome. Also, it is clear that most, but certainly not all, patients have spike-and-wave abnormalities and that the name spike-wave stupor has obvious limitations as a description for the overall syndrome of petit mal status.

Another EEG criterion for this syndrome is the definitive change from the preictal state. The concept of petit mal status assumes a change from the normal or resting EEG at the time of the ictal event (6). Although this criterion may seem obvious, some reports have shown confusion in this regard, especially with children who have continuous generalized EEG abnormalities and either mental retardation or behavioral abnormalities or both. This problem is not new; it was addressed by Kellaway and Chao (19) in 1955. In describing the phenomenon of petit mal status, they stated that "this clinical pattern should be distinguished from a condition more commonly observed in children in which the mental deterioration is not reversible." Presumably, the EEG abnormalities in children with Lennox-Gastaut syndrome, for example, are a reflection of a fixed, or at least continuing, deficit of the brain and are not a temporary difficulty, as is characteristic of petit mal status. Brett (7) evaluated a number of children in whom such distinguishing features were less distinct and reported status lasting 4 min to months in various patients. He noted that treatment was most effective in those patients whose EEG changes correlated with their clinical states.

RESPONSIVENESS: PETIT MAL STATUS VERSUS COMPLEX PARTIAL STATUS

It has been appreciated that patients vary greatly in responsiveness during spike-wave stupor, but it has only anecdotally been reported that such patients show moment-to-moment variations in their abilities to respond. This is well documented in the following case report of petit mal (absence) status, in which responsiveness is graphically depicted in Fig. 2.

Case 1: Petit Mal Status

A 20-year-old woman had a history of seizures since age 10, when brief staring spells first began. These came without warning and lasted 2 to 3 sec. They were preceded by normal consciousness and were followed immediately by a normal preictal level of performance. A diagnosis of absence seizures was made. In spite of medication therapy, these spells occurred at least every day, and over several years they became longer, sometimes lasting 10 to 45 min. In addition to unresponsiveness and staring, the patient would have some fluttering of the eyelids and nodding of the head. Occasionally she would fall to the floor, and rarely she would be incontinent of urine. Even with the longer attacks she was immediately alert on cessation of the seizure activity. The patient had also experienced about 12 generalized tonic-clonic seizures, usually following a brief staring spell.

There was no family history of epilepsy. The patient developed normally, both intellectually and socially, until age 10. After that time, however, she began to do poorly in school, and although she

graduated from high school, she was a below-average student. Both general physical and neurological examinations were normal. The CT scan was normal.

Several EEGs showed 2.5 to 3/sec spike-and-wave discharges, especially during hyperventilation. Intensive monitoring (simultaneous telemetered EEG, video recording, and continuous verbal testing) documented absence status with onset of 5 to 6/sec spike-and-wave discharges, changing in 2 to 4 sec to 2.5 to 3/sec spike-and-wave discharges. The patient was treated with increased doses of ethosuximide, the addition of valproic acid and phenytoin (the latter for the generalized tonic-clonic attacks), and decreased doses of phenobarbital. Her brief attacks diminished dramatically, but some longer spells persisted.

The responsiveness during petit mal status is contrasted with that seen in complex partial status (Fig. 3).

Case 2: Complex Partial Status

A 23-year-old man was well until age 8. While on summer vacation, he vomited, complained of a headache, and then had a generalized tonic-clonic convulsion. He was hospitalized and remained unconscious for a week. The diagnosis was encephalitis of uncertain origin. When discharged after 4 weeks, he was taking three anticonvulsants. The seizures have continued since that time.

The most common seizure consists of staring, with the head turning to the left. There is some clonic jerking, followed by a variety of automatic motions. He may smile, get up, run, chew, pick at his clothes, undress, or pound his hand. After the episode, he feels weak.

There was no family history of seizures. Prior to the encephalitis, the patient was in the third grade and received average grades; since then he has been in special classes, but his learning ability has not progressed.

The general physical examination was normal. The neurological examination was also normal except for the mental status. He was able to carry on a normal conversation, but was unable to perform serial subtractions of 7 or 3. The CT scan was normal.

Several EEGs showed epileptiform activity bilaterally, with independent right and left hemispheric discharges with shifting localization. The background was slow and disorganized. Intensive

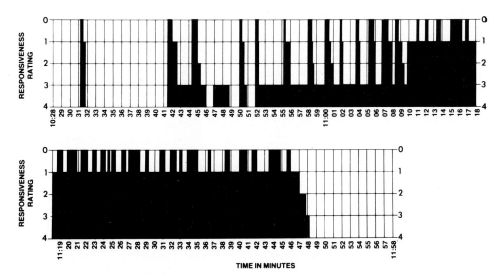

FIG. 2. Responsiveness during petit mal status. The patient had a brief absence attack at 10:31 a.m., then a series of attacks beginning at 10:41 a.m., with intervening periods of normal responsiveness. She had severe impairment of responsiveness from 11:10 a.m. to 11:48 a.m. and then made a sudden recovery without postictal abnormality or complaint. The verbal responsiveness rating is as follows: O = no response; 1 = minimal response; 2 = comprehends, follows simple directions, identifies receptively, cannot answer verbally, anomia may be present; 3 = partial responsiveness, responds appropriately with one or two words and rote phrases, abnormal affect, some anomia; 4 = accurate and immediate response, normal affect, responds to others, comments and initiates conversation, responds with more than one or two words.

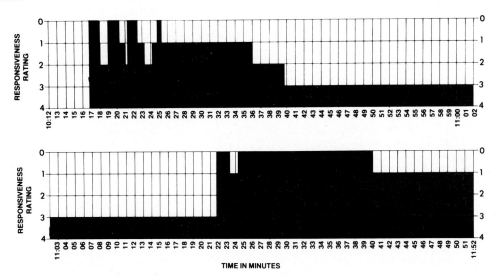

FIG. 3. Responsiveness during complex partial status. The patient had a complex partial seizure at 10:17 a.m. and did not return to normal consciousness until several hours later. He had several attacks at the onset of the status (10:17–10:25 a.m.), then appeared to be gradually recovering, but had another series of attacks beginning at 11:22 a.m. Recovery occurred gradually. The responsiveness rating is the same as in Fig. 2.

monitoring, as in the preceding case, documented complex partial seizures, with generalized 2 to 3/sec slow activity on the EEG without definite localization at onset.

Increased doses of phenytoin and carbamazepine were prescribed with equivocal results.

The clinical difference between petit mal and complex partial status helps to differentiate the two disorders. The former ends abruptly, without postictal abnormality; the latter is associated with postictal depression, confusion, or general malaise. In the petit mal status case, the patient suddenly recovered in less than 2 min from total unresponsiveness for more than 30 min to normal, alert responsiveness. This type of rapid recovery does not occur with complex partial status. Definitive discussion of complex partial status is presented in Chapter 7.

THERAPY

The therapy for petit mal status is pharmacological, assuming avoidance of precipitating factors. Many patients with single attacks of petit mal status have identifiable causes, such as structural or metabolic disease, and treatment of these problems is clearly paramount. In other patients with recurrent attacks of petit mal status, the need for antiepileptic drugs is clear. The use of antiabsence drugs is usually correct, and these should be tried to the fullest before being abandoned for phenytoin, carbamazepine, or phenobarbital. Antiabsence drugs are very effective against absence seizures. Therefore, to the extent that petit mal status resembles absence status, these drugs should be given maximal trial. Further, because the two major antiabsence drugs, ethosuximide and valproic acid, are nonsedative and are well tolerated by most patients, every effort should be made to assure response to these drugs before others are tried. It should be noted, however, that the acute attack often can be terminated by intravenous diazepam, if this is believed to be urgent.

The drug of first choice is ethosuximide, because of the small but definite risk of liver toxicity with valproic acid. Ethosuximide may be needed in rather high doses, and plasma levels (before the morning medication) in excess of 120 μg/ml may be required for seizure control in some patients. If valproic acid is used, plasma levels of 100 μg/ml may be necessary for seizure control. Ethosuximide and valproic acid can be used together with excellent effect in resistant patients.

Secondary antiabsence drugs include the benzodiazepine clonazepam or the oxazolidinedione trimethadione. If all antiabsence drugs fail, then the physician has no choice except to try phenytoin, phenobarbital, or carbamazepine. Unfortunately, there have been no well-controlled clinical trials in the treatment of petit mal status.

SUMMARY

Petit mal status is a heterogeneous clinical syndrome of nonconvulsive status epilepticus. The EEG accompaniment is likewise heterogeneous. Petit mal status occurs at all ages. The characteristics of this syndrome are quite nonspecific and consist of (a) behavioral changes, usually associated with lethargy, slowness, and decreased mental function, (b) abnormal generalized continuous or nearly continuous epileptiform EEG activity, and (c) absence of gross tonic-clonic activity or highly lateralized clonic activity.

These criteria do not distinguish petit mal status from complex partial status. Clinical evidence for abruptness of recovery and EEG evidence for localization are required for this distinction, an important factor in therapeutic decisions.

REFERENCES

1. Andermann, F., and Robb, J. P. (1972): Absence status. A reappraisal following review of thirty-eight patients. *Epilepsia*, 13:177–187.
2. Assael, M. I. (1972): Petit mal status without impairment of consciousness. *Dis. Nerv. Syst.*, 33:526–528.
3. Bancaud, J., Henriksen, O., Rubio-Donnadieu, F., Seino, M., Dreifuss, F. E., and Penry, J. K. (1981): Proposal for revised clinical and electroencephalographic classification of epileptic seizures. *Epilepsia*, 22:489–501.
4. Bendix, T. (1964): Petit mal status. *Electroencephalogr. Clin. Neurophysiol.*, 17:210–211.
5. Böhm, M. (1969): Status epilepticus petit-mal: Further observation of an adult case. *Electroencephalogr. Clin. Neurophysiol.*, 26:277–236.
6. Bornstein, M., Coddon, D., and Song, S. (1956): Case report. Prolonged alterations in behavior associated with a continuous electroencephalographic (spike and dome) abnormality. *Neurology (Minneap.)*, 6:444–448.
7. Brett, E. M. (1966): Minor epileptic status. *J. Neurol. Sci.*, 3:52–75.
8. Browne, T. R., Penry, J. K., Porter, R. J., and Dreifuss, F. E. (1974): Responsiveness before, during, and after spike-wave paroxysms. *Neurology (Minneap.)*, 24:659–665.
9. Crews, J., and Sidell, A. D. (1973): The clinical significance of spike and wave abnormalities in the adult. *Bull. Los Angeles Neurol. Soc.*, 38:60–68.
10. Dyro, F. M. (1977): Petit mal status epilepticus in a pregnant adult. *J. Maine Med. Assoc.*, 68:179–181, 185.
11. Friedlander, W. J., and Feinstein, G. H. (1956): Petit mal status. Epilepsia minoris continua. *Neurology (Minneap.)*, 6:357–362.
12. Gall, M. von, Scollo-Lavizzari, G., and Becker, H. (1978): Absence status in the adult. New results including computerized transverse axial tomography. *Eur. Neurol.*, 17:121–128.

13. Gastaut, H., Naquet, R., Poiré, R., and Tassinari, C. A. (1965): Treatment of status epilepticus with diazepam (Valium). *Epilepsia*, 6:167–182.
14. Goode, D. J., Penry, J. K., and Dreifuss, F. E. (1970): Effects of paroxysmal spike-wave on continuous visual-motor performance. *Epilepsia*, 11:241–254.
15. Hajnšek, F., and Dürrigl, V. (1970): Some aspects of so-called "petit mal status." *Electroencephalogr. Clin. Neurophysiol.*, 28:322.
16. Heathfield, K. W. G. (1972): Isolated petit-mal status presenting de novo in middle age. *Lancet*, 1:492 (letter).
17. Hess, R., Scollo-Lavizzari, G., and Wyss, F. E. (1971): Borderline cases of petit mal status. *Eur. Neurol.*, 5:137–154.
18. Hosokawa, K., and Booker, H. E. (1970): Spike-wave stupor. *Folia Psychiatr. Neurol. Jpn.*, 24:37–47.
19. Kellaway, P., and Chao, D. (1955): Prolonged status epilepticus in petit mal. *Electroencephalogr. Clin. Neurophysiol.*, 7:145.
20. Lion, P. (1967): A case of post-traumatic petit mal status. *Electroencephalogr. Clin. Neurophysiol.*, 22:96–97.
21. Lipman, I. J., Isaacs, E. R., and Suter, C. G. (1971): Petit mal status. A variety of non-convulsive status epilepticus. *Dis. Nerv. Syst.*, 32:342–345.
22. Male, C. J., and Allen, E. M. (1977): Methohexitone-induced convulsions in epileptics. *Anaesth. Intensive Care*, 5:226–230.
23. Mann, L. B. (1954): Status epilepticus occurring in petit mal. *Bull. Los Angeles Neurol. Soc.*, 19:96–109.
24. Merlis, S. (1960): Status epilepticus in petit mal. A case report. *Pediatrics*, 26:654–656.
25. Moe, P. G. (1971): Spike-wave stupor. Petit mal status. *Am. J. Dis. Child.*, 121:307–313.
26. Niedermeyer, E., and Khalifeh, R. (1965): Petit mal status ("spike wave stupor"). An electro-clinical appraisal. *Epilepsia*, 6:250–262.
27. Novak, J., Corke, P., and Fairley, N. (1971): "Petit mal status" in adults. *Dis. Nerv. Syst.*, 32:245–248.
28. Penry, J. K. (1973): Behavioral correlates of generalized spike-wave discharge in the electroencephalogram. In: *Epilepsy: Its Phenomena in Man*, edited by M. A. B. Brazier, pp. 171–188. Academic Press, New York.
29. Penry, J. K., and Dreifuss, F. E. (1969): Automatisms associated with the absence of petit mal epilepsy. *Arch. Neurol.*, 21:142–149.
30. Penry, J. K., Porter, R. J., and Dreifuss, F. E. (1975): Simultaneous recording of absence seizures with video tape and electroencephalography. A study of 374 seizures in 48 patients. *Brain*, 98:427–440.
31. Porter, R. J., and Penry, J. K. (1973): Responsiveness at the onset of spike-wave bursts. *Electroencephalogr. Clin. Neurophysiol.*, 34:239–245.
32. Rennick, P. M., Perez-Borja, C., and Rodin, E. A. (1969): Transient mental deficits associated with recurrent prolonged epileptic clouded state. *Epilepsia*, 10:397–405.
33. Schwab, R. S. (1953): A case of status epilepticus in petit mal. *Electroencephalogr. Clin. Neurophysiol.*, 5:441–442.
34. Schwartz, M. S., and Scott, D. F. (1971): Isolated petit-mal status presenting de novo in middle age. *Lancet* 2:1399–1401 (letter).
35. Thompson, S. W., and Greenhouse, A. H. (1968): Petit mal status in adults. *Ann. Intern. Med.*, 68:1271–1279.
36. Tucker, W. M., and Forster, F. M. (1950): Petit mal epilepsy occurring in status. *Arch. Neurol. Psychiatry*, 64:823–827.
37. van Leeuwen, W. S., Jennekens, F., and Sterk, C. E. (1969): A case of petit mal status with myoclonus. *Epilepsia*, 10:407–414.
38. Vignaendra, V., Ghee, L. T., and Lee, L. C. (1976): Petit mal status in a patient with chronic renal failure. *Med. J. Aust.*, 2:258–259.
39. Vignaendra, V., Frank, A. O., and Lim, C. L. (1977): Clinical note. Absence status in a patient with hypocalcemia. *Electroencephalogr. Clin. Neurophysiol.*, 43:429–433.
40. Vizioli, R., and Magliocco, E. B. (1953): Clinical and laboratory notes. A case of prolonged petit mal seizures. *Electroencephalogr. Clin. Neurophysiol.*, 5:439–440.

Advances in Neurology, Vol. 34: Status Epilepticus, edited by A.V. Delgado-Escueta, C.G. Wasterlain, D.M. Treiman, and R.J. Porter. Raven Press, New York © 1983.

7

Complex Partial Status Epilepticus

David M. Treiman and Antonio V. Delgado-Escueta

Nonconvulsive status epilepticus is characterized by the occurrence of prolonged epileptic fugue states manifested by confusion, speech arrest, automatic behavior, and amnesia. Two types of nonconvulsive status have been recognized. Petit mal status, or spike-wave stupor, is not uncommon (see Chapter 6). Since 1966, over 400 cases have been reported in the North American and western European literature (4). Complex partial status, on the other hand, is a rare condition. Since first described by Gastaut et al. (15) in 1956, only about 50 possible cases have been reported, including 24 in individual reports (2–5,10,12,13,15,17, 18,20,22–24,26,28–30,33,35,36) and the remainder in three reviews (14,19,36). Not all cases have been verified by EEG, and most have not completely fulfilled the criteria we shall propose for diagnosis.

One problem that may have contributed to the paucity of reports has been the lack of a precise definition of complex partial status epilepticus. This chapter will review what is currently known about the clinical and electrographic features of complex partial status and its differential diagnosis and treatment.

DEFINITION

Complex partial seizures are defined as seizures in which the initial clinical and electroencephalic changes are focal in onset and consciousness is impaired during the attack (7). Gastaut and Tas-

sinari (16) have suggested that two types of complex partial status epilepticus can be distinguished. One type consists of frequently recurring complex partial seizures that display classic psychomotor, psychosensory, or psychoaffective symptoms, but with interictal recovery of consciousness to nearly normal. The second form of complex partial status, according to Gastaut and Tassinari, consists of continuous long-lasting episodes of mental confusion and/or psychotic behavior with or without automatic behavior.

We would suggest that there is no fundamental difference between these two forms of complex partial status, but rather that they constitute two ends of a continuum of clinical behavior. As long as a patient is having repeated or continuous complex partial seizures and does not fully recover between seizures to a completely normal state, with no sign of residual deficits, then the patient can be considered to be in status. Wieser (35) has recently reported transition from repeated discrete seizures, during which his patient remained fully conscious and oriented, to a continuous epileptic clouded state.

DIAGNOSIS

Table 1 outlines our criteria for the diagnosis of complex partial status epilepticus. The fundamental characteristic of complex partial seizures, and the characteristic that allows differentiation from other causes of twilight states, is the cyclicity of

TABLE 1. *Criteria for diagnosis of complex partial status epilepticus*

1. Recurrent complex partial siezures without full recovery of consciousness between seizures, or a continuous "epileptic twilight state," with cycling between unresponsive and partially responsive phases
2. Ictal EEG with recurrent epileptiform patterns like those seen in isolated complex partial seizures
3. A prompt observable effect of intravenous antiepileptic drug on both ictal EEG and clinical manifestations of the status
4. Interictal EEG with a consistent epileptiform focus, usually in one or both temporal lobes

clinical behavior observed during complex partial status.

We have observed two separate behavioral phases during complex partial status in 11 patients (Fig. 1): (a) a continuous twilight state, with partial and amnestic responsiveness, partial speech, and quasi-purposeful complex automatisms, frequently interrupted by (b) staring, total unresponsiveness, speech arrest, and stereotyped automatisms. During the staring phase, temporal lobe discharges were always present on the EEG. During the twilight phase, the EEG pattern was different from that during the staring phase. In most cases, bilateral slow waves appeared, frequently intermixed with low-voltage fast activity; in 1 patient, the background was normal, and left anterior-temporal triangular slow waves were seen. Clinically and electroencephalographically, the phases observed in these 11 cases of complex partial status epilepticus were identical with the three clinical phases described for individual complex partial seizures by Delgado-Escueta and his colleagues (stare, stereotyped automatisms, reactive automatisms) (9,11). This suggests that complex partial status epilepticus consists of continuously recurring cycles of the clinical phases of complex partial seizures. Initially, discrete serial seizures may occur. Eventually the patient fails to completely recover from the longer state of partial and amnestic responsiveness before the next cycle of staring and stereotyped automatisms begins. At this point the patient

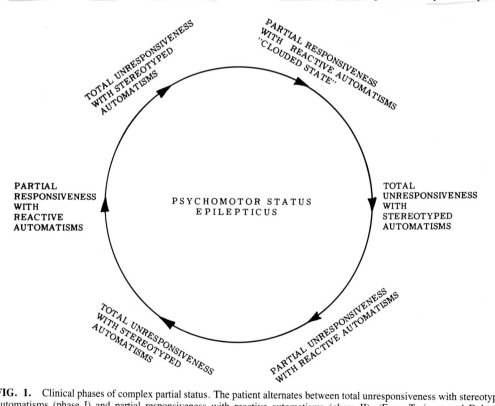

FIG. 1. Clinical phases of complex partial status. The patient alternates between total unresponsiveness with stereotyped automatisms (phase I) and partial responsiveness with reactive automatisms (phase II). (From Treiman and Delgado-Escueta, ref. 32).

should be considered to be in complex partial status. The frequency of the cycles may increase until the patient appears to be in a continuous epileptic twilight or fugue state. However, even in the most severe forms of complex partial status, careful observation should allow detection of the clinical phases and concomitant cycling of the EEG patterns.

The following case illustrates in detail the type of cyclicity of clinical and electrical activity we have seen (3): This patient had generalized major motor convulsions at age 2 years. At age 16, "blackout" spells occurring once a month and lasting 2 to 5 min were preceded by a sensation of fear, as if he were startled. Radiological examinations revealed a right posterior parietotemporal arteriovenous malformation and mild central atrophy.

Ten days before admission, at age 31 years, he had numerous generalized tonic-clonic seizures, despite oral anticonvulsant medication. Three generalized tonic-clonic seizures were witnessed in the emergency room. Between these major motor attacks, he was confused. In addition, episodes of blinking and total unresponsiveness alternated with periods of partial and amnesic responsiveness.

Sixty-eight sequences of total unresponsiveness with stereotyped automatisms and partial responsiveness with reactive automatisms were captured on the videotape during 6 hr of recording.

Total unresponsiveness occurred every 4 to 5 min. He stared and was motionless for 5 to 6 sec. Low-voltage 20-Hz fast rhythms in the right hemisphere were best seen in the lateral midtemporal (T4), central (C4), and medial temporal (NP2) regions. These coincided with the onset of the initial stare. During the first 16 sec, he did not respond to pinprick or deep pain (Fig. 2). Corneal reflexes were absent. Over the next 10 sec, 20-Hz rhythms increased in amplitude and subsequently changed into rhythmic 40- to 60-μV 16-Hz sharp waves and spikes that spread to both the lateral and medial aspects of the right temporal region. By this time, the patient responded to pain but appeared confused and did not speak. After a few seconds, frequencies slowed to 8 to 9 Hz. As low-voltage fast spikes appeared on the right side, 3- to 4-Hz irregular waves built up in the left hemisphere. These were best seen in the medial temporal areas (Fig. 2). The activities in the left hemisphere slowed further to 2 to 2.5 Hz as right medial 8- to 9-Hz sharp waves continued. As this stage continued,

he did not respond to verbal commands and looked from side to side. When 7-Hz and low-voltage 1- to 3-Hz activity appeared dominant in the right hemisphere, 2- to 2.5-Hz activity continued in the left hemisphere. At this time, behavior appeared quasi-purposeful, and verbal responses varied. He turned and sat up (Fig. 3). At times he was completely oblivious to commands and spoken communication. Occasionally, he responded appropriately and quickly to simple commands, such as "Open your mouth." As this state of amnesic responsiveness and complex purposeful behavior continued, the EEG showed diffuse, bilateral low-voltage fast activity and polymorphic medium-voltage 4- to 6-Hz waves. There were also frequent bursts of synchronous high-voltage 100- to 250-msec slow waves; these lasted 3 to 10 sec and occurred bilaterally and symmetrically. Right medial temporal spikes also appeared (Fig. 4).

In only a few other cases has this cyclicity been adequately documented (10,13,20,29,33,35). In the discrete or serial form of complex partial status, such as first described by Gastaut et al. (15), cyclicity can be easily identified because the patient has a series of complex partial seizures, with partial clearing of mentation between the seizures. However, others (17,26) have observed a waxing and waning of alertness during apparently continuous confusion, and definite cycles have not been identified. Henriksen (18) reported a 39-year-old woman who experienced a prolonged state of anxiety that frequently rose to bouts of maximal fear, without definite impairment of consciousness. The EEG showed almost continuous irregular spike activity in the right sphenoidal lead. Every 8 to 10 sec there was a spread of spike activity that was followed by generalized desynchronization and cessation of spike activity for 2 to 3 sec. The patient was asked to signal with her hand at the height of the fear sensation. Maximum fear always occurred in the middle of a period of desynchronization. Other studies have reported continuous confusion and disorientation, with no mention of variability in clinical status during the prolonged attack (2,22,24,28,36).

Engel et al. (13) reported fluctuations of consciousness in four attacks of complex partial status in a 20-year-old girl. During the attacks, which lasted several days to 2 weeks, the patient cycled between brief periods of deep coma, in which she was responsive only to deep pain, and a more prolonged trancelike state, during which she ex-

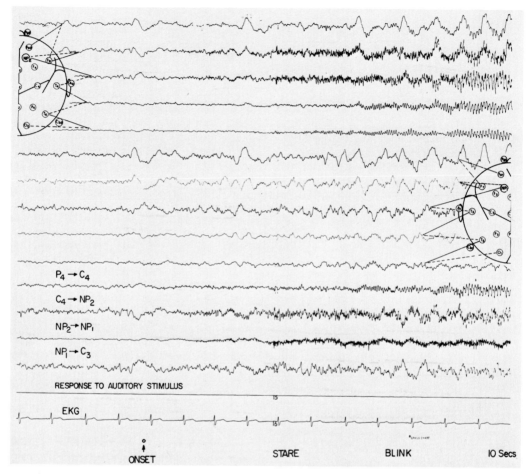

FIG. 2. Right-hemisphere 20-Hz rhythms best developed at T4, C4, and NP2 appear at the onset of stare. (From Belafsky et al., ref. 3, with permission).

hibited reactive automatisms. The EEG showed similar fluctuations, although there was no clear-cut correlation between clinical activity and EEG activity such as we observed in our case described earlier. Continuous epileptiform temporal-occipital abnormalities were recorded on the EEG. Individual cycles showed a sequential pattern of EEG abnormalities similar to those reported for individual complex partial seizures reported from medically intractable patients being considered for temporal lobe resection (34). Low-voltage 12- to 14-Hz discharges on one side evolved after seconds or minutes to higher-voltage 4- to 6-Hz sharp waves, followed by low-voltage slowing. Such cycles were repeated throughout the attack, except for one 13-min period of transient interruption after administration of 5 mg of diazepam. However,

there was no consistency in the side of onset of the low-voltage discharges, even though the EEGs obtained after the attack of complex partial status was resolved showed a left occipital-temporal focus. This alternation of sides of onset is similar to a pattern we have seen in a 57-year-old man with prolonged complex partial status (33). One week after the onset of waxing and waning confusion, he alternated between brief periods of total unresponsiveness and a confused, partially reactive twilight state for which he was subsequently amnestic. His EEG showed paroxysmal bursts of rhythmic 6-Hz sharp waves, with phase reversal around the sphenoidal electrodes, alternating between the left and right sides, superimposed on high-voltage delta activity during the unresponsive periods (Figs. 5 and 6). Low-voltage theta and

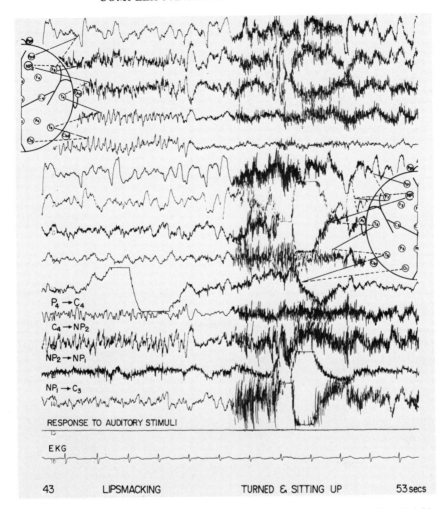

FIG. 3. Transition from stereotyped automatisms to quasi-purposeful complex automatisms. (From Belafsky et al., ref. 3.)

alpha activity was seen during the periods of reactive automatisms. Subsequent EEGs showed a right temporal lobe focus.

The ictal EEG patterns reported for complex partial status are essentially those reported for individual complex seizures by Ajmone Marsan and Van Buren (1), Walter (34), and Klass (21). The specific pattern seen in an individual case appears to be determined by the frequency with which the individual cycles repeat and the overall duration of the attack at the time of the recording. Thus, in several of our cases (Figs. 2 and 7) and in Heintel's cases (17) and Engel's cases (13), low-voltage fast activity was seen at the start of the cycle, followed by rhythmic buildup of higher-amplitude but lower-frequency discharges, just as

is seen in isolated complex partial seizures. In cases of longer duration before the EEG is recorded, as in another of our cases (33), no low-voltage fast activity is seen, but rather recurrent paroxysms of rhythmic sharp waves from one or the other sphenoidal electrode superimposed on a generally slow background (Figs. 5 and 6). Still others have described continuous sharp- and slow-wave discharges (2,24) or continuous spikes, polyspikes, or sharp waves (18,26,28) from the temporal regions.

There has been only one report of depth-electrode recording during complex partial status. Wieser (35) described a 22-year-old woman with medically intractable complex partial seizures who was evaluated for temporal lobectomy with deep elec-

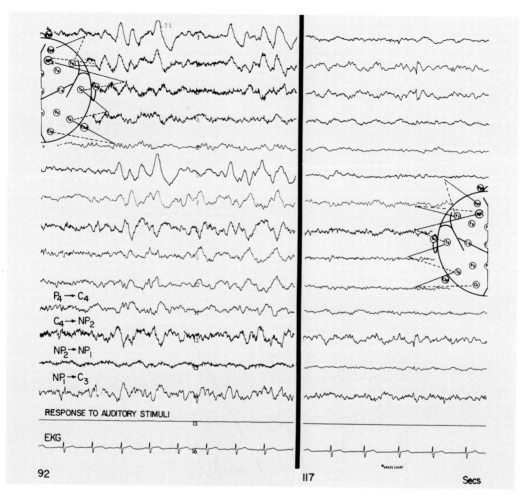

FIG. 4. Diffuse paroxysmal slow waves alternate with low-voltage fast activities during the continuous twilight state, with reactive automatic behavior. Right medial temporal spikes also appeared at this time. (From Belafsky et al., ref. 3.)

trodes. During the last 2 days of the recording period, she developed "psychomotor status." The episode began as frequently recurring focal seizures characterized by "strange feeling, anxiety, and sometimes . . . visceral symptoms" and associated with right hippocampal discharges that usually started in the amygdala. During the focal attacks, the patient remained fully conscious and oriented. The seizures progressed to produce impairment of consciousness and more elaborate psychosensory seizures. When consciousness was clouded, bilateral hippocampal discharges were seen. Ultimately the patient developed continuous electrical status of the right transverse gyrus of Heschl. When the right-sided hippocampal electrical activity became

more and more monotonous, it triggered activity of the left hippocampus, and the patient became increasingly anxious and stopped her animated conversation. During more tonic seizure activity, which recurred crescendolike at the beginning of the continuous status, the patient stared with fixed gaze and frozen face and then usually brought her left hand to her heart and turned her face slightly to the left. The stare and repeated stereotyped automatisms described here may correspond with phases I and II of isolated complex partial seizures previously described by Delgado-Escueta et al. (11). Wieser (35) suggested that the continuous form of complex partial seizures may best be thought of as a prolonged localized afterdischarge.

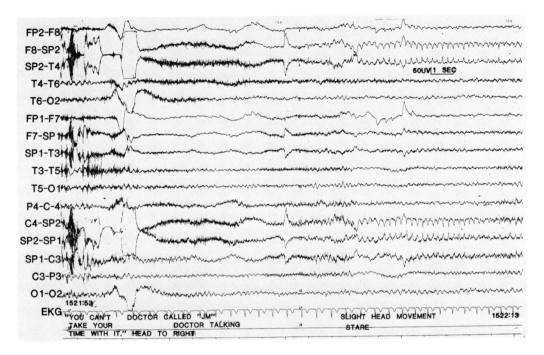

FIG. 5. Rhythmic 5-Hz sharp waves with phase reversal around right sphenoidal electrode appearing at onset of unresponsive phase and stare.

In most reported cases of complex partial status epilepticus the interictal EEG has exhibited spikes, spike-waves, or sharp waves from one or both temporal lobes, similar to the interictal epileptiform discharges usually associated with a temporal lobe epileptic focus. A few cases have shown temporal-occipital foci in the interictal EEG after temporal-occipital discharges during the episode of status (13,17,24).

Identification of interictal epileptiform discharges from a region of the brain known to produce complex partial seizures should be considered an essential element in the diagnosis of complex partial status epilepticus. However, EEG recording techniques adequate to capture interictal temporal spikes or sharp waves, if they are present, must be used. Delgado-Escueta (8) observed 3 to 1,200 temporal spikes per hour during prolonged EEG recording in a group of patients with known complex partial seizures when nasopharyngeal or sphenoidal electrodes were used during stage II sleep. Thus, a minimum of 30 min of recording in stage II sleep should result in the recording of at least one temporal lobe spike discharge to confirm the presence of an interictal temporal lobe focus.

DIFFERENTIAL DIAGNOSIS

When complex partial status epilepticus presents as a prolonged twilight or confusional state, there are many conditions with which it may be confused. The differential diagnosis of complex partial status epilepticus is outlined in Table 2.

Absence status epilepticus or petit mal status is the most common cause of an epileptic twilight state and may be difficult to distinguish from complex partial status epilepticus. However, there are several clinical and electrical characteristics by which these two forms of epileptic twilight states may be differentiated (Table 3). Complex partial status epilepticus is manifested by recurring cycles of two separate phases, whereas petit mal status appears to consist of only one continuous twilight state, with partial responsiveness of variable intensity. Total unresponsiveness does not occur in petit mal status, in contrast to the phase of staring, total unresponsiveness, and stereotyped automatisms that reoccurs in cyclical fashion in complex partial status epilepticus. Although stereotyped automatisms, such as blinking and chewing, appear in both petit mal status and complex partial status, they last longer in complex partial status and may be somewhat more complex. The EEG of petit mal

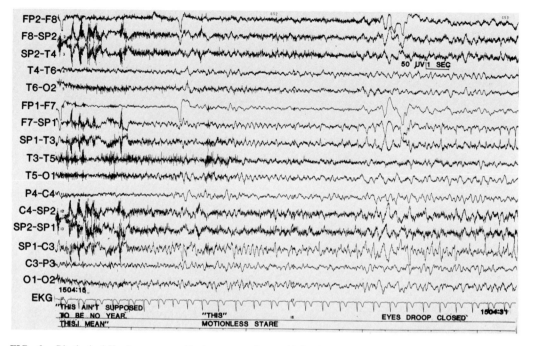

FIG. 6. Rhythmic 6-Hz sharp waves with phase reversal around left sphenoidal electrode appearing at onset of another cycle of total unresponsiveness and stare (same patient as in Fig. 5).

TABLE 2. *Differential diagnosis of complex partial status epilepticus*

1. Absence status epilepticus or spike-wave stupor
2. Other "epileptiform" causes of confusion
   Prolonged postictal confusion
   Delirium in cerebral infarction
   Confusion associated with PLEDs
   Poriomania
3. Organic encephalopathies
   Toxic-metabolic encephalopathies, especially hypoglycemia
   Alcohol and other drug intoxication or withdrawal
   Transient ischemic attacks
   Transient global amnesia
   Posttraumatic amnesia
4. Psychiatric syndromes
   Dissociative reactions
   Hysterical conversion reactions
   Acute psychotic reactions

status is characterized by diffuse spike-wave rhythms of 1 to 3 Hz or 4 to 6 Hz that may be continuous, intermittent, or irregular in their appearance. There is no exact correlation between variations in the EEG pattern and in clinical behavior. On the other hand, in complex partial status there is good correlation between the EEG changes and the cycling between the two clinical phases. During the staring phase, with stereotyped automatisms, EEG patterns like those seen at the onset of individual complex partial seizures, such as rhythmic spikes, sharp waves, or low-voltage fast activity, are always seen. During the twilight state, with partial responsiveness and reactive automatisms, there is normalization of the EEG and appearance of EEG patterns like those seen at the end of an individual complex partial seizure or in the immediate postictal phase. Various patterns have been observed during this twilight phase (Table 3).

Penfield and Jasper (31) have described prolonged postictal confusional states in which the EEG is diffusely slow. Such cases usually follow a well-documented generalized tonic-clonic seizure, and there is no cycling between two clinical phases as in complex partial seizures and no change in the EEG or clinical behavior following administration of diazepam intravenously. Passouant et al. (30) reported three episodes of confusion, agitation, and disorientation in a 57-year-old woman with general paresis. The third episode, which lasted 2 weeks, did not follow a convulsion and was believed to be an example of complex partial status epilepticus. However, the initial EEG showed rhythmic sharp waves in the left temporal region, which occurred approximately once per second and

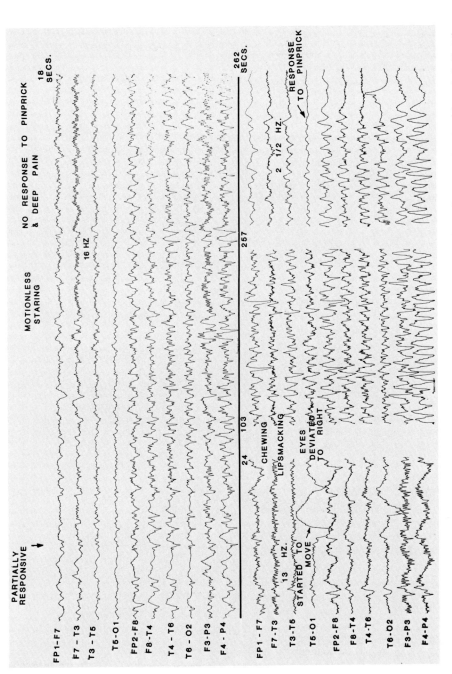

FIG. 7. Psychomotor status epilepticus in a 53-year-old patient. 16-Hz rhythms appear in the left anterior temporal region (channels 1–3) at the onset of stare and phase of total unresponsiveness. The phase of partial responsiveness is characterized by chewing, lip smacking, and deviation of the eyes to the right. Rhythmic slow waves are seen on the EEG bilaterally. (From Treiman and Delgado-Escueta, ref. 32.)

TABLE 3. *Clinical characteristics of prolonged twilight states*

Petit mal status		Complex partial status
	Clinical	
Prolonged state of one attack rather than repeated attacks		Continuous series of repeated attacks
Present	Phase of responsiveness with confusion, disorientation, speech arrest, amnesia, and automatisms	Present
Absent	Phase of total unresponsiveness with stereotyped automatisms	Present
	EEG	
Continuous or noncontinuous diffuse irregular 1.5–4-Hz multi-spike-wave complexes; no patterns are time-locked with automatisms	Phase of partial unresponsiveness and reactive automatisms	1. Low-voltage fast activities with bursts of diffuse slow waves, or 2. Rhythmic bilateral diffuse spokes or slow waves or both most evident anteriorly, or 3. Anterior temporal sharp waves with normal background
	Phase of total unresponsiveness and stereotyped automatisms	1. Correlates with bimedial temporal waves or lateralized to 8–20-Hz spikes

From Belafsky et al. (3).

had the appearance of periodic lateralized epileptiform discharges (PLEDs). PLEDs occur in patients with acute focal cerebral lesions, usually of vascular cause, and frequently are associated with confusion and lethargy, and they may superficially resemble other epileptic twilight states (6,25). Delirium and confusion may occasionally occur in association with cerebral infarction, even in the absence of PLEDs, but the clinical course following the infarction, the presence of focal or lateralizing neurological abnormalities, and the absence of cycling between two clinical phases should allow differentiation from complex partial status epilepticus without significant difficulty.

A variety of other organic encephalopathies may also give rise to acute confusional states that may occasionally be difficult to distinguish from a prolonged epileptic twilight state. Various metabolic encephalopathies, especially hypoglycemia, alcohol abuse, other drug intoxication or withdrawal, and head trauma all can give rise to prolonged confusional states. Although some waxing and waning of the level of consciousness may occur in these conditions, there is never a clearly cyclical pattern of alternation between partial responses associated with reactive automatisms and total unresponsiveness associated with stereotyped automatisms, as seen in complex partial status epilepticus. Furthermore, the EEG in these conditions is quite different from that seen in complex partial

status and does not show periodic ictal discharges, as are associated with the unresponsive phase of complex partial status.

Complex partial status epilepticus must be differentiated from several different psychiatric syndromes. This is especially important in patients with documented preexisting complex partial seizures, because many of these patients also have psychiatric disorders. The observation of interictal temporal lobe spike discharges is not sufficient to prove that a prolonged fugue state is indeed an epileptic twilight state. Apparent confusion due to psychotic episodes or due to psychogenic fugue states may occur in epileptic patients as well as nonepileptic patients. In these instances it is necessary to document ictal epileptiform abnormalities at the time of the fugue in order to establish the diagnosis of an epileptic twilight or fugue state. The diagnosis of complex partial status and its differentiation from absence status are then, as discussed earlier, based on the presence of clinical and EEG cycling between two distinct phases.

Poriomania represents a special type of dissociation reaction or fugue state that refers specifically to prolonged ambulatory behavior in epileptic patients for which they are amnestic.

Mayeux and his colleagues (27) recently reported 3 cases of poriomania recurring in patients with apparent complex partial seizures and interictal mesial temporal spike discharges on the EEG.

These authors suggested that poriomania is a prolonged postictal automatism and not psychogenic in origin. Unfortunately, EEGs could not be obtained at the time of attack for any of these 3 patients. In none of them was cycling between partial and total unresponsiveness described. Poriomania may be a special case of the postictal confusional state, but it should not be considered a type of complex partial status epilepticus unless it can be shown to fulfill the criteria for the diagnosis of complex partial status outlined in Table 1.

CONSEQUENCES OF COMPLEX PARTIAL STATUS

The role of the hippocampus in the acquisition of new memories has been well documented. There is increasing experimental evidence that repeated electrical discharges may produce profound neuronal damage, even in the absence of convulsive activity. Brown and Babb (Chapter 15), Söderfeldt et al. (Chapter 16), Meldrum (Chapter 24), and Collins et al. (Chapter 25) have presented evidence for focal neuronal damage following experimental status epilepticus. Clinically, Engel and his colleagues (13) have described a patient with a prolonged memory deficit following complex partial status epilepticus. We also have seen 2 patients who developed profound memory deficits following prolonged complex partial status (33).

The first patient was a 53-year-old man with a brief history of seizures. Carbamazepine caused a desquamating rash and was stopped abruptly, precipitating decreased consciousness and confusion. After 1 week he was transferred to our hospital in a continuous epileptic fugue state, and the diagnosis of complex partial status epilepticus was made. The patient was treated with intravenous diazepam, which stopped the episode of status. Following recovery to full consciousness, he had a significant deficit in mental function, particularly in short-term memory. Although the scores on the Wechsler Adult Intelligence Scale were normal 2 months later, the Wada test of memory, given after 4 months, showed that he was able to remember only one of three items in the left hemisphere and none of the items in the right hemisphere.

The second patient was a 53-year-old woman who worked as a bookkeeper until she had sudden onset of generalized tonic-clonic status epilepticus. After antiepileptic drug treatment, the status converted to a prolonged epileptic fugue state, during which she exhibited cycling between a clinical phase of immobile staring, with no response to the external environment, and a phase characterized by complex reactive automatic behavior. The patient was treated with a variety of anticonvulsant drugs, and finally with 2 g of intravenous phenobarbital, which stopped the episode of complex partial status epilepticus. Three weeks after the patient's first seizure, she awoke with no recent or remote memory. Since that time, she has had a persistent memory deficit and has continued to have intractable complex partial seizures, as well as several further episodes of complex partial status epilepticus. The cause of this patient's seizures was never ascertained.

TREATMENT

Responses to treatment have only infrequently been described in reports of complex partial status, and the details frequently have been lacking. Lugaresi et al. (24) reported that continuous sharp-and-slow-wave discharges in the right temporal-occipital region disappeared when the clinical episode of complex partial status ended, but they did not comment on treatment. Intravenous diazepam has been most frequently mentioned in those reports that have discussed treatment at all, but it has only sometimes been successful at stopping status at the dosages used. Wolf (36), in his first case, reported that diazepam improved both the clinical and EEG manifestations, but he gave no further details. Engel et al. (13) reported a transient interruption of continuous temporal-occipital epileptiform EEG abnormalities after administration of diazepam, but only gradual improvement after phenobarbital and phenytoin. In Wieser's case (35), diazepam produced a decrease in the frequency of the recurrent tonic discharges. Wolf (36), in his second case, and more recently Behrens (2), reported improvement the next day after treatment with diazepam or with diazepam and phenytoin.

Only two recent reports have documented definite responses to diazepam. Mayeux and Lueders (28) administered 2 mg of diazepam, which promptly stopped the epileptiform discharges on EEG, after which the patient slept for 5 min and then awoke alert and able to follow commands. Markand et al. (26) also reported that administration of diazepam promptly stopped both the clinical and electrical manifestations of status.

The ease and rapidity of response to intravenous anticonvulsant medication may be partially determined by the duration of status at the time of treatment. We have recently seen a 57-year-old man who had been in a stuporous twilight state for 8 days after cardiac surgery. The EEG showed continuous epileptiform discharges from both temporal regions. Four milligrams of diazepam promptly normalized the EEG, but full recovery of mental alertness required several days. If complex partial status is sufficiently prolonged before adequate treatment, permanent changes in mental status may occur, as described earlier.

Two patients with complex partial status who underwent temporal lobectomy have experienced no further seizures and no episodes of status following surgery (18,35).

The need for rapid and vigorous treatment of complex partial status epilepticus has only recently been recognized. In the past, the assertion was made that nonconvulsive status and focal convulsive status need not be treated with the same urgency as generalized tonic-clonic status. However, increasing evidence has amply demonstrated that profound neural damage can occur as a result of repeated electrical discharges in the brain, even in paralyzed ventilated animals. Therefore, it is imperative to treat all forms of status, with either primary or secondary engagement of the cerebral cortex, as quickly as possible to prevent permanent neuronal damage. However, in order to avoid inappropriate administration of large doses of potentially toxic drugs, it is essential to establish the diagnosis of status epilepticus prior to initiating treatment. In the cases of nonconvulsive status, the choice of drugs will be influenced by whether the epileptic fugue represents petit mal status or complex partial status. Thus a patient suspected of having complex partial status should be observed under EEG control sufficiently long to identify the patterns of clinical and EEG cyclicity described earlier. Treatment should then be initiated with intravenous diazepam and phenytoin. Intravenous diazepam should be given at a rate no faster than 2 mg/min until the status stops or to a total dose of 20 mg. Simultaneously or immediately after the diazepam is given, infusion of phenytoin should be initiated at a rate no faster than 50 mg/min to a total dose of 18 mg/kg.

REFERENCES

1. Ajmone Marsan, C., and Van Buren, J. M. (1958): Epileptiform activity in cortical and subcortical structures in the temporal lobe of man. In: *Temporal Lobe Epilepsy*, edited by M. Baldwin and P. Bailey, pp. 78–108. Charles C Thomas, Springfield, Ill.
2. Behrens, J. M. (1980): Psychomotor status epilepticus masking as a stroke. *Postgrad. Med.*, 68:223–226.
3. Belafsky, M. A., Carwille, S., Miller, P., Waddell, G., Boxley-Johnson, J., and Delgado-Escueta, A. V. (1978): Prolonged epileptic twilight states: Continuous recordings with nasopharyngeal electrodes and videotape analysis. *Neurology (Minneap.)*, 28:239–245.
4. Celesia, G. G. (1976): Modern concepts of status epilepticus. *J.A.M.A.*, 235:1571–1574.
5. Celesia, G. G., Messert, B., and Murphy, M. J. (1972): Status epilepticus of late adult onset. *Neurology (Minneap.)*, 22:1047–1055.
6. Chatrian, G. E., Shaw, C. M., and Leffman, H. (1964): The significance of periodic lateralized epileptiform discharges in EEG: An electrographic, clinical and pathological study. *Electroencephalogr. Clin. Neurophysiol.*, 17:177–193.
7. Commission on Classification and Terminology of the International League against Epilepsy (1981): Proposal for revised clinical and electroencephalographic classification of epileptic seizures. *Epilepsia*, 22:489–501.
8. Delgado-Escueta, A. V. (1979): Epileptogenic paroxysms: Modern approaches and clinical correlations. *Neurology (Minneap.)*, 29:1014–1022.
9. Delgado-Escueta, A. V., Enrile-Bascal, F., and Treiman, D. M. (1981): Complex partial seizures on the CCTV-EEG: A study of 682 attacks in 79 patients. *Ann. Neurol. (in press)*.
10. Delgado-Escueta, A. V., Boxley, J., Stubbs, N., Waddell, G., and Wilson, W. A. (1974): Prolonged twilight state and automatisms: A case report. *Neurology (Minneap.)*, 24:331–339.
11. Delgado-Escueta, A. V., Kunze, U., Waddell, G., Boxley, J., and Nadel, A. (1977): Lapse of consciousness and automatisms in temporal lobe epilepsy: A video tape analysis. *Neurology (Minneap.)*, 27:144–155.
12. Dreyer, R. (1965): Zur Frage des Status Epilepticus mit psychomotorischen Anfällen: Ein Beitrag zum temporalen Status Epilepticus and zu atypischen Dämmerzuständen und Verstimmungen. *Nervenarzt*, 36:221–223.
13. Engel, J., Jr., Ludwig, B. E., and Fettell, M. (1978): Prolonged partial complex status epilepticus: EEG and behavioral observations. *Neurology (Minneap.)*, 28:863–869.
14. Gastaut, H. (1980): *L'epilepsie temporale*. Le Concours Médical, Paris.
15. Gastaut, H., Roger, J., and Roger, A. (1956): Sur la signification de certaines fugues épileptiques: état de mal temporal. *Rev. Neurol. (Paris)*, 94:298–301.
16. Gastaut, H., and Tassinari, C. (1975): Status Epilepticus. In: *Handbook of Electroencephalography and Clinical Neurophysiology, Vol. 13A*, edited by A. Redmond, Elsevier, Amsterdam.
17. Heintel, H. (1969): Status von tonischen Dämmerattacken. *Arch. Psychiatr. Nervenkr.*, 212:117–125.
18. Henriksen, G. F. (1973): Status epilepticus partialis with fear as clinical expression. *Epilepsia*, 49:39–46.

19. Karbowski, K. (1980): *Status Psychomotoricus*. Hans Huber, Berne.
20. Kitagawa, T., Takahashi, K., Matsushima, K., and Kawahara, R. (1979): A case of prolonged confusion after temporal lobe psychomotor status. *Folia Psychiatr. Neurol. Jpn.*, 33:279–284.
21. Klass, D. W. (1975): Electroencephalographic manifestations of complex partial seizures. In: *Advances in Neurology, Vol. II*, edited by J. K. Penry and D. D. Daly, pp. 113–140. Raven Press, New York.
22. Kroth, N. (1967): Status with psychomotor attacks. *Electroencephalogr. Clin. Neurophysiol.*, 23:183 (abstract).
23. Kroth, H., and Hopf, H. C. (1966): Status psychomotorischer Aufälle. *Dtsch. Z. Nervenheilk*, 189:67–78.
24. Lugaresi, E., Pazzaglia, P., and Tassinari, C. A. (1971): Differentiation of 'absence status' and 'temporal lobe status.' *Epilepsia*, 12:77–87.
25. Markand, O. N., and Daly, D. D. (1971): Pseudoperiodic lateralized paroxysmal discharges in electroencephalogram. *Neurology (Minneap.)*, 21:975–981.
26. Markand, O. N., Wheeler, G. L., and Pollack, S. L. (1978): Complex partial status epilepticus (psychomotor status). *Neurology (Minneap.)*, 28:189–196.
27. Mayeux, R., Alaxander, M. P., Benson, D. F., Brandt, J., and Rosen, J. (1979): Poriomania. *Neurology (Minneap.)*, 29:1616–1619.
28. Mayeux, R., and Lueders, H. (1978): Complex partial status epilepticus: Case report and proposal for diagnostic criteria. *Neurology (Minneap.)*, 28:957–961.
29. Oana, Y., Matsuda, H., and Miura, S. (1979): Electroencephalographic study of status epilepticus. *Folia Psychiatr. Neurol. Jpn.*, 33:285–289.
30. Passouant, P., Duc, N., and Cadilhac, J. (1957): Accès confusionnel de longue durée et décharge épileptique temporale au cours de l'évolution d'une paralysie générale. *Rev. Neurol. (Paris)*, 96:329–332.
31. Penfield, W. P., and Jasper, H. H. (1954): *Epilepsy and the Functional Anatomy of the Brain*. Little, Brown, Boston.
32. Treiman, D. M., and Delgado-Escueta, A. V. (1980): Status epilepticus. In: *Critical Care of Neurologic and Neurosurgical Emergencies*, edited by R. A. Thompson and J. R. Green, pp. 53–99. Raven Press, New York.
33. Treiman, D. M., Delgado-Escueta, A. V., and Clark, M. A. (1981): Impairment of memory following prolonged complex partial status epilepticus. *Neurology (Minneap.)*, 31:109 (abstract).
34. Walter, R. D. (1973): Tactical considerations leading to surgical treatment of limbic epilepsy. In: *Epilepsy: Its Phenomena in Man*, edited by M. A. B. Brazier. Academic Press, New York.
35. Wieser, H. G. (1980): Temporal lobe or psychomotor status epilepticus: A case report. *Electroencephalogr. Clin. Neurophysiol.*, 48:558–572.
36. Wolf, P. (1970): Zur Klinik und Psychopathologie des Status Psychomotoricus. *Nervenarzt*, 41:603–610.

Advances in Neurology, Vol. 34: Status Epilepticus, edited by A.V. Delgado-Escueta, C.G. Wasterlain, D.M. Treiman, and R.J. Porter. Raven Press, New York © 1983.

8

Nonconvulsive Status Epilepticus in Childhood: Clinical Aspects and Classification

Hermann Doose

The classification of nonconvulsive status epilepticus in childhood is difficult. In adults, two well-defined conditions represented by the classic petit mal status and the status of psychomotor seizures can be distinguished. In children, however, the situation is more confusing. Typical petit mal status, also recognized in adulthood, is almost exclusively observed in older children. In early childhood this classic condition is rather rare. Far more frequent in young children is the nonconvulsive status epilepticus associated with the West syndrome and the so-called Lennox syndrome. This has been described as minor epileptic status (4) or myoclonic astatic petit mal status (6,20). Still lacking, however, is a really satisfactory classification of the various types of nonconvulsive status of the early childhood epilepsies. Probably, this is because the corresponding epileptic syndromes themselves have not been sufficiently differentiated nosographically. The remarkable disagreement in this field may be caused by the fact that the clinical and EEG phenomena in the different types of early childhood epilepsies with minor seizures are relatively uniform. Nevertheless, we must attempt to classify these epileptic conditions into primary and secondary types, as has been done for the epilepsies of adolescents and adults. Only then can a clear classification of nonconvulsive status epilepticus in early childhood evolve.

In view of the strong age dependence of the childhood epilepsies, the nonconvulsive status epilepticus of infancy and early childhood and of older children will be discussed separately.

NONCONVULSIVE STATUS IN INFANCY AND EARLY CHILDHOOD

West Syndrome (Infantile Spasms)

The West syndrome, or infantile spasms, belongs to the secondary generalized epilepsies of multifocal origin. It has no relationship to the primary generalized epilepsies of the corticoreticular type.

By definition, series of myoclonic jerks, as well as tonic seizures, are not categorized as nonconvulsive status epilepticus. Infants with hypsarrhythmia, however, can show conditions that have to be defined as nonconvulsive status. Their diagnosis is often difficult, because fluctuations in vigilance and attentiveness are hard to differentiate in severely retarded children. In less retarded children there can be observed a decrease or even a loss of visual and affective contact with the onset of hypsarrhythmia. These children become stuporous or apathetic and show salivation, oral automatisms, and eye blinking. In some children the diagnosis of status can be established only retrospectively on the basis of abrupt improvement after hypsarrhythmia has ceased. This type of status can be defined as twilight state in hypsarrhythmia.

When definite clinical symptoms are missing or cannot be exactly identified for the reasons mentioned earlier, hypsarrhythmia must be regarded as a bioelectrical status. This also applies to cases in which continuous hypsarrhythmia without clinical symptoms can be observed only during sleep *(vide infra)*.

Lennox Syndrome (Primary and Secondary Generalized Myoclonic-Astatic Epilepsies)

In no other field of pediatric epileptology does there exist such a confusion in terms as in the epileptic syndromes of early childhood with minor seizures. This confusion becomes evident in the different synonyms for these syndromes (Table 1). All of these syndromes are characterized by their strong tendency to develop long-lasting status epilepticus. The exact classification of these status episodes, however, depends on the classification of the underlying types of epilepsy. For a review of the literature about these syndromes, see Doose et al. (6), Kurse (20), and Ohtahara et al. (29).

The severe epilepsies have been summarized by Gastaut et al. (13) as the Lennox syndrome or, as it has been called by Niedermeyer (27), the Lennox-Gastaut syndrome, i.e., "childhood epileptic encephalopathy with diffuse slow spike waves." The syndrome is characterized by astatic and myoclonic fits, atypical absences, tonic-clonic grand mal, and tonic seizures. Most of these children are severely retarded mentally. The EEG shows pseudorhythmical diffuse slow spikes and waves, mostly with multifocal accentuation.

Despite an extensive literature on the Lennox syndrome, its classification remains indeterminate. As rightly pointed out by Aicardi (1), Loiseau et al. (25), and Jeavons (16), the syndrome represents a collection of heterogeneous epilepsies. These epilepsies doubtlessly share common clinical and EEG symptoms; however, they can be differentiated clinically, pathogenetically, and pathophysiologically into primary and secondary types. The work of Gastaut et al. (13), as well as the very detailed monograph of Kruse (20) and finally our own studies (6), shows clearly that the Lennox syndrome includes at least two subgroups: (a) secondary epilepsies in mostly severely retarded children and (b) a much rarer type of primary epilepsy that Doose et al. (6) proposed to call primary generalized myoclonic astatic epilepsy. Such differentiation between secondary generalized epilepsies and primary or "centrencephalic" epilepsies with minor seizures in early childhood is useful and necessary for successful classification of the nonconvulsive status episodes. Certainly, it must be admitted that the differentiation of these types of severe epilepsies can be extremely difficult and can be established in some cases only by longer observation of the clinical course.

Primary Generalized Myoclonic-Astatic Epilepsy

This rare type of epilepsy (6) occurs mostly in normally developed children at 1 to 5 years of age (Table 2). Boys are three times more often affected than girls. The epilepsy is characterized by myoclonic and astatic seizures, absences, and grand mal. The EEG shows bilateral, synchronous, irregular 2- to 3-Hz spikes and waves, as well as monofrequent theta rhythms. A genetic predisposition pathogenetically plays a decisive role (6).

In 30% to 40% of patients with primary generalized myoclonic-astatic epilepsy, a nonconvulsive status can be observed (6). The condition is

TABLE 1. *Symptoms for the epilepsies of early childhood with minor siezures*

Symptom	Reference
Static seizures	Hunt (15)
Akinetic epilepsy	Lennox (22)
Astatic epilepsy or drop seizures	Lennox and Davis (23)
Severe myokinetic epilepsy	Sorel (31)
Lennox syndrome	Gastaut el al. (13)
Myoclonic-astatic petit mal	Kruse (20)
Primary generalized myoclonic-astatic petit mal	Doose to al. (6)

TABLE 2. *Characteristics of primary generalized myoclonic-astatic epilepsy of early chilhood*

Age at onset	1–5 years
Boys:girls	3:1
Etiology	Brain lesions less important; mostly normal development before onset; regularly genetic predisposition (EEG in relatives)
Seizures	Myoclonic and astatic fits, absences, grand mal
EEG	Bilateral, synchronous slow spike waves; theta rhythms
Prognosis	Poor, often with dementia

characterized by apathy or even stupor. Careful observation reveals irregular twitching of the facial muscles and the extremities. The myoclonus is often easier to palpate than to see. Astatic seizures and head nodding can appear serially. The facial expression is slack, saliva drools, and speech is slurred or disappears completely. In severe cases, these children lie stuporous in bed. The status may last for hours or even days and weeks. In some cases there is a marked dependence on the sleeping-waking cycle, as short episodes of status occur mostly or even regularly after awakening. The EEG shows 2- to 3-Hz spikes and waves, rarely in regular groups, usually interrupted by slow waves (Fig. 1). In contrast with the multifocal epilepsies, there is a strong correlation between the EEG and the level of consciousness: Longer spike-wave series are constantly accompanied by a clouding of consciousness. As shown by a long-term followup of 95 cases in 1979, repeated, long-lasting status can lead to severe dementia in children who have developed normally so far (7).

Secondary Generalized Myoclonic-Astatic Epilepsy

This type of epilepsy forms the main group of the so-called Lennox syndrome; for review, see Gastaut et al. (13) and Kruse (20). Children at the age of 1 to 7 years, and sometimes older children, are affected. With few exceptions, these children are more or less severely retarded. Besides all other kinds of organic brain lesions, the causative factors are neurometabolic and degenerative diseases, e.g., tuberous sclerosis. A genetic predisposition plays a less important role. The clinical symptoms are more complex than in primary generalized myoclonic astatic epilepsy. They include drop seizures, head-nodding fits, myoclonic jerks, and tonic seizures, as well as atypical absences. Besides generalized seizures, different types of partial seizures can be observed. The EEG shows focal (more often multifocal) sharp slow waves, bilateral synchronous sharp slow waves, generalized spike-wave variants, and sometimes hypsarrhythmia. The Lennox syndrome of this multifocal type is often preceded by infantile spasms. As correctly pointed out by Jeavons (16) and Beaumanoir-Roger and Guediche (3), the West syndrome and this type of Lennox syndrome are to be understood as different age-dependent expressions of one syndrome.

The clinical symptoms of the status are similar to those of the primary generalized myoclonic-astatic epilepsy (20). They include stupor, astatic fits, slight head nodding, myoclonic jerks, and

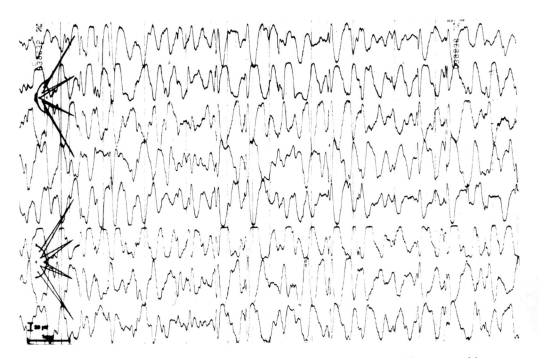

FIG. 1. EEG of a 3-year-old boy with primary generalized myoclonic-astatic epilepsy during nonconvulsive status.

polytopic myoclonias of the facial muscles and the extremities. The EEG (Fig. 2) shows generalized sharp slow waves and hypsarrhythmia or spike-wave variants, often with changing multifocal accentuation. In some cases a largely regular slow spike-wave pattern can be seen. In contrast with primary generalized myoclonic-astatic epilepsy, however, the correlation between the EEG and the clinical symptoms is less pronounced. There are children who show no definite seizure symptoms despite continuous generalized bilateral synchronous slow spike-waves in the EEG. Other patients appear only somewhat slow, moody, listless to play, or a little confused, as far as that can be ascertained in these mostly severely retarded children.

NONCONVULSIVE STATUS IN LATER CHILDHOOD

As compared with the epilepsies of early childhood, the nosology of the epilepsies in older children and the associated types of status are relatively clearly defined. As a rule, the primary generalized

and partial epilepsies can be easily differentiated, although there are some borderline cases that can be difficult to classify with certainty. A rather clear picture of the status exists in epilepsies with absences; for a review, see Andermann and Robb (2), Kruse (21), and Niedermeyer and Khalifeh (28).

Nonconvulsive Status in Epilepsies with Absences (Absence Status, Petit Mal Status)

The category of petit mal includes the prolonged continuous spike-wave stupor (28) as well as serial spike-wave absences. Both conditions can be seen in school-age children, but they occur predominantly in adolescents and adults. Because petit mal status in childhood actually presents no special problems, and because it has been discussed in Chapter 6, it will be excluded here.

Epilepsies with Complex Partial Seizures

The status of complex partial seizures in adults has been described by several authors (8–10,

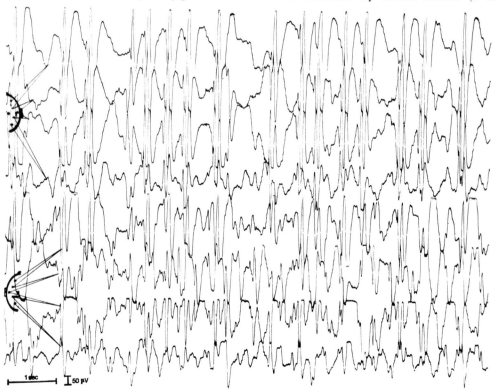

FIG. 2. EEG of a 3-year-old boy with secondary generalized myoclonic-astatic epilepsy (Lennox syndrome) during nonconvulsive status.

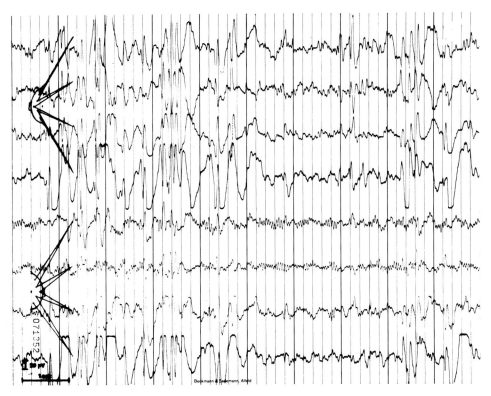

FIG. 3. EEG of a 7-year-old girl with psychomotor epilepsy and nonconvulsive status. Multifocal generalizing sharp slow waves are shown interictally.

12,14,17), but studies of this phenomenon in childhood epilepsy have been remarkably neglected. We know the different types of minor status in early childhood, as discussed earlier, as well as the typical petit mal status in older children. There have been no reports about the status of complex partial seizures in children, however, except the study of Mayeux and Leuders (26) and the questionable case history of Kroth and Hopf (19). In my experience, nonconvulsive status in severe partial epilepsies of childhood is by no means rare. Such a condition may be exemplified by a case history:

A 10-year-old girl who had suffered prenatal dystrophy had had several long-lasting tonic-clonic grand mal seizures with focal symptoms at the age of 3 to 6 years. At 7 years of age she had frequent psychomotor attacks and prolonged confusional states. Consciousness was not obviously impaired. The main symptoms were inattentiveness, inability to concentrate, a decrease in spontaneity, and memory deficit. These symptoms fluctuated in expression and persisted for hours and even days.

The interictal EEG showed focal sharp waves over the posterior regions, with intermittent generalization (Fig. 3). During the confusional state the EEG showed generalized sharp slow waves, sometimes resembling hypsarrhythmia (Fig. 4). During status, the girl was hardly able to write. It took hours to get down some words, and the writing was grossly deformed. On the other hand, she was able to sing a little song or recite a familiar poem, although the EEG showed generalized spike-wave variants (Fig. 5). During the last 3 years, repeated psychological investigations have shown a slowly decreasing IQ, although the girl, besides the confusional states and isolated psychomotor attacks, had no grand mal seizures.

Another girl had severe partial epilepsy and confusional states. The interictal EEG showed focal slowing over the left hemisphere (Fig. 6). During the confusional state (Fig. 7) it showed generalized hypersynchronous activity similar to hypsarrhythmia.

In summary, confusional states can also be observed in children with severe partial epilepsies.

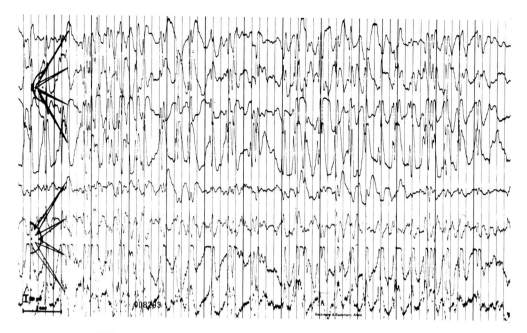

FIG. 4. Same patient as in Fig. 3 at 9 years old. EEG during twilight state.

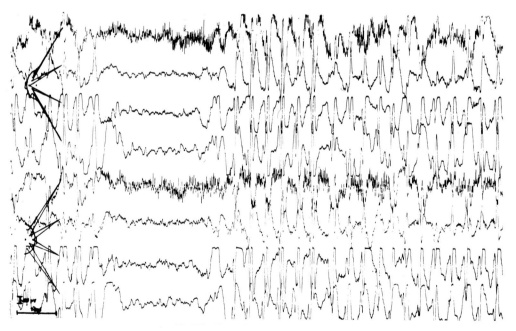

FIG. 5. Same patient as in Fig. 3 at 10 years old. During generalized spike-wave variants, the girl was able to sing a little song.

The main symptoms are only slightly impaired or even unimpaired consciousness, emotional and affective disturbances, a decrease in spontaneity, disturbances of orientation, irritability, often foolish behavior, inability to concentrate, to perform, and to react normally, and, conversely, unimpaired

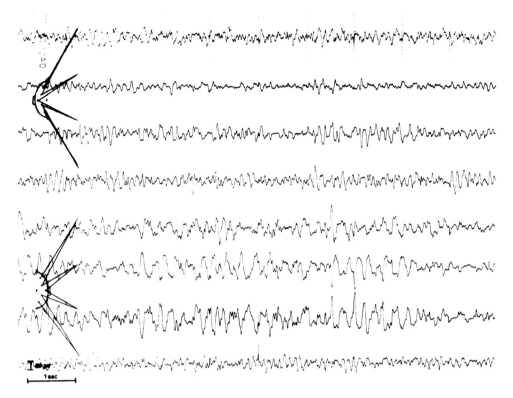

FIG. 6. EEG of an 8-year-old girl with psychomotor epilepsy and nonconvulsive status. Left temporal slowing and sharp waves are shown interictally.

or only slightly decreased ability to perform well-trained automatic activities. Characteristically, all of these symptoms show great fluctuation in expression. In contrast with the predominantly focal abnormalities that accompany confusional states in adults, the EEG mostly shows generalized, irregular, hypersynchronous activity during the status. The confusional or twilight state may last for hours or even days. There seems to be no doubt that this type of nonconvulsive status can also lead to mental deficit.

BIOELECTRICAL STATUS AND STATUS DURING SLEEP

Very little attention has been devoted to bioelectrical status without definite clinical symptoms. In the primary generalized epilepsies, there is generally a strong correlation between the EEG and the clinical symptoms. In the multifocal generalized epilepsies of childhood, these correlations are far less strong, as mentioned earlier. Even in cases with continuous generalized EEG changes such as sharp slow waves or hypsarrhythmia, clinical symptoms can be completely absent.

Patry et al. (30), Tassinari et al. (32), Dalla Bernadina et al. (5), Yamamoto et al. (33), Ohtahara et al. (29), and Fukuyama et al. (11) have described children in whom sleep, night after night, induced continuous generalized hypersynchronous activity that persisted throughout non-REM sleep and disappeared during REM sleep. According to our own experience from all-night EEG records, status during sleep in severe childhood epilepsy is far more frequent than previously assumed. Tassinari et al. (32) have suggested that this condition can lead to severe mental deterioration and psychic disturbances in some children.

CLASSIFICATION

With respect to the foregoing discussion, nonconvulsive status in childhood epilepsy can be classified as follows:

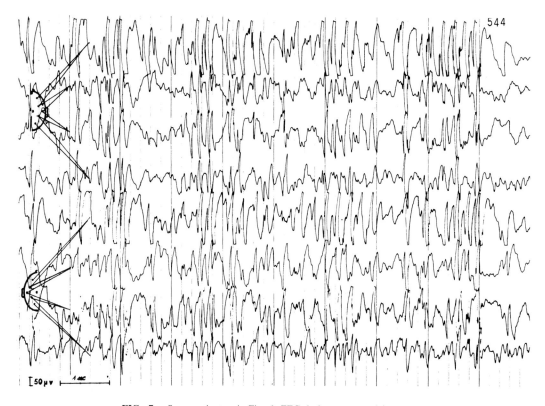

FIG. 7. Same patient as in Fig. 6. EEG during nonconvulsive status.

Primary generalized epilepsies
  Nonconvulsive status in:
    Primary generalized myoclonic-astatic epilepsy of early childhood (subgroup of Lennox syndrome)
    Epilepsies with absences (absence status, petit mal status)
Partial epilepsies with or without secondary generalization
  Nonconvulsive status in:
    West syndrome
    Secondary generalized myoclonic-astatic epilepsy (subgroup of Lennox syndrome)
    Epilepsies with complex partial seizures
    Bioelectrical status; sleep status

NONCONVULSIVE STATUS AND DEMENTIA

Brain damage and especially dementia occurring in the course of epilepsy are supposed to be mainly related to prolonged, frequently recurring grand mal seizures or grand mal status. It is generally not considered to be possible that dementia can result from nonconvulsive status. In 1956, Livingston et al. (24) first described the development of dementia following petit mal status in 6 of 11 mentally normal patients. Also, Brett (4) discussed the possibility that dementia could be associated with minor epileptic status. Doose et al. (6) reported such a correlation in children with primary myoclonic-astatic epilepsy. In a more detailed study with 117 children suffering from this type of epilepsy, the correlation between petit mal status and dementia was proved to be very likely (7). Dementia was found to be significantly more frequent in children with normal development before the onset of epilepsy when petit mal status occurred during the course.

Apparently, the same correlations apply to infants with infantile spasms and hypsarrhythmia, as well as to older children with nonconvulsive status in the course of multifocal myoclonic-astatic epilepsy or so-called Lennox syndrome (4,29,33). Also, prolonged confusional states with generalized hypersynchronous activity in older children can cause dementia, as exemplified by the history of a school-age girl *(vide supra)*. In this context, furthermore, the aphasic epilepsies in children with bioelectrical status must be mentioned; for a review, see Kellermann (18). The question of how we should interpret memory deficits following nonconvulsive status in adults, as reported by Engel et al. (9), is still unanswered.

Finally, all of these considerations must be examined with respect to the reported bioelectrical epileptic status during sleep, a condition that may last for hours or even the whole night. From the observations of several authors (5,30–33), it seems to be very likely that, at least in young children, these sleep status episodes can lead to cerebral damage or disturbance of brain development.

Conceptions about the responsible pathogenetic mechanisms can only be gained from animal experiments (see Chapters 17 and 33). Applied to the conditions in humans, the results of these experiments must appear even more significant, as the generalized seizure activity during nonconvulsive status in children does not continue for only hours but in some cases for days and even weeks. Such extreme conditions have never been investigated in animal experiments.

REFERENCES

1. Aicardi, J. (1973): The problem of the Lennox syndrome. *Dev. Med. Child Neurol.*, 15:77–80.
2. Andermann, F., and Robb, J. P. (1972): Absence status. A reappraisal following review of thirty-eight patients. *Epilepsia*, 13:177–187.
3. Beaumanoir-Roger, A., and Guediche, A. (1972): Syndromes de West et de Lennox, étude comparative. *Pädiatr. Fortbildungskurse Prax.*, 26:57–80.
4. Brett, E. M. (1966): Minor epileptic status. *J. Neurol. Sci.*, 3:52–75.
5. Dalla Bernadina, B., Tassinari, C. A., Dravet, C., Bureau, M., Beghini, G., and Roger, J. (1978): Epilepsie partielle bénigne et état de mal electroencéphalographique pendant le sommeil. *Rev. Electroencephalogr. Neurophysiol. Clin.*, 8:350–353.
6. Doose, H., Gerken, H., Leonhardt, R., Völzke, E., and Völz, C. H. (1970): Centrencephalic myoclonic-astatic petit mal. *Neuropaediatrie*, 2:59–78.
7. Doose, H., and Völzke, E. (1979): Petit mal-status and dementia. *Neuropaediatrie*, 10:10–14.
8. Dreyer, R. (1965): Zur Frage des Status epilepticus mit psychomotorischen Anfällen. *Nervenarzt*, 5:221–223.
9. Engel, J., Ludwig, B. I., and Fetell, M. (1978): Prolonged partial complex status epilepticus: EEG and behavioral observations. *Neurology (Minneap.)*, 28:863–869.
10. Escueta, A. V., Boxley, J., Stubbs, N., Waddell, G., and Wilson, W. A. (1974): Prolonged twilight state and automatisms: A case report. *Neurology (Minneap.)*, 24:331–339.
11. Fukuyama, Y., Shionaga, A., and Iida, Y. (1979): Polygraphic study during whole night sleep in infantile spasms. *Eur. Neurol.*, 18:302–311.
12. Gastaut, H., Roger, J., and Roger, A. (1956): Sur la signification de certaine fugues épileptiques. À propos d'une observation électroclinique d'état de mal temporal. *Rev. Neurol.*, 94:298–301.
13. Gastaut, H., Roger, J., Soulayrol, R., Tassinari, C. A., Regis, H., and Dravet, C. (1966): Childhood epileptic encephalopathy with diffuse slow spike-waves (otherwise known as "petit mal variant") or Lennox-syndrome. *Epilepsia*, 7:139–179.
14. Hedenström, J. von, and Schorsch, G. (1959): EEG-Befunde epileptischen Dämmer- und Verstimmungszuständen. *Arch. Psychiatr. Nervenkr.*, 99:311–329.
15. Hunt, J. R. (1922): On the occurrence of static seizures. *J. Nerv. Ment. Dis.*, 56:351–356.
16. Jeavons, P. M. (1977): Nosological problems of myoclonic epilepsies in childhood and adolescence. *Dev. Ment. Child Neurol.*, 19:3–8.
17. Karbowski, K. (1980): *Status psychomotoricus und seine Differentialdiagnose.* Hans Huber, Bern.
18. Kellermann, K. (1979): Recurrent aphasia with subclinical bioelectric status epilepticus during sleep. *Eur. J. Pediatr.*, 128:207–212.
19. Kroth, H., and Hopf, H. C. (1966): Status psychomotorischer Anfalle. *Dtsch. Z. Nervenheilk.*, 189:67–78.
20. Kruse, R. (1968): *Das myoklonisch-astatische Petit mal*, pp. 25–27. Springer-Verlag, Berlin.
21. Kruse, R. (1976): Absenzen-Status (typische Formen). *Aktuel. Neurol.*, 2:155–170.
22. Lennox, W. G. (1945): The petit mal epilepsies; their treatment with Tridione. *J. A. M. A.*, 129:1069–1074.
23. Lennox, W. G., and Davis, J. P. (1950): Clinical correlates of the fast and slow spike-wave electroencephalogram. *Pediatrics*, 5:626–644.
24. Livingston, S., Torres, I., Pauli, L., and Rider, R. V. (1956): Petit mal epilepsy. *J. A. M. A.*, 194:227–232.
25. Loiseau, P., Legroux, M., Grimond, P., du Pasquier, P., and Henry, P. (1974): Taxometric classification of myoclonic epilepsies. *Epilepsia*, 15:1–11.
26. Mayeux, R., and Leuders, H. (1978): Complex partial status epilepticus: Case report and proposal for diagnostic criteria. *Neurology (Minneap.)*, 28:957–961.
27. Niedermeyer, E. (1969): The Lennox-Gastaut-Syndrome—A severe type of childhood epilepsy. *Dtsch. Z. Nervenheilk.*, 195:263–282.
28. Niedermeyer, E., and Khalifeh, R. (1965): Petit mal status ("spike wave stupor"). *Epilepsia*, 6:250–262.
29. Ohtahara, S., Oka, E., Yamatogi, Y., Ohtsuka, Y., Ischida, T., Ischiba, N., Ischida, S., and Miyake, S. (1979): Nonconvulsive status epilepticus in childhood. *Folia Psychiatr. Neurol. Jpn.*, 33:345–351.
30. Patry, G., Lyagoubi, S., and Tassinari, C. A. (1971): Subclinical "electrical status epilepticus" induced by sleep in children. *Arch. Neurol.*, 24:242–252.
31. Sorel, M. L. (1964): L'épilepsie mykinetique grave de la première enfance avec pointe-onde lent (petit

mal variant) et son traitement. *Rev. Neurol. (Paris)*, 110:215–223.

32. Tassinari, A. C., Dravet, C., and Roger, J. (1977): Encephalopathy related to electrical status epilepticus during slow sleep. *Electroencephalogr. Clin. Neurophysiol.*, 43:529–530.

33. Yamamoto, N., Inoue, H., and Ohtahara, S. (1978): Subclinical electrical status epilepticus induced by sleep. *Nerv. Syst. Children*, 2:425–432 (in Japanese).

Advances in Neurology, Vol. 34: Status Epilepticus, edited by A.V. Delgado-Escueta, C.G. Wasterlain, D.M. Treiman, and R.J. Porter. Raven Press, New York © 1983.

9

Status Epilepticus in Newborns: A Perspective on Neonatal Seizures

Peter Kellaway and Richard A. Hrachovy

The high morbidity and mortality associated with neonatal seizures appear to be cogent evidence for the prevailing view that seizures are bad for the brain and that status epilepticus may be devastating, particularly to the developing nervous system. However, any discussion of status epilepticus in the newborn, the consequences of such status, and the treatment thereof must be conducted in the context of the special character of neonatal seizures, the etiological spectrum of these seizures, and the change that has occurred in this spectrum during the last 10 years.

AGE AT ONSET AND ETIOLOGICAL FACTORS

Analysis of the age at onset of seizures on a month-to-month basis throughout the entire period of infancy provides a perspective of the unique circumstances of the neonatal period. Figure 1 shows the ages at onset of seizures, with and without associated febrile illness, for 1,110 infants born at Baylor College of Medicine's teaching hospitals or referred during the 10-year period from January 1962 through December 1971. The striking feature of this age distribution is the remarkably high incidence of seizure onset in the first month of life in comparison with any other period in the first 36 months. About 80% of the seizures occurring in the first 2 months of life had their onset in the first

month, and of these, 85% began in the first 15 days (Fig. 2).

The cytoarchitectural and myelinogenetic development of the central nervous system is quite limited in the newborn (9), and experimental studies in animals have indicated that the brain exhibits a much lesser degree of epileptogenicity in the newborn period than at later stages of development (15). The implication, therefore, is that it is the particular circumstances of the perinatal period that are responsible for the high seizure incidence among neonates.

The general pattern of age distribution has not changed significantly since 1971, but there have been some changes in the overall incidence of infantile seizures, particularly in the first month of life. Figure 3 shows the ages at onset of seizures from birth through 36 months for 494 infants who were born at Baylor's teaching or referral hospitals between January 1972 and December 1977. In comparison with the 1962–1971 figures, there was an overall decrease of about 12% in the incidence of seizures; more important, the incidence in the first month of life decreased by about 33%.

The etiological factors in neonatal seizures reported in various studies from 1958 to 1977 are shown in Table 1. In our 1962–1971 series, metabolic factors (notably, hypocalcemia) accounted for about 31% of the seizures, which is consistent with the findings of other studies dating from 1969

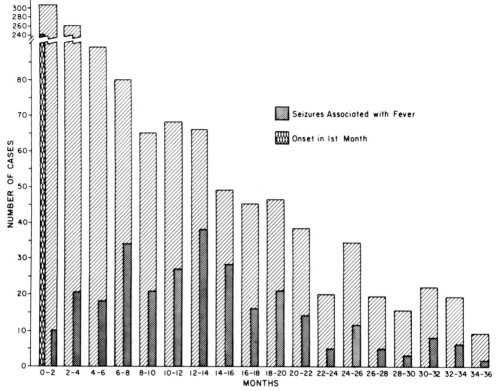

FIG. 1.   Age at first seizure for 1,110 infants (up to 3 years old) studied between 1962 and 1971.

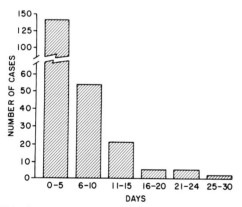

FIG. 2.   Age at first seizure for 228 infants having seizures during the first month of life.

through 1973. The incidences of primary and secondary hypocalcemia and of various other metabolic causes of neonatal seizures in our two series are illustrated in Table 2. The percentage of seizures associated with infection and with unknown causes increased in the 1972–1977 series, whereas metabolic causes, primarily hypocalcemia, decreased. Central nervous system infection (predominantly β-streptococcal meningitis) increased threefold (from 4% to 12%), thus equaling the incidence of metabolic causes in this period. Hypoxia accounted for 36% of cases in both time periods. These changes in the etiological profile have reduced the number of cases with relatively benign outcomes and have changed the percentage incidences of specific seizure types.

MORBIDITY AND MORTALITY

A compilation of the published figures for morbidity and mortality from neonatal seizures is shown in Table 3. Clearly, the predominant factor determining outcome is the destructive nature of the pathological process, not the seizures themselves. Before the recognition in the late 1960s that hypocalcemia was a common cause of clonic seizures, clonic status was the most frequent type of status epilepticus in newborns. Yet most infants (85%) left the hospital with no obvious signs of neurological impairment (Table 3).

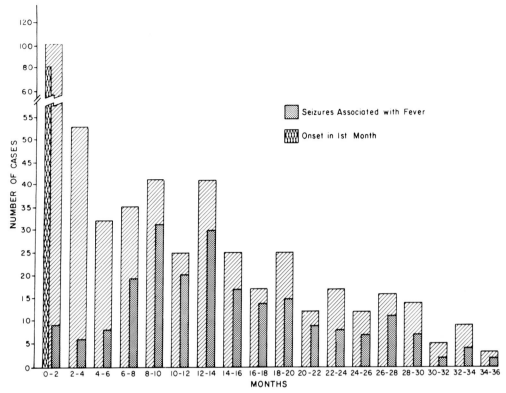

FIG. 3. Age at first seizure for 494 infants (up to 3 years old) studied between 1972 and 1977.

SEIZURE TYPES AND THEIR FREQUENCIES

The literature concerning the character of neonatal seizures and their significance is difficult to evaluate because the majority of seizures are not witnessed by physicians or others specially trained to interpret infant behavioral phenomena. Often the initial features of the attack are not seen or recognized. Seizures often are described as "grand mal" or tonic-clonic, but probably are neither.

On the basis of concomitant EEG and/or polygraphic recording and visual analysis of multiple seizures in more than 1,000 infants, a classification system for infant seizures has been developed (Table 4). In this series, no seizures of tonic-clonic type were recorded. Seizures were either clonic or tonic from onset. Pronounced tonic seizures often were accompanied by tremor of the hypertonic extremities, but no clonic movements. Clonic seizures were always clinically and electrographically unilateral at onset, and when they became bilateral, they were asynchronous on the two sides. Some seizures were predominantly autonomic, but most of these were associated with automatisms or with tonic postural movements, which could be quite subtle.

Table 4 shows the frequency of occurrence for each of the various seizure types in the two time periods studied. In the 1972–1977 series, tonic seizures replaced clonic seizures as the most common seizure type, and this has continued to be true to date. In our experience, clonic status is now a rarity, but prolonged and serially repeated tonic seizures are commonly seen. Tonic seizures and automatisms have a high association with the same etiological factors (Table 3), which involve a poor prognosis (particularly hypoxia), but are not seen in primary metabolic disorders. Tonic seizures are most commonly seen in infants with both clinical and EEG evidence of "depressed" brain function.

PHYSIOLOGICAL MECHANISMS OF SEIZURE ACTIVITY

Since 1969, we have recorded and observed more than 400 tonic seizures in 120 infants. In 102 of these infants the tonic seizures were not accom-

TABLE 1. *Etiological factors in neonatal seizures*

Reference	Year	Hypoxia (%)	↓ Calcium (%)	↓ Glucose (%)	Congenital (%)	Infection (%)	Unknown (%)
Ribstein and Walter (16)	1958	63				4	
Craig (4)	1960	66					
Schulte (19)	1966	54				7	23
Massa and Niedermeyer (11)	1968	40				50	
McInerny and Schubert (13)	1969		30	7	4	10	13
Rose and Lombroso (17)	1970	31	20	6	8	8	22
Kellaway (7)	1971	36	31[a]	5	6	4	23
Hopkins (5)	1972[b]	57	36	39		11	
Brown (2)	1973	45	55[c]				
Keen and Lee (6)	1973	13	41	3	1	1	33
Rossier et al. (18)	1973		21	22	6		4
Combes et al. (3)	1975	77	10	11			9
Kellaway (8)	1977	36	12[d]	4	5	12	30

[a]Primary metabolic, 16%.
[b]First week of life only.
[c]With ↓ magnesium.
[d]Primary metabolic, 3%.

TABLE 2. *Neonatal seizures of metabolic origin (1962–1971 versus 1972–1977)*

Age (days)	1962–1971 (N = 1,110)	1972–1977 (N = 494)
1	A,A,A,A,A,A[a]	A,C,D,D
2	A,A,A,B,C,D,D,D	A
3	B,C,C,D,D,D	A
4	A,B,C,D,D	
5	C	A,B
6	C,C,C	D
7	B,C,C,C,C	C
8	A,C	
9	B,C,C,C	
10	C	
11		
12		
13	C,C	
14	B,B	A,A
15		
16		
17		
18	C	
19		A
20		
21		D

[a]A = ↓ calcium + hypoxia ± other metabolic or nonmetabolic abnormality. B = ↓ calcium + other metabolic or nonmetabolic abnormality. C = ↓ calcium only. D = other metabolic abnormality.

TABLE 3. *Prognosis for neonatal seizures in relation to etiology[a]*

	Dead (%)	Neurological Deficits (%)	Normal (%)
Congenital anomalies	80	20	0
CNS infection	50	29	21
Perinatal hypoxia, ischemia, hemorrhage	17	47	36
Hypoglycemia	12	40	48
Hypocalcemia	6	8	86
Unknown cause	10	35	55

[a]Data from Schulte (19), McInerny and Schubert (13), Rose and Lombroso (17), and Rossier et al. (18).

panied by seizure activity on the electroencephalogram. This observation makes it necessary to reexamine the concept that all so-called tonic seizures are consequent to epileptic discharges in the brain. Certainly there are physiological mechanisms (Fig. 4) that could explain these types of seizures without recourse to an epileptic process, evidence of which is not forthcoming in the EEG recordings of 85% of our cases. We suggest that tonic seizures without EEG epileptiform activity are better explained as "brainstem release" phenomena. "Brainstem release" is the term used by early workers to characterize the hypertonic state produced by decortication in animals. The tonic seizures similarly may be conceived as expressions of disinhibition of normal tonic brainstem facilitory mechanisms consequent to depression of forebrain inhibitory influences.

Bonvallet and Hugelin (1) showed, by microelectrode recording, that as increasing hypoxia progressively depressed and ultimately abolished

TABLE 4. *Classification of infantile clinical seizure types*

	Before 1972 (%)	1972–1977 (%)
I. Motor		
A. Clonic	64.5	32.5
1. Focal clonic		
2. Hemiclonic: unilateral clonic jerking of extremities and face		
3. Alternating focal clonic		
4. Bilateral clonic of lateralized onset		
B. Tonic	17	42
1. Minor posturing (focal or lateralized)		
2. Hyperextension; usually of lower extremities and trunk, with flexion of upper extremities		
3. Tonic version of eyes, neck, and trunk		
C. Atonic: arrest of movement, limp and unresponsive	13	17
D. Infantile spasms	0.5	0.5
E. Motor automatisms: movement of head from side to side, thrashing about, smiling, grimacing, and other oral, buccal-lingual repetitive movements	5	8
F. Slow bilateral myoclonus		
II. Autonomic		
A. Respiratory: abrupt changes in rate and depth, apnea, grunting		
B. Ocular: pupillary dilatation or constriction, nystagmus		
C. Vasomotor: flushing, pallor, cyanosis		
D. Salivation		
III. Miscellaneous: eye opening, staring (fixed gaze), rhythmic blinking		

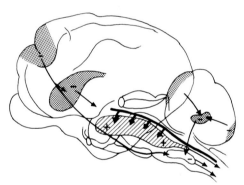

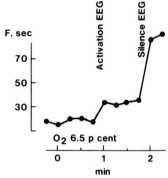

FIG. 4. Reconstruction of the cat's brain showing suppressor and facility pathways regulating spinal motor mechanisms. (Adopted from Lindsley et al., ref. 10.) The rich afferent collateral input to the brainstem reticulum demonstrated by Starzl et al. (21) is also shown. Cortical descending influences exert tonic inhibitory action on brainstem reticular tonic facility impulses acting on spinal motor systems via the reticulospinal tract.

FIG. 5. Progressive increase in the frequency of discharge over time of a single reticular neuron in a curarized cat breathing 6.5% O_2. Note the marked increase in rate of firing at the point that the EEG shows electrocortical silence.

cortical neuronal activity, neural activity of the brainstem reticulum was enhanced (Fig. 5). Parallel observations in humans (12) have demonstrated that transient anoxic depression of cortical activity, as evidenced by absence of electrical activity, is associated with hyperextension of the neck, trunk, and extremities (Fig. 6). The asymmetry and crossed flexor extension sometimes observed in tonic seizures can be understood in terms of the

observation in animals that stimulation of the reticulum at intensities just above the threshold for evoking movement may produce motor patterns consisting of flexion of ipsilateral limbs, extension of contralateral limbs, and turning of the head toward the side of the stimulation (20). Asymmetry of the pattern of disinhibition or of sensory input to the reticular core could explain such tonic movements. Furthermore, experimental studies have demonstrated that there is a topography of regions within the brainstem reticular core that exert opposing facility and inhibitory effects on the spinal

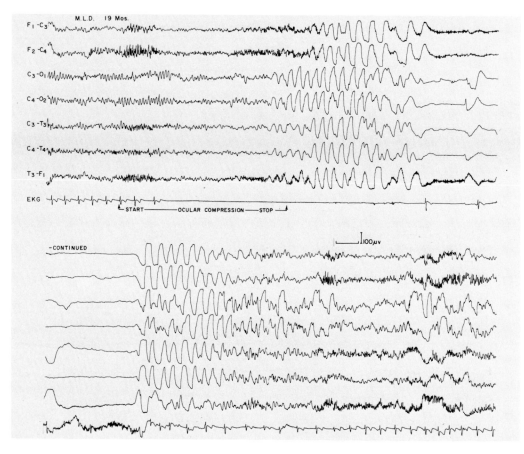

FIG. 6. Transient ischemic hypoxia produced by 11.5 sec of asystole results in an initial generalized slowing of the EEG, followed by a brief period of profound generalized voltage attenuation that in turn is followed by another episode of generalized slow activity, then a quick return to the prehypoxic pattern. Clinically, the child became limp and unconscious with the onset of slow activity, then showed hyperextension of the trunk, flexion of the arms, and hyperextension of the legs during the period of virtual electrocortical silence. The child then relaxed, with return of the slow activity, but remained unresponsive until the EEG returned to normal.

stepping motor system (14), thus providing a substrate for the pedaling automatisms that often are mistaken for seizures. The episodic occurrence of these tonic movements, which gives them the appearance of seizures, may be engendered by fluctuation of interoceptive and proprioceptive sensory input to the brainstem reticular facilitating system, which receives a rich input of collaterals from ascending spinal sensory pathways (21) (Fig. 4). It is a common observation that diverse stimuli can trigger tonic seizures and that proprioceptive stimuli, such as passive flexion of the trunk, can elicit tonic postural and pedaling movements.

The parsimonious approach would be that all tonic seizures involve the same brain mechanisms.

Is it necessary to invoke a different functional mechanism for the tonic seizures that are accompanied by electrical signs of seizure activity? The 15% of tonic seizures that are accompanied by epileptiform activity on the EEG are indistinguishable from those that are not, except that they more often have autonomic features. Both occur in infants with EEG and clinical evidence of depressed forebrain function, and the ictal EEG seizure discharges are of a type characteristic of this state. It is not difficult to conceive how a seizure discharge arising in functional forebrain neurons could further disrupt tonic descending inhibitory mechanisms and release brainstem reticular facilitating influences on spinal motor neurons.

CONCLUSION

The significance of these conjectures is three-fold: (a) Because tonic seizures now constitute the greater portion of neonatal "seizures" and account for most of the cases of status, and because they are apparently evidence of forebrain depression or damage, the inclusion of such seizures in the morbidity and mortality statistics weights the prognosis heavily on the adverse side. (b) If more than 42% of seizures in newborns are not, in fact, epileptic, the incidence of epileptic seizures is not much higher in the first month of life than in any other similar period in the first 6 months of life. (c) If tonic seizures are not epileptic but are evidence of forebrain depression, then the appropriateness of anticonvulsant drug treatment, particularly with depressant drugs such as phenobarbital, must be reexamined.

ACKNOWLEDGMENT

Supported by grant NS-11535 from the National Institute of Neurological and Communicative Disorders and Stroke, National Institutes of Health, U. S. Public Health Service.

REFERENCES

1. Bonvallet, M., and Hugelin, A. (1961): Influence de la formation reticulaire et du cortex cerebral sur l'excitabilité motrice au cours de l'hypoxie. *Electroencephalogr. Clin. Neurophysiol.*, 13:270–284.
2. Brown, J. K. (1973): Convulsions in the newborn period. *Dev. Med. Child Neurol.*, 15:823–846.
3. Combes, J. G., Rufo, M., Vallade, M. J., Pinsard, N., and Bernard, R. (1975): Les convulsions neonatales. Circonstances d'apparition et critères de pronostic. *Pediatrie*, 30:477–492.
4. Craig, W. S. (1960): Convulsive movements occurring in the first 10 days of life. *Arch. Dis. Child.*, 35:336–344.
5. Hopkins, I. S. (1972): Seizures in the first week of life. A study of etiological factors. *Med. J. Aust.*, 2:647–651.
6. Keen, J. H., and Lee, D. (1973): Sequelae of neonatal convulsions. *Arch. Dis. Child.*, 48:542–546.
7. Kellaway, P. (1971): unpublished data (presented to the American Epilepsy Society symposium, December 1971).
8. Kellaway, P. (1977): unpublished data.
9. Larroche, J. C. (1966): The development of the central nervous system during intrauterine life. In: *Human Development*, edited by F. Falkner, pp. 257–276. W. B. Saunders, Philadelphia.
10. Lindsley, D. B., Schreiner, L. H., and Magoun, H. W. (1949): An electromyographic study of spasticity. *J. Neurophysiol.*, 12:197–205.
11. Massa, T., and Niedermeyer, E. (1968): Convulsive disorders during the first three months of life. *Epilepsia*, 9:1–9.
12. Maulsby, R., and Kellaway, P. (1964): Transient hypoxic crises in children. In: *Neurological and Electroencephalographic Correlative Studies in Infancy*, edited by P. Kellaway and I. Petersén, pp. 349–360. Grune & Stratton, New York.
13. McInerny, T. K., and Schubert, W. K. (1969): Prognosis of neonatal seizures. *Am. J. Dis. Child.*, 117:261–264.
14. Mori, S., Nishimura, H., and Aoki, M. (1980): Brain stem activation of the spinal stepping generator. In: *The Reticular Formation Revisited*, edited by J. A. Hobson and M. A. B. Brazier, pp. 241–259. Raven Press, New York.
15. Purpura, D. P. (1964): Relationship of seizure susceptibility to morphologic and physiologic properties of normal and abnormal immature cortex. In: *Neurological and Electroencephalographic Correlative Studies in Infancy*, edited by P. Kellaway and I. Petersén, pp. 117–157. Grune & Stratton, New York.
16. Ribstein, M., and Walter, M. (1958): Convulsions du premier mois. *Rev. Neurol. (Paris)*, 99:91–99.
17. Rose, A. L., and Lombroso, C. T. (1970): Neonatal seizure states. *Pediatrics*, 45:404–425.
18. Rossier, A., Caldera, R., and le Oc Mach, A. (1973): Les convulsions neo-natales: étude de 53 cas. *Ann. Pediatr.*, 20:869–876.
19. Schulte, F. J. (1966): Neonatal convulsions and their relation to epilepsy in early childhood. *Dev. Med. Child Neurol.*, 8:381–392.
20. Sprague, J. M., and Chambers, W. W. (1954): Control of posture by reticular formation and cerebellum in intact, anesthetized and unanesthetized and in decerebrated cat. *Am. J. Physiol.*, 176:52–64.
21. Starzl, T. E., Taylor, C. W., and Magoun, H. W. (1951): Collateral afferent excitation of reticular formation of the brain stem. *J. Neurophysiol.*, 14:479–496.

Advances in Neurology, Vol. 34: Status Epilepticus, edited by A.V. Delgado-Escueta, C.G. Wasterlain, D.M. Treiman, and R.J. Porter. Raven Press, New York © 1983.

10

Prognosis in Neonatal Seizures

Cesare T. Lombroso

Few would disagree with the statement that seizures in newborns usually are powerful indicators of future neurological dysfunction. Reports of their incidence have varied from 1.5 to 3.5 in 1,000 live babies. Their epidemiology is thus uncertain and variable according to the degree of sophistication in intensive neonatal care and in the detection of seizures. We have more data about their relationship to long-term global outcome. The figures vary between earlier studies and more recent series: Mortality has been reported as high as 40% to 60% in earlier reports and as low as 16% in our latest prospective study (18). Morbidity has also varied from a high of 70% to about 35%.

In spite of such changing trends over the past three decades, the end results still indicate a remarkably poor outlook for neonates who develop seizures. Only about 50% seem to escape significant sequelae. This outcome stands in contrast to the outcomes for seizures occurring at most other ages.

Figure 1 summarizes the results of a few retrospective and prospective series published over the past 30 years. The earlier ones indicate greater mortality and morbidity than subsequent series, a reflection of variables such as the changes in etiological factors, the use of retrospective rather than prospective investigations, the gestational ages of the population, the duration of clinical follow-up, the definitions of quality and degree of the sequelae, and the radical changes in obstetrical and perinatal care.

Although mortality has decreased, morbidity following neonatal seizures has not, despite dramatic improvements in obstetrical and perinatal care. From these data it seems logical to assume that the brain of the newborn has a special vulnerability to sequelae from seizures, far greater than that in infants and children.

From the data of Spielmeyer (33), Gastaut et al. (14), Norman (25), Aicardi and Baraton (1), and Falconer (11), to name only a few, we know well the adverse effects that "status epilepticus convulsivus" or chronic epileptic syndromes may have on the brain in children and adults.

From the elegant laboratory data of Plum et al. (28) to those of Meldrum and Horton (21) and Wasterlain and Duffy (38), which are more pertinent to the neonatal period, strong evidence has emerged that this damage is far greater in the developing brain. Thus, Wasterlain and Plum (36) showed reductions in brain weight and cell numbers in brains of newborn rats subjected daily for 10 days to electroconvulsive attacks, both reductions being much less evident in postmitotic rat brains. Further, single 2-hr convulsions in 4-day-old rats markedly inhibited DNA, RNA, protein, and cholesterol synthesis, even without the increase in DNA breakdown or the occurrence of neuronal necrosis (the usual findings in conditions where energy demands in the brain overcome the supply). Behavioral milestones were affected as well. Similar maneuvers in older animals did not produce the same effects.

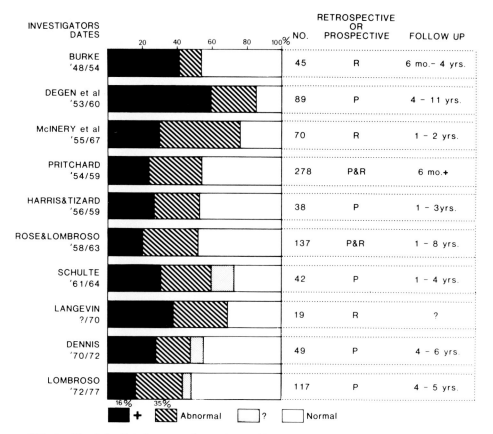

FIG. 1. Trends in clinical outcome for newborns with seizures from 1948 to 1977. On the whole, only modest improvements in mortality and morbidity have occurred over a span of about 30 years. Note that several studies were retrospective, the lengths of follow-up varied considerably, and only a few of the series contained more than 100 cases. The high mortality in the series of Degen et al. and Burke may be attributed to their inclusion of preterm infants.

Other evidence has been reported in this volume to persuade one and all that many factors can be potential conspirators in disrupting the processes necessary for the developmental schedule during a uniquely vulnerable time for the CNS. Neonatal animals are less apt to suffer from the cardiac, respiratory, and renal complications characteristic of "status epilepticus" in older animals, and the degree of lactic acidosis due to intensive convulsive activity is usually lower. In neonatal animals, the immaturity of glial cells and therefore the less efficient activation of phosphorylase enzymes, the apparently less efficient blood-brain transport of glucose, the inability to utilize ketones during hypoxic states, and the high dependence on glucose availability all conjoin in inhibiting the defenses available to older animals. In addition, it is possible that immature brain may also have less efficient autoregulation of cerebral blood flow, a

further potential for reduced adaptability and homeostasis. Thus the data reported from these animal models with variously induced convulsive states would seem to indicate clearly why seizures in the human newborn produce such high incidence of severe sequelae.

But as we look at the real world of clinical seizures in human infants, we are confronted by the following observations that do not fit with the laboratory data: (a) Almost 50% of newborns with seizures have normal global outcomes. (b) The severity and the duration of the ictal phenomena do not seem to correlate with outcome. (c) There is as yet no good evidence to indicate that anticonvulsant treatment in newborns with seizures has a direct effect in protecting them from long-term sequelae. The best correlations with good or poor outcomes lie within the causes of neonatal seizures and with neurophysiological measures. How does one reconcile these contrasting results between induced seizures in animal models and those occurring in a clinical context?

First, we might mention that most cerebral mitotic activity, elaboration of axonal and dendritic ramifications, and hence morphological, chemical, and bioelectrical connectivities in the rat (and some of the other animal models) occur mainly in the first 3 weeks of life, whereas in the human they continue at a significant rate for more than 24 months. These differences may provide one explanation. They also could explain the differences between patterns of seizures that occur in human infants and those obtained in animal newborns, in whom true epileptic status convulsivus can readily be induced by bicuculline, fluorothyl, or supramaximal electroshock (36,37).

EPILEPTIC STATUS

Status epilepticus convulsivus (SEC), as we define it, is a rare event in the human neonate and is a crucial issue. Recently I had the opportunity to ask Mme. Nicole Monod how often she saw SEC in newborns. "Almost never," was her answer. As recently as 1972, Monod and Dreyfus-Brisac and Monod (9) wrote a chapter on neonatal status epilepticus. I reread it carefully, and I shall quote now from their text: *"Neonatal status epilepticus* [NSE] is characterized by the repetition of clinical or even subclinical seizures, in a baby having abnormal neurological symptoms between them." Further: "The identification of NSE (often difficult in the neonate) depends upon the recognition of seizures occurring in already *severely neurologically damaged babies*." Further: "Hence, the gravity of prognosis of NSE is the same regardless of the state of consciousness," and "the poorest prognosis exists when *NSE begins after* the [baby has sunk into] coma." Also, the "results of treatment are disappointing as NSE seems to be beyond therapeutic resources. *Most cases seem to involve pre-existing lesions*."

These statements, written in 1972, are identical in substance with our earliest conclusions (15). These have not been modified basically after investigations covering a span of almost 20 years and a cohort of approximately 300 neonates, even though our own data on outcome are less pessimistic, and we believe that there are therapeutic interventions capable of decreasing this sinister outlook (16,18,20,30).

The main message here is the crucial difference between neonatal seizures and those occurring in older infants or children. In neonates, true SEC is a rare event, and neurological compromise seems to precede the onset of seizures in cases that show a nefarious outcome. In older infants, in whom true status epilepticus is more apt to occur, SEC can, indeed, induce significant CNS compromises or add to preexisting ones. Distinctions between the clinical consequences of SEC in human newborns and those in infants, children, and adults do not seem to have been taken into consideration by most investigators who have worked with animal models. It is often assumed that the pathogeneses of brain damage induced by SEC are the same in neonates, infants, and adults. Laboratory data obtained in newborn animals are often extrapolated to human situations by means of references to the consequences of status epilepticus in infants and children. Often cited are the reports of Aicardi and associates (1,5).

These important observations were made not on newborns but on infants and children who had undergone convulsive seizures lasting 1 hr or more or on other older patients with repeated SEC. Our experiences have been similar within these age groups, but we doubt that they can be extrapolated to the newborn period.

Now, a few words regarding seizure patterns. Because of the immaturities in morphological, chemical, and bioelectrical connectivities involving cortical and subcortical structures, ictal phenomena in the newborn lack many of the pathophysiological and clinical expressions that characterize an "epileptic" attack. Hence, we had to develop a clinical classification that has little in common with those proposed for older age groups. Table 1 summarizes the most common neonatal seizure types.

This classification, proposed about 12 years ago, has changed only in regard to the frequencies of some types of seizure patterns. For instance, the focal clonic pattern once very common in full-term neonates now is much less so, reflecting the almost complete disappearance of some etiological factors such as late-onset hypocalcemia. Instead, the groups of subtle and tonic patterns have become more frequent, especially if one includes preterm babies. Nonetheless, this classification seems to have achieved wide consensus (7,12,13).

Significant numbers of all neonatal seizures are transitory phenomena. This seems to be true even

TABLE 1. *Classification of most common seizure patterns in newborns*

Subtle (or minimal)	Abnormal eye movements; mild posturing; oral, lingual, etc.; pedaling, rowing movements; brief tremors; apneas (difficult to diagnose without EEG)
Clonic	
Focal	(Rarely imply focal brain lesion)
Multifocal	(Fragmentary, anarchic; must be differentiated from jitteriness)
Hemiconvulsive	(Rare in newborns; more frequent in young infants)
Tonic	Focal or generalized (may resemble decerebrate posturing; often accompanied by abnormal eye movements, apnea, cyanosis; more common in preterm newborns)
Myoclonic	(Often fragments of infantile spasms that are seen in later infancy; must be differentiated from Moro startles of NREM sleep)
Tonic-clonic	(Rare in newborns)

when they are not treated with anticonvulsants and also when they seem to be epiphenomena of anatomical cerebral insults. To be sure, others persist or more often reemerge later in life as various epileptic syndromes. In our overall data, approximately 20% of cases belong to this category. But should one classify as "epileptic" the other nonrecurrent neonatal seizures?

ETIOLOGICAL FACTORS

Because seizures in the newborn are mostly symptomatic, the cause should correlate with the prognosis. Thus, careful assessment of the cause is crucial. However, multiple problems are characteristic in the histories of many babies with seizures. For example, a newborn with asphyxia may have suffered an intracranial hemorrhage and also may suffer from early hypocalcemia or hypoglycemia. It is obvious that double or triple coding will result. Some authors (4) have tried to circumvent this problem by adopting a very simple classification: one group labeled "brain-damaged," the other, "metabolic by exclusion." This tends to put the cart before the horse, because the brain-damaged group is defined by evidence of clear neurological involvement in the newborn period and by the emergence of deficits at follow-up. This defeats the purpose of searching for correlations between all possible etiological factors and long-term prognosis. Worse, by not emphasizing the presence of multiple risk factors in the pathogenesis of neonatal seizures, one tends to miss therapeutic measures to simultaneously treat these various causes, some of which may well be preventable. To use our earlier example, for instance, we cannot tell for sure if the clinical outcome will be dictated by the asphyxia, the bleeding, or the hypoglycemia. We have followed the approach of

listing all presumptive etiological factors, well aware that multiple coding results.

During our prospective study covering almost two decades, now including a cohort of approximately 300 neonates, we have witnessed significant changes in the incidences of some etiological factors (15,16,18,30). These changing trends have been due to improvements in prenatal care and obstetrical techniques, particularly to the increasing sophistication in intensive perinatal interventions.

Table 2 lists the incidences of etiological factors in a study carried out from 1958 to 1968 and another study between 1969 and 1979. It shows that some factors have changed significantly, whereas others have remained about the same. Direct birth traumas have decreased, whereas asphyxia and intracranial hemorrhages have increased. Late-onset hypocalcemia has almost disappeared. "Dysmaturity" has also decreased. In contrast, infections, congenital CNS malformations, and cryptogenic factors have shown no great changes in incidence.

What do these variable trends in etiological factors mean in terms of prognosis? They appear to have had only a moderate impact. In fact, changes in early feeding trends have practically eliminated late-onset hypocalcemia, with its most benign prognosis. The increasing incidences of encephalopathies due to anoxic-ischemic insults occurring *in utero* and after birth, together with the increasing numbers of surviving premature infants with subependymal and intraventricular hemorrhages, have increased the numbers of infants neurologically at risk. Many of them develop seizures either from the primary condition or from early-onset hypocalcemia and hypoglycemia.

Nevertheless, our more recent series (Fig. 1) shows that overall mortality has decreased from about 20% to about 16%. There is no clear trend

TABLE 2. *Changing trends in main etiological factors in newborns with seizures*

	Presumptive causes				
	221 Newborns (1958–1968)		210 Newborns (1969–1979)		
	(No.)	(%)	(No.)	(%)	
Asphyxia[a]	25	11.5	51	24.5	$p < 0.01$
Intracranial hemorrhage					
Cryptogenic[a]	11	5	25	12	$p < 0.02$
Direct trauma[a]	22	10	9	4.5	$p < 0.02$
Infections					
Intrauterine	9	4	6	3	
Perinatal[a]	23	10.5	19	9	NS
	14	6.5	18	8.5	NS
CNS dysgenesis (recognized)					
Metabolic	17	8	29	14	NS
Early-onset hypocalcemia[a]	29	13	6	3	$p < 0.01$
Late-onset hypocalcemia	4	2	7	3.5	NS
Hypomagnesemia	13	6	18	8.5	NS
Transient hypoglycemia[a]	11	5	9	4.5	NS
Persistent hypoglycemia[a]	7	3	9	4.5	
Hypo-hypernatremia[a]	9	4	12	6	
Inborn errors of metabolism	10	4.5	5	2.5	NS
Postmaturity[a]	5	2.5	8	4	
Familial neonatal	6	3	4	2	
Drug withdrawal	9	4	12	5.5	
Miscellaneous	61	27.5	48	23	NS
Cryptogenic					

[a]Multiple factors often coexist.

to suggest that more sophisticated perinatal care has had significant impact on the incidence of later sequelae, which remains at about 35%. The only change discernible in more recent prospective investigations is a decrease in the severity and multiplicity of handicaps. For example, perinatal asphyxia, which caused seizures to persist or recur in our earlier series (30), has shown less tendency in our more recent study (18) to cause either persistence or recurrence of seizures, regardless of antiepileptic treatment.

A few words should be said regarding the almost one-fourth of cases classified as cryptogenic. This obviously represents a mixed group of seizure disorders, including some that escape our efforts to define diagnostic criteria. It includes many, probably about half, of what may be called benign neonatal seizures. They are often familial, suggesting an autosomal dominant inheritance with variable penetrance. Characteristically, these infants develop vigorous seizures several days after birth, with a peak at the fifth or sixth day. Their convulsions tend to resolve within the neonatal period. Somewhat less than one-half of these infants will later develop generalized epilepsies, but only a minority will exhibit other neurological sequelae.

In the prognosis of neonatal seizures, four factors have emerged as useful indicators for prognostic profiles. First, as a generalization, the earlier the onset of seizures, the worse the prognosis. In the majority of these infants, the seizures are related to severe prenatal and perinatal asphyxia (mainly those with ischemic insults, with or without concomitant metabolic aberrations) and intrauterine infections, some with acquired encephalitis (herpes) or bacterial meningitis. Direct brain trauma producing laceration of the tentorium or falx also leads to early onset of seizures. Some congenital metabolic defects (such as pyridoxine dependence), local anesthetic injections, and early drug withdrawal also may lead to early seizures. Seizure onset after 2 to 3 days of life most commonly results from asphyxia, intracranial hemorrhages (IVH, SAH, IPH), infections (sepsis and meningitis), congenital CNS malformations, or congenital metabolic defects (such as nonketotic hyperglycinemia, propionic acidemia, urea cycle disorders). After 2 to 4 days the common causes are infections, CNS dysgenesis, sepsis with electrolyte imbalances, and kernicterus; some cases of less severe postnatal asphyxia coincide with seizure onset. Later occurrences of seizures were often secondary to "tetany," but the latter has practically been eliminated. Infections, late sequelae of milder hypoxic insults, metabolic enzymatic disorders, and dysgenetic factors, as well as cryptogenic causes, prevail at this later onset, together with a miscellaneous group of rare disorders.

The second factor useful as an index for prognosis is the prevailing seizure pattern (Table 1). In general, the less obvious the peripheral manifestations of an ictal event, the worse the prognosis; conversely, the more vigorous and sustained the ictal manifestations, the better the long-term prognosis.

The third useful factor in delineating prognostic profiles is the EEG. Much has been written regarding neonatal EEGs, both normal and abnormal. The interested reader is referred to some reports on this subject (3,8–10,17,19,20,23,27,29, 34,39,40). Table 3 summarizes some correlations that have been found between specific EEG patterns and outcomes for newborns with seizures.

The fourth factor for prognosis is the neonatal neurological assessment. Predictions of long-term outcomes for infants with seizures have generally been considered hazardous (2,12,16,24,26,31,32). As neurobehavioral assessment of newborns at risk becomes more sophisticated, better predictive results can be foreseen. At present, the most reliable indices for long-term prognosis deriving from neonatal neurological assessment fall within two extremes: at one extreme are those infants profoundly compromised at most levels of cerebral function; at the other are those infants who consistently show signs of normality throughout the neonatal period. However, a significant percentage, close to half of the total population, falls between these extremes. These are the infants for whom neurophysiological measures and determination of etiological factors can be of help for outcome predictions.

Thus, we now have a fifth prognostic factor: the correlations between various etiological factors and long-term outcome. These are summarized in Table 4. It should be noted that "abnormal" refers to the presence of significant motor deficits, developmental delays, and continuation or reemergence of seizure syndromes. Relatively less severe sequelae, such as specific learning disabilities, "soft" motor deficits, and behavioral problems, are not included. Note that there are several etiological subgroups whose numbers are too small for χ^2 tests. This applies to the various types of intra-

TABLE 3. *Correlations between EEG patterns and clinical outcomes for newborns with seizures*

	Clinical outcome at 4–7 ± 2 years				
Neonatal EEG	Normal	Abnormal	Dead	Total	Level of significance by χ^2 test
Ictal abnormalities					
Focal discharges (spikes or sharp waves) with normal background	38	26	3	67	NS
Multifocal discharges with abnormal background	10	23	8	41	$p < 0.001$
Beta-, alpha-, theta-, deltalike discharges	5	14	6	25	$p < 0.004$
Repeated sharp waves at low frequencies, usually over a low-voltage background	3	8	3	14	$p < 0.05$
No recordable discharges during clinical ictus	—	2	3	5	NS[a]
Interictal abnormalities					
Isoelectric	—	4	6	10	$p < 0.002$
Paroxysmal or "burst-suppression"					
Both awake and asleep	1	12	7	20	$p < 0.001$
In REM and NREM sleep only	2	11	4	17	$p < 0.002$
Low voltage throughout REM and NREM sleep	1	7	1	9	$p < 0.04$
Persistent severe dysmaturity for CA	6	12	—	18	NS
Rolandic positive sharp transients	2	2	2	6	NS
Normal EEG	92	10	1	103	$p < 0.001$
Total	160	131	44	335	

[a]The χ^2 test did not reach a significant level because of the small number of patients, although none of the children were normal.

TABLE 4. *Correlations between etiological factors and clinical outcomes at age 5 ± 2 years in 213 newborns with seizures (1967–1977)*

	No. of patients	Dead (No.)	Abnormal (No.)	Dead and abnormal (%)	Normal (No.)	Normal (%)	Predictability
Asphyxia[a]	51	11	29	80	11	20	$p < 0.01$
Intracranial hemorrhage							
Cryptogenic[a]	30	6	15	70	9	30	$p < 0.025$
Trauma[a]	9	3	3	70	3	30	
Infections							
Intrauterine	7	1	5	90	1	10	
Postnatal	20	5	8	65	7	35	NS
CNS dysgenesis	19	6	12	95	1	5	$p < 0.005$
Metabolic							
Early-onset hypocalcemia[a]	32	8	12	66	12	36	NS
Late-onset hypocalcemia	10	0	1	10	9	90	$p < 0.025$
Transient hypoglycemia[a]	19	1	4	27	14	73	
Persistent (idiopathic) hypoglycemia	10	2	5	72	3	28	
Hypomagnesemia[a]	8	1	2	40	5	60	
Hypo-hypernatremia[a]	10	2	2	40	6	60	
Inborn errors of metabolism	13	1	9	80	3	20	$p < 0.05$
Postmaturity[a]	6	0	5	85	1	15	
Familial (benign)	9	0	1	8	8	92	$p < 0.025$
Drug-induced							
Iatrogenic	2	0	0	0	2	100	
Withdrawal	5	0	1	16	4	84	
Miscellaneous[a]	18	1	10		7		
Cryptogenic	54	3	14	32	37	68	$p < 0.01$

[a]Multiple factors often coexist.

cranial hemorrhages. Recent data (6) indicate that some "cryptogenic" hemorrhages reach predictability levels for outcome. Conversely, early-onset hypocalcemia, which has increased in incidence, has shown greater variability in clinical outcome in some recent series.

As mentioned earlier, our last series (1972–1977) indicates that one may still expect close to 16% mortality and a 35% incidence of long-term sequelae, whereas about 50% of newborns with seizures escape significant neurological involvement. This remarkable dichotomy in global outcome has been noted in all other series published before and after ours.

The discrepancy between the results obtained in animal models and those observed in human infants raises the question whether ictal phenomena per se may induce measurable neurophysiological effects in the latter. Indeed, we have at times observed some changes in EEG parameters occurring after seizures, sometimes even a single one. These changes belong to what we have called "regression in maturational levels," as measured by very simple parameters (17,18). We have studied these changes extensively in a large population of newborns at risk and have seen that whereas some exhibit what we call "transient dysmaturity," others show "persistent dysmaturity." Without going into details, I shall only say that infants with transient dysmaturity effects from any noxae usually show few, if any, measurable long-term sequelae. Those infants with persistent dysmaturity (those who on serial testings continue to lag behind expected age norms) have not as yet shown clear statistical evidence for significant neurological sequelae in the group of infants with seizures, although a trend is apparent. In a group of newborns at risk because of intracranial hemorrhages, it has been shown that persistence of dysmaturity in bioelectrical parameters appears to correlate significantly with long-term outcome (6). A recent study by Tharp et al. (35) has confirmed that some of these persistent dysmaturity features are poor prognostic indices for small prematures.

I can only briefly illustrate here some effects on bioelectrical parameters in neonates with seizures.

Figures 2 through 5 show EEGs from a full-term baby with uneventful history and existence until on the sixth day of life he developed vigorous clonic focal seizures. Figure 2 shows an epoch of his REM (active) sleep at CA of 41 weeks before (upper tracing) and a few minutes after (lower tracing) one of his seizures. All maturational parameters were normal before the attack, but afterward the concordance was clearly off, and there were about 10 times more spindle/delta bursts (a hallmark of dysmaturity). Figure 3 shows what happened in NREM (quiet) sleep. Again, the upper tracing shows an epoch before the seizure. In the lower tracing, just after the attack, the interhemispheric synchrony is clearly altered, and the spindle/delta bursts are 54 versus an expected range of 0.2. Figures 4 and 5, taken from an EEG 3 days later (when all seizures had stopped for 42 hr), show that his bioelectrical behavioral schedule was at the expected level for his CA in both REM and NREM sleep states. On clinical follow-up this baby was found to be normal.

The next case involves an instance of persistent dysmaturity in serial EEGs. This was a baby who had a history of asphyxia and seizures. Figures 6 and 7 are from one of the many recordings made,

all exhibiting clear retardation of the bioelectrical parameters we have been using. His clinical outcome was unfavorable when he was reexamined at 14 months. Thus, it is evident that seizures per se may affect neurophysiological mechanisms even at this age. What is not evident, however, is whether or not these perturbations signify some degree of brain damage irrespective of the underlying neurological disease responsible for the seizures.

We tried to find possible correlations between clinical outcome and the severity and duration of various types of neonatal seizures. Logically, if we extrapolate the experimental data that demonstrate profound alterations in neuronal and behavioral parameters when newborn animals are induced to convulse, then the more vigorous and prolonged ictal phenomena in human newborns should lead to greater disruption in their neurological functions, in contrast to babies who have either very short or barely recognizable ictal manifestations.

The number of babies we could assess in this way was necessarily small, because close monitoring was needed to achieve reliable data. The grading itself, in terms of assessing duration and severity of prevailing seizures, was somewhat em-

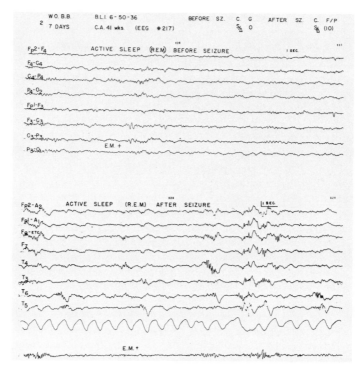

FIG. 2.

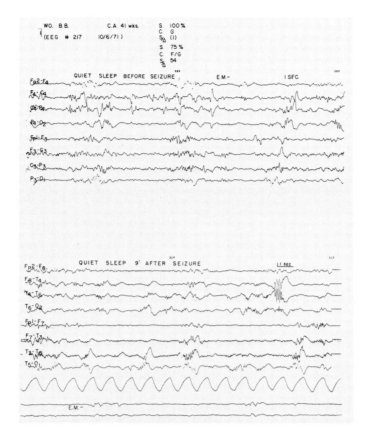

FIG. 3.

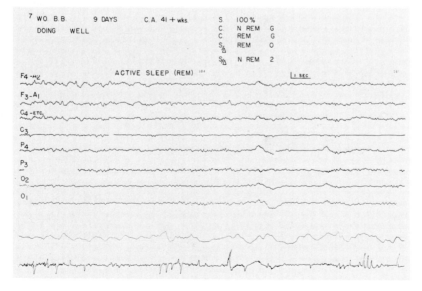

FIG. 4.

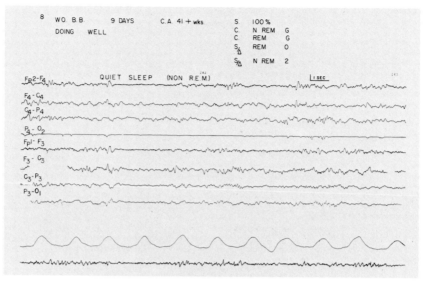

FIG. 5.

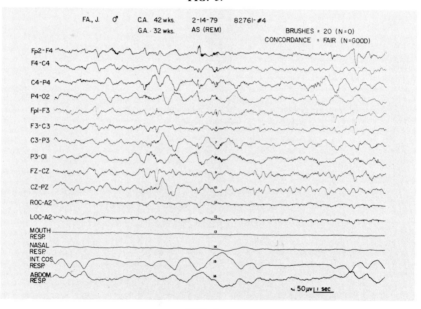

FIG. 6.

pirical. However, it seems adequate to test the hypothesis. Table 5 summarizes these data. We chose babies with mainly focal seizures lasting significantly longer than 4 min (group A) or less than 4 min (group B). Group C is composed of newborns with very short ictal phenomena. Group D is a group of babies with subtle seizures. The results of this analysis suggest a negative correlation between clinical outcome and the duration and severity of seizures, because it would appear from these data that the longer and more vigorous the seizure, the better the long-term outcome. These results run contrary to common sense. They are most likely due to the correlation with etiological factors. We know that seizures of a "subtle" pattern or with only brief myoclonic events occur mainly in newborns in whom cerebral function has already been significantly compromised before the onset of seizures. In contrast, the more vigorous, well-organized clinical seizures suggest a relatively in-

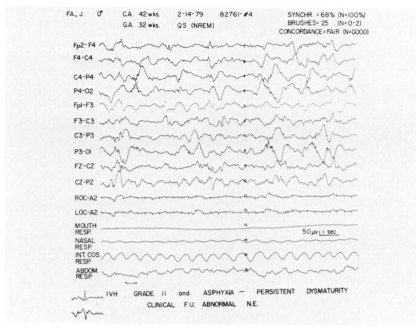

FA., J. ♂   C.A. 42 wks.   2-14-79   82761-#4   SYNCHR. = 68% (N=100%)
              G.A. 32 wks.   QS (NREM)   BRUSHES= 25   (N=0-2)
                                                           CONCORDANCE = FAIR (N=GOOD)

IVH   GRADE II   and   ASPHYXIA —   PERSISTENT   DYSMATURITY
CLINICAL   F.U. ABNORMAL   N.E.

FIG. 7.

TABLE 5. *Relationship between severity of seizures and neurological deficits (including IQ of 80 or below) at age 6 ± 1.3 years*

Group[a]	No. of patients	Normal	Deficits (No.)	Deficits (%)
A	14	9	5	35.7
B	16	10	6	37.5
C	6	2	4	66.7
D	10	2	8	80.0
Total	46	23	23	50.0

[a]A = focal or diffuse clonic seizures lasting ≥ 4 min; B = focal or diffuse clonic seizures lasting < 4 min; C = myoclonic seizures (lasting seconds); D = "minimal" seizure patterns, with least convulsive activity and electrical discharges.

tact CNS. Thus, in this analysis we would be comparing apples and oranges. However, if we look only at groups A and B, these presumably represent a more homogeneous group in which the main difference is, indeed, the duration of the prevailing convulsive episodes. No differences between them emerged in regard to long-term outcome (Table 5). These observations are strengthened by the benign outcome for a significant percentage of the cryptogenic group of convulsing newborns who develop with no detectable neurological sequelae.

Obviously, this does not contradict the fact that a newborn who persists having seizures, in spite of appropriate treatment, is a cause for concern.

In conclusion, the outcome for convulsing newborns correlates best with the presumptive causes, the findings on serial EEGs, and repeated neurobehavioral assessments. This conclusion does not deny *a priori* that more subtle long-term sequelae may still be found in cohorts of newborns with seizures. It only indicates that the profound cerebral insults observable in newborn animals subjected to induced convulsive states do not appear to be comparable to what happens in the human newborn.

Similar discrepancies have emerged from the experimental studies of others. An example is provided by the contrasting results obtained by Meldrum et el. (22), Meldrum (Chapter 40), and Brown and Babb (Chapter 15). For instance, Meldrum found significant pathological changes in adolescent *Papio papio* baboons subjected to epileptic status, even when the confounding variables of hypoxia, hypotension, hypoglycemia, hypopyrexia, and peripheral motor activity were controlled, but Brown and Babb failed to confirm these pathological changes as long as metabolic homeostasis was maintained. These striking differences apparently were not due to methodological variables, such as differences in anesthesia, nor to other apparent experimental variables.

If such different results occur within the highly controllable context of experimental investigations, it is not surprising that there are differences between the convulsive states induced in animal models and those spontaneously appearing in human neonates.

What we need to do, if possible, is to progress from group predictions to single-case predictions, as well as to clarify whether or not neonatal seizures per se add to underlying brain abnormalities and may cause long-term, relatively mild, though possibly important, deficits in cognitive, behavioral, and other abilities.

We need to determine why seizures are such relatively common events in this age group. This will require a better understanding of the multiplicity of perturbations that can modify neuronal excitability to induce epileptogenic tendencies in cortical and subcortical immature systems, in which *a priori* one would expect relatively high seizure thresholds. Although at present the clinical prospective data on newborns with seizures do not support the idea that these perturbations in the developing CNS represent a major factor for later epileptic syndromes, the latter may still prove to have their roots within early alterations in neuronal, synaptic, and neurotransmitter modulators and receptors that might prepare, so to speak, the necessary substrata for later onset of epileptic syndromes.

REFERENCES

1. Aicardi, J., and Baraton, J. (1971): A pneumoencephalographic demonstration of brain atrophy following status. *Dev. Med. Child Neurol.*, 13:660–667.
2. Amiel-Tison, C. (1979): Birth injury as a cause of brain dysfunction in full-term newborns. In: *Advances in Perinatal Neurology, Vol. 1*, edited by R. Korobkin and G. Guilleminault, pp. 57–83. Spectrum, New York.
3. Anders, T., Emde, R., and Parmelee, A. H. (1971): *A Manual of Standardized Terminology, Techniques and Criteria for Scoring of States of Sleep and Wakefulness in Newborn Infants*. U.C.L.A. Brain Information Service, Los Angeles.
4. Brown, J. K., Cockburn, F., and Forfar, J. O. (1972): Clinical and chemical correlations in convulsions in the newborn. *Lancet*, 1:135–139.
5. Chevrie, J. J., and Aicardi, J. (1975): Duration and lateralization of febrile convulsions' etiological factors. *Epilepsia*, 16:787–789.
6. da Costa, J. C., and Lombroso, C. T. (1980): Neurophysiological correlates of neonatal hemorrhages. *Electroencephalogr. Clin. Neurophysiol.*, 50:183–187.
7. Dennis, J. C. (1978): Neonatal convulsions: Etiology, late neonatal status and long-term outcome. *Dev. Med. Child Neurol.*, 20:143–158.
8. Dreyfus-Brisac, C. (1964): The electroencephalogram of the premature and full-term newborn. Normal and abnormal development of waking and sleeping patterns. In: *Neurological and Electroencephalographic Studies in Infancy*, edited by P. Kellaway and I. Petersen, pp. 186–197. Grune & Stratton, New York.
9. Dreyfus-Brisac, C., and Monod, N. (1972): Neonatal status epilepticus. *Electroencephalogr. Clin. Neurophysiol.*, 15:38–52.
10. Ellingson, R. J. (1979): The EEGs of premature and full-term newborns. In: *Current Practice in Clinical Electroencephalography*, edited by D. D. Daly and D. W. Klass, p. 149. Raven Press, New York.
11. Falconer, M. A. (1968): The significance of mesial temporal sclerosis (Ammon's horn sclerosis) in epilepsy. *Gary's Hospital Reports*, 117:1–12.
12. Fenichel, G. M. (1980): Seizures in newborns. In: *Neonatal Neurology*, Chapter 2. Churchill Livingstone, New York.
13. Freeman, J. M., and Leitman, P. S. (1973): A basic approach to the understanding of seizures and the mechanism of action and metabolism of anticonvulsants. *Adv. Pediatr.*, 20:291–311.
14. Gastaut, H., Pinsard, N., and Genton, P. (1980): Electroclinical correlations of CT-scans in secondary generalized epilepsies. In: *Advances in Epileptology*, edited by R. Canger, F. Angeleri, and J. K. Penry, pp. 45–52. Raven Press, New York.
15. Lombroso, C. T. (1965): Neonatal seizure states. In: *Proceedings of the Ninth International Congress of Pediatrics*, pp. 38–59. University of Tokyo Press, Tokyo.
16. Lombroso, C. T. (1973): Seizures in the newborn period. In: *Handbook of Clinical Neurology, Vol. 15*, pp. 189–218. North-Holland, Amsterdam.
17. Lombroso, C. T. (1975): Neurophysiological observations in diseased newborns. *Biol. Psychiatry*, 10:527–558.
18. Lombroso, C. T. (1978): Convulsive disorders in newborns. In: *Pediatric Neurology and Neurosurgery*, edited by R. A. Thompson and J. R. Green, pp. 205–239. Spectrum, New York.
19. Lombroso, C. T. (1979): Quantified electroencephalographic scales on 10 pre-term healthy newborns followed up to 40–43 weeks CA by serial polygraphic recordings. *Electroencephalogr. Clin. Neurophysiol.*, 46:460–473.
20. Lombroso, C. T. (1982): Neonatal electroencephalography. In: *Electroencephalography: Basic Principles, Clinical Applications and Related Fields*, edited by E. Neidermeyer and P. Lopes da Silva, pp. 599–637. Urban and Schwatzenburg, Baltimore.
21. Meldrum, B. S., and Horton, R. W. (1973): Physiology of status epilepticus in primates. *Arch. Neurol.*, 28:1–9.
22. Meldrum, B. S., Horton, R. W., and Brierly, J. B. (1974): Epileptic brain damage in adolescent baboons following seizures induced by allyl-glycine. *Brain*, 97:407–418.
23. Monod, R., Pajot, N., and Guidasci, S. (1972): The neonatal EEG: Statistical studies and prognostic value

in full-term and pre-term babies. *Electroencephalogr. Clin. Neurophysiol.*, 32:529–544.

24. Nelson, K. B., and Broman, S. H. (1979): Perinatal risk factors in children with serious motor and mental handicaps. *Ann. Neurol.*, 2:371–388.

25. Norman, R. M. (1964): The neuropathology of status epilepticus. *Med. Sci. Law*, 4:46–51.

26. Parmelee, A. H., and Haber, A. (1973): Who is the "risk infant"? *Clin. Obstet. Gynecol.*, 16:376–381.

27. Petre-Quadens, O. (1972): Sleep in mental retardation. In: *Sleep and the Maturing Nervous System*, edited by C. D. Clemente, D. P. Purpura, and F. E. Mayer, pp. 383–396. Academic Press, New York.

28. Plum, F., House, D. C., and Duffy, T. E. (1974): Metabolic effects of seizures. In: *Brain Dysfunction in Metabolic Disorders*, edited by F. Plum, pp. 141–150. Raven Press, New York.

29. Prechtl, H. F. R., Theorell, K., and Blair, A. W. (1973): Behavioral state cycles in abnormal infants. *Dev. Med. Child Neurol.*, 15:606–615.

30. Rose, A. L., and Lombroso, C. T. (1970): Neonatal seizure states: A prospective study in 137 full-term babies. *Pediatrics*, 45:404–425.

31. Saint-Anne Dargassies, S. (1977): Long-term neurological follow-up studies of 286 truly premature infants: The positive and negative aspects of the outcome of prematurity. Part I. Neurological sequelae. *Dev. Med. Child Neurol.*, 19:462–478.

32. Saint-Anne Dargassies, S. (1979): The normal and abnormal neurological examination of the neonate: Silent neurological abnormalities. In: *Advances in Perinatal Neurology, Vol. I*, edited by R. Korobkin and G. Guilleminault, pp. 1–19. Spectrum, New York.

33. Spielmeyer, W. (1927): Die Pathogenese des epileptischen Krampfes. *Z. Ges. Neurol. Psychiatry*, 109:501–520.

34. Tharp, B. R. (1980): Pediatric electroencephalography. In: *Electrodiagnosis in Clinical Neurology*, edited by M. J. Aminoff, pp. 67–117. Churchill Livingstone, New York.

35. Tharp, B. R., Cukier, F., and Monod, N. (1981): The prognostic value of the electroencephalogram in premature infants. *Electroencephalogr. Clin. Neurophysiol.*, 51:219–236.

36. Wasterlain, C. G., and Plum, F. (1973): Vulnerability of developing rat brain to electroconvulsive seizures. *Arch. Neurol.*, 29:38–45.

37. Wasterlain, C. G. (1976): Effects of neonatal status epilepticus on rat brain development. *Neurology (Minneap.)*, 26:975–986.

38. Wasterlain, C. G., and Duffy, T. E. (1976): Status epilepticus in immature rats. *Arch. Neurol.*, 33:821–827.

39. Watanabe, K., Iwase, K., and Hara, K. (1974): Development of slow-wave sleep in low-birthweight infants. *Dev. Med. Child Neurol.*, 16:23–32.

40. Werner, S. S., Stockard, J. E., and Bickford, R. (1977): *Atlas of Neonatal Electroencephalography*. Raven Press, New York.

Advances in Neurology, Vol. 34: Status Epilepticus, edited by A.V. Delgado-Escueta, C.G. Wasterlain, D.M. Treiman, and R.J. Porter. Raven Press, New York © 1983.

11

Consequences of Status Epilepticus in Infants and Children

Jean Aicardi and Jean-Jacques Chevrie

In this chapter we shall review the available evidence on the neurological, mental, and epileptic sequelae of convulsive status epilepticus in children between the ages of 1 month and 15 years. Convulsive status epilepticus is defined as a series of motor seizures, generalized, unilateral or partial, without recovery of consciousness between the individual fits, or as a single prolonged convulsion (23,54). In neither type has the minimum seizure duration necessary to establish a diagnosis of status epilepticus been agreed on; in most recent works the minimum has been set at 30 min (8,14,46), but in several earlier studies 1 hr was the accepted limit (4,23).

A large proportion of the cases of status epilepticus observed in infants and children are unilateral in location and clonic in type, but generalized clonic or tonic status is also common (4). Myoclonic status is not considered in this review, because it seems to be closer in its consequences to nonconvulsive status epilepticus than to major convulsive episodes.

METHODOLOGICAL PROBLEMS

The study of the consequences of status epilepticus involves a number of difficulties. First, the definitions of status epilepticus have varied for different authors and different dates of publication. Second, the actual durations of episodes of status

often have not been known precisely, because the reported series have been compiled retrospectively, and the types, locations, and intensities of the convulsive phenomena have rarely been indicated. In addition, complicating factors that may be important in the production of brain damage, such as the degree of fever, blood pressure measurements, evidence of hypoxia, acidosis, or hypoglycemia, and serum electrolyte derangements, have rarely, if ever, been studied. Third, the treatments given have not been indicated, and their possible influences on sequelae (15) cannot be determined. Fourth, the criteria used in determining the cause of the status, which obviously has a bearing on the outcome, have varied from patient to patient, depending on the depth of the investigations performed. A fifth difficulty is that the reported series, whether involving children or adults, have been likely to be biased in favor of the severest cases, because of their retrospective character and their origin from specialized centers. Finally, the evaluation of sequelae has been dependent on the length of follow-up. In addition, it has often been difficult with young patients, who have not been examined before their episodes of status, to determine if any recognized abnormality has been a consequence of the status or has antedated it.

The findings presented in this review should be evaluated with these reservations in mind. Some sequelae, especially the gravest ones, are likely to be overrepresented, whereas less striking consequences, such as behavioral problems and learning disorders, are probably underestimated.

MORTALITY

The mortality from status epilepticus remains significant, even though it has decreased considerably over the past 50 years (27,28,32). In a series of 232 infants and children with convulsive status epilepticus lasting 1 hr or more, there were 27 deaths. Ten of these occurred acutely at the time of the first episode, whereas 17 deaths occurred months or years after the acute event (4). Approximately half the fatalities were attributed to status epilepticus itself (whether initial or recurrent), the rest being due to the causes of the seizures (e.g., meningitis, encephalitis). The long-term mortality may be higher, because many children were left with severe neurological and mental abnormalities, and the follow-up was relatively short in several cases. These figures are of the same order of magnitude as those reported in recent adult series, which have varied from 6.6% to 25% (30,32,33,55,63). The grave significance of status epilepticus is also attested by the poor long-term outcome for the 32 patients with epilepsy following status epilepticus reported by Lindsay et al. (36), 14 of whom died as children or were wholly dependent.

NEUROLOGICAL AND MENTAL CONSEQUENCES

The true incidence of neurological and mental abnormalities following status epilepticus in infants and children is not known, because almost all reported series have not distinguished between children and adults (12,28,30,55) or have been concerned only with sequelae such as acute acquired hemiplegia (2,22,24,53) or epilepsy (20).

In the one large series comprising exclusively children between 1 month and 15 years of age each having experienced an episode of convulsive status lasting 1 hr or more (4), gross neurological deficits were found in 88 of 239 patients (37%) (Table 1). These were apparently acquired at the time of status in 47 patients (20%). The neurological syndromes encountered included diplegia, extrapyramidal syndromes, choreoathetosis and other abnormal movements, bilateral pyramidal tract signs, cerebellar syndromes, and decorticate or de-

TABLE 1. *Sequelae in 239 patients with convulsive status epilepticus lasting 1 hr or more*

Sequela	Total	Acquired[a]
Permanent neurological signs	88 (37%)	47 (20%)
Mental retardation	114 (48%)	78 (33%)
Any mental or neurological disability	136 (57%)	82 (34%)
Epilepsy	104 (44%)	49 (21%)
Any disability	159 (67%)	85 (36%)

From Aicardi and Chevrie (4).
[a] Acquired at the time of the episode of status in previously well children.

cerebrate rigidity. Microcephaly often was associated with the neurological signs and occasionally was the only abnormality found. Hemiplegia was especially common, being present in 28 patients, and it was always acquired at the time of the status. These global figures, however, are of only limited significance, because not all patients in this study were followed up, and part of them were referred after the first episode of status for evaluation of established sequelae. When only those 118 patients seen at the time of the first acute attack of status and followed for at least 1 year (referred to as "acute cases") are considered, the incidence of neurological abnormalities is less: 47 of 118, or 40%. Fifty-nine of these 118 patients belonged to the cryptogenic group, i.e., they had no known abnormalities prior to their status episodes, and no causes were discovered for their attacks. Twelve of these 59 patients had neurological signs after their acute episodes (20%), 12 in the form of acute hemiplegia.

Mental deficits, defined as an IQ under 80, but usually of a severe grade, were observed in 114 of 239 cases (48%). The deficits apparently were acquired at the time of status epilepticus in 78 (33%). In these 78 children, acute encephalopathy of known cause was deemed to be the origin of the intellectual defect in 23 cases; in the remaining 55 cases, no cause could be found for either the status or the mental deficit. Among the 118 acute cases, mental deficits were present in 51 (43%), as well as in 14 of the 59 cryptogenic acute cases (24%).

Neurological and mental abnormalities were almost always associated with one another and with epilepsy. Thus the total incidence of mental and/or neurological abnormalities was 57% (136 of 239) in the whole series (Table 1), of which 34% (82) appeared to have been acquired at the time of status epilepticus. In the subgroup of 118 acute cases, the incidence was 45% (53 of 118), and when only the 59 cryptogenic acute cases are considered, it is 25% (15 of 59). In an occasional patient, however, mental retardation, apparently acquired, was found in isolation.

The occurrence of acquired neurological and mental defects following prolonged convulsive seizures in childhood has often been reported (4,35,37,47). Fujiwara et al. (20) found mental and/or neurological sequelae in 40 of 79 children with status lasting 1 hr or more. Twenty-five of these patients had hemiplegia. Special attention has been paid to acute acquired postconvulsive hemiplegia (2,22,24,29), also known as the hemiconvulsion-hemiplegia (HH) syndrome (21,22). This syndrome occurs almost exclusively in young children and infants, 57% of the cases appearing before 2 years of age and 72% before 3 years (54). Its onset is marked by unilateral or predominantly unilateral convulsions, usually of a mainly clonic type. The seizures go on to unilateral status in 80% of patients (22). The seizures are generally associated with coma and are immediately followed by the appearance of hemiplegia, initially flaccid, which becomes eventually spastic and persists indefinitely in approximately 80% of cases, although its intensity often tends to decrease. Fever is present at the onset of seizures in 75% of cases. The course is severe. Mental retardation is associated with the hemiplegia in 68% of patients (2). Epilepsy is a complicating feature in 65% to 70% of patients (2,22,53).

The syndrome of acquired postconvulsive hemiplegia, like other forms of status epilepticus, has multiple causes. It may occur during the course of severe disorders such as meningitis, encephalitis (44), acute dehydration, pyogenic ear infections, and mastoid infections (22). In the majority of cases, however, the syndrome follows an undefined, apparently common, upper respiratory infection occurring in a previously well infant, and it can therefore be regarded as a form of cryptogenic status epilepticus. It has often been assumed that vascular mechanisms, especially arterial (11,61) or venous (22) thrombosis, play a prominent role in its genesis. In fact, cerebral angiograms were normal in all of our 35 patients submitted to this procedure, as well as in those of Isler (29) and Greer and Waltz (25). There have been very few

reports of postconvulsive hemiplegia with definite arterial occlusion (2,61) or with demonstrated venous thrombosis (9,44). Pathologically, there is diffuse dropout of neurons throughout the involved hemisphere, often in a laminar distribution and without relation to the arterial or venous territories (44).

EPILEPTIC CONSEQUENCES

Epileptic seizures frequently follow status epilepticus, especially in children, in whom status occurs as the first epileptic manifestation in 77% to 80% of cases (4,20,53). In our own series of 239 patients with status lasting 1 hr or more (4), only 55 (23%) had had one or several seizures before their episodes of status. In about a third of these (18/55), the number of antecedent seizures was less than three and usually one (Table 2). The antecedent seizures were generalized in 48 cases, unilateral in 13 cases, and partial motor or partial with complex symptoms in 14 cases (several types of seizures could occur in any given patient). On the other hand, seizures were commonly observed following status epilepticus. One hundred and four patients (44%) were known to have had subsequent seizures, and the proportion was 57% (82) in those followed for 1 year or more after their status episodes. The ictal manifestations following status differed from those preceding it both in frequency (73% had three seizures, and usually many more) and in type. Partial seizures and secondary generalized seizures (West and Lennox-Gastaut syndromes) accounted for 80% of all ictal phenomena.

TABLE 2. *Types of seizures preceding and following status epilepticus in 239 children*

Types of seizure	Before status N[b]	Before status Percent[a]	Following status N[c]	Following status Percent[a]
Tonic-clonic generalized	48	64.0	43	29.4
Clonic unilateral	13	17.4	16	11.0
Partial motor	7	9.3	16	11.0
Partial complex	7	9.3	30	20.5
Lennox syndrome	0	0	16	11.0
Infantile spasms	0	0	10	6.8
Iterative status	—	—	15	10.3

From Aicardi and Chevrie (4).
[a]Percentage of type of seizures.
[b]75 types of seizures in 55 patients.
[c]146 types of seizures in 104 patients.

Thus epilepsy after status epilepticus, in this series, was usually of the kind associated with organic damage to the brain, either focal or diffuse, whereas these particular types were rare prior to prolonged convulsive episodes.

Among 79 children with epilepsy following convulsive status epilepticus reported by Fujiwara et al. (20), 27 had secondarily generalized seizures, and 52 had partial seizures (21 with elementary symptoms and 31 with complex symptoms). Other workers have reported similar findings in series of patients with prolonged unilateral convulsions. Gastaut et al. (22) found that most patients with the HH syndrome developed partial motor or psychomotor seizures within a few years of the initial ictal event, a condition they termed the hemiconvulsion-hemiplegia-epilepsy (HHE) syndrome. Roger et al. (54), in a study of 100 cases of hemiclonic status, found that the subsequent seizures were mainly partial complex seizures (44%), either pure or combined with unilateral clonus, pure clonic seizures involving all or part of one side of the body (18%), and secondarily generalized seizures (18%). Aicardi et al. (2) recorded seizures in 58 of 89 patients with postconvulsive hemiplegia. The seizures were of a partial motor type in 29 patients, a partial complex type in 28 patients, and iterative status in 11 patients. Only 18 of their 89 infants (20%) had had seizures prior to the unilateral status.

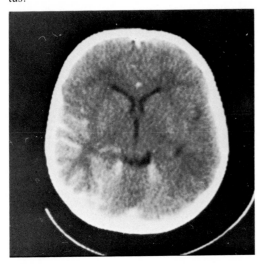

FIG. 1. Enhanced CT scan from a 2-year-old patient 4 days after right-sided partial status epilepticus. Increased vascularity in the left occipital region is evident. A repeat CT scan 1 month later was normal, as was angiography.

Likewise, in series of children with partial epilepsy, especially of the temporal lobe, a history of status epilepticus or of "prolonged or severe" infantile convulsions is common. Ounsted et al. (48) found that 32 of their 100 patients with temporal lobe epilepsy had status as the first ictal event. Falconer and his colleagues (17,18,38) reported that a history of severe infantile convulsions was present in as many as half their patients operated on for temporal lobe epilepsy, especially when the onset was under 10 years of age. Although such a high frequency of antecedent infantile convulsions has not been found in other neurosurgical series of partial epilepsy (31,52), the evidence linking status epilepticus in infancy with later epilepsy, especially of a partial type, is strong, even though the nature of this relationship cannot be inferred from retrospective studies.

PATHOLOGICAL AND NEURORADIOLOGICAL CONSEQUENCES

Pathological changes in the brains of children dying at various times following status epilepticus have been documented in several reports (19,38,45,48,49,57). As compared with those described in adults (see Chapter 12), the lesions tend to be more extensive and are more often predominantly unilateral (51). It appears that the period of status that will produce extensive damage in a child is shorter than that for an adult (40). The acute lesions are venous congestion and small petechial hemorrhages with variable signs of edema. The most evident histological abnormality is ischemic cell change, followed, with survival of 1 to 14 days, by proliferation of microglia, neuronophagia, cell loss, and proliferation of reactive astrocytes. The regional distributions of such changes are similar in adults and children and broadly involve the areas and cell types that are affected in systemic hypoxia. At a late stage, the nerve cell dropout and the retractile gliosis are responsible for marked atrophy of the involved structures.

This pathological sequence of events is reflected in the results of neuroradiological examinations performed at various times after status epilepticus. Increases in vascularization, especially venous, in the brain areas involved in the seizure activity have been reported on the basis of angiograms obtained shortly following episodes of prolonged convulsions (34,39,65). This hypervascularization may also be seen on CT scans, as shown in Fig. 1. It is probably accompanied by an increase in the permeability of the blood-brain barrier, as demonstrated by localized uptake of radioactive tracers (50,65) or by areas of increased density on CT scans (56). Pneumoencephalograms obtained within 1 or 2 weeks following status usually show a marked swelling of the hemisphere involved in the epileptic activity in unilateral or predominantly unilateral seizures. A shift of the median structures toward the more normal side is evident, and signs of increased pressure, such as suture splitting, may be seen. In pneumoencephalograms performed weeks or months after the episode of status, ventricular dilatation is demonstrated in many cases and predominates in, or is limited to, the hemisphere that was initially swollen. This results in a reversal of the shift of the median structures away from the more normal side, often associated with evidence of cortical atrophy (3,22,24,29) (Fig. 2).

For 19 children with various types of status epilepticus we performed two consecutive pneumoencephalograms, the first one within 10 days of the attack, the second during the following months (usually within 2 months). In 17 cases, significant degrees of ventricular dilatation appeared between the two examinations, resulting from atrophy, not from hydrocephalus. The localization of atrophy corresponded closely, as a rule, to that of the status epilepticus, being unilateral in all but 1 case of unilateral seizures and bilateral in all 3 cases of generalized status. No specific encephalopathy could be diagnosed in any of these patients. Eight of them had three or more seizures antedating the status attack. In these children, the antecedent convulsions did not differ clinically from the severe seizure, except in duration. It would be difficult to assume that the cause of the status episode was not the same as that of the antecedent seizures and thus to attribute the postconvulsive atrophy to anything other than the long-lasting seizure itself (3). Similar results can now be obtained by computerized tomography, which better demonstrates brain edema and more clearly shows cortical atrophy (21). The sequence of events using this technique is illustrated in Fig. 3.

More limited lesions, not demonstrable by neuroradiological examinations, may result from less severe episodes of status. In such cases, Ammon's horn, amygdala, and related structures are pref-

A,B

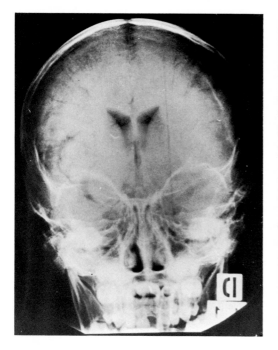 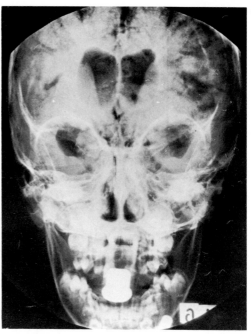

FIG. 2. **A:** Pneumoencephalogram from a 3-year-old girl 2 days after generalized status epilepticus. Normal-size ventricles. **B:** Repeat pneumoencephalogram in same patient 3 months after status. There is marked dilatation of both lateral ventricles and sulci.

A,B

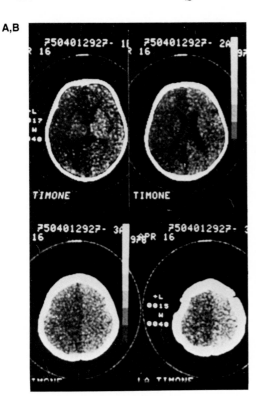
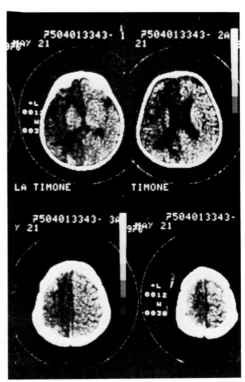

FIG. 3. **A:** CT scan obtained 2 days after right unilateral status epilepticus. The whole left hemisphere is hypodense; the left ventricle is slightly shifted to the right. **B:** Repeat CT scan 1 month later in same patient. Ventricular dilatation is now evident, as well as cortical atrophy. Residual hypodensity of the left hemisphere is seen.

erentially affected (Ammon's horn sclerosis or mesial temporal sclerosis). The relationships of this lesion to temporal lobe epilepsy, on the one hand, and to prolonged and/or repeated seizures, on the other hand, have been extensively discussed in the literature (26,38,49,57) and are reviewed elsewhere (Chapter 12).

MECHANISMS OF THE SEQUELAE OF STATUS AND THEIR RELATIONSHIPS TO INFANTILE CONVULSIONS

The brain damage responsible for the majority of clinical sequelae of status epilepticus can result from several causes. First, the lesions may antedate the attack of status, this being only one manifestation of a chronic encephalopathy of various possible origins. Second, both the status and the brain damage clinically expressed as sequelae may be due to an acute encephalopathy (e.g., meningoencephalitis, brain trauma). Third, the prolonged seizures may be responsible for brain damage, regardless of their cause, the long-lasting

epileptic activity, and/or the associated physiopathological events (e.g., hypotension, anoxia, fever) inducing an epileptic encephalopathy (44, 45,48). This may occur in a structurally intact brain, in the case of cryptogenic status epilepticus, or may supervene as a complication of a lesional epilepsy, with a resultant increase in the extent of the original lesions. The extent of the damage will vary with the topography and intensity of the episode of status—from diffuse damage involving the whole brain to the more limited lesions of mesial temporal sclerosis. The high incidence of unilateral damage may result from the common lateralization of prolonged convulsions (13). There is, in fact, good correlation between the localization of the initial attack of status and that of the epileptic and other sequelae (1).

The first two of these mechanisms are undoubtedly common. They accounted for approximately half the cases in our 1970 series (4). Moreover, the real incidences of acute and chronic encephalopathies as causes of status are likely to be underestimated, because (a) some acute neurological disorders (e.g., encephalitis) can be misdiagnosed as cryptogenic status when the CSF remains normal, and (b) cases classified as cryptogenic may, in fact, result from unrecognized chronic encephalopathies, especially when the episode of status occurs in a young infant, in whom development prior to the acute attack is difficult to assess retrospectively. The third mechanism, however, is of special importance, because prompt and effective treatment of the status in such cases should prevent brain damage or limit its extent.

There are a number of arguments to support the hypothesis that prolonged seizures can produce brain damage, irrespective of their cause.

1. In a high proportion of these patients, amounting to more than half in one large series (4), no cause can be discovered for the episode of status. In such cases the incidence of sequelae remains high (of the order of 25%), even though it is lower than in symptomatic cases.

2. The sequelae following status epilepticus do not differ clinically with the cause of the episode, as exemplified by the syndrome of acute acquired hemiplegia, which can result from several different disorders.

3. The pathological findings are nonspecific. They are mainly of an anoxic-ischemic type and are not related to arterial or venous territories, but rather to the localization of the epileptic discharges, thus suggesting a mechanism of consumption anoxia (41). In this regard it is worth mentioning that diffuse neuronal loss and glial proliferation of an anoxic type were regularly found in hemispherectomy specimens from patients with acquired, mainly postconvulsive hemiplegias, whereas cystic softening of arterial territories, usually the middle cerebral artery, was encountered in specimens from children with congenital hemiplegias not consequent to an acute infantile illness (10,64).

4. Experimental evidence has amply confirmed that epileptic activity does produce neuronal damage similar in appearance and localization to that observed in humans after status epilepticus. The lesions produced in animal models by prolonged induced convulsive activity are partly the result of the systemic changes associated with the seizures, such as hypotension, hypoxia, or fever (7,40,41). However, more limited brain damage is also seen in animals with prolonged convulsions, even when the systemic changes are prevented,

thus showing that the epileptic discharge itself is an essential factor (42).

If the hypothesis that even cryptogenic seizures occurring in normal brain can induce lesions is correct, the role of prolonged febrile convulsions in the genesis of postictal brain damage should be examined, because febrile seizures are by far the most common type in children. Febrile seizures have been reported to last 30 min or more in about 4% of cases (43), and 59 of 239 status episodes in our 1970 series (4) were apparently febrile convulsions lasting more than 1 hr. Residual brain damage following febrile convulsions has been mentioned in pathological studies (19,66) and clinical studies (5,35), and it is especially expressed in the form of temporal lobe epilepsy. Prospective studies of children with febrile convulsions, however, have revealed low incidences of acquired hemiplegia and mental retardation (6,43). Likewise, these studies have not indicated a higher proportion of epilepsies with partial complex seizures, as opposed to other types of epilepsy, in children who had had febrile seizures than in the general population of epileptic patients in the same age range (6,16). However, Wallace (62) found that in children with spontaneous seizures following febrile convulsions, partial complex seizures were electively observed in those who had had prolonged febrile convulsions.

In order to evaluate the role of long-lasting febrile seizures (30 min or more) in the genesis of sequelae, we compared 131 patients whose febrile seizures had been followed by sequelae (114 with epilepsy) and 86 children with uncomplicated febrile seizures (controls). All patients were followed up for at least 3 years, and the criteria defining febrile convulsions were uniform. The results appear in Tables 3 and 4. Patients who developed sequelae were mostly those who had long and unilateral seizures, whereas these were uncommon in the controls. The duration of seizures was the important factor, and brief lateralized seizures were not associated with sequelae. A young age at onset of the first febrile seizure was also linked to the occurrence of later disturbances. Eighty-one of the 109 children with classifiable residual epilepsy had partial or secondarily generalized seizures of a type usually associated with brain damage, whereas 28 had generalized seizures, probably of a nonlesional nature. Comparison of these two subgroups showed that only partial and secondarily generalized epilepsy was associated with the earlier occurrence

TABLE 3. *Febrile convulsions: comparison between patients with sequelae and controls*

Factor studied	Controls (N = 86)	All sequelae[a] N = 131	p	Epilepsy N = 114	p
Age at first febrile convulsion (months)	20.3	16.2	<0.05	16.3	<0.05
Seizure ≥ 30 min	15 (17.4)[b]	66 (50.4)	<0.001	53 (46.5)	<0.001
Lateralized seizure	15 (17.4)	57 (43.5)	<0.001	50 (43.9)	<0.001
Female sex	40 (46.5)	67 (51.1)	NS	60 (52.6)	NS
Abnormal pregnancy	5 (5.8)	15 (11.4)	NS	11 (9.6)	NS
Abnormal delivery	19 (22.1)	19 (14.5)	NS	15 (13.2)	NS
Birth weight (g)	3,195	3,178	NS	3,205	NS
Positive family history	29 (33.7)	44 (33.6)	NS	40 (35.1)	NS

From Aicardi and Chevrie (5).
[a]Includes neurological, mental, and epileptic sequelae.
[b]In each column, the first figure indicates the number of cases with the factor; the second figure (in parentheses) indicates the percentage of patients with the factor.

TABLE 4. *Comparison between 81 partial and 28 generalized epilepsies following febrile convulsions*

Factor studied	Partial epilepsy	Generalized epilepsy	p
Age at first febrile convulsion (months)	14.2	20.7	<0.001
Seizure ≥ 30 min	49 (60.5)[a]	1 (3.6)	<0.001
Lateralized seizure	46 (56.8)	1 (3.6)	<0.001
Female sex	44 (54.3)	8 (28.6)	<0.05
Positive family history	30 (37.0)	8 (28.6)	>0.40
Frequency of mental retardation	42 (51.8)	4 (14.3)	<0.001
Frequency of neurological sequelae	25 (30.9)	1 (3.6)	<0.001

[a]In each column, the first figure indicates the number of cases with the factor; the second figure (in parentheses) indicates the percentage of patients with the factor.

of long and/or lateralized febrile convulsions. In addition, mental retardation and neurological abnormalities were very significantly more common in this subgroup (5). These data are consistent with the hypothesis that febrile seizures, when prolonged in status epilepticus, are able to produce significant brain damage that may in turn become epileptogenic. However, only those epilepsies manifested by partial or multifocal seizures can be interpreted as resulting from such a mechanism.

FACTORS AFFECTING THE OUTCOME IN STATUS EPILEPTICUS

Cause of the Status

The cause of the status is, as expected, the most important factor that affects the outcome. As shown

in Table 5, the outcome in symptomatic status epilepticus is very significantly poorer than that in cryptogenic cases. Moreover, some of the cases classified as cryptogenic may, in fact, be caused by undemonstrated lesions, because the early development of infants and young children is difficult to assess retrospectively.

TABLE 5. *Incidence of neurological and mental sequelae according to etiology in 118 acute cases followed 1 year or more*

Etiology	Patients with sequelae	All patients	Percent
Cryptogenic status	15	59	25
Symptomatic status	38	59	64
Total	53	118	45

p < 0.001

Age

Death and all types of sequelae of status epilepticus are significantly more common in younger infants. Among 179 of our patients with convulsive status (4) who were followed long enough to determine the frequency of sequelae, the incidence of death and severe sequelae declined from 77% (27/35) for infants less than 6 months of age to 58% (55/94) for children aged 6 months to 3 years and 46% (23/50) for patients older than 3 years. The higher incidence of severe sequelae is not entirely due to the more frequent occurrence of symptomatic status in younger patients. Table 6 indicates that the proportion of sequelae following cryptogenic status in children less than 3 years of age is also greater than that in older patients. In a recent series of 40 infants under 1 year of age with afebrile convulsive status epilepticus, defined as any convulsion lasting longer than 30 min, we found a mortality of 22%; 38% of 35 infants surviving to 1 year of age or more had neurological residua, and 83% were mentally retarded, 60% severely so. Sixteen of those infants had cryptogenic status, 27% of whom were left with neurological defects and 67% with mental defects (14).

Sex

The outcome in status epilepticus does not vary significantly according to the sex of the patients. There is, however, a trend for girls to develop cryptogenic status epilepticus more commonly than boys. Thus, 41 of 67 patients with febrile cryptogenic status were female (4), whereas boys have outnumbered girls in most studies of febrile convulsions (35).

Prenatal and Perinatal Antecedents

The effect of an abnormal prenatal or perinatal history on the prognosis in status epilepticus has not been investigated. However, the high incidences of low birth weights and of abnormal perinatal periods in children with acquired hemiplegia following status are remarkable, with approximately 20% of such children in two large series weighing less than 2,500 g at birth (2,53).

Duration of Status Epilepticus

Little information is available on the relationship between the precise length of an episode of status and the occurrence of residua. The minimum duration of convulsive activity that is able to produce clinical sequelae is not known. Seizures lasting 30 min or more (but not briefer ones) are associated with abnormalities in the functioning of the blood-brain barrier (58) and with abnormal CSF lactate-pyruvate ratios suggestive of brain damage (59,60). Much longer seizures, however, sometimes appear to be well tolerated. Postconvulsive hemiplegia almost always follows very long seizures. Roger et al. (53) noted that no case of hemiplegia was observed after seizures lasting less than 2 hr. In the series of Aicardi et al. (2) involving 73 cases in which the lengths of the seizures were known, the durations of the attacks of status leading to hemiplegia were longer than 24 hr in 31 cases and longer than 6 hr in another 20 cases. No case was observed with status lasting less than 90 min. The relationship between length of seizures and the occurrence of complications other than hemiplegia has not been studied.

CONCLUSIONS

Status epilepticus in infants and children is a serious condition that requires immediate and ef-

TABLE 6. *Status epilepticus: incidence of neurological and mental sequelae according to age and etiology in 118 cases followed for 1 year or more*

	Cryptogenic status (N = 59)		Symptomatic status (N = 59)	
	< 3 years	≥ 3 years	< 3 years	≥ 3 years
Sequelae	13 (35%)[a]	2 (9%)	31 (65%)	7 (64%)
No sequelae	24 (65%)	20 (91%)	17 (35%)	4 (36%)
Total	37	22	48	11

[a]The first figure in each column indicates the number of patients: the second figure (in parentheses) indicates the percentage of patients with or without sequelae in each age group.

fective treatment. Its frequency is higher in infancy and childhood than in any other period of life, and it often constitutes the first epileptic manifestation. Sequelae are frequent, even when the episode of status is not the result of a primary brain lesion. Febrile convulsions probably are a common cause of status epilepticus. A more precise evaluation of the risks attendant to status epilepticus and the possible means of preventing brain damage is highly desirable. Such an evaluation will necessitate a uniformly accepted definition of status and collection of detailed data on the seizures, the associated systemic changes, the populations studied, and the methods of assessment.

REFERENCES

1. Aicardi, J. (1977): Post-natal sejzures. Clinical effects. In: *Brain/Fetal and Infant*, edited by S. R. Berenberg, pp. 295–301. Martinius Nijhoff, The Hague.
2. Aicardi, J., Amsili, J., and Chevrie, J. J. (1969): Acute hemiplegia in infancy and childhood. *Dev. Med. Child Neurol.*, 11:162–173.
3. Aicardi, J., and Baraton, J. (1971): A pneumoencephalographic demonstration of brain atrophy following status epilepticus. *Dev. Med. Child Neurol.*, 13:660–667.
4. Aicardi, J., and Chevrie, J. J. (1970): Convulsive status epilepticus in infants and children. A study of 239 cases. *Epilepsia*, 11:187–197.
5. Aicardi, J., and Chevrie, J. J. (1976): Febrile convulsions: Neurological sequelae and mental retardation. In: *Brain Dysfunction in Infantile Febrile Convulsions*, edited by M. A. B. Brazier and F. Coceani, pp. 247–257. Raven Press, New York.
6. Annegers, J. F., Hauser, W. A., Elveback, L. R., and Kurland, L. T. (1979): The risk of epilepsy following febrile convulsions. *Neurology (Minneap.)*, 29:297–303.
7. Blennow, G., Brierley, J. B., Meldrum, B. S., and Siesjo, B. K. (1978): Epileptic brain damage. The role of systemic factors that modify cerebral energy metabolism. *Brain*, 101:687–700.
8. Brown, J. K. (1976): Fits in childhood. In: *A Textbook of Epilepsy*, edited by J. Laidlaw and A. Richens, pp. 66–108. Churchill Livingstone, Edinburgh.
9. Byers, R., and Hass, G. (1933): Thrombosis of the dural venous sinuses in infancy and in childhood. *Am. J. Dis. Child*, 45:1161–1183.
10. Carmichael, E. A. (1966): Current status of hemispherectomy for infantile hemiplegia. *Clin. Proc. Child. Hosp. Wash.*, 22:285–293.
11. Carter, S., and Gold, A. P. (1967): Acute infantile hemiplegia. *Pediatr. Clin. North Am.*, 14:851–864.
12. Celesia, G. G. (1976): Modern concepts of status epilepticus. *J.A.M.A.*, 235:1571–1574.
13. Chevrie, J. J., and Aicardi, J. (1975): Duration and lateralization of febrile convulsions. Etiological factors. *Epilepsia*, 16:781–789.
14. Chevrie, J. J., and Aicardi, J. (1978): Convulsive disorders in the first year of life: Neurological and mental outcome and mortality. *Epilepsia*, 19:67–74.
15. Duffy, F. H., and Lombroso, C. T. (1978): Treatment of status epilepticus. In: *Clinical Neuropharmacology, Vol. 3*, edited by H. L. Klawans, pp. 41–56. Raven Press, New York.
16. Ellenberg, J. H., and Nelson, K. B. (1978): Febrile seizures and later intellectual performance. *Arch. Neurol.*, 35:17–21.
17. Falconer, M. A. (1971): Genetic and related aetiological factors in temporal lobe epilepsy. A review. *Epilepsia*, 12:13–21.
18. Falconer, M. A., Serafetinides, E. A., and Corsellis, J. A. N. (1964): Etiology and pathogenesis of temporal lobe epilepsy. *Arch. Neurol.*, 10:233–248.
19. Fowler, M. (1957): Brain damage after febrile convulsions. *Arch. Dis. Child.*, 32:67–76.
20. Fujiwara, T., Ishida, S., Miyakoshi, M., Sakuma, N., Moriyama, S., Morikawa, T., Seino, M., and Wada, T. (1979): Status epilepticus in childhood: A retrospective study of initial convulsive status and subsequent epilepsies. *Folia Psychiatr. Neurol. Jpn.*, 33:337–344.
21. Gastaut, H., Pinsard, N., Gastaut, J. L., Regis, H., Michel, B., and Dravet, C. (1977): Étude tomodensitométrique des accidents cérébraux responsables des hémiplégies aigues de l'enfant. *Rev. Neurol. (Paris)*, 133:595–607.
22. Gastaut, H., Poirier, F., Payan, G., Salamon, G., Toga, M., and Vigouroux, M. (1960): H. H. E. syndrome: Hemiconvulsions, hemiplegia, epilepsy. *Epilepsia*, 1:418–447.
23. Gastaut, H., Roger, J., and Lob, H. (1967): *Les états de mal épileptiques*. Masson, Paris.
24. Gastaut, H., Vigouroux, M., Trevisan, C., and Regis, H. (1957): Le syndrome hémiconvulsion-hémiplégie-épilepsie. *Rev. Neurol. (Paris)*, 97:37–52.
25. Greer, H. D., and Waltz, H. G. (1965): Acute neurologic disorders of infancy and childhood. *Dev. Med. Child Neurol.*, 7:507–517.
26. Hanefeld, F., and Crome, L. (1979): Beziehungen zwischen Epilepsie und neuropathologischen Befunden im Kindesalter. In: *Epilepsia 1978*, edited by H. Doose and G. Gross-Selbeck, pp. 66–77. Thieme, Stuttgart.
27. Heintel, H. (1972): *Der Status epilepticus*. G. Fisher, Stuttgart.
28. Hunter, R. A. (1959): Status epilepticus: History, incidence and problems. *Epilepsia*, 1:162–188.
29. Isler, W. (1971): *Acute Hemiplegias and Hemisyndromes in Childhood*. Heinemann, London.
30. Janz, D., and Kautz, G. (1964): The aetiology and treatment of status epilepticus. *Ger. Med. Mon.*, 9:451–456.
31. Jensen, I. (1976): Temporal lobe epilepsy. Etiological factors and surgical results. *Acta Neurol. Scand.*, 53:103–118.
32. Kas, S., and Orszagh, J. (1976): Clinical study of status epilepticus: Review of 111 statuses. *Acta Univ. Carol. [Med.] (Praha)*, 22:133–178.
33. Ketz, E., and Meier, H. R. (1979): Verlauf- und prognosebestimmende Faktoren beim Grand-mal-Status. *Aktuel. Neurol.*, 6:233–239.

34. Lee, S. H., and Goldberg, H. I. (1977): Hypervascular pattern associated with idiopathic focal status epilepticus. *Radiology*, 125:159–163.
35. Lennox-Buchthal, M. A. (1973): *Febrile Convulsions. A Reappraisal.* Elsevier, Amsterdam.
36. Lindsay, J., Ounsted, C., and Richards, P. (1979): Long-term outcome in children with temporal lobe seizures. I. Social outcome and childhood factors. *Dev. Med. Child Neurol.*, 21:285–298.
37. Lyon, G., Dodge, P. R., and Adams, R. D. (1961): The acute encephalopathies of obscure origin in infants and children. *Brain*, 84:680–708.
38. Margerison, J. H., and Corsellis, J. A. N. (1966): Epilepsy and the temporal lobes: A clinical, electroencephalographic and neuropathological study of the brain in epilepsy with particular reference to the temporal lobes. *Brain*, 89:499–530.
39. McDonald, E. J., Goodman, P. C., Nielsen, S. L., and Winestock, D. P. (1975): Cerebral hypervascularity and early venous opacification in status epilepticus. *Neuroradiology*, 117:87–88.
40. Meldrum, B. S. (1976): Neuropathology and pathophysiology. In: *A Textbook of Epilepsy*, edited by J. Laidlaw and A. Richens, pp. 314–354. Churchill Livingstone, Edinburgh.
41. Meldrum, B. S. (1978): Physiological changes during prolonged seizures and epileptic brain damage. *Neuropädiatrie*, 9:203–212.
42. Meldrum, B. S., Vigouroux, R. A., and Brierley, J. B. (1973): Systemic factors and epileptic brain damage: Prolonged seizures in paralyzed, artificially ventilated baboons. *Arch. Neurol.*, 29:82–87.
43. Nelson, K. B., and Ellenberg, J. H. (1978): Prognosis in children with febrile seizures. *Pediatrics*, 61:720–727.
44. Norman, R. M. (1962): Neuropathological findings in acute hemiplegia in childhood. In: *Acute Hemiplegia in Childhood*, edited by M. Bax and R. Mitchell, pp. 37–48. Heinemann, London.
45. Norman, R. M. (1964): The neuropathology of status epilepticus. *Med. Sci. Law*, 4:46–51.
46. O'Donohoe, N. V. (1979): *Epilepsies of Childhood.* Butterworth, London.
47. Ounsted, C. (1971): Some aspects of seizure disorders. In: *Recent Advances in Paediatrics*, edited by D. Gairdner and D. Hull, pp. 363–400. Churchill Livingstone, London.
48. Ounsted, C., Lindsay, J., and Norman, R. (1966): *Biological Factors in Temporal Lobe Epilepsy.* Heinemann, London.
49. Peiffer, J. (1963): *Morphologische Aspekte der Epilepsien.* Springer, Berlin.
50. Prensky, A. L., Swisher, C. N., and Devivo, D. C. (1973): Positive brain scans in children with idiopathic focal epileptic seizures. *Neurology (Minneap.)*, 27:798–807.
51. Radermecker, J., Guazzi, G. C., Toga, M., and Payan, H. (1967): Les lésions cérébrales en rapport avec les crises épileptiques graves prolongées et notamment avec les états de mal chez l'homme. In: *Les états de mal épileptique*, edited by H. Gastaut, J. Roger, and H. Lob, pp. 287–325. Masson, Paris.
52. Rasmussen, T. B. (1977): Temporal lobe seizures in children. Surgical aspects. In: *Topics in Child Neurology*, edited by M. Blaw, I. Rapin, and M. Kinsbourne, pp. 143–171. Spectrum, New York.
53. Roger, J., Bureau, M., Dravet, C., Dalla Bernardina, B., Tassinari, C. A., Revol, J., Challamel, J., and Taillandier, P. I. (1972): Les données EEG et les manifestations épileptiques en relation avec l'hémiplégie cérébrale infantile. *Rev. Electroencephalogr. Neurophysiol. Clin.*, 1:5–28.
54. Roger, J., Lob, H., and Tassinari, C. A. (1974): Status epilepticus. In: *Handbook of Clinical Neurology, Vol. 15, The Epilepsies*, edited by P. J. Vinken and G. W. Bruyn, pp. 145–188. North-Holland, Amsterdam.
55. Rowan, A. J., and Scott, D. F. (1970): Major status epilepticus. *Acta Neurol. Scand.*, 46:573–584.
56. Rumack, C. M., Guggenheim, M. A., Fasules, J. W., and Burdick, D. (1980): Transient positive postictal computed tomographic scan. *J. Pediatr.*, 97:263–264.
57. Sano, K., and Malamud, N. (1953): Clinical significance of sclerosis of the cornu Ammonis. *Arch. Neurol. Psychiatry*, 70:40–53.
58. Siemes, H., Siegert, M., and Hanefeld, F. (1978): Febrile convulsions and blood-cerebrospinal fluid barrier. *Epilepsia*, 19:57–66.
59. Simpson, H., Habel, A. H., and George, E. L. (1977): Cerebrospinal acid-base status and lactate and pyruvate concentrations after convulsions of varied duration and aetiology in children. *Arch. Dis. Child*, 52:844–849.
60. Simpson, H., Habel, A. H., and George, E. L. (1977): Cerebrospinal fluid acid-base status and lactate and pyruvate concentration after short (< 30 minutes) first febrile convulsions in children. *Arch. Dis. Child.*, 52:836–843.
61. Solomon, G. E., Hilal, S. K., Gold, A. P., and Carter, S. (1970): Natural history of acute hemiplegia of childhood. *Brain*, 93:107–120.
62. Wallace, S. J. (1977): Spontaneous fits after convulsions with fever. *Arch. Dis. Child.*, 52:192–196.
63. Whitty, C. W. M., and Taylor, M. (1949): Treatment of status epilepticus. *Lancet*, 2:591–594.
64. Wilson, P. J. E. (1970): Cerebral hemispherectomy for infantile hemiplegia. A report of 50 cases. *Brain*, 93:147–180.
65. Yarnell, P. R., Burdick, D., Sanders, B., and Stears, J. (1974): Focal seizures, early veins, and increased flow. A clinical, angiographic and radioisotopic correlation. *Neurology (Minneap.)*, 25:512–516.
66. Zimmerman, H. M. (1938): The histopathologia of convulsive disorders in children. *J. Pediatr.*, 13:859–890.

Mechanisms of Brain Damage

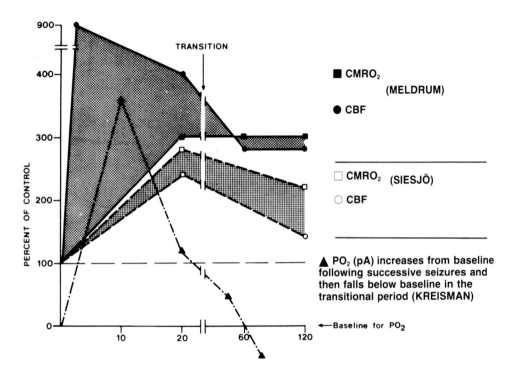

Convulsive status epilepticus should be controlled before the transitional period begins (within 20–60 min) to prevent metabolic consequences and selective cell damage. Meldrum and Siesjö both have documented significant increases in cerebral blood flow (CBF) and metabolic rate (CMR_{O_2}) with convulsive status epilepticus. They agree that excessive enhancement of local metabolic rate causes selective cell death within 60 min. Kreisman also has emphasized that the regional oxygen insufficiency that occurs during the transitional period (i.e., after 20 min) further contributes to cell damage.

Advances in Neurology, Vol. 34: Status Epilepticus, edited by A.V. Delgado-Escueta, C.G. Wasterlain, D.M. Treiman, and R.J. Porter. Raven Press, New York © 1983.

12

Neuropathology of Status Epilepticus in Humans

J. A. N. Corsellis and C. J. Bruton

In 1880, Sommer (4) published an intriguing and now largely forgotten paper entitled "Disease of Ammon's Horn as an Aetiological Factor in Epilepsy." In that study he established the pattern of histological damage now widely known as Ammon's horn sclerosis or hippocampal sclerosis, and he identified a particularly vulnerable segment of hippocampal neurons that was later named the Sommer sector. But that was by no means the origin of the subject. There were other pioneers before that time, and we refer to Sommer's work only as a way of emphasizing the considerable efforts that have been made in the neuropathology of convulsive disorders for well over 100 years. Perhaps largely because of this considerable time and the fact that efforts seem to have reached a dead end (3), little formal neuropathological research on the human epileptic brain is now being carried out. This means, unfortunately, that we have little new to offer. Having spent many years trying to fathom the pathological processes in the brain in epilepsy, we thought that it might be useful to investigate the case material available to us in relation to the occurrence and the nature of cerebral damage in all patients who had died, irrespective of age, following attacks of status epilepticus.

We have emphasized the age factor because of the question of the vulnerability of the adult brain in these circumstances. In 1964, Norman (2) wrote that "neurologists who are familiar with adult patients recovering completely after protracted bouts of serial fits are often sceptical about the damage of the fits *per se*." He also wrote that "the high incidence of brain lesions in children as contrasted with adults is not understood." It may be because of this apparent lack of damage in adults that so much of the published work on the pathology of status epilepticus is concerned, as Norman (2) was, with small children.

PATIENTS AND METHODS

In order to make a comparison between the two age groups we began the present study of 290 epileptic patients whose clinical histories and whose brains we have been able to investigate over a period of some 25 years. The cases have derived mainly from residential hospitals for psychiatric and mentally retarded patients, with a leavening from general hospitals and neurological and neurosurgical centers.

TABLE 1. *Number and ages of patients with status epilepticus*

	No. of patients	Ages
Epileptic patients	290	5 months to 88 years
One or more episodes of status epilepticus	52 (18%)	5 months to 88 years
Died in status epilepticus	20 (7%)	5 months to 60 years

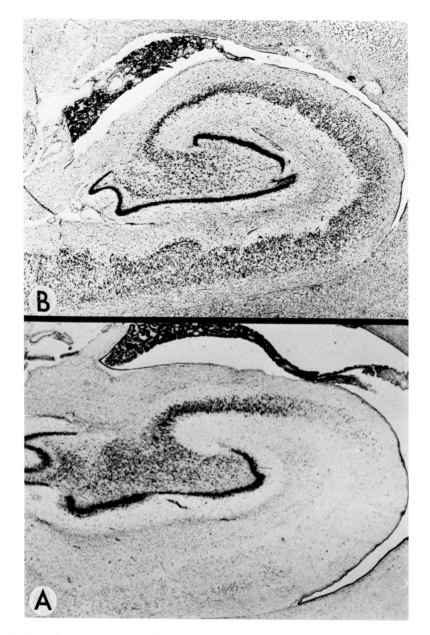

FIG. 1. **A:** Severe degree of acute neuronal loss present in the swollen Sommer sector (H1 field) of the hippocampus. This may be compared with the normal appearance (**B**). Cresyl violet. × 11.

Of the 290 epileptic patients, 52 (18%) had at some time in their lives suffered from one or more recorded episodes of status epilepticus, and 20 of these 52 (7% of the total) had died during or shortly after an attack (Table 1). We adhered as far as we could to accepting as evidence of status epilepticus convulsions that had occurred without intervening periods of consciousness for 1 hr or more. Only 2 patients were known to have had more than one attack, and 18 therefore died in relation to the first and only episode.

The ages of the 20 patients at death ranged from 5 months to 60 years; there were 8 children and 12 adults, with a slight overall preponderance of

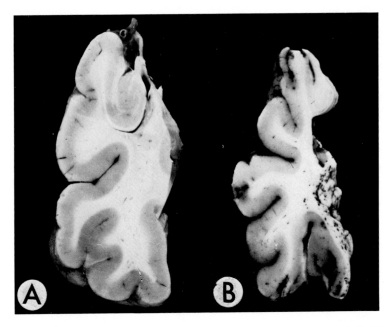

FIG. 2. Naked-eye coronal views of two human temporal lobes. **A:** The specimen is normal. **B:** This temporal lobe had been removed surgically from an adult epileptic patient. There is marked atrophy of the hippocampus and to a lesser extent of the adjacent gyri. Cresyl violet. × 1.4.

males (12 males to 8 females). This, however, is in no sense a statistical study, and the case material was studied in order to establish the pattern of abnormalities and its possible variations. In examining this material, it is necessary first to recall the main features of the classic neuropathological changes that are liable to occur in association with the epilepsies and following status epilepticus (2).

Insofar as the gross appearance of the brain is concerned, no striking abnormality is found in most cases, the obvious exception being when the epilepsy is symptomatic of some visible lesion such as a tumor or a malformation. The brain, in the absence of such a gross lesion, may appear swollen, but according to Norman (2), and from our own experience, this is not a constant feature, and the brain not infrequently appears normal, apart from some congestion. Evidence of either transtentorial or cerebellar herniation is therefore often absent; when present, it is seldom gross. Similarly, the gray matter, and particularly the cerebral cortex, usually appears intact to the naked eye, even though there may be extensive neuronal destruction with reactive glia at the histological level. An occasional exception to this, which we shall illustrate later, is the hippocampus, which in the acute stages may be visibly swollen, whereas with longer

survival it can shrink down to a small white scar. In general, those areas such as the cerebellum, the thalamus, and the cerebral cortex that are particularly vulnerable in the acute stages of a fatal attack of status epilepticus are also the areas liable to suffer from neuronal loss, gliosis, and atrophy in the brains of patients with long-standing epilepsy.

RESULTS

The nature of the neurohistological damage is best illustrated by reviewing the findings from the 20 patients in the present study.

Children

Six of the 8 children had died within 3 years of birth; the remaining 2 children were older, having died at the ages of 12 and 13. These last 2 children had been epileptic for years—one from the age of 5 years. The second, whose brain was malformed, had suffered from convulsions since birth. Neither, however, showed evidence of acute neuronal or glial changes that could have been related to the fatal episodes of status, although the second child, with polymicrogyria, also had evidence of scarring, presumably a sequel to the earlier attacks in infancy.

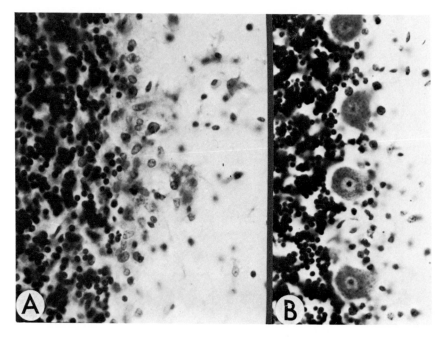

FIG. 3. **A:** Section of cerebellar cortex from the brain of an infant dying in status epilepticus. All the Purkinje cells have disappeared, and there is an intense glial reaction. **B:** Similar area from another infant also dying in status. In this case, however, the cerebellum has been spared. Cresyl violet. ×400.

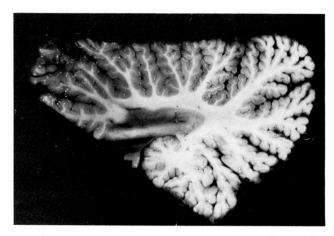

FIG. 4. Naked-eye appearance of the cerebellum of an adult patient with long-standing epilepsy. The folia on the oblique undersurface are pale and atrophied, whereas those along the dorsal border appear unaffected. This is an example of the patchy cerebellar atrophy that is sometimes seen in one or another part of the cerebellum. ×1.4.

Acute cerebral changes were present in all 6 of these patients who died in infancy, but the extent of the damage varied considerably. One of those more severely affected was a 6-month-old infant with a history of normal birth who developed a chest infection accompanied by an attack of status epilepticus, from which he died 4 days later. At autopsy, the brain was not appreciably swollen, and no macroscopic abnormality was detected. At the histological level, however, extensive destruction of hippocampal nerve cells was seen. Both sides were affected (as they were in the other 5 infants). The almost complete loss of neurons in the swollen Sommer sector shows up as a curved,

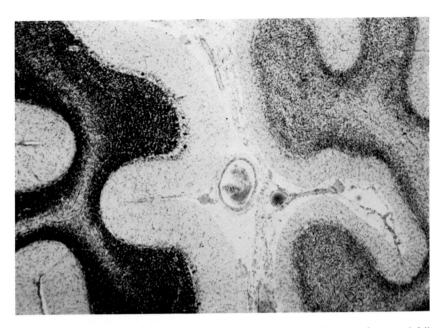

FIG. 5. The same cerebellum as in Fig. 4. This photograph was taken at the junction of a normal folium and an abnormal folium. The gross cell loss in the granular and Purkinje cell layer is seen on the right of the photograph; the more normal appearances are on the left. Cresyl violet. × 30.

broad, pale, acellular strip (Fig. 1A), which may be compared with the appearance of a normally populated hippocampus (Fig. 1B). It should be emphasized that this is an acute lesion, for the classical Ammon's horn or hippocampal sclerosis is seen only when the patient has survived long enough for the "scar tissue" and the atrophy to develop. Figure 2A illustrates the gross appearance of the normal hippocampus and the adjacent temporal lobe in coronal section for comparison with the same region of brain obtained after a temporal lobectomy that had been carried out on an epileptic person. The marked whiteness, atrophy, and loss of definition are seen in Fig. 2B, which also suggests more widespread cortical narrowing.

After the hippocampus, the next most vulnerable part of the brain is the cerebellar cortex, in which degeneration and destruction of Purkinje cells, accompanied by an acute glial reaction, can range from widespread and severe to no appreciable alteration. This range is illustrated in two specimens from infants who died in status epilepticus. In Fig. 3A, all the Purkinje cells have disappeared, and proliferating glia have taken their place. In contrast, a remarkably intact strip of Purkinje cells is seen in Fig. 3B.

As with the hippocampus, the sequel to an acute lesion, if the patient survives long enough, is gradual atrophy of the cerebellum. Figure 4 shows the typical appearance of the cerebellum of a chronic epileptic patient in which the cortex on the obliquely running undersurface of the specimen looks pale and atrophied, whereas the cerebellar folia on the upper or dorsal surface are well preserved. In a lesion of this severity, not only the layer of Purkinje cells but also the granular layer lose much of their neuronal population. Figure 5 shows these appearances in two adjoining folia in the same cerebellum. The right half is grossly pathological; the left approaches the normal.

In the gray matter of the cerebral hemisphere, the thalamus is particularly vulnerable. As with the cerebellum, the extent of damage may not only vary from one infant to another but also vary within the thalamus of a given child. Figure 6 shows the range of damage in one infant. Massive neuronal destruction and gliosis occur in one part of the thalamus (Fig. 6B), whereas the nearby area is relatively intact (Fig. 6A). The corpus striatum may also be severely damaged in some cases (Fig. 7A), whereas in others the identical area will have a normal population of cells (Fig. 7B).

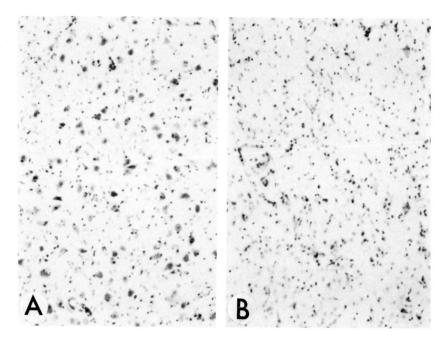

FIG. 6. A: Relatively normal neuronal and glial population in one part of the thalamus of a child who had died in status epilepticus. **B:** Adjacent area taken from the same section in which massive neuronal loss and a marked glial reaction may be seen. Cresyl violet. × 130.

Finally, acute neuronal necrosis may lead to almost complete erasure of many cortical nerve cells, particularly in the middle cortical layers, stretching over wide areas of the cerebral mantle or being only patchily distributed. This is illustrated in similar specimens of cortex from 2 infants who died in status epilepticus. The specimen shown in Fig. 8B was taken from an infant with only mild cortical damage; Fig. 8A shows the same anatomical area with marked cortical pallor in the stained section that is due to massive loss of nerve cells. This loss, together with the accompanying proliferation of glial cells, is more clearly seen in Fig. 9, in which the normal arrangement of nerve cells streams horizontally across the field (Fig. 9A), but is completely broken up by the mixture of neuronal loss and gliosis (Fig. 9B).

Adults

Of the 12 adults who had died during or shortly after a bout of status epilepticus, 7 had been diagnosed as suffering clinically from cryptogenic epilepsy, and 5 belonged to the symptomatic group. The unusually high proportion of cryptogenic cases in this small series is probably a consequence of the siting of the neuropathological laboratories in a residential hospital that has long had a special responsibility for patients with intractable epilepsy.

Acute cerebral damage was found in 3 patients in the symptomatic group. The first case involved a schizophrenic man 36 years of age who died in the wake of insulin treatment. The brain was slightly swollen, but without evidence of herniation. Histologically, scattered areas of acute neuronal necrosis with occasional laminar loss were seen in the frontal, occipital, and insular cortex and to a lesser extent in both hippocampi. These changes are the same as those that may be found in relation to status epilepticus or severe hypoglycemia.

The second symptomatic case involved a 30-year-old schizophrenic woman who died after 2 days in status epilepticus, the cause of which could not be clinically established. The brain showed no gross abnormality apart from a slight grayness of the white matter in the temporal lobes. The histological findings were of an acute widespread encephalitis that was most marked in the medial temporal regions and the cerebellum. Although both hippocampi were severely damaged in a way that

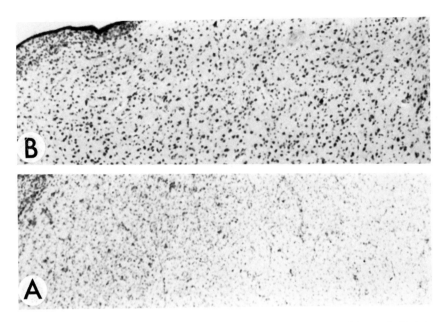

FIG. 7. The head of the caudate nucleus adjacent to the ventricle. **A:** Severe neuronal loss and gliosis in one infant who died in status epilepticus. **B:** Another infant dying in status in whom the caudate nucleus had been spared. Cresyl violet. ×65.

bore a superficial resemblance to the other cases, the nature of the underlying process, with marked perivascular cuffing, was inflammatory.

The third symptomatic patient was a 57-year-old woman with a frontal meningioma who, after several sporadic convulsions, went into status epilepticus and died 24 hr later. The brain was swollen, and the midline was displaced laterally. No tentorial herniation was seen, but both hippocampi showed scattered ischemic nerve cells and slight patchy neuronal loss.

No acute changes were found in the remaining 2 patients with symptomatic epilepsy. Classification of the first was uncertain, because she started in childhood in the cryptogenic category, being severely epileptic and disturbed for no identifiable reason. After 20 years, a prefrontal leukotomy was carried out that seemed to benefit both her convulsive attacks and her personality. Eighteen months later, however, she lapsed into serial seizures that passed into status epilepticus, bronchopneumonia, and death. The only cerebral abnormality was the result of the leukotomy.

The last of the symptomatic patients had a lifelong history of epilepsy, with cerebral injury at birth. She died in status epilepticus at age 26. No acute changes were found in the brain; the old damage consisted of cortical scarring in both occipital lobes and both cerebellar hemispheres.

Only 2 of the 7 cases in the cryptogenic category were found to show acute cerebral damage. The most striking example, and the one that stimulated us to begin this study, involved a woman of 56 who started to have grand mal attacks that were considered, after full investigation, to be "idiopathic." She died 4 years later as a sequel to an episode of status epilepticus, having had three similar attacks in the intervening years. Extensive clinical investigation over this period never identified a cause, and neither extracerebral nor intracerebral abnormality was found at autopsy. The brain appeared normal to the naked eye, but histological examination revealed acute hypoxic-ischemic changes that were at their most severe in both hippocampi. One side is shown in Fig. 10, in which the Sommer sector (or H1 field) appears slightly swollen and blurred and is unusually pale because of loss of most of its nerve cells. The end folium, and to a less clear extent the dentate fascia, also shows considerable neuronal depletion. Although it is not visible at low power, there was an intense proliferation of microglial cells and astrocytes in the affected areas. The rest of the cerebral gray matter was less severely damaged, and neuronal loss, although identifiable in places, was much less

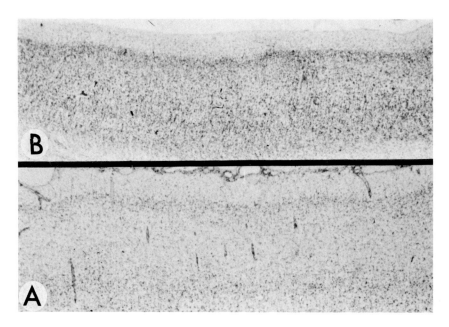

FIG. 8. Comparable strips of cerebral cortex from 2 infants, both dying in status epilepticus. **A:** Marked pallor, particularly in the middle layers of the cortex, that is due to the extensive necrosis and loss of nerve cells. **B:** A much milder lesion. The cortex appears normal at this magnification, but a slight degree of neuronal loss could be seen at higher power. Cresyl violet. ×25.

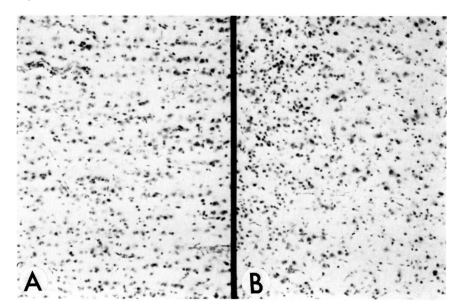

FIG. 9. Views taken from different cortical areas in the case illustrated in Fig. 8A. **A:** On the left half, the normal pattern of nerve cells streams horizontally across the field. **B:** On the right side the cortical architecture is disrupted by the mixture of neuronal loss and an acute glial reaction. Cresyl violet. ×130.

extensive than that seen in affected infants. Widespread neuronal changes of the hypoxic-ischemic type were nevertheless seen in many parts of the cerebral and cerebellar cortex and to a lesser extent in the deep gray matter, including the thalamus and striatum.

The only other cryptogenic case showing acute changes involved a man of 46 who had suffered from convulsive attacks since the age of 12. He started to have serial seizures that developed into status epilepticus and he died 3 days later. The complication, however, was that pulmonary tuberculosis had been diagnosed a month before his death, and he had been receiving antituberculous drugs, including isoniazid and streptomycin. The brain appeared slightly atrophic but was otherwise normal. Under the microscope the right hippocampus showed extensive neuronal necrosis, with an acute glial reaction. A segment of the affected Sommer sector is shown in Fig. 11A for comparison with the normal appearance at the same magnification in Fig. 11B. No other evidence of acute cerebral damage was identified, although the end folium on the opposite side showed considerable neuronal loss and a dense fibrous gliosis, the origin of which must have been well in the past.

The remaining cryptogenic case involves five epileptic patients, each of whom died following an isolated episode of status epilepticus. They had been having major attacks of unknown origin for an average of 34 years (range 27–37 years). All were men whose ages at death ranged from 37 to 58 years (mean 46 years). In the brains of 3 of these men there was clear evidence of old scarring, with neuronal loss and heavy gliosis, that mainly affected the cerebellum and the hippocampus. In a fourth case, an old contrecoup cortical erosion of one temporal lobe was probably the result of a head injury sustained in a fall during a major attack. In none of these five brains, however, was evidence found of acute neuronal necrosis or glial reaction that was in any way comparable to that described in the other cases.

CONCLUSION AND SUMMARY

If this study has achieved nothing more, it may at least remind us of the nature of the acute damage to the brain that may develop in association with status epilepticus, particularly when it occurs in the early years of life and even in the apparent absence of any previous disease. The possible var-

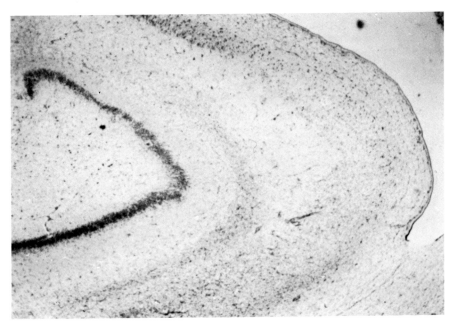

FIG. 10. Neuronal necrosis and loss in the Sommer sector and the end folium of the hippocampus in a woman of 56. Cresyl violet. ×25.

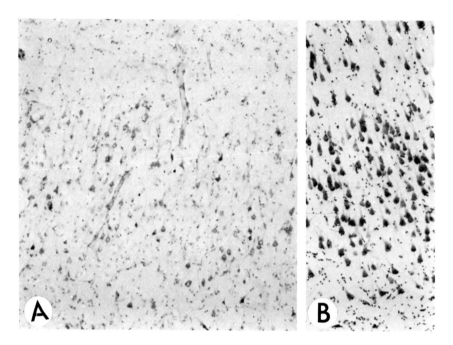

FIG. 11. **A:** Neuronal loss and shrinkage with an acute glial reaction in the Sommer sector of an epileptic man of 46 who had died in status epilepticus. **B:** The normal appearance. Cresyl violet. ×80.

iations in severity and in the topography of the lesions from infant to infant have been mentioned.

In this study we have also tried to establish the extent to which the brains of adult patients dying in relation to status epilepticus might also be affected. The results are largely those that might have been expected, although the numbers are small, and it would be rash to generalize. Briefly, acute neuronal and glial changes were identified in 3 of the adult patients in whom the attacks were found to have been symptomatic of some gross cerebral or metabolic abnormality. However, in 2 of the 3 patients the changes were those of the underlying disorder, one of which was an acute inflammatory reaction, whereas the other could be attributed to hypoglycemia during insulin treatment for a psychosis. In a third patient, with a meningioma and a swollen brain, acute neuronal changes of the ischemic-hypoxic type were found, essentially in the hippocampi. No acute changes were found in the 2 chronic epileptic patients classified as belonging to the symptomatic group. One of them had been considered to belong to this group as a consequence of injury at birth. The other was an epileptic transferred to the group following a leukotomy (1).

These last two negative observations are consonant with the remarkable fact that no evidence of acute cerebral damage could be found in the 5 members of the cryptogenic group who had died as a sequel to status epilepticus. All 7 members of this group had suffered convulsions over many years, and some had shown evidence of old hippocampal or cerebellar scarring. In all but 2 patients, however, the lethal attacks of status epilepticus led to no histological evidence of acute damage, even though the patients usually survived their attacks for days, long enough to develop terminal bronchopneumonia. Thus, Norman's comment, quoted earlier, about the lack of manifest damage in adult patients recovering from status epilepticus might be extended to include the fact that demonstrable damage to the brain is far from certain, even if the patient does not recover.

It does not seem possible to go further than this on the available data, and the unimaginative morbid anatomist is left with the hope that others will explain what has been observed. Anyone trying to understand the abnormalities of the brain in epilepsy seems sooner or later to get caught in a vicious cycle in which it is accepted that brain damage can lead to seizures and that the physiological components of the seizure can also lead to brain damage. Now, added to this long-established idea, there is the proposal by Meldrum (Chapter 24) and others that the relentless overactivity of certain nerve cells may lead them into destruction and thus add to, or even initiate, a further sequence of structural changes in the brain.

Fortunately, this is now the realm of the experimental worker, and this is where, in our view, the future lies. We are reminded, though, of the difficulties by the remark of a cab driver when we complained of the insoluble mess that London traffic was in: "It's a vicious snowball," he said.

REFERENCES

1. Janz, D. (1961): Conditions and causes of status epilepticus. *Epilepsia (Amst.)*, 2:170–177.
2. Norman, R. M. (1964): The neuropathology of status epilepticus. *Med. Sci. Law*, 4:46–51.
3. Peiffer, J. (1970): Zur Neuropathologie der Epilepsie. *Mod. Probl. Pharmacopsychiatry*, 4:42–70.
4. Sommer, W. (1880): Erkrankung des Ammonshornes als aetiologisches Moment der Epilepsie. *Arch. Psychiatr. Nervenkr.*, 10:631–675.

Advances in Neurology, Vol. 34: Status Epilepticus, edited by A.V. Delgado-Escueta, C.G. Wasterlain, D.M. Treiman, and R.J. Porter. Raven Press, New York © 1983.

13

Regional Brain Metabolism During Seizures in Humans

Jerome Engel, Jr., David E. Kuhl, and Michael E. Phelps

Epileptic seizures represent pathological alterations in cerebral function that may or may not be related to significant abnormalities in brain structure. Even in those patients with clearly defined cerebral lesions underlying their epileptic disorders, the transition from the interictal state to the ictal state appears to reflect a pure alteration in function, as opposed to structure. Consequently, in order to investigate the anatomical substrates and basic mechanisms of seizures in humans, it is necessary to use methods that allow *in vivo* measurements of local neuronal function. Of the standard clinical diagnostic techniques available to neurologists, only EEG and related procedures such as evoked potentials have provided sufficient functional information to be useful in studies of epileptic phenomena. Therefore, our knowledge of human epilepsy has been largely confined to electrophysiological descriptions. There are, however, significant limitations to the validity of extrapolating from these descriptions to conclusions regarding neuronal activity in specific parts of the brain. This is in part due to the sampling error introduced by the inability of the EEG to record activity occurring beyond the cerebral cortex immediately below the scalp. Although depth electrodes and evoked-potential techniques allow measurements of subcortical activity, they still place restrictions on the number and delineation of brain sites that can be examined.

Investigations of human brain function have also been pursued with the use of radioactive tracers. Earlier nuclide methods limited brain study to global measurements of cerebral metabolism or blood flow (10) and to regional assessments of blood-brain barrier permeability (18) or perfusion (9). Small but significant local alterations could easily be obscured. A major improvement occurred with the introduction of the transverse section scan (11) combined with mathematical reconstruction (12, 13,20), a process now called emission computed tomography (ECT). ECT made possible quantitative three-dimensional mapping of local cerebral function (17), just as X-ray CT has displayed cerebral structures. Further refinements in the capability to measure local cerebral function have occurred through the advent of positron-labeled tracers and the use, in our laboratory, of the ECAT tomograph (19). The relative distribution of local cerebral blood flow (LCBF) can be examined with $^{13}NH_3$ (21), and quantitative measurements of local cerebral metabolic rate for glucose (LCMR$_{glc}$) can be made by using ^{18}F-fluorodeoxyglucose (FDG) (8,22,24) in a manner analogous to the ^{14}C-2-deoxyglucose (2-DG) autoradiographic method of Sokoloff et al. (25). With positron-emission computed tomography (PECT) it is now possible to perform noninvasive clinical investigations that provide multiple images of the entire brain, displaying patterns of LCBF and LCMR$_{glc}$. We have found that

[13]NH_3 measurements do not faithfully follow small alterations in LCBF that may be associated with interictal or ictal epileptiform activity, but that patterns of $LCMR_{glc}$ provided by FDG are extremely useful for studying epilepsy (14–16).

INTERICTAL STUDIES

Patients with partial epilepsy commonly demonstrate zones of decreased $LCMR_{glc}$ that correspond anatomically to the site of their epileptogenic lesions as determined by EEG studies (2,4,5,14–16). There is also strong correlation between the location and degree of decreased $LCMR_{glc}$ as seen with PECT and the location and severity of the pathological abnormalities as found in the resected specimens from patients who have undergone surgical treatment for epilepsy (4). The functional abnormality displayed with PECT, however, is invariably larger than the structural lesion seen under the light microscope (4). PECT has now demonstrated its clinical usefulness as an important confirmatory test for localizing epileptic lesions, and at UCLA it now provides one of the criteria for electing surgical therapy for patients with intractable partial epilepsy (5).

It is of particular interest that interictal PECT investigations have shown no clear correlation between the degree of metabolic dysfunction observed in the presumed epileptogenic lesion and the appearance, frequency, or amplitude of epileptiform electrical events recorded simultaneously from the same area with scalp, sphenoidal, and intracerebrally implanted depth electrodes (2). Thus, the data obtained from PECT and EEG are not redundant, and therefore they are complementary with respect to understanding the neurophysiological processes under investigation. PECT measurements of $LCMR_{glc}$ reflect the average temporal intensity of activity in all the cellular elements that constitute each cerebral structure measured and is weighted primarily according to energy requirements, whereas the EEG measures the spatiotemporal relationships of specific excitatory and inhibitory neuronal events within these structures and are weighted according to the degree of synchrony of these events. Consequently, the use of these two tests in combination should provide more information regarding basic mechanisms and the distributions in time and space of the involved structures than can either test alone.

Although most of our PECT investigations in epilepsy have been concerned with interictal ab-

normalities, these findings are presented here only as background for the description of our initial attempts to use PECT to study the human ictal state.

ICTAL STUDIES

Ictal PECT scans obtained with FDG are still not numerous because of the technical and logistical problems involved in producing the positron-labeled tracer and the temporal limitations imposed by the 2-hr half-life of [18]F. Ictal scans can be obtained only when a seizure fortuitously occurs shortly after the FDG injection, when a patient is in partial status, or when seizures can be safely induced. We have reported preliminary results obtained from ictal FDG scans in partial epilepsy (3), and to date, we have performed 18 ictal scans in all: six studies in 5 patients with partial seizures and one each in 2 patients with generalized seizures, all occurring spontaneously during the course of FDG uptake; one study in a patient during a partial seizure induced by eye closure; one study in each of 6 patients during absence seizures induced by hyperventilation; three studies in 2 patients during electroconvulsive therapy.

The absolute accuracy of the measured $LCMR_{glc}$ with FDG is not known, because this method is based on the 2-DG autoradiography method of Sokoloff et al. (25), which assumes a constant rate of glucose metabolism during the course of the study (i.e., steady-state condition). In PECT studies, the patients are injected intravenously with FDG, and "arterialized blood" (22,24) is drawn at regular intervals to determine the rate of delivery of FDG to the brain. The scan is performed approximately 40 min after injection to measure specifically the FDG that has been phosphorylated and trapped within cells, using a tracer kinetic model (8,22). If, during the time between injection and the scan, the patient has one or more seizures that produce transient changes in glucose metabolism, the final tomographically measured value of $LCMR_{glc}$ will represent an average value weighted by the magnitude and duration of the metabolic rates. In addition, the final value of $LCMR_{glc}$ is weighted more toward the metabolic rate shortly after injection, when the blood FDG concentration is high. Consequently, seizures of short duration occurring immediately after FDG injection will have the largest impact on the calculated value of $LCMR_{glc}$, whereas short-duration seizures occurring 5, 10, or 20 min after injection will have progressively smaller influences. Also, a very brief seizure may induce such a transient alteration in cerebral metabolism that the cellular uptake of FDG will be insufficient to produce a significant alteration in the $LCMR_{glc}$ calculated from data obtained over the full time from the injection to the scan. Furthermore, an ictal event does not represent a step function in neuronal activity, but usually consists of an ictal phase followed by a postictal phase, each presumably involving very different anatomical and physiological processes. The relative contributions of these two influences on the average $LCMR_{glc}$ cannot be adequately determined, and they could conceivably cancel each other in some regions of the brain, resulting in no specific alteration in the final measurement.

Experimentally, epilepsy has been studied with the 2-DG autoradiographic technique by producing seizure states that are continuous over a 40- to 60-min period (1) or by sacrificing the animal shortly after injection (6). The first technique is not applicable to most clinical situations, and the second provides no quantitative information. Mathematical approaches are available to solve the problem for transient changes that last for several minutes or more (7), and methods are being developed that may provide a solution to studying the complex problems presented by ictal events. In the meantime, however, ictal PECT studies will help to elucidate anatomical patterns of alterations in $LCMR_{glc}$ associated with specific types of seizures, although the absolute values of $LCMR_{glc}$ derived from the studies are only approximate estimates of the metabolic rate of the ictal focus.

The use of FDG as an "energy-specific stain" for defining the metabolic anatomy of specific behavioral events, without quantitative measurements of $LCMR_{glc}$, can still be of value for understanding the basic mechanisms of epileptogenesis. It is anticipated that these studies will help to identify the anatomical substrates of various ictal and postictal behaviors and may provide insight into the initiation and spread of ictal events. In addition, ictal patterns of relative decreases, as well as increases, in FDG uptake may reflect neuronal mechanisms that act to confine or terminate ictal events.

Scans obtained during partial seizures have generally demonstrated a zone of hypermetabolism that roughly corresponds to the hypometabolic area seen on the interictal scan. This phenomenon is evident in the scans of a 5-year-old boy with fre-quent partial seizures involving the right face and arm (Fig. 1). In comparison with the interictal scan, the ictal scans seem to show an increase in metabolic activity at the site of the epileptogenic focus and a relative decrease in metabolic activity peripheral to it. A corresponding ictal EEG is shown in Fig. 2. We have observed other relative reductions in metabolic activity ipsilateral and also contralateral to the epileptogenic focus on ictal scans obtained from several patients with partial epilepsy. Unfortunately, nothing can be said about the temporal course of these apparent alterations in cerebral metabolism. Although it is tempting to speculate that the pattern of peripheral hypometabolism reflects surround inhibition (23), it is equally possible that the reduction of $LCMR_{glc}$ occurred after the ictal event and is the result of more diffuse postictal depression.

Ictal scans also give unreliable information concerning the site of origin of an ictal event, because the area of hypermetabolism most likely includes all or most of those structures recruited during the entire ictal behavior displayed by the patient. This fact is made apparent by the scan of a 12-year-old girl with right-sided tonic-clonic seizures and hemiparesis resulting from a porencephalic cyst in the left parietal area (Fig. 3). The electrographic seizure originated at the site of the porencephalic cyst and spread into more normal brain. The PECT scan appears to reveal all the structures of the left hemisphere that were involved in the ictal event, and the spread to frontal areas may have resulted in greater increases in metabolic activity there, because the hemispheric damage is presumably greater posteriorly. Consequently, when epileptiform activity spreads away from the primary focus, the ictal scan is less useful than the interictal scan in providing information regarding the actual site of the epileptogenic lesion. Because the cells in the primary focus itself may be damaged, or theoretically could be much more efficient at generating the neuronal activity necessary to initiate the ictal event than the surrounding brain is at sustaining it, it is conceivable that the contribution of the primary focus to the overall metabolic changes accompanying the seizure could be so small that it would not appear in the scan at all.

As seen in Fig. 4, 2-DG autoradiography studies of amygdaloid kindled rats showed increased 2-DG uptake in the direct projection fields of the stimulated amygdala when stimulation led to partial seizures, but not when it led to generalized

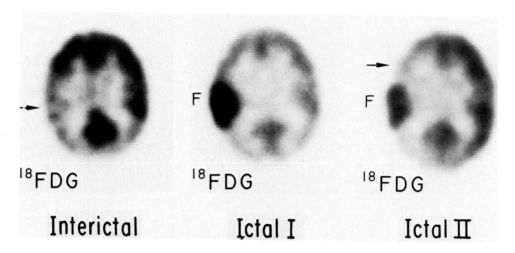

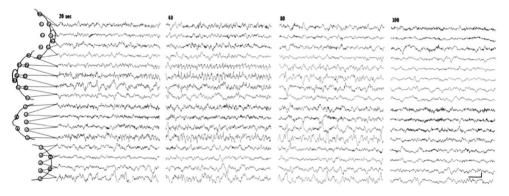

FIG. 1. One interictal (left) and two ictal PECT scans of FDG from a 5-year-old boy with partial seizures involving the right face and arm, with aphasia and normal consciousness. Interictally there is a zone of hypometabolism involving the left temperocentral region (*broken arrow*). The middle ictal scan shows an area of focal hypermetabolism (F) that conforms roughly to the hypometabolic zone seen interictally. The ictal scan on the right shows, in addition to the hypermetabolic focus (F), an anterior and posterior region of hypometabolism (*arrow*). (From Kuhl et al., ref. 16, with permission.)

FIG. 2. Segments of an EEG recording made during FDG uptake in ictal scan I shown in Fig. 1. The numbers in the upper left-hand corner of each segment indicate the time interval, in seconds, after FDG injection. The seizure begins with low-voltage fast activity in the left midtemporal region 20 sec after injection and evolves into higher-voltage 5/sec sharp waves more prominent in the frontotemporal region (40 sec), followed by irregular spike-wave discharges (80 sec) and, finally, focal slowing (100 sec). Calibration: 1 sec, 100 μV.

seizures (6). Presumably the ictal EEG discharge initiated and recorded at the site of amygdaloid stimulation during the generalized seizure was insufficient to produce a significant alteration in $LCMR_{glc}$ relative to the changes that occurred in other cerebral structures that actually mediated the tonic-clonic convulsion. Consequently, it must be realized that the metabolic anatomy revealed by the PECT scan may not be a faithful picture of the actual anatomical substrates of the ictal event being studied, and certainly the degree of metabolic change

from one area to another may bear no relationship to the importance of these areas in the initiation of the seizure or the manifestation of the overall behavior observed. Clearly, simultaneous EEG and PECT measurements are necessary in order to begin to approach an understanding of the significance of the observations made during ictal studies.

The fact that the ictal scans in Figs. 1 and 3 show hypermetabolism in areas that were hypometabolic interictally suggests that the interictal hypometabolism may not be due entirely to neu-

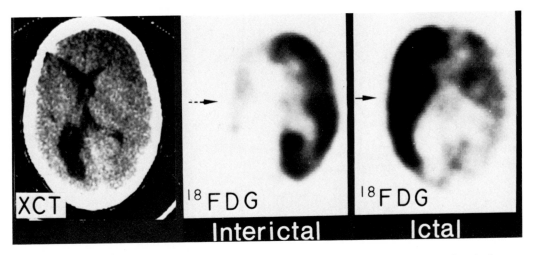

FIG. 3. X-ray CT scan and interictal and ictal PECT scans of FDG from a 12-year-old girl with a left parietal porencephalic cyst, atrophy of the left hemisphere, right-sided tonic-clonic seizures, and hemiparesis. The interictal FDG scan shows the entire left hemisphere to be hypometabolic (*broken arrow*), but this is most marked in the parietal region where the interictal EEG spike focus was noted. When a seizure originating in the left parietal area occurred during FDG uptake, the ictal PECT scan showed the entire left hemisphere to be hypermetabolic (*arrow*). The hypermetabolism is more marked anteriorly, presumably because there is less neuronal damage. (From Kuhl et al., ref. 16, with permission.)

ronal destruction. This conclusion is supported by the observation that pathological lesions are smaller than the corresponding zones of hypometabolism seen on PECT scans (4). Although these observations in no way prove the existence of a purely functional component to interictal hypometabolism, the ictal hypermetabolism can only represent a functional alteration. The actual causes of decreased $LCMR_{glc}$ at the site of the epileptogenic lesion and the nature and magnitude of the ictal events necessary to produce the observed increase in $LCMR_{glc}$ during a seizure are subjects for further study. It is also not clear from our work thus far whether or not any increased metabolic activity is a necessary concomitant of ictal events. One PECT scan obtained with FDG during a prolonged visual aura actually showed a zone of hypometabolism in the left occipital lobe. Unfortunately, this patient has refused to return for a repeat control scan, and the significance of this finding is not clear. The same area may be even more hypometabolic interictally.

To study the relative contribution of postictal versus ictal events in the observed patterns of $LCMR_{glc}$, we are obtaining PECT scans from patients undergoing electroconvulsive therapy. Our preliminary findings indicate that the cerebral metabolic rate is generally increased over control values when FDG is injected just before the shock is delivered and is decreased well below control values when FDG is injected during the postictal depression, at the termination of the ictal event (Fig. 5). Differences in patterns of $LCMR_{glc}$ also exist among ictal, interictal, and postictal scans, and this work is being pursued.

Several other studies of regional brain metabolism during seizures are in progress. Children with newly diagnosed absence seizures are being investigated. An initial PECT scan is performed during hyperventilation in order to produce absence attacks following FDG injection. Several months after anticonvulsant medication has been instituted and the patient is seizure-free, a second scan is obtained during hyperventilation without absence seizures. Preliminary data indicate a generalized increase in cerebral metabolic rate with absence seizures that does not occur with hyperventilation alone. Another study aimed at identifying the spatiotemporal parameters of electrical afterdischarge necessary to produce alterations in the pattern of $LCMR_{glc}$ utilizes patients undergoing electrical stimulation of implanted depth electrodes as part of the routine evaluation for surgical therapy for epilepsy. FDG is injected just prior to electrical stimulation, and prolonged afterdischarge has been observed with variable changes in $LCMR_{glc}$. Finally, in order to develop methods that might overcome the technical difficulties in-

A   B

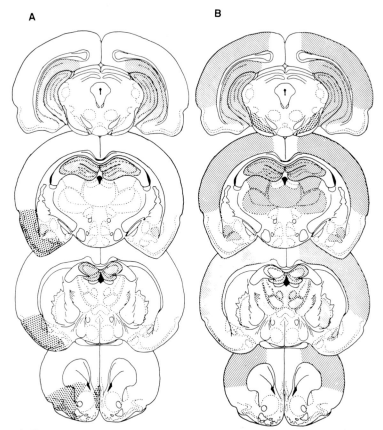

FIG. 4. Schematic diagrams summarizing autoradiographs of ^{14}C-labeled 2-DG uptake in amygdaloid kindled rats during partial seizures **(A)** and generalized seizures **(B)** induced by left amygdala stimulation. Dotted areas indicate structures that always showed increased uptake in each group; cross-hatched areas indicate structures that showed increased uptake in only some animals of each group. (From Engel et al., ref. 6, with permission.)

troduced by the steady-state requirements of the FDG method, studies are also being carried out using single-photon-emission computed tomography with the Mark IV system (13). Currently, technetium-labeled red blood cells are used to obtain images of alterations in cerebral blood volume at 50-sec intervals in patients who are having relatively frequent seizures. Plans are in progress to develop other radiopharmaceuticals that will allow us to better visualize cerebral structures with more dynamic techniques.

This description of our work in regional brain metabolism during seizures is necessarily brief, because the methods are new and the results are still preliminary. It is anticipated, however, that with the great interest in the application of 2-DG autoradiography to experimental models of epilepsy, and with the increase in the number of centers planning to develop capabilities for PECT and/or

single-photon-emission computed tomography, the next few years will witness significant contributions of these techniques to our understanding of the basic mechanisms of epileptogenesis in humans.

SUMMARY

PECT has been used to investigate patterns of $LCMR_{glc}$ associated with epileptic disorders. Interictal scans from patients with partial epilepsy demonstrate zones of hypometabolism that correspond anatomically to the site of the epileptogenic focus as determined by both EEG studies and pathological evaluation of resected specimens from patients who undergo surgical therapy. FDG scans and electrophysiological recordings provide complementary information on altered neuronal function in epilepsy. Many difficulties are encountered in the use of PECT for ictal investigations, and at

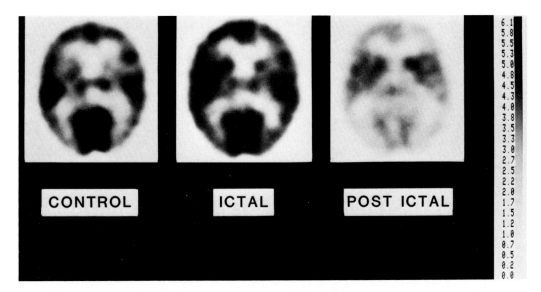

FIG. 5. PECT scans of FDG obtained from a patient undergoing a series of electroconvulsive treatments for depression. These scans display actual calculated LCMR$_{glc}$ (mg/100 g tissue per minute), as indicated on the gray scale at the right.

present, this technique is more useful for identifying anatomical patterns of metabolism during seizures than for obtaining quantitative values of LCMR$_{glc}$. Ictal patterns reflect the spread of epileptic discharge to those brain areas involved in the ictal behavior observed and are not reliable for identifying the site of ictal origin. Ictal FDG scans also reveal areas of hypometabolism that could represent mechanisms that act to confine or terminate the seizure or may reflect a more diffuse postictal depression. In FDG scans obtained from patients undergoing electroconvulsive therapy, the postictal depression appears as a generalized decrease in LCMR$_{glc}$. The use of this relatively new and powerful technique for displaying functional alterations in the human brain associated with seizures has barely begun, and significant contributions from the many centers worldwide developing the capability for PECT investigations of epilepsy should be forthcoming in the near future.

ACKNOWLEDGMENTS

This work was supported by grants NS-02808 and NS-15654 from the National Institute of Neurological and Communicative Disorders and Stroke, by grant GM-4839 from the National Institute of General Medical Sciences, and by contract DE-AMO 3-76-SF0012 from the Department of Energy.

REFERENCES

1. Collins, R. C., Kennedy, C., Sokoloff, L., and Plum, F. (1976): Metabolic anatomy of focal motor seizures. *Arch. Neurol.*, 33:536–542.
2. Engel, J., Jr., Kuhl, D. E., and Phelps, M. E. (1981): A comparison of electrical and metabolic studies of brain function in epileptic patients: Simultaneous EEG and positron emission computed tomography. *Trans. Am. Neurol. Assoc.*, 105:74–76.
3. Engel, J., Jr., Kuhl, D. E., and Phelps, M. E. (1981): Patterns of local metabolism during partial seizures in man. *Neurology*, 31 (Part 2); 31:130.
4. Engel, J., Jr., Kuhl, D. E., Phelps, M. E., Crandall, P. H., and Brown, W. J. (1981): Pathological correlates of focal temporal lobe hypometabolism in partial epilepsy. *Epilepsia*, 22:236.
5. Engel, J., Jr., Rausch, R., Lieb, J. P., Kuhl, D. E., and Crandall, P. H. (1981): Correlation of criteria used for localizing the epileptic foci in patients considered for surgical therapy of epilepsy. *Ann. Neurol.*, 9:215–224.
6. Engel, J., Jr., Wolfson, L., and Brown, L. (1978): Anatomical correlates of electrical and behavioral events related to amygdaloid kindling. *Ann. Neurol.*, 3:538–544.
7. Huang, S. C., Phelps, M. E., Hoffman, E. J., and Kuhl, D. E. (1980): Sensitivity analysis of the fluorodeoxyglucose method for the measurement of local cerebral metabolic rate of glucose. *J. Nucl. Med.*, 21:21–22.
8. Huang, S. C., Phelps, M. E., Hoffman, E. J., Sideris, K., Selin, C. E., and Kuhl, D. E. (1980): Non-invasive determination of local cerebral metabolic rate of glucose in man. *Am. J. Physiol.*, 238:E69–E82.

9. Ingvar, D. H., and Lassen, N. A. (1962): Regional blood flow of the cerebral cortex determined by krypton-85. *Acta Physiol. Scand.*, 54:325.

10. Kety, S. S., and Schmidt, C. G. (1945): The determination of cerebral blood flow in man by the use of nitrous oxide in low concentrations. *Am. J. Physiol.*, 143:53–66.

11. Kuhl, D. E., and Edwards, R. Q. (1963): Image separation radioisotope scanning. *Radiology*, 80:653–662.

12. Kuhl, D. E., Edwards, R. Q., Ricci, A. R., and Reivich, M. (1973): Quantitative section scanning using orthogonal tangent correction. *J. Nucl. Med.*, 14:196–200.

13. Kuhl, D. E., Edwards, R. Q., Ricci, A. R., Yacob, R. J., Mich, T. J., and Alavi, A. (1976): The Mark IV system for radionuclide computed tomography of the brain. *Radiology*, 121:405–413.

14. Kuhl, D. E., Engel, J., Jr., and Phelps, M. E. (1980): Emission computed tomography: Applications in stroke and epilepsy. In: *Cerebral Circulation and Neurotransmitters*, edited by A. Bes and G. Geraud, pp. 37–43. Excerpta Medica, Amsterdam.

15. Kuhl, D. E., Engel, J., Jr., Phelps, M. E., and Kowell, A. P. (1978): Epileptic patterns of local cerebral metabolism and perfusion in man: Investigations by emission computed tomography of ^{18}F-fluorodeoxyglucose and ^{13}N-ammonia. *Trans. Am. Neurol. Assoc.*, 103:52–53.

16. Kuhl, D. E., Engel, J., Jr., Phelps, M. E., and Selin, C. (1980): Epileptic patterns of local cerebral metabolism and perfusion in man determined by emission computed tomography of ^{18}FDG and ^{13}NH$_3$. *Ann. Neurol.*, 8:348–360.

17. Kuhl, D. E., Reivich, M., Alavi, A., Nyary, I., and Staum, M. (1975): Local cerebral blood volume determined by three-dimensional reconstruction of radionuclide scan data. *Circ. Res.*, 36:610–619.

18. Moore, G. E. (1953): *Diagnosis and Localization of Brain Tumors: A Clinical and Experimental Study Employing Fluorescent and Radioactive Tracer Methods.* Charles C Thomas, Springfield, Ill.

19. Phelps, M. E., Hoffman, E. J., Huang, S. C., and Kuhl, D. E. (1978): ECAT: A new computerized tomographic imaging system for positron emitting radiopharmaceuticals. *J. Nucl. Med.*, 19:635–647.

20. Phelps, M. E., Hoffman, E. J., Mullani, N. A., and Ter-Pogossian, M. M. (1975): Application of annihilation coincidence detection to transaxial reconstruction tomography. *J. Nucl. Med.*, 16:210–213.

21. Phelps, M. E., Hoffman, E. J., and Raybaud, C. (1977): Factors which affect cerebral uptake and retention of ^{13}NH$_3$. *Stroke*, 8:694–702.

22. Phelps, M. E., Huang, S. C., Hoffman, E. J., Selin, C. E., and Kuhl, D. E. (1979): Tomographic measurement of local cerebral glucose metabolic rate in man with ^{18}F-fluorodeoxyglucose: Validation of method. *Ann. Neurol.*, 6:371–388.

23. Prince, D. A., and Wilder, B. J., (1967): Control mechanisms in cortical epileptogenic foci. *Arch. Neurol.*, 16:194–202.

24. Reivich, M., Kuhl, D., Wolf, A., Greenberg, J., Phelps, M. E., Ido, T., Casella, V., Fowler, J., Hoffman, E., Alavi, A., and Sokoloff, L. (1979): The ^{18}F-fluorodeoxyglucose method for the measurement of local cerebral glucose utilization in man. *Circ. Res.*, 44:127–137.

25. Sokoloff, L., Reivich, M., Kennedy, C., Des Rosiers, M. H., Pattak, C. S., Pettigrew, K. D., Sakurada, O., and Shinohara, M. (1977): The [^{14}C] deoxyglucose method for the measurement of local cerebral glucose utilization: Theory, procedure and normal values in the conscious and anesthetized albino rat. *J. Neurochem.*, 28:897–916.

*Advances in Neurology, Vol. 34: Status
Epilepticus*, edited by A.V. Delgado-Escueta,
C.G. Wasterlain, D.M. Treiman, and R.J. Porter.
Raven Press, New York © 1983.

14

Experimental Models of Status Epilepticus and Mechanisms of Drug Action

Dixon M. Woodbury

The purpose of this chapter is to discuss experimental models of status epilepticus and their usefulness in the development of new drugs for the treatment of status epilepticus. A previous report from this laboratory (10) discussed the general application of experimental models of epilepsy to the evaluation of anticonvulsant drugs, but this chapter will be directed specifically at the problem of models potentially useful for the assay of drugs useful in status epilepticus. Status epilepticus has been defined as an "epileptic seizure which is so prolonged or so frequently repeated as to create a fixed and lasting epileptic condition" (2). Usually when status is present, the patient does not recover consciousness between the seizures. The concept of status epilepticus is not limited to generalized tonic-clonic (grand mal) status, for there are as many types of this condition as there are types of epileptic seizures. Therefore, the medications recommended for the treatment of status are numerous and usually are the same drugs as used for the treatment of epilepsy of the same type that results in status. However, there is no single drug that will always help patients in status epilepticus. Presumably this is because the mechanisms for producing the continuous seizures involve different actions for each type of status, and none of these are known. The mechanisms appear to be due to either excessive excitatory drive or loss of the intrinsic mechanisms involved in arrest of seizures,

i.e., loss of inhibitory input or lack of glial cell homeostatic regulation. Consequently, to develop new drugs for status epilepticus, it is essential to elucidate the processes that inactivate the arrest mechanisms of seizures and lead to status. This requires development of models of status epilepticus that can be used to evaluate the causes of continuous seizures in humans and to predict drugs effective for the various types of status.

RELEVANCE OF EXPERIMENTAL MODELS

Experimental models are essential, because the initial phases of testing cannot be carried out in humans. Also, there is a great need for new drugs effective in status epilepticus, because the current drugs do not control all seizures in any one type of status epilepticus or fail to control all the different types of status; i.e., they are not selective in their actions, or the presence of side effects limits their use in many patients. Thus, it is necessary to evaluate whether or not experimental models can accurately predict drugs of value in human epilepsy, and it is imperative that experimental models of status be developed for evaluation of drugs because of the potential hazards of testing new therapeutic agents in humans. The relevance of such screening procedures is clearly related to the degree to which the experimental models approximate the disease in humans. The ideal model for testing the effects of potential status drugs would closely resemble human status, would be simple and inexpensive, and would yield rapid results. At present, no model meets all these criteria, but all models are potentially useful for evaluation of anticonvulsant activity for status epilepticus of one kind or another. The models currently used represent compromises; those that are simple and rapid may not be as closely related to status epilepticus in humans, whereas those that are more expensive and provide less rapid answers probably are more closely related to the disorder.

It is obvious, of course, that the best approach to the development of new antiepileptic drugs is to elucidate the mechanisms of action of the drugs currently used in the different types of epilepsies. Once the mechanism by which a drug prevents seizures is known (which also implies that the mechanism of seizure induction by the model used is also understood), a model can be set up to find new drugs that may exert the same effect on status epilepticus. Thus, new drugs for status can be tailor-made by this approach, as has been the case, for example, in the development of allopurinol for the treatment of gout, based on its ability to interfere with the synthesis of uric acid.

Other problems in the use of experimental models for evaluation of drugs useful for status epilepticus in humans involve differences in absorption, distribution, biotransformation, and excretion of the drugs in animals as compared with humans. However, if the Brodie and Reid hypothesis (1) that humans are not unique in their responses to drugs is correct, then these pharmacokinetic differences may not be a problem. Brodie and Reid postulated that animals and humans will exhibit the same effects at the same plasma levels of the drug being tested. Such factors as species, age, and genetic differences also generate problems in the use of animals for simulating human disease. It is pertinent to point out that two criteria must be met in order for an experimental model to be classified as a status-epilepticus-like model and to be used as a method for evaluation of drugs useful in status: (a) electrographic studies must show the presence of statuslike activity in the EEG (e.g., continuous spiking activity); and (b) clinical status-seizure-like activity must be manifested (e.g., continuous motor movements such as clonus and tonus). Once

these criteria have been established, a particular procedure is a potentially useful model of status epilepticus, and anticonvulsant drugs can be assayed in it to assess its value and to evaluate its selectivity.

It is now pertinent to examine the various tests and assess their validity as experimental models of status useful for drug evaluation. Before doing so, however, it is of value to look at the spectrum of actions of current antiepileptic drugs against various status seizure types in humans (Table 1). This list of human epilepsies tells us the various types of animal models that are necessary and which of the anticonvulsants can be used as standards for testing those models. Once the standards have been evaluated and the model validated, then new drugs can be tested against the model. It is evident from Table 1 that some of the drugs are effective against several seizure types, whereas others are effective against only one type. The more selective drugs are more useful standards than the nonselective wider-spectrum drugs for studies of mechanisms of action.

MECHANISMS OF CONVULSANT DRUG ACTION

In order to understand the various experimental models, it is essential to know the different mechanisms by which convulsant drugs act. A summary of their actions has been presented elsewhere (11). A summary of the potential mechanisms for convulsant drug actions is presented in Table 2. Two potential mechanisms are seen: increased excitation or block of inhibition. Effects can be noted on the transmitter action, on the receptors, or on the membrane. With respect to transmitters, increased excitation can be produced by enhanced release of an excitatory transmitter per se or synchronization of excitatory feedback, and block of inhibition can result from a decrease in the amount of inhibitory transmitter available or a decrease in its release. Examples of these actions can be seen in Table 2. Stimulation of postsynaptic excitatory receptors per se, or enhanced activity of the excitatory transmitter, can cause seizures as a result of an effect on the receptors. Blockade of postsynaptic inhibitory receptors or reduced activity of presynaptic inhibitory transmitter, as shown in Table 2, can cause blockade of inhibition and result in seizures. Finally, effects on the membrane can

TABLE 1. *Drug treatment of epilepsy based on classification of seizures*

	Primary drugs	Secondary drugs
Partial seizures		
With elementary symptoms (focal) (motor, sensory, autonomic)	Carbamazepine	
With complex symptoms (complex partial seizures, psychomotor)	Phenytoin Primidone	Mephenytoin
Partial seizures with secondary generalization (tonic-clonic seizures beginning focally)	Phenobarbital	
Generalized Seizures		
Tonic-clonic (grand mal)		
Simple absences	Ethosuximide	Clonazepam Valproate
Complex absences		Trimethadione Methsuximide Nitrazepam
Atonic and akinetic		
Myoclonic jerks		
Infantile spasms		

From Sherwin (9).

TABLE 2. *Potential mechanisms for convulsant drug action*

Increased excitation	Block of inhibition
Transmitters	
Increased release of excitatory transmitter *per se* or synchronization of excitatory feedback	Decrease in the amount of inhibitory transmitter available or decrease in release, e.g., allylglycine, thiosemicarbazide, tetanus toxin, 3-mercaptopropionic acid
Receptors	
Stimulation of postsynaptic excitatory receptors *per se* or enhanced activity of excitatory transmitter	Block of postsynaptic inhibitory receptors, e.g., strychnine, picrotoxin, penicillin, bicuculline; block of presynaptic inhibitory transmitter, e.g., picrotoxin, bicuculline, pentylenetetrazol, bemegride, penicillin
Membrane	
Direct increased excitability of postsynaptic membrane, e.g., pentylenetetrazol	Block of membrane changes initiated by receptor activation, e.g., D-tubucurarine, tetramethylenedisulfotetramine (TETS), pentylenetetrazol, picrotoxin

be expressed as a direct increased excitability of the postsynaptic membrane (as with pentylenetetrazol) or a block of membrane changes initiated by receptor activation (e.g., as with pentylenetetrazol, picrotoxin, or others shown in Table 2).

A summary of the actions of convulsant drugs is shown in Table 3. The different types of mechanisms by which the convulsant drugs act are shown in the left column, and the proposed actions of these drugs are shown in the right column. The main mechanisms are enhancement of excitatory systems, blockade of inhibitory systems, blockade of energy metabolism, and inhibition of ion transport. Many of the convulsant drugs act on inhibitory GABA synapses to prevent GABA interactions with the receptor or the chloride ionophore (picrotoxin, pentylenetetrazol, penicillin, bicuculline) or inhibit its synthesis (allylglycine, pyridoxal antagonists, etc.). Fewer known drugs act on the inhibitory glycine synapses (strychnine, brucine). Others block cation or anion transport (ouabain, thiocyanate, perchlorate) or metabolic processes (fluoroacetate, deoxyglucose, methionine sulfoximine) or have direct stimulatory effects on excitatory glutamic acid (kainic acid) or acetylcholine (anticholinesterases) synapses or act directly on neurons

TABLE 3. *Proposed mechanisms of action of convulsant drugs*

Drugs	Proposed actions
Enhance excitatory systems	
Pentylenetetrazol	Selectively antagonizes GABA-mediated postsynaptic inhibition by blocking effect of GABA to increase chloride conductance; direct effect on membrane properties to increase spontaneous discharge by altering ionic conductance
Anticholinesterases	Inhibit acetylcholinesterase and cause accumulation of acetylcholine
Fluorothyl (hexafluorodiethyl ether)	Opens up Na^+ channels by an effect on membranes
Convulsant barbiturates (CHEB, DMBB)	Increase Ca^{2+} influx into nerve terminals and thereby increase release of excitatory transmitters
Homocysteic acid, kainic acid, *N*-methyl aspartic acid, ibotenic acid	Stimulate excitant amino acid receptors (glutamate, aspartate); appear to increase Na^+ permeability by displacing Ca^{2+} from the surface of the membrane
Substance P	Unknown; probably same as glutamic acid
Block inhibitory systems	
Block effect of GABA at receptor	
Picrotoxin, penicillins, bicuculline	Block interaction of GABA with postsynaptic receptor; direct effect on chloride channel to prevent enhanced conductance of Cl^- induced by GABA; GABA-mediated presynaptic and postsynaptic inhibition is blocked
Block GABA synthesis or release	
Tetanus toxin	Blocks release of inhibitory transmitter in spinal cord
Allylglycine	Inhibits GAD (probably acts via its metabolite, 2-keto-4-pentenoic acid); also inhibits γ-glutamylcysteine synthetase and cystathionase
3-Mercaptopropionic acid	Inhibits GAD competitively; enhances GABA-aminotransferase
Oxygen at high pressure	Inhibits GAD and thereby decreases brain GABA
Thiosemicarbazide, semicarbazide, and other pyridoxal phosphate antagonists (see text)	Decrease the synthesis of GABA by inhibiting GAD in presynaptic endings via an action on pyridoxal phosphate
Block effect of glycine at receptor	
Strychnine, brucine	Block postsynaptic inhibition at glycine receptor-ionophore complex probably by preventing glycine-induced increase in chloride conductance
Block energy metabolism	
Fluoroacetate, fluorocitrate, 2-deoxyglucose	Interfere with energy metabolism and thereby inhibit ion transport
Methionine sulfoximine	Inhibits glutamine synthetase, γ-glutamylcysteine synthetase, and also protein synthesis; also promotes formation of abnormal methylated excitatory substances or enhances breakdown of *S*-adenosyl homocysteine to the excitatory substances homocysteine or homocysteic acid
Ion transport inhibitors	
Cations, ouabain	Inhibits Na^+-K^+-ATPase and thereby alters ion distribution across neurons
Anions, SCN^-, ClO_4^-	Inhibit glial cell anion transport system and HCO_3^--ATPase

From Woodbury (11).

to open up sodium channels (fluorothyl, pentylenetetrazol). It is evident that there is a wide variety of convulsant actions; hence, potentially there is a multitude of agents to choose from in selecting a model for status epilepticus and for testing the effects of anticonvulsant drugs. Also, because the mechanisms by which these drugs produce convulsions are known, the mechanisms by which anticonvulsant drugs act to prevent such seizures can also be understood, particularly if the drug acts by competitive blockade of the convulsant agent. This aspect will be discussed later.

MECHANISMS OF ANTICONVULSANT DRUG ACTION

In order to show that anticonvulsant action may be the opposite of convulsant drug action, Table 4 illustrates the multiple nature of anticonvulsant drug action. The neurophysiological, biochemical, and biophysical effects of the anticonvulsants are shown, and the proposed mechanisms are given. The effects are related to actions on the membrane to alter either potassium, sodium, or calcium permeability or are exerted on synapses to affect the synthesis, release, or presynaptic and postsynaptic actions of transmitter substances such as GABA, acetylcholine, epinephrine, and serotonin.

Actions on membrane-active transport of ions also may occur. These various effects of anticonvulsants illustrate the possible experimental models that could be set up to test anticonvulsant drug actions. Such tests as effects on membrane permeability, transport, calcium uptake, neurotransmitter actions, synthesis and uptake, and effects on glial cell function could all be evaluated as models.

EXPERIMENTAL MODELS OF EPILEPSY

Table 5 summarizes the various experimental models of epilepsy that have been most used for the study of seizure mechanisms and therefore the

TABLE 4. *Summary of possible mechanisms of action of antiepileptic drugs*

Drug	Neurophysiological effects	Biochemical and biophysical effects	Proposed mechanisms
Phenytoin	↓ Spread of seizure discharge ↑ Cerebellar discharge ↓ PTP ↓ Threshold in neonatal animals	↑ Na transport ↓ Na permeability ↑ Na permeability ↓ Protein synthesis ↑ Liver cell EM ↑ K efflux ↓ Ca^{2+} influx	Stimulate Na transport ↑ Na permeability ↓ Na permeability ↓ Ca influx into synaptic endings ↓ Synthesis of excitatory transmitter
Phenobarbital	↓ Spread of seizure discharge ↑ Convulsive inhibition by threshold for electrical stimulation of brain	↓ CO_2 of brain ↓ ACh production ↑ K permeability of Aplysia neurons	↑ K permeability of neurons and thereby cause hyperpolarization
Trimethadione	↓ Repetitive discharge ↑ Convulsive threshold for electrical and (PTZ) stimulation ↓ SCC ↑ by PTZ	↓ Permeability to K of epithelial cell membrane Alters metabolism of GABA	↓ Permeability of glial cells to K ↑ GAD activity and reverse isoniazid
Primidone	↓ Spread of seizure discharge ↑ Convulsive threshold	?	?
Ethosuximide	↑ PTZ convulsive threshold ↓ SCC ↑ by PTZ	↓ Permeability to K Alters GABA metabolism	↓ Permeability to K ↑ GAD activity and reverse inhibition by isoniazid
Diazepam	↑ Convulsive threshold to PTZ ↓ SCC ↑ by PTZ	↓ K permeability Alters GABA metabolism	↓ K permeability ↑ GAD activity and reverse inhibition by isoniazid
Acetazolamide	↓ Spread of seizure discharge ↓ CO_2-induced seizures and withdrawal seizures ↓ Monosynaptic action potential in spinal cord	↓ Carbonic anhydrase activity in brain and choroid plexus ↑ Total CO_2 in brain ↓ Na uptake in brain ↓ CSF flow	↓ Carbonic anhydrase activity of glial and choroid plexus cells ↑ CO_2 in brain ↓ CSF flow
Na valproate	↑ Convulsive threshold for electrical, PTZ, picrotoxin, and strychnine seizures	Inhibits GABA-T activity in brain ↑ K^+ permeability in Aplysia neurons ↑ GAD activity	↑ Brain GABA concentration hyperpolarizes Aplysia neurons by increase in K^+ permeability

drive with loss of inhibitory drive would be the best model of status epilepticus. The models to be discussed here have this attribute and would seem to be potentially useful models of status epilepticus.

COMPARISON OF ANTICONVULSANT DRUG ACTIVITIES

One approach to discovering drugs that may be of value in status epilepticus is to examine new drugs that fit into the same category as the drugs that are currently used in this condition. An example of this method is shown in Fig. 1. It is readily observed from these two simple tests of anticonvulsantdrug activity that several groups or clusters of drugs can be identified, each group of which contains drugs effective against a different type of epilepsy in humans. Those efficacious against MES but not against PTZ (infinite value for ED_{50} versus S.C. MET) are drugs useful in generalized tonic-clonic and focal seizures. Those highly efficacious against PTZ and poorly effective against MES relative to toxicity (ethosuximide, trimethadione, dimethadione, and paramethadione in one group and the benzodiazepines in another group) are drugs useful in absence seizures. These two types of actions clearly sort out into three clusters on this scatter plot of the data. The remainder of the points, that is, those drugs with intermediate effectiveness against both PTZ and MES, appear to be drugs useful in simple partial (focal) seizures, complex partial seizures, and myoclonic seizures in children. More discrete clusters can be elicited by also including the TD_{50} values in the analysis, as has been done, for example, by Krall (5). Also sorted out by this type of plot are the carbonic-anhydrase-inhibitor sulfonamides. The plot puts this group in a separate cluster. The point of this type of plot is that new types of drugs may be identified by comparing them with the standard drug clusters or determining if they form a new cluster. For example, by this method two types of sulfonamides have been identified as having anticonvulsant activity of different patterns. Even greater differentiation of anticonvulsants can be made by examining the profile against a number of different convulsants having different mechanisms of action, as will now be discussed.

COMPARISON OF MECHANISMS OF ACTION

In the long range, the most rational method for testing anticonvulsant drugs in experimental models is by use of the mechanism-of-action approach. The model in this case is a drug in which the mechanism of its convulsant effect is known, e.g., picrotoxin, which blocks presynaptic and postsynaptic GABA receptors. Thus, a potential anticonvulsant drug that is being tested can be ascertained to act in the same way as the convulsant used as a model if it competitively blocks the convulsions produced by the convulsive agent. Thus, anticonvulsant drugs could be developed on the basis of their mechanisms of action and their effects against various types of epilepsy in humans. This would then yield a spectrum of actions in humans and help to elucidate the mechanisms of different types of epilepsy. This approach is illustrated in Table 6, which indicates the various mechanisms by which the convulsant drugs act. Thus, the convulsant drug can be used as an experimental model for the action that it produces. Anticonvulsant drugs at different dose levels can then be tested against each of these models (mechanisms) and their spectra and type of inhibition determined. Profiles of actions can then be constructed, and hopefully new drugs can be determined from these profiles. Examples of this approach are shown in Fig. 2. The MES test is shown for comparison. It is evident that drugs used in absence seizures have similar profiles (ethosuximide and trimethadione) and are quite selective for PTZ, whereas the wider-spectrum anticonvulsants, phenobarbital and diazepam, are about equally effective in all tests, except strychnine, and have completely different spectra from the other drugs. Their spectra are also different from that of valproate, which appears to be more selective for PTZ but also protects against strychnine in nontoxic doses. The carbonic anhydrase inhibitors, acetazolamide and sulthiame, are similar to each other but different from all the other drugs shown, but like the others they are more selective against PTZ-induced convulsions. These profiles are limited in the numbers of models tested and also by the fact that some of the convulsants used have the same effects on the GABA system. However, PTZ and to a lesser extent picrotoxin, in contrast to the more selective action of bicuculline to block the GABA receptor, have direct actions on the neuronal membrane to increase so-

TABLE 6. *Proposed experimental models of epilepsy based on mechanisms of action*

Mechanism	Anti-ChE	Fluro-thyl	Convulsant barb.	Kainic acid, etc.	PTZ	Picrotoxin Bicuculline Penicillins	Allyl glycine	3-Mercapto propionic acid	Isoniazid etc.	Strychnine	MSO	Ouabain	SCN^- ClO_4^-
Enhance excitatory systems													
ACh effects													
Block receptors													
Block metabolism	X												
Increase Na permeability		X			X								
Increase Ca^{2+} influx			X										
Glutamic acid effects													
Receptor stimulus				X									
Block synthesis													
Block inhibitory systems													
Block GABA effects													
Block receptor					X	X							
Block synthesis													
B6 antagonist									X				
Inhibit GAD							X	X					
Block glycine effects													
Block receptor										X			
Block energy metabolism													
Inhibit glutamine synthetase											X		
Block ion transport													
Cations												X	
Anions													X

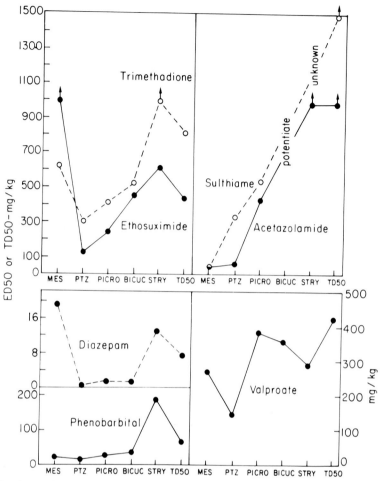

FIG. 2. Profiles of various anticonvulsant drugs on a variety of experimental models of epilepsy. On the ordinate is the ED_{50} or TD_{50} (mg/kg) of the drug being tested. On the abscissa: MES = maximal electroshock seizure test; PTZ = pentylenetetrazol test; PICRO = picrotoxin test; BICUC = bicuculline test; STRY = strychnine test. TD50 = toxic dose 50 in rotorod test used to assess neurotoxicity. Data from unpublished observations of E. A. Swinyard and H. Kupferberg.

dium permeability in addition to their GABA receptor blocking action. Thus, these data suggest that the direct effects of trimethadione, ethosuximide, phenobarbital, sulthiame, acetazolamide, and even valproate may be more prominent than their effects on GABA receptors, because the ED_{50} values are lower for PTZ than for picrotoxin and bicuculline. In the case of the carbonic anhydrase inhibitors, any GABA effect is unlikely, because both the agents tested potentiated bicuculline-induced seizures. These data suggest direct membrane effects, as do other data from our laboratory. Valproate, as has already been postulated, may also have some GABA receptor blocking effects. The GABA-mimetic agent SL76002 (6) is more potent against bicuculline and picrotoxin than against PTZ, as would be expected from its GABA effect. Thus, these profiles are a useful way of screening drugs on the basis of their mechanisms of action.

Phenytoin, if plotted on this graph, would show effectiveness only against MES, because it potentiates all other chemical seizures. Its profile and therefore its mechanism are thus quite different. Because phenytoin blocks ouabain-induced seizures, its effects on transport mechanisms as well as on membrane Na^+ and Ca^+ channels appear likely to be effects we have demonstrated on the toad bladder, gut, and choroid plexus.

Finally, of the drugs shown in Fig. 2, only valproate showed protection against strychnine in nontoxic doses, and its mechanism appears to differ from those of all the other drugs shown. This suggests a generalized effect to block seizures regardless of their cause. This is probably due to an influence on the membranes or myelin. The effects of valproate against other models should be assessed to determine if it is indeed a general anticonvulsant drug and, if so, whether or not it will be effective in status epilepticus, as are diazepam and phenobarbital.

POTENTIAL EXPERIMENTAL MODELS OF STATUS EPILEPTICUS

Table 7 summarizes some potential experimental models of status epilepticus. None of these models has been completely tested to determine if it can serve as a model for developing drugs useful in status epilepticus, but they are included here because they seem to be potentially capable of elucidating not only the drugs useful in treating this condition but also the mechanisms by which status epilepticus is produced. Both acute and chronic models are considered. The acute models use convulsant agents that stimulate excitatory sys-

TABLE 7. *Summary of potential experimental models of status epilepticus*

Acute models
  Stimulate excitatory systems
    Glutamic acid (10-day-old rats)
      Kainic acid
      Fluorothyl
  Block inhibitory systems
    Picrotoxin + phenytoin
    Pentylenetetrazol + 100% oxygen
    Pentylenetetrazol + phenytoin
  Block ion transport mechanisms
    Ouabain, applied locally or given to neonatal rats
Spontaneous (genetic) models
  Gerbils
  Photosensitive baboons
  Audiogenic-seizure mice
  Photosensitive chickens
  Single-locus recessive mutations in mice
    Partial motor seizures
      Lethargic
      Ducky
      Tottering
    Generalized convulsions
      Dilute (lethal)
      Quaking
      Wabbler (lethal)
Chronic models
  Alumina cream in monkeys
  Cobalt, applied bilaterally to frontal or parietal cortex

tems, such as kainic acid, glutamic acid, and fluorothyl, and agents that decrease inhibitory activity, such as picrotoxin, bicucullin, and penicillin, or better still a combination of these two effects, such as PTZ or picrotoxin combined with phenytoin. The combination of phenytoin, which stimulates both excitatory and inhibitory systems, with picrotoxin, which blocks GABA-induced presynaptic and postsynaptic inhibition, produces prolonged seizures resembling status epilepticus. The picrotoxin blocks the stimulation of inhibitory mechanisms by phenytoin and hence allows its excitatory effects to predominate. Phenytoin is known to have both inhibitory and excitatory effects on neurons, and the overall expression of its effects depends on the relative balance between the excitatory and inhibitory effects. In neonatal animals the excitatory effects predominate, and phenytoin increases excitability, whereas in adult animals the inhibitory systems predominate, and therefore the inhibitory effects of phenytoin predominate. Thus, the continuous seizures produced by the combination of phenytoin and picrotoxin are due to release of inhibition imposed by the picrotoxin effect overcoming the phenytoin stimulation, plus excessive excitatory drive resulting from the stimulatory effects of phenytoin. Diazepam, valproate sodium, phenobarbital, and methsuximide protect against such seizures, but ethosuximide, trimethadione, and phensuximide do not. It is therefore a promising model. Kainic acid, which produces continuous statuslike seizures, may also be useful, as might glutamic acid in 10-day-old rats. At this age, glutamic acid can cross the blood-brain barrier and induce prolonged seizures (3). Ouabain, an inhibitor of Na^+,K^+-ATPase, also produces prolonged seizures in neonatal rats and may be a useful model as well.

Chronic models of various types of status can be produced by implantation of heavy metals (e.g., tungstic acid, cobalt, alumina cream) into different areas of the brain. Such models have been inadequately examined, and no systematic studies of drugs useful in therapy for status (diazepam, phenytoin, phenobarbital) have been performed on them. That changes in the concentrations of the substrates of the brain, glucose and oxygen, may be important in precipitating status epilepticus is evident from examination of one model (pentylenetetrazol plus 100% oxygen) listed in Table 6. Providing oxygen to the brain during convulsions, where oxygen may be limited in the *in vivo* situation, provides sufficient substrate to allow the seizures to continue indefinitely. Therefore, the PTZ plus 100% oxygen model, which results in seizures that last as long as the PTZ is in the body, is a potentially useful model for status. The effects of various drugs should be tested on this model. The spontaneous (genetic) models offer potentially useful models of status, because the seizures are recurrent and paroxysmal, as is human epilepsy. However, status does not generally occur, and some evocative agent might have to be used if the model is to be useful. Particularly interesting are the single-locus recessive mutations in mice described by Noebels (7). Mice with partial motor or generalized types of seizures have been described (Table 7). Status could be produced by giving agents that decrease the threshold for seizures, such as glucocorticosteroids, thyroxine, and a low-sodium diet.

Unfortunately, no well-characterized models of status epilepticus are extant that can be used for assessing mechanisms of continuous seizures and for assay of potentially useful drugs. Such models, and studies of them, are urgently needed.

ACKNOWLEDGMENTS

This work was supported by program project 1PO1-NS-15767, and the author is the recipient of a research career award (5-K6-13,828), both from the National Institute of Neurological and Communicative Disorders and Stroke.

REFERENCES

1. Brodie, B. B., and Reid, W. D. (1969): Is man a unique animal in response to drugs? *Am. J. Pharm.*, 141:21–17.

2. Fröscher, W. (1979): *Treatment of Status Epilepticus.* University Park Press, Baltimore.

3. Johnston, G. A. R. (1973): Convulsions induced in 10-day-old rats by intraperitoneal injection of monosodium glutamate and related amino acids. *Biochem. Pharmacol.*, 22:137–139.

4. Krall, R. L., Penry, J. K., White, B. G., Kupferberg, H. J., and Swinyard, E. A. (1978): Antiepileptic drug development: II. Anticonvulsant drug screening. *Epilepsia*, 19:409–428.

5. Krall, R. L. (1980): Quantitative structure-activity relationships of anticonvulsant drugs. *Adv. Neurol.*, 27:233–248.

6. Lloyd, K. G., Worms, P., Depoortere, H., and Bartholini, G. (1978): Pharmacological profile of SL76002, a new GABA-mimetic drug. In: *GABA Neurotransmitters: Pharmacochemical, Biochemical and Pharmacological Aspects*, edited by P. Krogsgaard-Larsen, J. Scheel-Kruger, and H. Kofod, pp. 308–325. Munksgaard, Copenhagen.

7. Noebels, J. L. (1979): Analysis of inherited epilepsy using single locus mutations in mice. *Fed. Proc.*, 38:2405–2410.

8. Purpura, D. P., Penry, J. K., Tower, D. B., Woodbury, D. M., and Walter, R. D. (editors) (1972): *Experimental Models of Epilepsy.* Raven Press, New York.

9. Sherwin, A. L. (1978): Pharmacological principles in the management of patients with epilepsy. In: *Advances in Epileptology, 1977: Psychology, Pharmacotherapy, and New Diagnostic Approaches*, edited by H. Meinardi and A. J. Rowan, pp. 211–219. Swets and Zeitlinger, Amsterdam.

10. Woodbury, D. M. (1972): Applications to drug evaluations. In: *Experimental Models of Epilepsy*, edited by D. P. Purpura, J. K. Penry, D. B. Tower, D. M. Woodbury, and R. D. Walter, pp. 557–583. Raven Press, New York.

11. Woodbury, D. M. (1980): Convulsant drugs: Mechanisms of action. *Adv. Neurol.*, 27:249–303.

Advances in Neurology, Vol. 34: Status Epilepticus, edited by A.V. Delgado-Escueta, C.G. Wasterlain, D.M. Treiman, and R.J. Porter. Raven Press, New York © 1983.

15

Effects of Repeated Seizures on Hippocampal Neurons in the Cat

W. Jann Brown and T. L. Babb

Seizures have been evoked by changes in cerebral metabolism (14), by modifications in neural structures (11,12,23), by alterations in the external or internal milieu of the neuron (22), and, of course, by disease (3,24). The structural basis for the ictus in humans is still puzzling; hence, we continuously use experimental models to help understand human seizure phenomena. At the University of California at Los Angeles (6), more than 100 cases of human temporal lobe epilepsy have been studied with direct recordings from electrodes placed in the temporal lobes by the use of stereotactic coordinates. The resected tissues from some of those cases studied by Golgi techniques (19) or electron microscopy have shown various changes such as degenerations and contractions of axons and dendrites, development of varicosities on axons, and loss of dendritic spines. The findings of these studies have caused us to consider an active disease process, and it is possible that alterations are under way in the opposite hippocampus. We cannot study such changes in humans, especially because we cannot examine the remaining temporal lobe except by remote techniques such as electrical recordings. We have tested two methods of inducing repeated convulsions that might cause injury to temporal lobe neurons. These recurrent seizures could lead to structural changes and result in the development of new seizure-sensitive cortex, e.g., a "mirror focus" (17). Focal cobalt-induced hip-

pocampal seizures have resulted in no neuronal abnormalities in contralateral homotypic hippocampal cortex, despite repeated synaptic driving of the cortex during numerous clinical seizures that ranged from 60 to 144 attacks in 8 hr. These seizures were characterized by bilateral hippocampal discharges, although contralateral discharges were never found to be independent. Synaptic bombardment of the contralateral homotypic cortex, then, did not induce a "mirror focus," and structural alterations secondary to metabolic stress were not found. Status epilepticus, induced for as long as 300 min by intravenous bicuculline, similarly did not cause structural alterations, provided homeostasis was maintained in the animal. This indicates that continuously increasing synaptic activity during generalized seizures did not cause structural damage under these conditions.

MATERIALS AND METHODS

Eleven healthy young adult cats, male and female, were studied. In 5 cats, under general anesthesia (sodium pentobarbital 35 mg/kg intraperitoneally), a 20-gauge cannula was stereotactically introduced through a burr hole into the right ventral hippocampus (A 8.0, L 11.0, H -50) (21). After 7 to 10 days, 4.6 mg of hexahydrate cobaltous chloride ($CoCl_2 \cdot 6H_2O$) dissolved in 2 μl of distilled water was injected into each of 4 cats from

TABLE 1. *Cobalt treatment of right hippocampus: time intervals and summary of results for each experimental animal*

Cat no.	Cobalt chloride dose	No. of clinical seizures	Average duration of clinical seizures (sec)	Perfusion after cobalt	Tissue alterations Right hippocampus	Left hippocampus
1 2B	4.6 mg/2 μl	Day 1 = 94	24	7 hr	4b + [a]	0
2 Y	4.6 mg/2 μl	Day 1 = 144	22	5 days[b]	4d −	0
3 Al	4.6 mg/2 μl (day 1)	Day 1 = 60	25	23 days[b]	4c +	0
	4.6 mg/2 μl (day 5)	Day 5 = not recorded				
4	4.6 mg/2 μl	Day 1 = not recorded	Not recorded	18 hr[c]	4d +	0
5	Control (saline 2 μl)		0	24 hr[b]	000	0

From Brown et al. (4).

[a]Necrosis 1–5 (5 = worst); gliosis a–e (e = most extensive); inflammation (+ , −).

[b]Seizures were controlled by injection of sodium pentobarbital or diazepam, then perfusion intravitam.

[c]Perfused while comatose.

a microsyringe with a long 26-gauge needle that could be inserted into the end of the cannula; for details see Babb et al. (1). Saline only was injected into 1 cat. Electrical activity was recorded from the chronically implanted cannula and other stainless-steel electrodes in the opposite hippocampus and anterior ventral nucleus of the thalamus and bilaterally over the somatosensory cortex. Continuous recording was carried out for 18 hr after application of cobalt salt. The animals were then anesthetized overnight with sodium pentobarbital. Daily recordings 2 hr in duration were made from each animal to determine that no clinical or EEG seizure activity persisted beyond the first day.

Injections were made into the right ventral hippocampus while the cat was painlessly restrained in a canvas bag. EEG recordings were taken 2 hr before injection and continuously up to the time of vital perfusion (Table 1).

TABLE 2. *Summary of drug dose, seizure duration, and structural alterations of hippocampus with bicuculline HCl*

Cat no.	Total drug dose (mg)	Duration of continuous seizures (min)	Delay of perfusion from seizure onset (min)
6	6.4	250[a]	250
7	4.8	120[a]	120
8	8.0	275[a]	275
27A	6.68	275[a]	995
24A	10.80	94[b]	120
9	8.0	300[b]	510

From Brown et al. (4).

[a]Gallamine triethiodide administered.

[b]Gallamine not administered.

Six cats were given bicuculline HCl (pH 5.8). The compound was prepared according to Brown et al. (4). Approximately 1.6 mg was initially injected intravenously to cause irregular EEG spikes in about 90 sec. Neocortical EEG recordings were taken from skull screws overlying the suprasylvian gyri bilaterally. Hippocampal recordings were not made.

Four bicuculline-treated cats were artificially ventilated after paralysis with gallamine (5 mg/kg intravenously). Wound margins were locally anesthetized by applying a 2% lidocaine HCl solution. The restrained animal was intubated with an endotracheal tube coated with lidocaine gel. Room air was administered by respirator. After peripheral limb nerve blocks using 2% lidocaine HCl, indwelling polyethylene catheters were placed in the femoral artery to sample blood for both pH and O_2 every 30 min and in the opposite femoral vein for intravenous administration of drugs and to maintain a continuously slow infusion of 5% glucose in 0.09% saline. Rectal temperature was continuously measured. Blood pH was maintained at 7.39 to 7.40 by intravenous 1-N sodium lactate solution. All bicuculline-treated cats received intravenous heparin (5 mg/kg i.v.). Two cats did not receive gallamine, but were restrained in an elevated canvas bag to allow artifact-free EEG recording (Table 2). In all animals, after seizures were terminated, general anesthesia (sodium pentobarbital 35 mg/kg i.p.) was given prior to perfusion (except cat 4, Table 1, which was comatose). The thorax was opened, and 0.8 ml of 1% $NaNO_2$ was injected into the left cardiac ventricle. A cannula was passed through the ventricle and tied into the ascending aorta. The right atrium was opened to allow return flow. The descending aorta was clamped, and the brain was perfused according to Brown et al. (4). The head was placed in a plastic bag at 4°C for 2 hr, the skull was removed, and the brain was immersed overnight in additional cold fixative (5). After fixation, slices were made across both ventral and dorsal segments of the hippocampus.

Segments of tissues from the ventral hippocampus of both sides were then selected in the manner depicted in Fig. 1. Blocks were further fixed, dehydrated, and embedded according to Brown et al. (4). Other blocks of hippocampus and cerebellum were embedded in paraffin and stained with luxol-blue/periodic-acid-Schiff stain.

RESULTS

Cobalt-treated Cats

After the cobalt salt was injected into the right hippocampus of the unanesthetized adult cat, focal hippocampal EEG spiking and seizures were seen. Eventually the hippocampal seizures spread to in-

volve all cortical and subcortical regions shown in Fig. 2. The only alterations in motor behavior during the seizures were series of marked masticatory movements, excessive salivation, occasional eye blinks, and slight turning of the head, although in later stages extremity clonus was also seen (Fig. 2B).

Abnormal electrical activity in all 4 cobalt-treated cats was observed on the EEG record within 60 to 90 min of the application of cobalt salt. A 5- to 10-min postictal interval of depression usually ensued before seizure activity was again seen. The periods of depression steadily shortened and the periods of spiking activity lengthened from 60 to 120 min. If either barbiturate or diazepam was given, seizure activity gradually eased. Seizures were allowed to continue unabated in 1 animal (cat 4, Table 1) until it was perfused after 18 hr.

Structural alterations in the pyramidal layer of right hippocampus included dark pyramidal cells, occasional macrophages, and lipid droplets. The increased density of the pyramidal cells is explained by the presence of large masses of pigment, probably related to cobalt. Profound gliosis

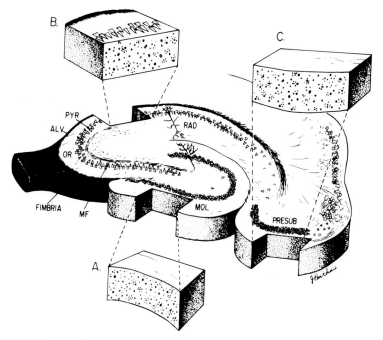

FIG. 1. Exploded diagram of ventral cat hippocampus showing three of several sites sampled in the study. This diagram shows the orientation of the apical dendrites of the pyramidal cell layers. It should be emphasized that regions other than those designated A, B, and C were also examined. Abbreviations: ALV, alveus; PYR, pyramidal cell; RAD, stratum radiatum; OR, striatum oriens; MOL, stratum moleculare; PRESUB, presubiculum; MF, mossy fibers. (From Brown et al., ref. 4, with permission.)

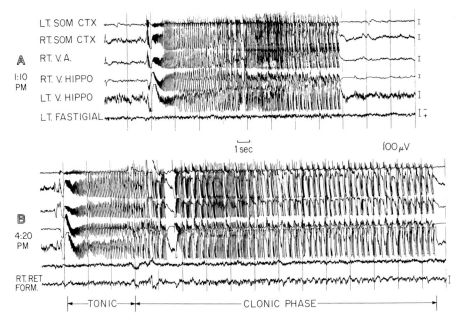

FIG. 2. Morphology of tonic and clonic components in short- and long-duration cobalt seizures. In **A**, a 16-sec seizure with a tonic phase just over 6 sec long. In the same cat, 190 min later (**B**), a 31-sec seizure occurred with a tonic phase of about 6 sec, indicating that the duration of the clonic phase alone increases with time. (From Babb et al., ref. 1, with permission.)

was also found intimately sheathing the basement membranes of the perithelial cells, capillaries, small arterioles, and venules. Some of the capillaries appeared to be newly developed. The most extensive alterations were found in pyramidal cells adjacent to the injection site. The contralateral hippocampus in both experimental and control cats showed neither light microscopic nor electron microscopic changes in neuronal architecture, dendritic geometry, or spine morphology, except for minimal alterations related to narrow-gauge recording electrodes.

Bicuculline-treated Cats

Approximately 90 sec after intravenous administration of 1.6 mg of bicuculline, irregular spikes were seen in the EEG (Fig. 3). Gallamine prevented any overt motor activity in 4 cats. In the 2 cats not given gallamine, tonic-clonic seizures involving the whole axial musculature and extremities were observed for the durations shown in Table 2. The spiking and electrical hyperactivity continued thereafter except for short (12- to 14-sec) periods of inactivity. The arterial blood pH, O_2, and body temperature were maintained at normal values. Seizures continued from 120 to 300 min be-

fore being halted with diazepam (0.25 mg/kg i.v.). The cats were then intravitally perfused under general anesthesia. One animal (cat 27A, Table 2) was maintained for an additional 12 hr and another (cat 9) for 8 hr after cessation of seizures to allow additional time for possible development of ischemic lesions (Figs. 5 and 6).

Neither light microscopic (Fig. 4) nor ultrastructural (Figs. 5 and 6) examination of various sectors of the right and left hippocampus revealed any abnormalities, nor were any found in the cerebellum by light microscopy.

In Fig. 3, portions of the EEG record from cat 27A are shown. This animal was treated in the same manner as cat 24A, except that gallamine was not given and the seizures continued for 275 min. The arterial blood pH was maintained at 7.4, although it increased occasionally to 7.46, but was never depressed. This cat was intravitally perfused 12 hr after seizures were controlled. The normal-appearing light microscopic structural status of the hippocampus of this cat is shown in Fig. 4. There was no evidence of ischemic necrosis in any blocks of the parts of the hippocampus, as depicted in Fig. 1. Ultrastructural examination of various parts of the hippocampus shown in Fig. 4 was carried

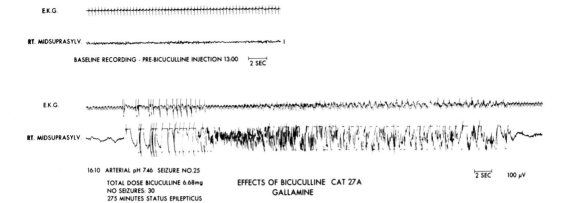

E.K.G.

RT. MIDSUPRASYLV.

BASELINE RECORDING - PRE-BICUCULLINE INJECTION 13:00   2 SEC

E.K.G.

RT. MIDSUPRASYLV.

16:10 ARTERIAL pH 7.46 SEIZURE NO.25

TOTAL DOSE BICUCULLINE 6.68mg
NO SEIZURES: 30
275 MINUTES STATUS EPILEPTICUS

EFFECTS OF BICUCULLINE CAT 27A
GALLAMINE

2 SEC   100 μV

FIG. 3. Sample of EEG record from cat 27A in which seizures were induced with 6.68 mg of bicuculline HCl. (From Brown et al., ref. 4, with permission.)

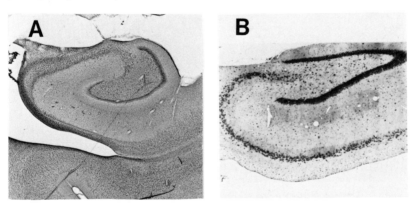

FIG. 4. Photomicrographs of hippocampi taken from cats following either cobalt-induced seizures (**A**) or bicuculline seizures (**B**). In **A**, 4.6 mg CoCl₂ was injected in the opposite, right hippocampus of cat 2B, and the left hippocampus, shown in **A**, had no abnormalities, despite 94 seizures with an average duration of 24 sec (Table 1). In **B**, the hippocampus of cat 27A had normal cytoarchitecture in all subfields, despite repeated seizures for 275 min and a delay to perfusion-fixation of 995 min (Table 2). (**A** from Babb et al., ref. 1, with permission.) (**B** from Brown et al., ref. 4, with permission.)

out because of the possibility that very early ischemic changes might be present in neurons. Extensive examination of many blocks of the hippocampus showed neurons with intact plasma membranes, synpases, dendrites, spines, and axons (Figs. 5 and 6). Montages of individual whole pyramidal and granule cells showed no degenerative alterations or increased glial profiles. An indication of the ultrastructural integrity of parts of the dendritic geometry is seen in Fig. 5. This longitudinal section of a terminal portion of an apical dendrite of a pyramidal cell showed intact presynaptic and postsynaptic membranes, microtubules, mitochondria, and spines (Fig. 6). Tangential sections of another segment of the pyramidal cell layer are seen in Fig. 6. In the cross sections of these

dendrites, the microtubules were still arrayed in a normally spaced distribution. Presynaptic and postsynaptic membranes showed no evidence of ischemic damage, nor was there any swelling of astrocyte profiles, either in Fig. 6 or in other similar electron micrographs of the pyramidal cell or granule cell layers.

DISCUSSION

Using two different models for inducing increased synaptic activity in the temporal lobe of the cat, no structural alterations were observed, despite the extended hyperphysiological drive of neurons. These results suggest that recurrent seizures themselves are not enough to induce the

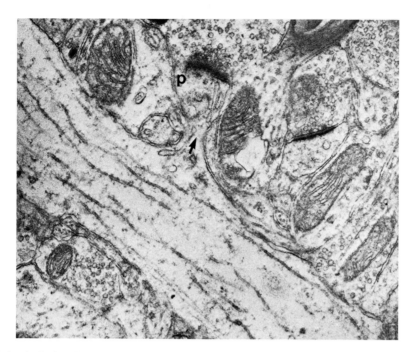

FIG. 5. A longitudinal section of a pyramidal cell apical dendrite near its periphery in sector CA3. Spinous processes (p) were numerous, and their integrity appeared to be maintained. There was a spine apparatus present *(arrow)*; mitochondrial organization and microtubules all appeared to be normal. There was no obvious change in synaptic vesicular population. Cat 27A. ×26,250. (From Brown et al., ref. 4, with permission.)

structural changes that may be seen in some primary seizure foci. Because seizures and increased neuronal metabolic demand probably operate in tandem, it is reasonable to assume that long episodes of seizure activity might well result in neuron loss due to ischemia or hypoxia, which is what Meldrum et al. (15) found in young baboons after long periods of seizure activity were initiated and maintained with bicuculline. In their optical study it is plainly evident that injured cells were diffusely distributed in the neocortex, limbic cortex, basal ganglia, and cerebellum. In our use of bicuculline, however, we closely monitored the animals to avoid intermittent apnea, depression of blood pH below 7.39 to 7.40, decreases in blood pressure, and elevations in body temperature above normal; intravenous fluid and glucose were continuously administered. We were therefore able to confirm a later study of Meldrum et al. (16) showing that if homeostasis is maintained, severe seizures need not lead to severe cell loss due to vascular insufficiency. Recently, Mouritzen-Dam et al. (18) gave rats tonic-clonic seizures at a rate of three per day to a total of 140 seizures by the use of electrical

shock, then allowed the animals to rest for either 14 or 72 days. They reported no changes in cell densities in any subfield of the hippocampus. Of additional interest in this regard is the recent study by Escobar and Nieto (8), who, in an attempt to produce neuronal damage in Ammon's horn, induced seizures with pentylenetetrazol (PTZ) in young rats that ranged in age from 8 days to 3 months. In one group, hyperthermia was also created by means of subcutaneous injection of a vaccine for human use. In that group, seizures were induced while the rats were hyperthermic. A second group was given PTZ only. The third group was protected with diazepam before PTZ was administered. A fourth group of seizure-free animals served as controls. At least one episode of several seizures was given each experimental animal. If the animals survived, they usually recovered within 12 hr and again were subjected to seizures at intervals of 36 hr each. After the fourth episode, the animals were killed and perfused. No lesions of the neurons in Ammon's horn were observed in any of the groups. The results, according to Escobar and Nieto (8), suggested that febrile exper-

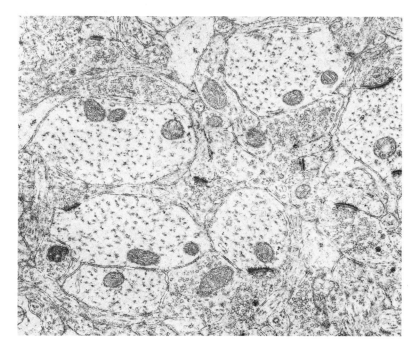

FIG. 6. Tangential section of region CA2 of cat 27A. The alveus was shaved off, leaving exposed the cross sections of other pyramidal cell dendrites. Note integrity of microtubules, mitochondria, synapses, and synaptic vesicles. ×15,750. (From Brown et al., ref. 4, with permission.)

imental seizures in the rat do not constitute a pathogenic mechanism for Ammon's horn sclerosis.

The application of cobalt to the hippocampal cortex produces "feline psychomotor" attacks (1), but it also causes a severe necrotizing injury at the site of injection, with indiscriminate damage to neurons, neuroglia, and endothelial cells. The local damage is of such magnitude as to preclude examination of many of the physiological parameters of the residual neurons, whose dendritic geometry is markedly changed because of both direct injury and evolving glial scar. The neomicrovasculature that is produced undoubtedly alters functional aspects of the blood-brain barrier in the immediate surround, permitting differential electrolyte flux and possibly inducing neuronal firing.

Light microscopic studies of cobalt damage to cortex showed local necrosis, inflammation, and gliosis. Local ultrastructural damage caused by cobalt (9) or alumina (10) has been reported. In an earlier study in which cobalt damage was examined for several time periods, indications were that there is continuing damage due to the presence of cobaltous salt, despite the fact that seizures were

not allowed to persist beyond 18 hr after the salt was applied (1).

Studies of the fine structure of tissues displaying hyperactivity remote from injection or application sites are not numerous; so we are uncertain about changes in such cortex. One report by Brennan et al. (2) indicated no evident injury in cortex after the induction of single electrically stimulated seizures in well-oxygenated animals. Schwartz et al. (20) similarly found no significant structural modifications in cat hippocampus after as long as 120 min of electrically induced focal seizures. The findings of De Robertis et al. (7) of swollen astrocytes around capillaries after PTZ-induced seizures in the rat can be attributed at least partially to artifact from immersion fixation. Although we sampled the contralateral cortex of the cat extensively, we were not aware of the presence of any unusual glial component, nor did there appear to be any in relation to whole pyramidal or granule cell surfaces in montages. Also, electron-dense presynaptic and postsynaptic structures were not apparent in our examination of the contralateral homotypic cortex.

Prevention of such various-size epileptogenic foci in the hippocampal cortex by support of homeostatic mechanisms in children with febrile convulsions is probably as important as was suggested by McLardy (13).

ACKNOWLEDGMENTS

This work was supported by grants HD-05615, NS-12054-03, NS-02808, and NS-4-2331 from the U.S. Public Health Service.

REFERENCES

1. Babb, T. L., Mitchell, A. G., and Crandall, P. H. (1974): Fastigiobulbar and dentatothalamic influences on hippocampal cobalt epilepsy in the cat. *Electroencephalogr. Clin. Neurophysiol.*, 36:141–154.
2. Brennan, R. W., Petito, C. K., and Porro, R. S. (1972): Single seizures cause no ultrastructural changes in brain. *Brain Res.*, 45:574–579.
3. Brown, W. J. (1973): Structural substrates of seizure foci in the human temporal lobe (A combined electrophysiological optical microscopic and ultrastructural study). In: *Epilepsy, Its Phenomena in Man*, edited by M. Brazier, pp. 339–374. Academic Press, New York.
4. Brown, W. J., Mitchell, A. G., Jr., Babb, T. L., and Crandall, P. H. (1980): Structural and physiologic studies in experimentally induced epilepsy. *Exp. Neurol.*, 69:543–562.
5. Brown, W. J., and Palay, S. L. (1972): Acetylcholinesterase activity in certain glomeruli and Golgi cells of the granular layer of the rat cerebellar cortex. *Z. Anat. Entwicklungsgesch.*, 137:317–334.
6. Crandall, P. H. (1973): Developments in direct recordings from epileptogenic regions in the surgical treatment of partial epilepsies. In: *Epilepsy, Its Phenomena in Man*, edited by M. Brazier, pp. 287–310. Academic Press, New York.
7. De Robertis, E., Alberici, M., and Arnaiz, G. R. (1969): Astroglial swelling and phosphohydrolases in cerebral cortex of metrazol convulsant rats. *Brain Res.*, 12:461–466.
8. Escobar, A., and Nieto, D. (1980): Absence of lesions in Ammon's horn neurons following metrazol induced seizures in the hyperthermic rat. In: *Advances in Epileptology*, edited by J. A. Wada and J. K. Penry, p. 494. Raven Press, New York.
9. Fischer, J. (1969): Electron microscopic alterations in the vicinity of epileptogenic cobalt-gelatine necrosis in the cerebral cortex of the rat (A contribution to the ultrastructure of "plasmatic infiltration" of the central nervous system). *Acta Neuropathol.*, 14:201–214.
10. Harris, A. B. (1973): Ultrastructure and histochemistry of alumina in cortex. *Exp. Neurol.*, 38:33–63.
11. Keith, H. M., and Bickford, R. G. (1954): Observations on the properties of an electrical focus induced by freezing the animal cortex. *Am. J. Physiol.*, 179:650–651.
12. Kopeloff, L. (1960): Experimental epilepsy in the mouse. *Proc. Soc. Exp. Biol. Med.*, 104:500–504.
13. McLardy, T. (1969): Ammon's horn pathology and epileptic dyscontrol. *Nature*, 221:877–878.
14. Meldrum, B. S., and Brierley, J. (1973): Prolonged epileptic seizures in primates. *Arch. Neurol.*, 28:10–16.
15. Meldrum, B. S., Vigouroux, R. A., and Brierley, J. B. (1973): Systemic factors and epileptic brain damage. Prolonged seizure in paralyzed, artificially ventilated baboons. *Arch. Neurol.*, 29:82–87.
16. Meldrum, B. S., Vigouroux, R. A., Rage, P., and Brierley, J. B. (1973): Hippocampal lesions produced by prolonged seizures in paralyzed artificially ventilated baboons. *Experientia*, 29:561–563.
17. Morrell, F. (1960): Secondary epileptogenic lesions. *Epilepsia (Amst.)*, 1:538–560.
18. Mouritzen-Dam, A., Hertz, M., and Bolwig, T. G. (1980): The number of hippocampal neurons in rats after electrically induced generalized seizures. *Brain Res.*, 193:268–272.
19. Scheibel, M. E., and Scheibel, A. B. (1973): Hippocampal pathology in temporal lobe epilepsy. A Golgi survey. In: *Epilepsy, Its Phenomena in Man*, edited by M. Brazier, pp. 311–337. Academic Press, New York.
20. Schwartz, I. R., Broggi, G., and Pappas, G. D. (1970): Fine structure of cat hippocampus during sustained seizure. *Brain Res.*, 18:176–180.
21. Snider, R. S., and Niemer, W. T. (1961): *A Stereotaxic Atlas of the Cat Brain*. University of Chicago Press, Chicago.
22. Walker, A. E., Johnson, H. C., and Funderburk, W. H. (1945): Convulsive factor in commercial penicillin. *Arch. Surg.*, 50:69–73.
23. Ward, A. A., Jr. (1972): Topical convulsant metals. In: *Experimental Models of Epilepsy*, edited by D. P. Purpura, J. K. Penry, D. B. Tower, D. M. Woodbury, and R. D. Walter, pp. 13–35. Raven Press, New York.
24. Zimmerman, H. M. (1938): Histopathology of convulsive disorders in children. *J. Pediatr.*, 13:859–890.

Advances in Neurology, Vol. 34: Status
Epilepticus, edited by A.V. Delgado-Escueta,
C.G. Wasterlain, D.M. Treiman, and R.J. Porter.
Raven Press, New York © 1983.

16

Histopathological Changes in the Rat Brain During Bicuculline-Induced Status Epilepticus

Birgitta Söderfeldt, Hannu Kalimo, Yngve Olsson, and Bo Siesjö

Ischemic nerve cell changes and various degrees of edema are considered to be the two major neuropathological alterations that can be detected by classic neuropathological methods in patients dying after prolonged epileptic seizures or status epilepticus. The autopsy studies (during the last 30 years involving mostly children) have naturally involved patients in whom severe medical complications occurred during the seizures. It is therefore difficult to draw conclusions about the pathogenesis of the cell and tissue lesions from such material, because these patients may well have suffered from various degrees of hypoxia and circulatory disturbances apart from the direct effects of epilepsy.

Physiological parameters and tissue oxygenation can be controlled in animal experiments with pharmacologically induced status epilepticus. However, also in light microscopic (LM) studies of such material the progression of neuronal changes has been considered identical with that in hypoxia-ischemia. This type of nerve cell injury has been described by Brierley and associates in terms of three transitional stages: microvacuolation and ischemic nerve cell change with or without incrustations, eventually leading to dissolution and disappearance of the cell (6). In hypoxia-ischemia, electron microscopic (EM) studies have shown that the microvacuoles consist of swollen mitochondria (2). By analogy, the vacuoles seen in status epi-

lepticus have been considered to be swollen mitochondria.

EXPERIMENTAL STUDIES IN THE RAT

We have studied status epilepticus induced in artificially ventilated rats by intravenous injection of the GABA receptor blocking agent bicuculline. Seizure periods up to 2 hr in duration were studied. The rats were killed directly after the seizure period or after 2 hr of recovery, the seizures being arrested by injection of diazepam. The effect of the early ictal blood pressure increase was studied by comparing animals with such an increase and others in which the blood pressure was kept under 150 mm Hg by injection of an α-blocking agent. The brains were fixed by perfusion with glutaraldehyde and processed for LM and EM according to procedures previously described (1,5). The details of these procedures and results will be described in a forthcoming publication.

RESULTS

After 1 or 2 hr of EEG seizures we found pronounced changes in the cerebral cortex and hippocampus. Status spongiosus was observed in the middle cortical layers (Figs. 1 and 2) and in the hippocampus (Figs. 3 and 4). After 1 hr the status spongiosus was mostly localized to cortical layer 3, but as it became more pronounced after 2 hr

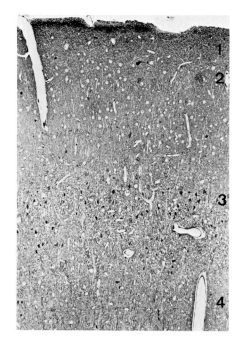

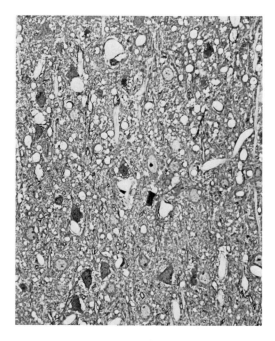

FIG. 1. Cerebral cortex after 1 hr of status epilepticus. Layer 3 is spongy with numerous darkly stained injured neurons. The outermost layers appear compact, as they also do after 2 hr of epilepsy. Epon + toluidine blue. ×82.5.

FIG. 2. Higher magnification of cortical layer 3 from the same animal as in Fig. 1 showing the status spongiosus (edema) with condensed dark-staining injured neurons surrounded by perineuronal vacuoles. Epon + toluidine blue. ×360.

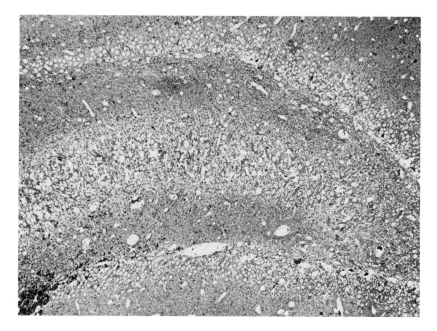

FIG. 3. Hippocampus after 2 hr of status epilepticus. Both the area CA4 and the inner layers of fascia dentata appear markedly spongy, principally because of swelling astrocytes. Epon + toluidine blue. ×120.

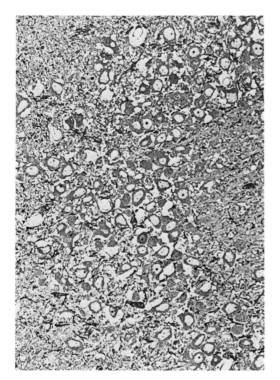

FIG. 4. Higher magnification of the hippocampal lesion in area CA1 (Sommer's sector) after 2 hr of epilepsy. The neurons are angular and somewhat condensed, with perineuronal vacuoles. These vacuoles, as also the pericapillary vacuolation, are due to the swelling of astrocytic processes. Epon + toluidine blue. ×255.

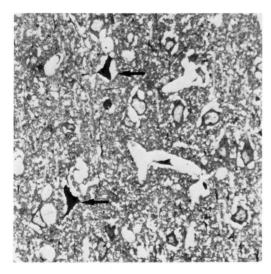

FIG. 5. After 2 hr of epilepsy, the status spongiosus in cortical layer 3 has become more pronounced, and the injured neurons appear more condensed, which makes it impossible to discern the nucleus in two cells (*arrows*). Epon + toluidine blue. ×323.

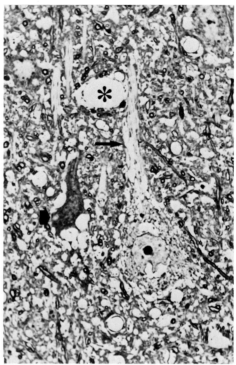

FIG. 6. After 2 hr of epilepsy, the edema also spreads into the deeper cortical layers, here layer 5. The large neuron shows the characteristic injury, with intracytoplasmic slit-formed vacuoles, which are often perinuclear and also extend into the dendrites (*thin arrow*). The smaller neuron (*thick arrow*) displays the other type of injury with darkly stained condensed cytoplasm and karyoplasm. The perineuronal vacuolation is due to swollen astrocytic processes, which also make the neuropil appear spongy. The astrocytic nucleus (*asterisk*) is markedly distended and watery. Epon + toluidine blue. ×816.

(Fig. 5) it spread also to the deeper layers (Fig. 6). Swollen astrocytes were seen both in areas with status spongiosus and in more normal-appearing neuropil.

Neuronal changes were conspicuous. By cell count, half of the neurons in the cerebral cortex appeared to be damaged after 1 hr of status epilepticus and two-thirds after 2 hr. There were principally two types of neuronal changes. The first and most frequent type was seen predominantly in areas with pronounced status spongiosus. The neurons were dark-staining, often with shrunken cytoplasm, and were surrounded by perineuronal vacuoles (Fig. 2). In the group with changes after 2 hr, about 50% of the neurons showed this alteration, and of those, about 10% had changes that were so pronounced that internal structures could not be discriminated (Figs. 2 and 5). In EM the

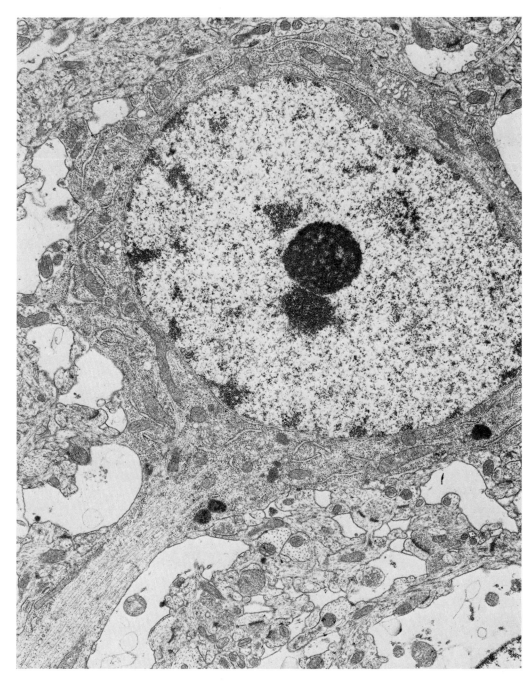

FIG. 7. Pyramidal neuron with slight condensation of cytoplasm and incipient widening of endoplasmic reticulum. The mitochondria look normal. Note the swollen astrocytic processes surrounding the neuron.

less severely injured neurons of this type showed up as electron-dense cells with slight dilatation of endoplasmic reticulum. The cells contained some vacuoles in their cytoplasm (Fig. 7). There was little indication that these vacuoles represented ballooned mitochondria. Instead, these organelles either looked normal or showed only slight loss of inner matrix. The neurons that in LM were more se-

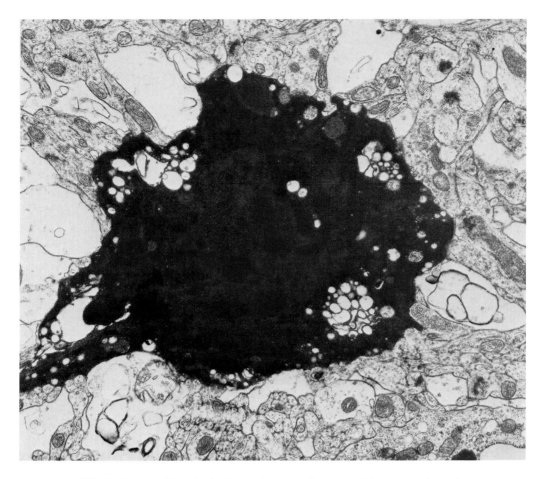

FIG. 8. Neuron with markedly electron-dense cytoplasm and multiple groups of vacuoles.

verely condensed and darkly stained had in EM a markedly electron-dense cytoplasm and contained multiple groups of vacuoles (Fig. 8). Some of these vacuoles may have been mitochondria, but most were so small that a mitochondrial origin seemed unlikely. Most probably they represented dilated Golgi cisternae.

The other type of neuronal alteration was mostly seen in deeper cortical layers and showed up in LM as normal-staining neurons with slit-formed cytoplasmic vacuoles (Fig. 6). In EM, the vacuoles proved to consist of widened portions of rough endoplasmic reticulum, including the nuclear envelope (Fig. 9). Apart from these large vacuoles, this type of neuron also contained small vacuoles, apparently diluted Golgi cisternae. Most mitochondria looked normal, but very rarely a few vacuoles with double membranes and cristalike material could be seen.

We also conducted LM studies of the cerebral cortex after 2 hr of recovery. Most of the edema had vanished, and most neurons looked normal. However, a few neurons appeared to be as severely damaged as at the end of the seizure period (Fig. 10), evidently indicating an irreversible injury of these cells. A curtailment of the blood pressure rise in the early ictal phase reduced the degree of status spongiosus, but some dark condensed neurons could also be seen in these animals.

DISCUSSION

Because the EM study indicated that most intraneuronal vacuoles were dilated portions of rough endoplasmic reticulum, our results fail to support the suggestion of Meldrum and Brierley (6) that status epilepticus is associated with the same type of microvacuolation observed in hypoxia-ischemia.

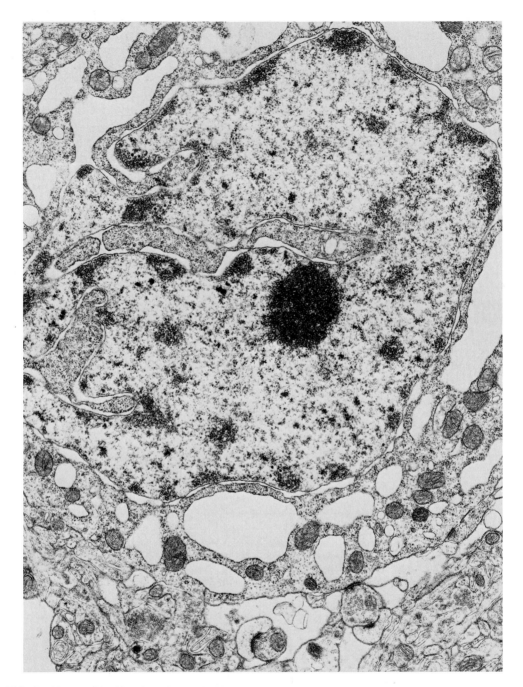

FIG. 9. Neuron with widened rough endoplasmic reticulum including the nuclear envelope. The mitochondria look normal.

Other studies have shown that status epilepticus can be associated with either minimal histopathological changes or none (3,7,8). In comparing different experimental studies, it is important to consider several variations in the experimental procedure. Because the lesions are largely reversible, killing the animal after a period of recovery may result in few conspicuous neuropathological changes

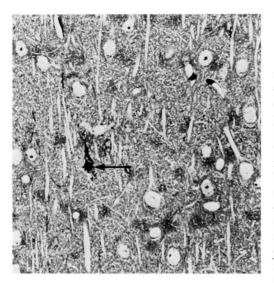

FIG. 10. Status epilepticus of 1 hr followed by diazepam-induced recovery for 2 hr. The edema in cortical layer 3 has practically disappeared. Among the mostly quite normal-appearing neurons there is one very darkly stained angular nerve cell (*arrow*) evidently undergoing disintegration. This suggests that a few cells may have become irreversibly injured. Epon + toluidine blue. × 404.

or none. Furthermore, as we have shown, the excessive blood pressure rise at the beginning of the seizure period aggravates the lesions. We have not studied the influence of compensation of the blood acidosis during bicuculline-induced seizures. Tentatively, acidosis could be a factor contributing to the lesions, and it should be taken into consideration when comparing our results with those of Brown et al. (3). Thus, in the experimental model used in that study, large amounts of bicarbonate were given during the seizures. Variations between species and even between different strains can be another factor of importance, as shown by Hicks and Coy (4).

CONCLUSIONS

Our study indicates that histopathological changes due to sustained bicuculline-induced seizures are different from the "ischemic nerve cell changes" with which the cell injury of status epilepticus was formerly considered identical. Instead, we observed pronounced structural alterations that were

of two types: (a) status spongiosus that evidently is caused mainly by swelling of the astrocytes and their processes; (b) two principal types of neuronal lesions characterized either by condensation of the neurons with perineuronal vacuoles or by intracytoplasmic slit-formed vacuoles, which are mainly dilated cisternae of the rough endoplasmic reticulum. Presumably the nerve cell changes are in some way linked to the edema developing during the seizures, and the nerve cell changes are largely reversible. However, some cells appear irreversibly damaged. Further, we cannot exclude the possibility that normal-appearing cells have suffered damages to structures remote from the cell body (e.g., their dendrites or the axon). However, a more precise evaluation of the entire neuron requires additional techniques like those of the Golgi methods or a combination of the Golgi methods and EM.

REFERENCES

1. Agardh, C.-D., Kalimo, H., Olsson, Y., and Siesjö, B. K. (1980): Hypoglycemic brain injury. I. Metabolic and light microscopic findings in rat cerebral cortex during profound insulin induced hypoglycemia and the recovery period following glucose administration. *Acta Neuropathol. (Berl.)*, 50:31–41.
2. Brown, A. W., and Brierley, J. B. (1972): Anoxic-induced cell change in rat brain. Light microscopic and fine-structured observations. *J. Neurol. Sci.*, 16:59–84.
3. Brown, W. J., Mitchell, A. G., Jr., Babb, T. L., and Crandall, P. H. (1980): Structural and physiologic studies in experimentally induced epilepsy. *Exp. Neurol.*, 69:543–562.
4. Hicks, S. P., and Coy, M. A. (1958): Pathologic effects of antimetabolites. *Arch. Pathol.*, 65:378–389.
5. Kalimo, H., Agardh, C.-D., Olsson, Y., and Siesjö, B. K. (1980): Hypoglycemic brain injury. II. Electron-microscopic findings in rat cerebral cortical neurons during profound insulin induced hypoglycemia and in the recovery period following glucose administration. *Acta Neuropathol. (Berl.)*, 50:43–52.
6. Meldrum, B. S., and Brierley, J. B. (1973): Prolonged epileptic seizures in primates: Ischemic cell change and its relation to ictal physiological events. *Arch. Neurol*, 28:10–17.
7. Purpura, D. P., and Gonzalez-Monteagudo, O. (1960): Acute effects of methoxypirdoxine on hippocampal end-blade neurons: An experimental study of "special pathoclisis" in the cerebral cortex. *J. Neuropathol. Exp. Neurol.*, 19:421–432.
8. Schwartz, I., Broggi, G., and Pappas, G. D. (1970): Fine structure of rat hippocampus during sustained seizures. *Brain Res.*, 18:176–180.

*Advances in Neurology, Vol. 34: Status
Epilepticus,* edited by A.V. Delgado-Escueta,
C.G. Wasterlain, D.M. Treiman, and R.J. Porter.
Raven Press, New York © 1983.

17

Mechanisms Underlying Interictal-Ictal Transitions

D. A. Prince, B. W. Connors, and L. S. Benardo

In this chapter we shall review some potential mechanisms for the development of isolated interictal neuronal discharges and their conversion to those that characterize ictal episodes. Although the continuum from normal neuronal activity to interictal activity, to ictal episodes, and finally to repeated ictal episodes or status epilepticus appears to be one of gradually increasing excitability, we should not assume that the same mechanisms are necessarily responsible for the transitions at all steps. In other words, the factors leading from normal to interictal discharge may be quite different from those that lead to repeated ictal episodes. We shall first discuss the development of interictal discharges and then some factors that might lead to interictal-ictal transitions.

DEVELOPMENT OF INTERICTAL DISCHARGES

By now it has been well established that large depolarization shifts (DSs) of the resting membrane potential, which are associated with bursts of spike activity, are the events that underlie interictal epileptiform discharges in neurons of a variety of experimental epileptiform foci; see the work by Prince (46) for a review. Recent data from slices of excised epileptogenic cortex in humans (51) suggest that similar depolarizing envelopes are characteristic of neurons in human epileptogenic

neocortex. The general similarities in the neuronal events underlying interictal epileptogenesis in chronic epileptiform foci of monkey neocortex studied *in vivo* (Fig. 1A), guinea pig neocortex studied during penicillin epileptogenesis *in vitro* (Fig. 1B), and human epileptiform neocortex studied *in vitro* (Fig. 1C) are consistent with the possibility that similar mechanisms give rise to such discharges. It is important to emphasize, however, that a variety of mechanisms could account for

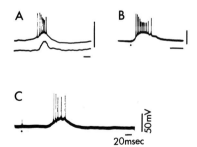

FIG. 1. Depolarization shifts during neocortical epileptogenesis. **A:** Intracellular recording (upper trace) and EEG (lower trace) from alumina-cream-induced epileptogenic focus in monkey neocortex. (From Prince and Futamachi, ref. 47, with permission.) **B:** Intracellular recording from neuron in neocortical slice exposed to penicillin. **C:** Intracellular recording from neuron in human epileptogenic slice. (From Prince and Wong, ref. 51, with permission.) Event in **A** was spontaneous. DSs in **B** and **C** evoked by orthodromic stimulation *(dots)*. Calibrations in **A** and **B:** 20 msec, 50 mV.

burst generation and that these may vary at different sites in the brain, as will be discussed later.

An analysis of data obtained over the last 5 years from neurons of hippocampal and neocortical slice preparations has led to identification of at least three principal underlying pathophysiological events that contribute to the conversion of normal neuronal activities to those of interictal discharges. These processes include alterations in the balance between inward Ca^{2+} and Na^+ currents and outward K^+ currents, disinhibition, and increases in the summated amplitude or duration of EPSPs in a population of neurons. These basic alterations in the regulation of neuronal excitability are intimately linked, for reasons that will be discussed later.

Mechanisms of Burst Generation in Hippocampal Pyramidal Neurons: Roles of Inward Ca^{2+} and Na^+ and Outward K^+ Currents

Studies of the effects of convulsant drugs on neuronal activities in hippocampal slices (52–54) have given rise to several important findings relevant to the mechanisms of epileptogenesis. First, as can be seen in Fig. 2, convulsant drugs such as penicillin can give rise to changes in extracellular field potentials (Fig. 2A) and intracellular activities (Fig. 2B1–2) that are very similar to those occurring in acute epileptiform foci *in vivo* (13). A second important point illustrated in Fig. 2 is that different regions within a single hippocampal slice appear to have different susceptibilities to the development of epileptiform discharge. For example, although extracellular burst activity can be seen in recordings from the CA3 and CA1 regions (Fig. 2A3), the pacemaker population for such discharges resides in the CA3 pyramidal cell region. This is supported by the observation that extracellular burst activity that results from synchronous DS generation in the population of CA3 cells is eliminated in the CA1 region, but persists in CA3, after the Schaffer collaterals that connect these two areas are cut (Fig. 2A4). Other observations have shown that the granule cell region in the dentate gyrus does not generate epileptiform field potentials under the same experimental circumstances (53). Intracellular recordings from granule cells have shown that these elements do not generate DSs when exposed to convulsant agents (18). Possible reasons for this variable involvement of different cell groups in epileptogenesis will be discussed later. A third and unexpected finding in hippocampal slice experiments is that, in some neurons, DSs associated with epileptiform field potentials (Fig. 2B1) can be blocked by hyperpolarizing current pulses (Fig. 2B2–4), suggesting that intrinsic membrane events contribute significantly to the generation of the slow membrane depolarization underlying the burst of spikes.

The CA3 pyramidal neurons, which serve as pacemakers for epileptiform discharges in the slice, tend to generate spontaneous asynchronous burst discharges under normal (nonepileptogenic) conditions (35,60). The mechanisms underlying this burst generation have recently been examined (60,62). Single fast spikes in CA3 pyramidal neu-

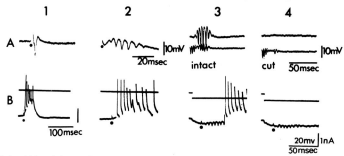

FIG. 2. Extracellular **(A)** and intracellular **(B)** activities from hippocampal slices. **A1–2:** Evoked responses in stratum pyramidale of CA1 following orthodromic stimulation in stratum radiatum *(dots)* before **(A1)** and after **(A2)** perfusion with solution containing penicillin. **A3:** Spontaneous epileptiform field potentials in CA1 (upper trace) and CA3 (lower trace) regions. **A4:** Following section of stratum radiatum between CA1 and CA3; epileptiform field potential persists in CA3 but disappears in CA1. **B1:** Orthodromically evoked DS in CA1 pyramidal neuron with succeeding hyperpolarization. **B2–4:** Intracellular recording in another CA1 neuron at resting membrane potential **(B2)** and during increasing intracellular hyperpolarizing current pulses that delay **(B3)** and block **(B4)** the DS and spike burst. Calibrations in **A2** for **A1–2,** in **A4** for **A3–4,** and in **B4** for **B2–4.** (**A** from Schwartzkroin and Prince, ref. 53, with permission; **B** from Schwartzkroin and Prince, ref. 52, with permission.)

rons are followed by a depolarizing afterpotential (DAP) (35) that seems to be mediated by inward movements of Ca^{2+} (62). Bursting occurs when DAPs following each fast spike summate until higher-threshold slow spikes are evoked. These latter events are primarily Ca^{2+}-mediated as well, although it is not clear whether or not two separate Ca^{2+} channels are involved in DAP and Ca^{2+} spike generation. The slow depolarization of the CA3 pyramidal cell burst is terminated by a hyperpolarization that presumably is due to a Ca^{2+}-activated K^+ conductance (1,30,62). When a Ca^{2+} blocker such as Mn^{2+} is used in the perfusion solution, the slow envelope of the normal CA3 burst is entirely blocked, although fast spikes can still be elicited with direct intracellular depolarization. These findings and the results of voltage clamp studies on CA3 neurons (34) show that spontaneous burst generation in CA3 neurons occurs as a result of voltage-dependent inward Ca^{2+} currents.

Depolarization in hippocampal CA1 pyramidal cells also activates presumed inward Ca^{2+} and Na^+ currents, as well as outward K^+ currents (32). Intrinsic burst tendencies are more variable in this population. In neurons with prominent outward currents, depolarization will not give rise to bursts; however, a change in the balance between inward and outward currents (i.e., an increase in inward current or a decrease in outward current) in a susceptible cell will allow it to generate bursts. Similar mechanisms for burst generation are well known in molluscan neurons (9,15,59). This leads to the prediction that burst behavior will be initiated in CA1 neurons by maneuvers that decrease outward (K^+) currents. It might also be suggested that if intrinsic burst-generating capacities play an important role in epileptiform burst generation, neurons such as granule cells of the dentate gyrus, which normally do not generate epileptiform bursts following convulsant drug exposure, will have a low capacity for intrinsic burst generation and will be less affected by K^+-channel blockers or facilitation of inward currents than will susceptible neurons such as CA3 or CA1 pyramidal cells. These predictions are confirmed by data from experiments shown in Figs. 3 and 4. Normal responses to synaptic (Fig. 3A1) and direct (Fig. 3A2) depolarization in hippocampal CA1 pyramidal cells are converted to prolonged depolarizing envelopes with multiple spike generation after intracellular injection of tetraethylammonium ions, whose pre-

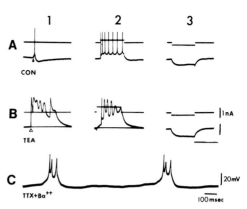

FIG. 3. A: Control responses to orthodromic stimulation (**A1**) and depolarizing and hyperpolarizing current pulses (**A2–3**) in a CA1 pyramidal neuron. **B:** Responses to antidromic stimulation (**B1**) and depolarizing and hyperpolarizing current pulses (**B2–3**) after intracellular injection of tetraethylammonium ions in another neuron. **C:** Rhythmic depolarizations and bursts of spikes from CA1 neuron in solution containing Ba^{2+} and tetrodotoxin. (**A** and **B** from Schwartzkroin and Prince, ref. 55, with permission; **C** adapted from Hotson and Prince, ref. 31.)

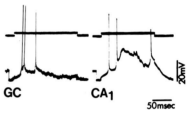

FIG. 4. Intracellular recordings from a granule cell of the dentate gyrus (GC) and a CA1-region pyramidal cell (CA1) recorded from the same slice in a solution containing 0.1-mM Ba^{2+}. Intracellular depolarization evokes a few spikes in the GC, and by contrast the CA1 pyramidal neuron generates a large depolarization shift unrelated to the current intensity. Calibration pulses are included at the onset of each sweep.

dominant action is to block voltage-dependent potassium conductance (gK) (Fig. 3B1-2). Ba^{2+} ions, which move through Ca^{2+} channels more readily than Ca^{2+} (24) and also block K^+ conductance (25,37,39), also give rise to burst generation in CA1 neurons, even in the presence of tetrodotoxin, which blocks voltage-dependent Na^+ conductances. Under these conditions the spontaneous slow depolarizations and bursts of spike potentials that occur must be mediated entirely by Ba^{2+} and Ca^{2+} (Fig. 3C). Other experiments (18) have shown that granule cells are much less susceptible to such maneuvers than are CA1 pyramidal cells. For instance, the granule cell and CA1 pyramidal cell shown in Fig. 4 were recorded in the same slice during exposure to 0.1-mM Ba^{2+}-containing medium. At this concentration of Ba^{2+}, depolarizing pulses in the CA1 neuron elicit large DS-like potentials and spontaneous burst responses (not shown), whereas granule cells show only small depolarizations and a few spikes during similar current pulses. Other maneuvers, such as increases in $[K^+]_o$ from levels of 3 or 5 mM to 10 mM, can regularly evoke bursts in populations of CA3 and CA1 pyramidal neurons, as judged by the multiphasic evoked field potentials and intracellular recordings (49,50), although similar increases in $[K^+]_o$ do not elicit burst generation in neocortical or dentate gyrus granule cells of *in vitro* slices (19). These effects of increasing $[K^+]_o$ on pyramidal neurons may be due to shifts in the equilibrium potential for K^+ that result in smaller outward currents, an effect that can in turn increase the net inward current underlying the DS slow envelope. A similar effect has been proposed to explain burst generation in motoneurons exposed to penicillin (56).

Burst generation in individual neurons through the mechanisms described will not be an adequate explanation for the synchronous bursting in groups of neurons that characterizes epileptogenesis. Additional mechanisms are required, as will be discussed.

Disinhibition

If, as suggested earlier, intrinsic burst-generating capabilities play a major role in the genesis of interictal epileptiform discharges in some neurons, one might question how a convulsant agent such as penicillin gives rise to synchronous DSs in populations of neurons. Recent experiments on CA1 pyramidal cells have shown that penicillin does not affect resting membrane properties (54) or intrinsic events mediated by Ca^{2+} or K^+ conductances (31). However, there have been repeated demonstrations that penicillin can antagonize the effects of γ-aminobutyric acid (GABA), as well as reduce presumed GABA-mediated synaptic inhibition in neurons of invertebrates (29,44) and vertebrates (12,14,28,54,61). After release of a population of neurons from some of the modulatory influences of synaptic inhibition, intrinsic bursting capabilities and excitatory interconnectivity may combine to produce synchronous, explosive paroxysmal events.

Some of the mechanisms underlying penicillin-induced DS generation have been examined by recording from dendrites of hippocampal CA1 and

CA3 neurons (61,63). Under normal circumstances, pyramidal cell dendrites generate EPSP-IPSP sequences following orthodromic (stratum radiatum) stimuli (Fig. 5B). However, direct depolarization of the same dendrite (by injecting current through the recording electrode) can lead to intrinsic burst generation associated with fast (Na^+) and slow (Ca^{2+}) spikes (Fig. 5A,C). Following application of penicillin, recordings from the same dendrite show that orthodromic stimuli become effective in evoking bursts identical with those previously produced only by intracellular depolarization (Fig. 5C–D). When the dendrite is hyperpolarized during the orthodromic stimulus under these conditions, the burst is blocked, and an underlying EPSP is uncovered (Fig. 5D, lower superimposed trace). Field-potential recordings have shown that penicillin has given rise to synchronous spontaneous (Fig. 5E) and orthodromically evoked (Fig. 5F) burst discharges in large groups of neurons. In other words, the EPSPs of penicillin-treated dendrites can trigger intrinsic bursts. The mechanism for this change in behavior lies in the blockade of the IPSP by penicillin (14,61). The IPSP, presumably by producing membrane hyperpolari-

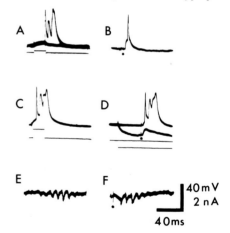

FIG. 5. Intracellular recordings from CA1 pyramidal cell dendrite. **A:** Intracellular depolarizing pulse evokes a burst of spikes at threshold. **B:** Orthodromic stimulation in stratum radiatum evokes an EPSP-IPSP with a single associated spike in the same dendrite. **C–D:** After penicillin application, both intracellular depolarization (**C**) and orthodromic stimulation (**D**) evoke burst discharges similar to those in the control sweep of **A**. Hyperpolarizing current pulse uncovers a long-lasting underlying EPSP in **D** (lower superimposed trace). The same penicillin application gives rise to spontaneous (**E**) and evoked (**F**) field-potential bursts. Calibrations in **F** for all sweeps. (Adapted from Wong and Prince, ref. 61.)

zation and increased conductance for Cl^-, diminishes the effectiveness of the orthodromic EPSP and shunts the inward currents carried by Ca^{2+} and Na^+ so that the threshold for burst generation is not normally reached.

Giant EPSPs

The hypothesis that "giant EPSPs" make significant contributions to generation of DSs has been critically reviewed elsewhere (46). One defining characteristic of epileptic events is that they are highly synchronous among a large proportion of neurons within a population. There is little doubt that excitatory synaptic interconnections form the major mechanism for such synchronization. As we have discussed, convulsant agents such as penicillin may cause a release from some synaptic inhibitions, but how this may affect the aggregate excitatory synaptic activity in a highly convergent network is difficult to predict. Certainly the functional bulk of interconnectivity (comprised of the number, location, and efficacy of interneuronal contacts) is decisively important, but other phenomena peculiar to the pathophysiology of the epileptic state probably also contribute. For example, bursts of action potentials arise in presynaptic terminals within epileptic foci (22,42); these may propagate orthodromically and antidromically and contribute to the spatial and temporal dissemination of paroxysms.

Whatever their origin, there are two basic properties of interictal synaptic drives that may distinguish them from the normal state: their synchrony and their size. Although synaptic synchrony would seem to be an absolute requirement for phase locking large numbers of cells, there is no strict *a priori* reason for such synaptic activity to be of abnormally large amplitude when viewed at the level of the single cell. The characteristic size of the interictal synaptic generator may vary critically between neuronal systems. For example, EPSPs recorded from somata of CA1 pyramidal cells do not grow in amplitude following penicillin treatment (54); yet dendritic recordings under these conditions reveal that increases in EPSP duration may be sufficient to trigger intrinsic burst discharges (61). Because hippocampal pyramidal cells retain large voltage-dependent inward currents, it is difficult to separate synaptic events from intrinsic events experimentally; however, portions of the DS envelope can be blocked with hyperpolarization, exposing apparent underlying EPSPs of variable size (52–54), some of which may be quite large in amplitude, e.g., Fig. 10 of Schwartzkroin and Prince (54). Recent studies in CA3 pyramidal cells (33) have also shown that large spontaneous synaptic events (termed giant EPSPs) underlie the penicillin-induced synchronized bursting. In these CA3 neurons, large inward Na^+ and Ca^{2+} currents activated by synaptic depolarization would serve to amplify and sustain membrane activity (34,60, 62).

The evidence favoring contributions of large-amplitude EPSPs to the envelope of slow depolarization in neocortical penicillin foci has been summarized elsewhere (2,45,46). Recent experiments in isolated slices of neocortex (21) have emphasized that the mechanisms of DS generation may be somewhat different from those in hippocampus. The response of a typical neocortical neuron in a penicillin-treated slice to orthodromic stimulation is shown in Fig. 1B. In neocortical neurons, spikes superimposed on DSs usually are of short duration, suggesting that Ca^{2+} spikes do not contribute to the burst. Tetrodotoxin-resistant, presumed Ca^{2+} spikes are extremely rare during intracellular depolarization in normal medium. In contrast to the situation in hippocampal pyramidal cells, where an important component of the DS slow envelope appears to derive from summation of spike depolarizing afterpotentials, DSs in penicillin-treated neocortical slices persist after all superimposed spikes are blocked during intense hyperpolarizations. Further, it has only rarely been possible to evoke a slow depolarizing envelope and burst in a neocortical neuron with depolarizing current pulses under normal recording conditions. This behavior stands in marked contrast to that of most hippocampal pyramidal cells and suggests that neocortical neurons have much less pronounced capacities for intrinsic burst generation. This is not to imply that slow Na^+ and Ca^{2+} currents are not present in neocortical cells. Ca^{2+}-dependent conductances can be easily revealed by appropriate pharmacological manipulations (21). Intracellular injections of Cs^+, which blocks some gKs, can lead to the development of slow spikes during DSs (Fig. 6, 0 nA) and on direct depolarization (not shown). These slow spikes are presumably mediated by Ca^{2+} and Na^+. Because of the blockade of gK and the resulting increase in input resistance, large changes in membrane potential are produced

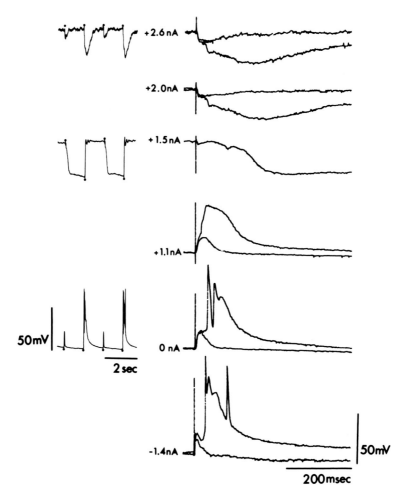

FIG. 6. Orthodromically evoked depolarization shift in penicillin-treated guinea pig neocortical slice. Recordings were made with a 1-M Cs⁺ acetate-filled microelectrode to block K⁺ conductances. Orthodromic stimuli alternately evoke large DSs and EPSPs. **Left:** Inkwriter traces of evoked DSs and EPSPs when membrane potential is at resting level (0 nA) and during application of constant depolarizing current through recording electrode (+1.5 and +2.6 nA). **Right:** Data from same experiment on expanded time scale. Two consecutive stimuli are superimposed in each case. At rest, burst is evoked by every other stimulus. At intermediate current levels, spikes are inactivated (+1.1 nA), and a region of instability is encountered (+1.5 nA), presumably because of the close balance between slowly inactivating inward and outward membrane currents. With electrode currents of +2.0 and +2.6 nA, the underlying synaptic potentials are inverted, and alternate stimuli evoked synaptic events of larger amplitude and longer duration that presumably are associated with DS generation.

in Cs⁺-filled neurons during intracellular current injections. Not only do neocortical neuronal DSs persist during intense hyperpolarization (Fig. 6, −1.4 nA), but also during intense depolarization it appears that orthodromically evoked DSs may be inverted to negative-going events at potentials close to 0 mV (Fig. 6, +2.6 nA). This suggests that EPSPs may play the major role in neocortical DS generation. Thus the relative contributions of intrinsic currents and excitatory synaptic potentials

to DS generation seem to vary considerably in different brain regions.

Although chemically mediated EPSPs provide the most obvious substrate for neuronal synchronization, recently described anatomical and physiological data show that cells of both hippocampus (38) and neocortex (23) are electrically coupled to each other. The extent to which this flexible but potentially powerful mechanism contributes to focal epileptogenesis is not yet known.

TRANSITIONS FROM INTERICTAL TO ICTAL DISCHARGE

The mechanisms that underlie the development of the ictal episode have not been as carefully examined as those responsible for interictal discharges; however, it is probable that certain events that are known to occur during this transition have an important role. Among such events are (a) changes in the ionic microenvironment, with increases in extracellular potassium concentration ($[K^+]_0$) and decreases in extracellular calcium ($[Ca^{2+}]_0$), (b) long-duration alterations in the balance between Ca^{2+}, Na^+, and K^+ currents, resulting in prolonged net inward currents, (c) axonal burst generation, and (d) effects on transmitters and modulators such as acetylcholine.

Intracellular recordings in neocortex have shown that the transition from interictal to ictal discharge is characterized by a gradual loss of post-DS afterhyperpolarizations, with subsequent development of prolonged afterdepolarizations that trigger multiple spike discharges, initiating the tonic phase of the ictal episode (3). Although it had previously been assumed that these transitions were the result of prolonged temporally summated EPSPs, other alternatives now seem equally likely.

Alterations in Ionic Microenvironment

Studies with ion-sensitive microelectrodes have shown that there are significant increases in $[K^+]_0$ during closely spaced interictal discharges (41, 48,57). Although such measurements suggested that there was no distinct threshold at which increases in $[K^+]_0$ led to generation of seizures in the hippocampus (16), experiments in hippocampal slices have clearly shown that iatrogenic increases in $[K^+]_0$ in the bathing medium similar to those that occur during interictal epileptiform discharges can provoke epileptiform discharges in "normal" slices or facilitate the development of penicillin-induced epileptiform discharges; see Figs. 2 and 3 of Prince and Schwartzkroin (50). Decreases in $[Ca^{2+}]_0$ also occur during interictal activity (7,27,58), and although these are not sufficiently large to block EPSPs, they could tend to destabilize the membrane by decreasing divalent cation screening effects (17). Although increases in $[K^+]_0$ might have effects on synaptic events and produce small depolarizations in neurons, such changes would also produce a positive shift in the equilibrium potential for K^+ and would decrease

K^+ currents, effects that might result in prolonged burst discharges akin to those that occur following application of Ba^{2+} (30,31) or tetraethylammonium (55) to hippocampal pyramidal neurons.

Cholinergic Modulation of Neuronal Properties

Recent *in vitro* experiments (4,5) have identified the muscarinic actions of acetylcholine (ACh) as another potential mechanism underlying both the transition from normal activity to interictal discharges and the subsequent progression to the ictal state. Brief ACh applications onto hippocampal CA1 neurons induce transient slow depolarization and long-term increases in cell membrane input resistance (R_N) (Figs. 7A and 8). This persistent increase in R_N has a prominent voltage-dependent component (Fig. 8) and is associated with the de-

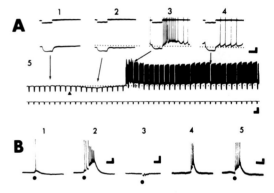

FIG. 7. Effects of ACh application on CA1 hippocampal pyramidal neurons. **A:** The response of one neuron to focal application of ACh (50 mM) is shown. Triangle in the chart record **A5** indicates the time of application. Sweeps in **A1**–4 were obtained at times indicated by arrows. Upper traces in 1–4 are current monitor; lower traces are intracellular records. Membrane potential hyperpolarizes by 4 mV, and R_N decreases from 40 MΩ (**A1**) to 29 MΩ (**A2**). **A3:** Membrane subsequently depolarizes by 10 mV with concomitant rapid firing. **A4:** R_N increases to 69 MΩ, and the cell remains depolarized by about 4 mV. **B:** Long-term effects of ACh exposure. Dots in **B1**–3: Orthodromic stimuli in stratum radiatum. **B2:** Same cell as **B1** 4 min following ACh application. **B3:** Field-potential recording from another experiment approximately 1 to 2 hr after ACh application. **B4:** Spontaneous burst from a neuron in an area previously exposed to ACh. **B5:** Burst evoked by 1-msec intracellular depolarizing pulse *(dot)* in same cell as **B4**. Calibrations in **A4** for sweeps of **A:** vertical bar, 10 mV and 0.5 nA; horizontal bar, 100 msec. Calibrations in **A5:** vertical bar, 10 mV and 0.5 nA; horizontal bar, 1 sec. **B2:** 10 mV and 60 msec for **B1** and **B2**. **B3:** 10 mV and 20 msec. **B5:** 10 mV and 60 msec for **B4** and **B5**. (Adapted from Benardo and Prince, ref. 5).

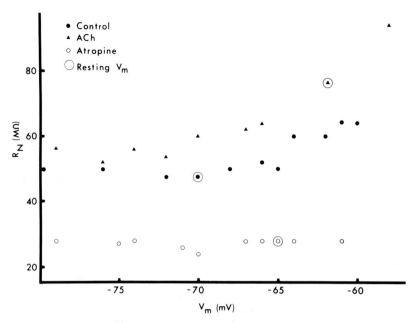

FIG. 8. Plots of input resistance (R_N) versus membrane potential (V_m) in one neuron before (filled circles) and after (filled triangles) an iontophoretic application of ACh and from a neuron in another slice bathed in solution containing 10^{-7}-M atropine (small open circles). Large circles indicate resting V_m for each neuron. Anomalous (inward) rectification is evident in data from typical control neuron (filled circle). Following ACh application to the same cell, increases in R_N occur, both in the range of anomalous rectification and at more hyperpolarized levels (filled triangles). Note also that the cell shown is depolarized by 8 mV from the control resting V_m. (From Benardo and Prince, ref. 5, with permission.)

velopment of burst generation (Fig. 7B2,4,5), which can occur synchronously in the population as evidenced by the appearance of multiphasic field potentials (Fig. 7B3).

Further studies (6) on the ionic mechanisms of ACh excitation have demonstrated that this substance acts to reduce both the Ca^{2+}-activated gK that is prominent in CA1 pyramidal neurons (30) and a voltage-dependent gK similar to that underlying the "m current" in sympathetic ganglion cells (8). The consequences of such effects are to shift the balance between inward and outward currents so that net inward movements of Ca^{2+} and Na^+ are favored, in the manner described earlier. DSs occurring during epileptogenesis resulting from the actions of ACh are therefore most likely due to alterations in intrinsic membrane properties. The actions of ACh are quite similar to those of Ba^{2+}; in fact, these two agents seem to act on the same ionophore (6,11). Thus the predictions from pharmacological studies of the effects of impeded K^+ currents on cell behavior (Fig. 3B) are corroborated by experiments examining the effects of ACh, an endogenous transmitter substance that decreases gK.

It has also been shown that these actions of ACh can be blocked by atropine, a muscarinic antagonist, and that the properties of normal hippocampal pyramidal neurons are altered by atropine (Fig. 8) and eserine in directions that suggest that a tonic effect of ACh to increase R_N is present under normal conditions (5). Thus, cholinergic activity may play an important role in epileptogenesis. If large amounts of ACh were released, or if some failure in hydrolysis due to deficiencies in acetylcholinesterase were present (26), epileptiform discharge could result. ACh release during any type of interictal activity would increase the effectiveness of other excitatory inputs. Such modulatory actions might give rise to ictal events, particularly in situations where increased epileptiform activity would in turn give rise to more ACh release. The long-term or tonic ACh effects would tend to make a large population of neurons vulnerable to additional seizure activity once frequent interictal discharge or an ictal episode had occurred.

Axonal Burst Generation

Although the foregoing discussion has been oriented toward activities in neuronal cell bodies and dendrites, it is important to note that the conductances in membranes of axonal terminal regions may be quite similar to those in dendrites. Terminals are known to have the capacity to generate Ca^{2+} spikes (40), and they have significant K^+ conductances (36). It is known that axonal terminals can be induced to generate burst discharges following exposure to some drugs (20) and possibly during alterations in the ionic milieu. Studies of the behavior of thalamocortical axons in acute epileptiform foci (22,42) and during electrically induced neocortical seizures (43) have shown that axonal terminals burst during interictal discharges and generate progressively longer runs of spike activity during interictal-ictal transitions. These bursts, which can be detected as antidromically invading spikes in the cell bodies of thalamocortical relay neurons, presumably propagate into axonal arborizations, where they result in intense release of transmitter. Because of the remarkable divergent distribution of axonal arborizations of relay cells onto cortical neurons (10), such terminal bursting might have an important synchronizing effect on cortical neuronal populations. It should be noted that bursts generated in axons would not be under inhibitory control of the remote somata. The reasons for development of these axonal burst discharges are not known; however, it might be suggested that the increases in $[K^+]_0$, decreases in $[Ca^{2+}]_0$, and potential influences of ACh on nonjunctional muscarinic receptors of axonal terminals might all be factors leading to this phenomenon.

CONCLUSIONS

The data currently available suggest that an interaction between intrinsic burst-generating capacities, disinhibition, and synchronous EPSPs in populations of neurons can convert normal neuronal activities to those characterized as interictal discharges, i.e., synchronous depolarization shifts in large groups of neurons. The extent to which each of these factors plays a role will vary in different neuronal cell groups. Processes that cause intense synchronization, prolonged depolarizations, and loss of intrinsic control mechanisms may facilitate transitions from interictal to ictal discharges. Among these, alterations in the extracellular microenvironment with large increases in $[K^+]_0$, or other processes that tend to decrease K^+ currents, allowing large Ca^{2+}- and Na^+-induced depolarizations to occur, probably are very im-

portant. Certain modulatory effects such as a muscarinic ACh action may produce large shifts in this balance between inward and outward currents that are very long lasting. We would speculate that both increases in $[K^+]_0$ and actions of ACh to decrease gK might underlie the development of prolonged burst discharges in axonal terminals. Such discharges, in turn, might account for massive releases of transmitter that facilitate the development of the avalanche of excitation that characterizes the ictal episode. Other mechanisms have been less carefully examined, but electrical coupling among large neuronal aggregates, and other processes that have not been investigated in neocortical neurons, might have important roles in transitions between interictal and ictal discharges. Whether or not these mechanisms, or others in addition, lead to the emergence of recurrent ictal activity (status epilepticus) is not known, but obviously this will be an issue of great importance in future studies.

ACKNOWLEDGMENTS

We thank R. Fricke, M. Gutnick, and R. Wong for their valuable contributions to the unpublished work cited here and Jay Kadis and Cheryl Joo for technical and secretarial assistance.

This work was supported by NIH grants NS-06477 and NS-12151 from the National Institute of Neurological and Communicative Disorders and Stroke (D.A.P.), NIH postdoctoral fellowship (B.W.C.), and NSF predoctoral fellowship (L.S.B.).

REFERENCES

1. Alger, B. E., and Nicoll, R. A. (1980): Epileptiform burst after hyperpolarization: Calcium-dependent potassium potential in hippocampal CA1 pyramidal cells. *Science*, 210:1122–1124.
2. Ayala, G. F., Dichter, M., Gumnit, R. J., Matsumoto, H., and Spencer, W. A. (1973): Genesis of epileptic interictal spikes: New knowledge of cortical feedback systems suggests a neurophysiological explanation of brief paroxysms. *Brain Res.*, 52:1–17.
3. Ayala, G. F., Matsumoto, H., and Gumnit, R. J. (1970): Excitability changes and inhibitory mechanisms in neocortical neurons during seizures. *J. Neurophysiol.*, 33:73–85.
4. Benardo, L. S., and Prince, D. A. (1980): Acetylcholine: A neuromodulator of hippocampal pyramidal neurons. *Neurosci. Abstr.*, 6:514 (abstract 178.3).
5. Benardo, L. S., and Prince, D. A. (1981): Acetylcholine induced modulation of hippocampal pyramidal neurons. *Brain Res.*, 211:227–234.
6. Benardo, L. S., and Prince, D. A. (1982): Ionic mechanisms of cholinergic excitation in mammalian hippocampal pyramidal cells. *Brain Res. (in press).*

7. Benninger, C., Kadis, J., and Prince, D. A. (1980): Extracellular calcium and potassium changes in hippocampal slices. *Brain Res.*, 187:165–182.

8. Brown, D. A., and Adams, P. R. (1980): Muscarinic suppression of a novel voltage-sensitive K^+ current in a vertebrate neurone. *Nature*, 283:673–676.

9. Carnevale, N. T., and Wachtel, H. (1980): Two reciprocating current components underlying slow oscillations in *Aplysia* bursting neurons. *Brain Res. Rev.*, 203:45–68.

10. Colonnier, M. L. (1966): The structural design of the neocortex. In: *Brain and Conscious Experience*, edited by J. C. Eccles, pp. 1–23. Springer, Berlin.

11. Constanti, A., Adams, P. R., and Brown, D. A. (1981): Why do barium ions imitate acetylcholine? *Brain Res.*, 206:244–250.

12. Curtis, D. R., Game, C. J. A., Johnston, G. A. R., McCulloch, R. M., and MacLachlan, R. M. (1972): Convulsant action of penicillin. *Brain Res.*, 43:242–245.

13. Dichter, M., and Spencer, W. A. (1969): Penicillin-induced interictal discharges from the cat hippocampus. I. Characteristics and topographical features. *J. Neurophysiol.*, 32:649–662.

14. Dingledine, R., and Gjerstad, L. (1980): Reduced inhibition during epileptiform activity in the *in vitro* hippocampal slice. *J. Physiol. (Lond.)*, 305:297–314.

15. Ducreux, C., and Gola, M. (1975): On des paroxysmales induites par le metrazol (PTZ) sur les neurones d'Helix p.: modele fonctionnel. *Pfluegers Arch.*, 361:43–53.

16. Fisher, R. S., Pedley, T. A., Moody, W. J., Jr., and Prince, D. A. (1976): The role of extracellular potassium in hippocampal epilepsy. *Arch. Neurol.*, 33:76–83.

17. Frankenhaeuser, B., and Hodgkin, A. L. (1957): The action of calcium on the electrical properties of squid axons. *J. Physiol. (Lond.)*, 137:218–244.

18. Fricke, R., and Prince, D. A. (1981): unpublished data.

19. Fricke, R., Wong, R. K. S., and Prince, D. A. (1981): unpublished data.

20. Grundfest, H. (1966): Some determinants of repetitive electrogenesis and their role in the electrical activity of the central nervous system. In: *Comparative and Cellular Pathophysiology of Epilepsy* (proceedings of a symposium held in Liblice near Prague), edited by A. Bischoff and F. Luthy, pp. 19–42. Czechoslovak Academy of Sciences, Prague and Exerpta Medica Foundation, New York.

21. Gutnick, M. J., Connors, B. W., and Prince, D. A. (1981): Mechanisms of depolarization shift generation in the penicillin-treated neocortical slice. *Neurosci. Abstr.* 7:629.

22. Gutnick, M. J., and Prince, D. A. (1972): Thalamocortical relay neurons: Antidromic invasion of spikes from a cortical epileptogenic focus. *Science*, 176:424–426.

23. Gutnick, M. J., and Prince, D. A. (1981): Dye-coupling and possible electrotonic coupling in the guinea pig neocortical slice. *Science*, 211:67–70.

24. Hagiwara, S., Fukuda, J., and Eaton, D. C. (1974): Membrane currents carried by Ca, Sr, and Ba in barnacle muscle fiber during voltage clamp. *J. Gen. Physiol.*, 63:564–568.

25. Hagiwara, S., Miyazaki, S., Moody, W., and Patlak, J. (1978): Blocking effects of barium and hydrogen ions on the potassium current during anomalous rectification in the starfish egg. *J. Physiol. (Lond.)*, 279:167–185.

26. Hebb, C. O., Krnjevic, K., and Silver, A. (1963): Effects of undercutting on the acetylcholinesterase and choline acetyltransferase activity in the cat's cerebral cortex. *Nature*, 198:692.

27. Heinemann, U., Lux, H. D., and Gutnick, M. J. (1977): Extracellular free calcium and potassium during paroxysmal activity in the cerebral cortex of the cat. *Exp. Brain Res.*, 27:237–243.

28. Hill, R. G., Simmonds, M. A., and Straughan, D. W. (1976): Antagonism of γ-aminobutyric acid and glycine by convulsants in the cuneate nucleus of the cat. *Br. J. Pharmacol.*, 56:9–19.

29. Hochner, B., Spira, M. E., and Werman, R. (1976): Penicillin decreases chloride conductance in crustacean muscle: A model for the epileptic neuron. *Brain Res.*, 107:85–103.

30. Hotson, J. R., and Prince, D. A. (1980): A calcium activated hyperpolarization follows repetitive firing in hippocampal neurons. *J. Neurophysiol.*, 43:409–419.

31. Hotson, J. R., and Prince, D. A. (1981): Penicillin and Ba^{++}-induced bursting in hippocampal neurons: Actions on Ca^{++} and K^+ potentials. *Ann. Neurol.*, 10:11–17.

32. Hotson, J. R., Prince, D. A., and Schwartzkroin, P. A. (1979): Anomalous inward rectification in hippocampal neurons. *J. Neurophysiol.*, 42:889–895.

33. Johnston, D., and Brown, T. H. (1981): Giant synaptic potential hypothesis for epileptiform activity. *Science*, 211:294–297.

34. Johnston, D., Hablitz, J. J., and Wilson, W. A. (1980): Voltage clamp discloses slow inward current in hippocampal burst-firing neurones. *Nature*, 286:391–393.

35. Kandel, E. R., and Spencer, W. A. (1961): Electrophysiology of hippocampal neurons. II. Afterpotentials and repetitive firing. *J. Neurophysiol.*, 24:243–259.

36. Katz, B., and Miledi, R. (1969): Tetrodotoxin-resistant electrical activity in presynaptic terminals. *J. Physiol. (Lond.)*, 203:459–487.

37. Krnjevic, K., Pumain, R., and Renaud, L. (1971): Effects of Ba^{2+} and tetraethylammonium on cortical neurones. *J. Physiol. (Lond.)*, 215:223–245.

38. MacVicar, B. A., and Dudek, F. E. (1980): Dye-coupling between CA3 pyramidal cells in slices of rat hippocampus. *Brain Res.*, 196:494–497.

39. Meech, R. W., and Standen, N. B. (1975): Potassium activation in *Helix aspersa* neurones under voltage clamp: A component mediated by calcium influx. *J. Physiol. (Lond.)*, 249:211–239.

40. Miledi, R., and Slater, C. R. (1966): The action of calcium on neuronal synapses in the squid. *J. Physiol. (Lond.)*, 184:473–498.

41. Moody, W. J., Jr., Futamachi, K. J., and Prince, D. A. (1974): Extracellular potassium activity during epileptogenesis. *Exp. Neurol.*, 42:248–263.

42. Noebels, J. L., and Prince, D. A. (1978): The development of focal seizures in cerebral cortex: Role of

axon terminal bursting. *J. Neurophysiol.*, 41:1267–1281.

43. Noebels, J. L., and Prince, D. A. (1978): Excitability changes in thalamocortical relay neurons during synchronous discharges in cat neocortex. *J. Neurophysiol.*, 41:1282–1296.

44. Pellmar, T. C., and Wilson, W. A. (1977): Penicillin effects on iontophoretic responses in *Aplysia californica. Brain Res.*, 136:89–101.

45. Prince, D. A. (1976): Cellular activities in focal epilepsy. In: *Brain Dysfunction in Infantile Febrile Convulsions*, edited by M. A. B. Brazier and F. Coceani, pp. 187–212. Raven Press, New York.

46. Prince, D. A. (1978): Neurophysiology of epilepsy. *Ann. Rev. Neurosci.*, 1:395–415.

47. Prince, D. A., and Futamachi, K.-J. (1970): Intracellular recordings from chronic epileptogenic foci in the monkey. *Electroencephalogr. Clin. Neurophysiol.*, 29:496–510.

48. Prince, D. A., Lux, H. D., and Neher, E. (1973): Measurement of extracellular potassium activity in cat cortex. *Brain Res.*, 50:489–495.

49. Prince, D. A., Pedley, T. A., and Ransom, B. R. (1978): Fluctuations in ion concentrations during excitation and seizures. In: *Dynamic Properties of Glia Cells*, edited by G. Frank, L. Hertz, E. Schoeffeniels, and D. B. Tower, pp. 281–303. Pergamon Press, Elmsford, N.Y.

50. Prince, D. A., and Schwartzkroin, P. A. (1978): Nonsynaptic mechanisms in epileptogenesis. In: *Abnormal Neuronal Discharges*, edited by N. Chalazonitis and M. Boisson, pp. 1–12. Raven Press, New York.

51. Prince, D. A., and Wong, R. K. S. (1981): Human epileptic neurons studied *in vitro. Brain Res.*, 210:323–333.

52. Schwartzkroin, P. A., and Prince, D. A. (1977): Penicillin-induced epileptiform activity in the hippocampal *in vitro* preparation. *Ann. Neurol.*, 1:463–469.

53. Schwartzkroin, P. A., and Prince, D. A. (1978): Cellular and field potential properties of epileptogenic hippocampal slices. *Brain Res.*, 147:117–130.

54. Schwartzkroin, P. A., and Prince, D. A. (1980): Changes in excitatory and inhibitory synaptic potentials leading to epileptogenic activity. *Brain Res.*, 183:61–73.

55. Schwartzkroin, P. A., and Prince, D. A. (1980): Effects of TEA on hippocampal neurons. *Brain Res.*, 185:169–181.

56. Schwindt, P. C., and Crill, W. E. (1980): Role of a persistent inward current in motoneuron bursting during spinal seizures. *J. Neurophysiol.*, 43:1296–1318.

57. Somjen, G. G. (1979): Extracellular potassium in the mammalian central nervous system. *Ann. Rev. Physiol.*, 41:159–177.

58. Somjen, G. G. (1980): Stimulus-evoked and seizure-related responses of extracellular calcium activity in spinal cord compared to those in cerebral cortex. *J. Neurophysiol.*, 44:617–632.

59. Wilson, W. A., and Wachtel, H. (1974): Negative resistance characteristic essential for the maintenance of slow oscillations in bursting neurons. *Science*, 186:932–934.

60. Wong, R. K. S., and Prince, D. A. (1978): Participation of calcium spikes during intrinsic burst firing in hippocampal neurons. *Brain Res.*, 159:385–390.

61. Wong, R. K. S., and Prince, D. A. (1979): Dendritic mechanisms underlying penicillin-induced epileptiform activity. *Science*, 204:1228–1231.

62. Wong, R. K. S., and Prince, D. A. (1981): Afterpotential generation in hippocampal pyramidal cells. *J. Neurophysiol.*, 45:86–97.

63. Wong, R. K. S., Prince, D. A., and Basbaum, A. I. (1979): Intradendritic recordings from hippocampal neurons. *Proc. Natl. Acad. Sci. U.S.A.*, 76:986–990.

Advances in Neurology, Vol. 34: Status Epilepticus, edited by A.V. Delgado-Escueta, C.G. Wasterlain, D.M. Treiman, and R.J. Porter. Raven Press, New York © 1983.

18

Physiological Basis of Chronic Epilepsy and Mechanisms of Spread

Arthur A. Ward, Jr.

Status epilepticus may occur during the course of many of the epilepsies, but our knowledge of basic mechanisms is largely derived from studies of epileptic processes of focal origin. It appears that the best experimental model of human epilepsy of focal cortical onset is the chronic primate model in which focal scarring is induced in the sensorimotor cortex (20). To understand how spontaneous propagating seizures occur, and to form a basis for identifying some of the factors that may play a role in the production of status, it is first useful to summarize some of the properties of neurons in the chronic focus. Much of the data to be discussed were obtained in the chronic primate model, but most of the major properties of the experimental model have also been confirmed in epileptic foci in humans.

THE FOCUS

The chronic epileptic focus in both monkeys and humans contains neurons that autonomously fire in bursts (29). They are intrinsically hyperexcitable. A single "epileptic" neuron with such properties obviously cannot generate clinical seizures, but an adequate population of such epileptic neurons in a circumscribed region of cortex appears to constitute the essential feature of an epileptic focus. The data obtained over many years indicate that chronic foci are composed of neurons that

show a spectrum of intrinsic abnormalities ranging from neurons having normal physiological properties through a sequence to those that are highly epileptic and appear to serve as pacemakers to the focus. Under these circumstances, the pacemaker neurons are responsible for the focal epileptogenicity, and periodic clinical seizures are induced by recruiting surrounding neurons into bursting activity, thereby producing the necessary critical mass to induce a propagating seizure.

In awake monkeys or humans it is unusual for normal precentral neurons to fire with interspike intervals less than 5 msec. Epileptic neurons in monkeys and humans, on the other hand, are characterized by high-frequency bursts of action potentials with interspike intervals commonly less than 5 msec. Consequently, the percentage of interspike intervals lasting less than 5 msec (measured in a 15-sec epoch) is a reliable, objective measure of abnormal firing patterns of pyramidal neurons. This percentage has been termed the burst index. Under waking conditions, normal neurons have mean burst indexes less than 10%, whereas epileptic neurons have burst indexes greater than 10%.

Epileptic neurons, in turn, can be divided into two groups. Group 1 neurons (strongly epileptic or pacemaker neurons) fire almost exclusively in bursts and thus have high burst indexes (Fig. 1). In addition, their activity is stereotyped, and the

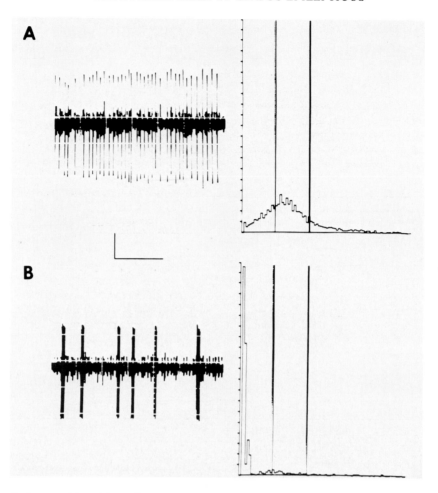

FIG. 1. Action potentials and interspike-interval histograms from a normal neuron (**A**) and an epileptic pacemaker neuron (**B**). Histograms are from 3 min of spontaneous activity. Calibration: 100 μV and 200 msec: cursors on histograms at 30 and 60 msec. (From Wyler et al., ref. 26, with permission.)

variability of their burst indexes is less than ± 10%, even when activities recorded during divergent behavioral states such as sleep and alert wakefulness are compared. Group 2 epileptic neurons have lower and extremely labile burst indexes, with a variablity greater than ± 10%. Foci are composed of a spectrum ranging from normal to pacemaker epileptic neurons.

Pacemaker neurons are believed to be intrinsically hyperexcitable, generating burst behavior as an all-or-nothing event. When a normal pyramidal neuron is antidromically activated, it responds with a single action potential. On the other hand, pacemaker epileptic neurons respond to such antidromic activation with a stereotyped high-frequency burst. Fetz (5) initially demonstrated that monkeys

could be operantly conditioned to increase or decrease the firing rates of single precentral neurons. In the epileptic focus, however, it has been shown that monkeys can operantly control the intervals between bursts but cannot control the interspike intervals that form the burst (28). Monkeys cannot operantly generate burst firing by increasing excitatory drive onto the neuron. Thus, it appears that although epileptogenic neurons may generate bursts intrinsically, the structure and occurrence of the burst are influenced by synaptic events.

Calvin et al. (4) have described neurons within the chronic monkey focus that fire with an unusual structured burst pattern. This burst, characterized by an initial action potential followed by an interval that is terminated by an extremely stereotyped "afterburst," has been called a long-first-interval burst. The long-first-interval epileptic bursts have been recorded only in animals with chronic foci induced in several ways. Subsequently, such bursts have been recorded from human epileptic cortex (3) (Fig. 2). In the monkey, it has been shown that such long-first-interval bursts are a property only of pyramidal tract neurons in the focus. There are other reasons to speculate that the mechanisms accounting for this very specialized type of burst firing require the geometry of dendritic arborizations that characterize such pyramidal cells (29).

Group 2 (weakly epileptic) neurons, in contrast, have lower mean burst indexes that vary significantly. Most important, the burst index is highly influenced by the behavioral state. When the monkey is attending to an operant task, the burst index may drop to zero, and the patterns of firing may be indistinguishable from those of a neuron in normal cortex. However, the same neuron during slow-wave sleep may exhibit dramatic burst firing, and the burst index may approach the same magnitude as for group 1 pacemaker neurons.

SEIZURE FREQUENCY AND PERCENTAGE OF PACEMAKER NEURONS

If, indeed, the epileptogenicity of the chronic focus is maintained by pacemaker epileptic neurons, it would be predicted that the proportion of such neurons within any one focus should correlate with the frequency of clinical seizures. To test this hypothesis, the activities of 1,617 neurons from 13 epileptic monkeys were systematically characterized (26). The spontaneous seizure frequencies in these animals represented a spectrum ranging from relatively infrequent seizures at one extreme to epilepsia partialis continua with continuous jerking of the contralateral hand in 2 animals. Of these 1,617 neurons, 25% were group 1 or pacemaker neurons; 32% were group 2 neurons, and 43% were normal. It should be noted that in animals with occasional seizures, almost half of the neurons in the electrographic focus were physiologically normal. Of those monkeys having less than one seizure per day, the percentage of group 1

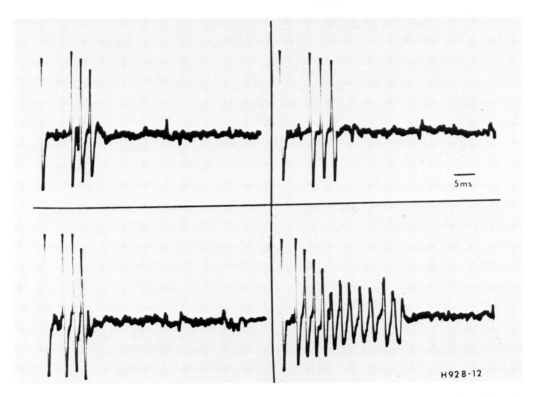

FIG. 2. Examples of structured epileptic burst activity from human epileptic foci. (From Calvin et al., ref. 3, with permission.)

highly epileptic neurons varied between 1% and 24%. The animal in whom only 1% of the recorded neurons were pacemaker neurons had, on the average, only one seizure every 10 days. The animal in whom 24% of the neurons were highly epileptic neurons was having slightly less than one seizure per day. At the other extreme were 2 animals with epilepsia partialis continua, with occasional secondarily generalized seizures as well. In these 2 highly epileptic animals, pacemaker neurons constituted 88% and 99% of all abnormal neurons recorded.

If one plots the percentage of epileptic neurons in the focus against seizure frequency (Fig. 3), the relationship is seen to be decidedly nonlinear and approximates a logarithmic function. The logarithmic correlation between this derived index of epileptogenicity and seizure frequency is highly significant ($r = 0.95$, $p < 0.001$). The fact that this relationship is logarithmic rather than linear is an indication of the power that pacemaker neurons exert on the recruitment of surrounding group 2 and normal neurons. It is apparent that only a small increment in the number of pacemaker neurons results in a much greater increase in clinical seizures. By the same reasoning, a modest reduction in the number of abnormally functioning neurons (e.g., by pharmacological means) could have major consequences in reducing seizure frequency.

These concepts may be relevant to strategies used in therapy for status epilepticus.

MECHANISMS OF SPREAD OF EPILEPTIC DISCHARGE

The foregoing factors may well account for the occurrence of epilepsia partialis continua, but they do not directly bear on the problem of status epilepticus consisting of repeated generalized seizures. Status requires frequent and rapid propagation of the seizure discharge widely through the brain.

The burst firing of epileptic neurons in the focus may have synaptic consequences not ordinarily considered in the usual models of transmission of signals in the central nervous system. The current conception of neuronal firing is that depolarizations of the neuronal membrane are converted into the firing rate of that neuron, which in turn induces net depolarizations at the next synapse. This "amplitude-to-frequency" model is supported by many studies of repetitive firing in cat motoneurons and studies of cortical neurons. A general theory of postsynaptic potential summation has been developed by Calvin (2), who has applied this theory to bursting synaptic inputs such as those generated by epileptic neurons.

The depolarization induced by a single synapse can be estimated from available data and usually attains a height of 0.5 mV (or less) and may decay

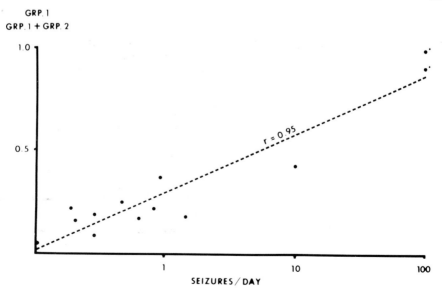

FIG. 3. Logarithmic plot of ratio pacemaker neurons to all epileptic neurons against seizure frequency for 13 epileptic monkeys. (From Wyler et al., ref. 26, with permission.)

exponentially with a 5-msec time constant. A typical active input can produce 20 spikes per second. Thus, in Calvin's computer-simulated model, the mean depolarization induced in the postsynaptic neuron from such activity in a single synapse would be only 50 mV (10% of the peak height). However, given 200 such synapses, a net average depolarization of 10 mV could be attained, which is about threshold for firing the postsynaptic cell. Thus, 2% of the 10,000 synapses on a motoneuron firing asynchronously could either elicit rhythmic firing from a previously silent cell or markedly increase a preexisting firing rate. Because group 1A afferents from muscle spindles account for only 2% of the synaptic inputs on a spinal motoneuron, the fact that a knee jerk can be obtained with ease indicates that this small number of synapses can be most effective. In addition, the data indicate that roughly four times this steady depolarization can often drive a cell to its high-frequency firing range. Thus, 8% of a motoneuron's synapses, firing at a nominal 20/sec each, could drive a normal cell to high firing rates. Because a neuron in the motor cortex has some 60,000 synapses, presumably 1.3% of its synapses firing at these nominal rates could generate high-frequency firing.

This is the situation for normal neurons. Epileptic neurons, on the other hand, instead of firing at 20/sec, often fire at rates of 200 to 900/sec during their bursts. Making the conservative assumption of only 200/sec rates within an epileptic burst, this output from an epileptic neuron need only project to 80 synapses on a normal neuron to cause high-frequency firing in that normal cell. Thus, only 0.13% of the 60,000 synapses on a normal cortical neuron need to be driven by burst firing from an epileptic neuron to convert this normal cell into one also generating high-frequency firing. It is apparent that this packaging of action potentials into bursts generates a much higher depolarization in the postsynaptic cell than the same number of action potentials from a normal cell firing randomly at 20/sec. Thus, with perhaps 40 to 100 bursting inputs, a bursting response is predicted in the normal postsynaptic neuron. The longer the input from the epileptic bursts, the greater the possibility of the responding bursts overlapping in time with them, and thus the greater the potential of the recruited neuron contributing to further burst recruitment of still other normal cells. It appears that this is one of the fundamental mechanisms by which the epileptic discharge propagates to an ever enlarging number of neurons in the brain during a generalized seizure.

MECHANISMS OF LOCAL SPREAD OF EPILEPTIC DISCHARGE

The population of bursting pacemaker neurons in the focus might be expected to have an appreciable density of synaptic connections to group 2 and normal neurons in the focus and possibly adjacent cortex, thereby allowing recruitment of additional neurons to widen the extent of the apparent "focus." A variety of factors should bias such recruitment. On this basis, the size of the "epileptic focus" should dynamically expand or shrink, depending on such factors as background synaptic activity, synchronizing factors, and local changes in the ionic environment (2). During the onset of a spontaneous seizure in the monkey, the frequency of bursts generated by the group 1 pacemaker neurons does not significantly change. So the critical factor in the occurrence of a seizure is the degree of recruitment of adjacent neurons to encompass a sufficiently large number of bursting neurons.

Many factors are presumably involved in this local recruitment of other neurons into bursting activity. The pacemaker neurons appear to be providing a relatively invariant bursting input to such nearby cells, but it is less clear why this synaptic input induces bursting activity in them at only infrequent intervals.

One factor of major interest is the extracellular ionic environment. Sugaya et al. (18) first reported that presumed glial cells undergo waves of depolarization during seizure activity evoked by local electrical stimulation. It was concluded that this glial depolarization reflected increases in extracellular potassium. It was then proposed (13,14) that the repetitive firing of neuronal aggregates of neurons during the initiation of a seizure would liberate excessive quantities of K^+ into the extracellular space, which might play a role in the recruitment of additional neurons into the repetitive firing mode. In normal cortex, potassium clearance is presumably accomplished by diffusion through extracellular channels and by transport of excess K^+ away from the neurons (by glia) to maintain normal neuronal excitability. The epileptic focus, in contrast to normal cortex, is characterized by a striking proliferation of astroglia. In addition, Glotzner (6) has shown that such reactive glia in the chronic epileptic focus are more effective than normal glia in removing interstitial K^+. This increased capacity of glia in the focus to spatially buffer K^+ would be consistent with the morphological data. Harris (8) has documented that the astrocytes in the chronic focus are characterized by a striking increase in connections of both desmosome and gap varieties. These findings would be consistent with the observations of Pedley et al. (15), as well as subsequent data presented by Lewis et al. (12), indicating that $[K^+]_0$ values in epileptogenic and normal cortex are very similar.

Although $[K^+]_0$ may be normal under steady-state conditions, the dynamic changes associated with the onset of a locally propagating seizure may be significantly different in chronic epileptogenic cortex than in normal cortex. Finally, in addition to changes in glial function that may alter K^+ transport when the system is stressed by the massive liberation of K^+ during the onset of a seizure, there are changes in the extracellular space in the chronic focus that may be equally important. Ultrastructural studies undertaken by Harris and Jenkins (9) have shown that the extracellular space in the chronic focus is compromised. Infusion of horseradish peroxidase (HRP) into the normal subarachnoid space rapidly fills the extracellular space in normal cortex. When HRP was infused into the subarachnoid space over a chronic epileptogenic focus in the monkey, penetration into the extracellular space of the focus was reduced to 67% of that in controls. This significant reduction of extracellular space in the focus may significantly modify the local ionic environment close to individual neurons in the focus, and this would lead to the conclusion that potassium clearance would be impaired, as Lewis et al. (12) have reported.

These factors are of more than theoretical interest, because one of the most striking histological changes that characterize cortical epileptic foci is striking gliosis. It has been proposed (21) that glial cells proliferate and increase their capability to transport K^+. These changes would be an appropriate adaptive biological response to transport excess K^+ away from the epileptic neurons to maintain normal neuronal excitability. However, this glial increase may be maladaptive. Although these reactive glia may be even more efficient than normal astrocytes in removing potassium, excessive glial processes may block the important extracellular routes of diffusion.

More recent data indicate that the role of calcium ions may be of even greater importance in epilep-

togenesis. Schwartzkroin and Wyler (17) have recently proposed a model of the epileptogenic neuron that incorporates these concepts. They proposed that epileptogenic neurons are characterized by dendritic alterations that include a shortening of the electronic length from dendrites to soma. This would give the dendrites a more active role in burst generation by mechanisms that might include a higher density of calcium channels in dendrites and a closer approximation to initial segment trigger zones. From studies with calcium-sensitive microelectrodes (10) it is known that there is a decrease in $[Ca^{2+}]_0$ during epileptiform events, suggesting that an inward calcium current contributes to the discharge. Furthermore, as Schwartzkroin and Wyler (17) pointed out, increases in $[K^+]_0$ would result in longer and larger membrane depolarizations due to calcium influx. Large inward calcium currents would trigger more potassium efflux and thus might develop a positive-feedback situation that could lead to sustained cellular depolarizations and thus to ictal activity.

In addition to ionic mechanisms, there are well-documented synaptic events that may play a role in the local recruitment of neurons into an ictal discharge. It is known that alterations in synaptic input associated with changing behavioral states can profoundly influence the recruitment of group 2 (weakly epileptic) neurons into burst firing. The best-studied factor is normal sleep (24). In the primate model of chronic epilepsy, the spontaneous activity of neurons in the focus has been recorded during the transition from wakefulness to sleep. Group 1 or pacemaker epileptic neurons pass from wakefulness into sleep with very little change in interburst intervals, consistent with the presumption that they are fairly autonomous units unaffected by surrounding activity. Group 2 or mildly epileptic neurons behave very differently. During wakefulness, their behavior may vary widely, ranging from normal patterns of firing to mild bursting activity. During sleep, their activity changes dramatically, with marked increases in their burst indexes, so that their patterns of burst firing may be indistinguishable from those of pacemaker neurons. This observation would correlate well with the well-recognized clinical observation that the majority of seizure disorders show EEG activation as well as increased frequency of ictal events during the early stages of non-rapid-eye-movement sleep. Conversely, the activity of such group 2 weakly epileptic neurons could be significantly reduced by certain behavioral tasks. Such cells lowered their burst indexes when placed on operant conditioning schedules (27), even before the animal demonstrated appropriate operant control of the neurons. Once cell activity was under operant control, the burst index was further suppressed, often decreasing to zero. This would be consistent with the clinical impression that seizures are less frequent when patients are busy and active, particularly when attending closely to complex tasks.

Presumably, hormonal factors also alter excitability, which may account for the increased frequency of seizures associated with menses in some patients and with estrus in epileptic monkeys. In the monkey, it can be shown that behavioral stress will increase seizure frequency, and there is an extensive clinical folklore relating seizure frequency and stress in humans.

MECHANISMS OF PROPAGATION OF SEIZURES THROUGHOUT BRAIN

It is known that seizures propagate through the brain over known projection pathways from the epileptogenic focus (22). It appears that the induction of a seizure discharge in distant circuits involves mechanisms that are the same regardless of the technique used to originate the discharge at a focus. Thus the propagation of electrical afterdischarge is an easily studied model of the process. The intracellular changes leading to involvement of a normal neuron in major propagated seizure phenomena after repetitive transcallosal stimulation have been well studied (13,16). These changes include loss of hyperpolarizing responses, gradual depolarization of the membrane, and an increase in slope conductance leading to spike inactivation. It is probable that large inward calcium currents play a significant role in this process as well (7). At the stage of spike inactivation, the axons of such cells are exhibiting bursts of high-frequency repetitive spikes (19) that are, of course, projecting onto the next relay cells. In this fashion the seizure discharge may spread to involve most of the brain (22).

SEIZURE TERMINATION

The mechanisms involved in seizure termination are less clear. In a given cluster of neurons, the sustained cellular depolarizations characteristic of the clonic phase are followed by postictal hyperpolarization consistent with elevated extracellular

K^+ and intracellular Na^+ (and Ca^+) in the face of a persisting increased membrane conductance. It has been proposed that the hyperpolarizing potential may be due to an electrogenic pumping mechanism within neuronal and glial membrane attempting to return extracellular and intracellular ionic environments to an interictal normal state. With return of resting membrane potential following the postictal hyperpolarization, there is slow recovery of normal EPSP and IPSP activity, as well as return of interictal slope conductance and return of spike afterhyperpolarizations. All these events indicate that the period of postictal hyperpolarization, which corresponds to the period of electrical silence in the EEG, is the period during which the cell returns to normal activity after a seizure (14).

Although models may thus be constructed that might account for the sequence of cellular events, it is less clear why the seizure propagating through the brain stops. In fact, it is well recognized that seizure activity occurring in many different parts of the brain may be abruptly and synchronously terminated. This has led to an obvious proposal: Either a central pacemaker is driving such clonic activity, and such pacemaker activity is suddenly terminated, or (more likely) there is activation of a widely projecting inhibitory system. Unfortunately, these phenomena have not been widely studied, and definitive information is lacking.

This is unfortunate, because an understanding of the mechanisms involved in seizure termination is crucial to an understanding of the physiological mechanisms involved in status epilepticus. Clearly, most seizures run their course and stop. It is not clear why, on rare occasions, the process should repeat itself some seconds or minutes later. The mechanisms that appear to underlie epilepsia partialis continua do not appear to be those that are responsible for production of status. Some combination of factors presumably comes into play, involving neuronal excitability throughout the brain, which accounts for status. These factors appear to be, in part, independent of those operating at the epileptogenic focus.

CONSEQUENCES OF SEIZURES

It is now well documented in both the monkey model and in humans that random clinical seizures result in neuronal death. This can be most definitively studied in epileptic monkeys. It has been shown that in epileptic monkeys, axonal degeneration in the focus and streaming out from it can be demonstrated as long as clinical seizures are occurring. If the clinical seizures are suppressed by anticonvulsant medications for a sufficient period of time, so that the degeneration products are removed, the histological evidence for neuronal death is no longer present. Similar evidence of neuronal damage associated with clinical seizures has been demonstrated in human material (1). If occasional spontaneous seizures can have such consequences, it would be predicted that significant anatomical changes should follow status epilepticus.

IMPLICATIONS FOR THERAPY OF STATUS EPILEPTICUS

Both clinical experience and experimental data indicate that repeated major seizures are undesirable and that there is a premium on achieving seizure control as rapidly as possible. Status is clearly not a benign biological process, and it should be treated aggressively.

Our current knowledge of epileptic mechanisms provides few explicit clues that point to new potential therapeutic approaches. However, there are some additional experimental observations that may be clinically relevant. Some years ago it was proposed (23) that dendritic deformation might play a role in the genesis of the epileptic discharge. Interest in the possible role of mechanosensitivity has been rekindled by two recent studies. Howe et al. (11) studied the mechanosensitivity of dorsal root ganglia and spinal roots in normal animals as well as in preparations where scarring has been induced in these structures. It was found that the production of chronic scarring led to marked mechanosensitivity, which induced sustained repetitive firing that was not seen with compression of normal roots. A study was then undertaken by Wyler (25) to study mechanosensitivity of neurons in the epileptic focus of the monkey, as compared with normal cortex. Wyler found that neurons recorded from epileptic cortex are more mechanosensitive than those recorded from normal cortex or penicillin-induced epileptic cortex. The data indicate that membrane deformation of neurons in a cortical scar augments the firing rate of that cell. It is known that neurons in the chronic focus in both monkey and human are embedded in a glial scar. Changes in glial geometry might thus influence neuronal burst firing by increasing membrane deformation. Under these circumstances, local glial

swelling induced by Na^+ accumulation (7) might augment neuronal firing rates by membrane deformation and also reduce the already compromised extracellular diffusion pathways and thereby trap extracellular ions and neurotransmitters and contribute to the establishment of tonic hyperexcitability. It is clear that mild water intoxication may precipitate seizures in epileptic patients, and these factors may be playing significant roles in the induction of the necessary cellular environment to sustain status epilepticus. This would lead to the suggestion that therapy directed at restoring water balance in the brain might be a useful adjuvant to conventional therapy.

Obviously, the best solution to the problem of status is to prevent its occurrence. There is reason to believe that the incidence of status is lower in those patients having rare seizures than in those having frequent seizures. Because seizure frequency appears to be related to the percentage of pacemaker neurons in the chronic focus, it is obviously desirable to minimize the number of pacemaker neurons. Unfortunately, it is not clear that this can be accomplished in the established focus by other than surgical means. There are hints that pharmacological prophylaxis may be effective in this regard, so that the administration of anticonvulsant drugs during the phase that the focus is developing may be the most effective way to reduce the incidence of status in the population. Once seizures are established, the evidence indicates that alterations in the behavior of pacemaker neurons do not precede the development of propagating seizures. Factors that are of major importance are those that are involved in the recruitment of additional neurons into the bursting mode. Finally, factors responsible for the propagation of seizures throughout the brain probably represent the point of intervention that is most effective therapeutically in status. As we gain more information about the interactions between various excitatory and inhibitory transmitters in this process and about alterations in the kinetics of transmitter metabolism, as well as local ionic changes, it may be possible to construct more rational therapeutic approaches.

ACKNOWLEDGMENT

This research was supported by NIH research grant NS-04053, awarded by the National Institute of Neurological and Communicative Disorders and Stroke, PHS/DHHS.

REFERENCES

1. Brown, W. J. (1973): Structural substrates of seizures focus in the human temporal lobe. In: *Epilepsy: Its Phenomena in Man*, edited by M. A. B. Brazier, pp. 339:374. Academic Press, New York.

2. Calvin, W. H. (1972): Synaptic potential summation and repetitive firing mechanisms: Input-output theory for the recruitment of neurons into epileptic bursting firing patterns. *Brain Res.*, 39:71–94.

3. Calvin, W. H., Ojemann, G. A., and Ward, A. A., Jr. (1973): Human cortical neurons in epileptogenic foci: Comparison of interictal firing patterns to those of "epileptic" neurons in monkeys. *Electroencephalogr. Clin. Neurophysiol.*, 34:337–351.

4. Calvin, W. H., Sypert, G. W., and Ward, A. A., Jr. (1973): Structured timing patterns within bursts from epileptic neurons in undrugged monkey cortex. *Exp. Neurol.*, 21:535–549.

5. Fetz, E. E. (1969): Operant conditioning of cortical unit activity. *Science*, 163:955–958.

6. Glotzner, F. L. (1973): Membrane properties of neuroglia in epileptogenic gliosis. *Brain Res.*, 55:159–171.

7. Grossman, R. G., and Seregin, A. (1977): Glial-neural interaction demonstrated by the injection of Na⁺ and Li⁺ into cortical glia. *Science*, 195:196–198.

8. Harris, A. B. (1975): Cortical neuroglia in experimental epilepsy. *Exp. Neurol.*, 49:691–715.

9. Harris, A. B., and Jenkins, D. P. (1975): Intercellular space in epileptic brain. *Neurosci. Abstr.*, 1:179.

10. Heinemann, U., Lux, H. D., and Gutnick, M. J. (1977): Extracellular free calcium and potassium during paroxysmal activity in the cerebral cortex of the cat. *Exp. Brain Res.*, 27:237–243.

11. Howe, J. F., Loeser, J. D., and Calvin, W. H. (1977): Mechanosensitivity of dorsal root ganglia and chronically injured axons: A physiological basis for radicular pain of nerve and root compression. *Pain*, 3:25–41.

12. Lewis, D. V., Mutsuga, N., Schuette, W. H., and Van Buren, J. (1977): Potassium clearance and reactive gliosis in the alumina gel lesion. *Epilepsia*, 18:499–506.

13. Oakley, J. C., Sypert, G. W., and Ward, A. A., Jr. (1972): Conductance changes in neocortical propagated seizure: Seizure initiation. *Exp. Neurol.*, 37:287–299.

14. Oakley, J. C., Sypert, G. W., and Ward, A. A., Jr. (1972): Conductance changes in neocortical propagated seizure: Seizure termination. *Exp. Neurol.*, 37:300–311.

15. Pedley, T. A., Fisher, R. S., and Prince, D. A. (1976): Focal gliosis and potassium movement in mammalian cortex. *Exp. Neurol.*, 50:346–361.

16. Sawa, M., Kaji, S., and Usuki, K. (1965): Intracellular phenomena in electrically induced seizures. *Electroencephalogr. Clin. Neurophysiol.*, 19:248–255.

17. Schwartzkroin, P. A., and Wyler, A. R. (1980): Mechanisms underlying epileptiform burst discharge. *Ann. Neurol.*, 7:95–107.

18. Sugaya, E., Goldring, S., and O'Leary, J. L. (1964): Intracellular potentials associated with direct cortical response and seizure discharge in cat. *Electroencephalogr. Clin. Neurophysiol.*, 17:661–669.

19. Sypert, G. W., and Reynolds, A. F. (1974): Single pyramidal-tract fiber analysis of neocortical propagated seizures with reference to inactivation responses. *Exp. Neurol.*, 45:228–240.

20. Ward, A. A., Jr. (1972): Topical convulsant metals. In: *Experimental Models of Epilepsy*, edited by D. P. Purpura, J. K. Penry, D. Tower, D. M. Woodbury, and R. Walter, pp. 1–35. Raven Press, New York.

21. Ward, A. A., Jr. (1978): Glia and epilepsy. In: *Dynamic Properties of Glia Cells*, edited by E. Schofeniels, G. Franck, L. Hertz, and D. B. Tower, pp. 413–427. Pergamon Press, Oxford.

22. Ward, A. A., Jr., McCulloch, W. S., and Kopeloff, N. (1948): Temporal and spatial distribution of changes during spontaneous seizures in monkey brain. *J. Neurophysiol.*, 11:377–386.

23. Ward, A. A., Jr., and Schmidt, R. P. (1961): Some properties of single epileptic neurons. *Arch. Neurol.*, 5:308–313.

24. Wyler, A. R. (1974): Epileptic neurons during sleep and wakefulness. *Exp. Neurol.*, 42:593–608.

25. Wyler, A. R. (1977): Discrimination between epileptic and injury-induced repetitive firing in chronic epileptic cortex. *Exp. Neurol.*, 55:603–617.

26. Wyler, A. R., Burchiel, K. J., and Ward, A. A., Jr. (1978): Chronic epileptic foci in monkeys: Correlations between seizure frequency and proportion of pacemaker epileptic neurons. *Epilepsia*, 19:475–483.

27. Wyler, A. R., and Fetz, E. E. (1974): Behavioral control of firing patterns of normal and abnormal neurons in chronic epileptic cortex. *Exp. Neurol.*, 42:448–464.

28. Wyler, A. R., Finch, C. A., and Burchiel, K. J. (1978): Epileptic and normal neurons in monkey neocortex: A quantitative study of degrees of operant control. *Brain Res.*, 151:269–281.

29. Wyler, A. R., and Ward, A. A., Jr. (1980): Epileptic neurons. In: *Epilepsy: A Window to the Brain*, edited by J. S. Lockard and A. A. Ward Jr., pp. 51–68. Raven Press, New York.

Advances in Neurology, Vol. 34: Status Epilepticus, edited by A.V. Delgado-Escueta, C.G. Wasterlain, D.M. Treiman, and R.J. Porter. Raven Press, New York © 1983.

19

Na$^+$K$^+$-ATPase Within Neurons and Glia in the Generation of Seizures

Thierry Grisar, Georges Franck, and Antonio V. Delgado-Escueta

Two theories are currently used to explain how glial cells limit the rise of extracellular potassium $[K^+]_0$ released by neurons during cell firing: (a) clearance by passive diffusion through either glial syncytium or extracellular space; (b) active accumulation of potassium mediated by the Na$^+$K$^+$-ATPase of glial cells; reviews have been published (10,30). Henn et al. (19), Grisar et al. (14), and Moonen and Franck (25) showed that glial Na$^+$K$^+$-ATPase was specifically activated by high K$^+$ ion concentrations (18–20 mM), whereas neuronal enzyme activity saturated at 3- to 6-mM K$^+$ (Fig. 1). Moreover, high K$^+$ ion concentrations increased the physiological efficiency (the ratio V_{max}/K_{mapp} for ATP) of glial Na$^+$K$^+$-ATPase while decreasing the same kinetic parameter in perikaryon and synaptosomal enzyme preparations (15,16). More specifically, kinetic and thermodynamic characteristics suggested that the physiological efficiency of the glial enzyme was enhanced by increasing $[K^+]_0$ from 5 to 20 mM (13,15,16). Glial and neuronal Na$^+$K$^+$-ATPases therefore appeared as two different molecular entities. From previous thermodynamic (2) and kinetic (27) data, two forms of Na$^+$K$^+$-ATPase in brain could be suggested. Although Kimmelberg et al. (21) did not find any fundamental differences, Sweadner (31) resolved two molecular forms of brain Na$^+$K$^+$-ATPase by gel electrophoresis in sodium dodecyl sulfate,

demonstrating differences in affinity to strophanthidin and sensitivity to digestion by trypsin and differences in the number or reactivity of sulfhydryl groups. The evolutionary significance of glial enzymes that increase efficiency as K$^+$ ion concentrations increase could be that K$^+$ is actively taken up by glial cells when concentrations of $[K^+]_0$ increase.

On the basis of a growing body of evidence linking changes in $[K^+]_0$ and seizures, Franck (9) and Pollen and Trachtenberg (28) independently proposed in 1970 the hypothesis that epilepsy could be the result of degradation of the $[K^+]_0$ spatial buffering function of glial cells. As a result, several electrophysiological studies measured the biophysical properties of glial cells and the variations of $[K^+]_0$ within glial scarred epileptogenic foci during ictal and interictal episodes. K$^+$-specific microelectrodes measured baseline levels of $[K^+]_0$ in normal and epileptogenic brains and found them to be identical, i.e., around 3 mM K$^+$ (24). Because of this observation, an impairment of glial spatial buffering function was considered an unlikely cause of paroxysmal depolarization shifts (PDSs) within neurons of the seizure focus. However, Dichter et al. (8) claimed that glial abnormalities could be responsible for the transition of interictal discharges to ictal episodes. In spite of this suggestion, electrophysiological data remain

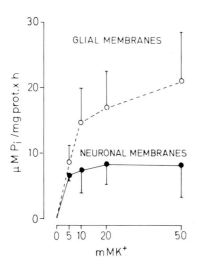

FIG. 1. Influence of K⁺ ions on the Na⁺K⁺-ATPase activities of bulk-isolated glial cells and perikaryon membranous fractions from adult rabbit brain. The cell fractions were isolated as previously reported (1,14). The membranes were prepared as previously described (17). ATPase activities were determined as reported elsewhere (4) and are expressed in μM Pi·mg prot⁻¹·hr⁻¹. Vertical bars represent $\pm$ SD (N = 6). Medium: ATP·Na$_2$ (vanadate-free) 1 mM, MgCl$_2$ 1 mM; NaCl 120 mM; KCl as indicated; EGTA 0.1 mM; TRIS chloride 10 mM; pH 7.4; 37°C.

conflicting, the glial cells within the epileptogenic focus being variously described as being more effective than (11), less effective than (23,28), or as effective as (24,26,30) normal glia in removing interstitial K⁺.

Our purpose in this chapter is to present new biochemical information to analyze the K⁺ activation mechanisms of glial and synaptosomal Na⁺K⁺-ATPase isolated from normal and epileptogenic tissue. The results favor the concept that glial enzyme characteristics are modified within actively firing epileptogenic tissue.

METHODS

Freeze Lesions

Freeze lesions (10-mm) were produced in adult cats (weighing between 2 and 4 kg) according to previously established procedures (5,6) after intraperitoneal injections of sodium pentobarbital (35 mg/kg). In control cats (C), no freeze lesions were produced (sham-operated).

Electrocorticograms (ECOGs) were performed 35 to 50 days later, as previously reported (5,6). Briefly, cats were paralyzed by gallamine triethiodide and supported by artificial respiration. They were mounted in stereotactic frames; the right and left hemispheres were fully exposed, and the presence of seizure discharges was verified by ECOG.

Three brain areas were selected (Fig. 2): (a) the primary focus (F), i.e., the 10-mm-diameter lesion and the adjacent cortex (left anterior suprasylvian gyrus); (b) the secondary or "mirror" focus (M), i.e., the homologous contralateral cortex (right anterior suprasylvian gyrus); (c) the homolateral posterior ectosylvian or posterior suprasylvian gyrus corresponding to the posterior perifocal or surround tissue (PF).

Both F and M ECOG recordings always showed 1/sec to 3/sec negative positive sharp waves or triangular slow waves, but this phenomenon was not seen in PF (Fig. 2). Brain cerebral cortex regions were dissected as far as 3 to 4 mm in depth, wet-weighed, and used for the preparation of glial and synaptosomal fractions.

Preparation of Glial and Synaptosomal Enriched Fractions

Glial, neuronal, perikaryon, and synaptosomal fractions were prepared according to the methods of Blomstrand and Hamberger (1,16). However,

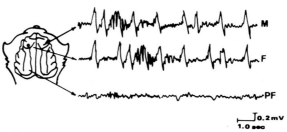

FIG. 2. ECOG recording of epileptogenic discharges within the primary (F) and secondary (M) foci. Note the absence of discharges in PF, i.e., the posterior suprasylvian gyrus homolateral to the lesion. The tracings were obtained in reference to nasion with a time constant of 0.8 sec. Relative negativity of grid 1 produces an upward deflection. See Dichter et al. (8) for details.

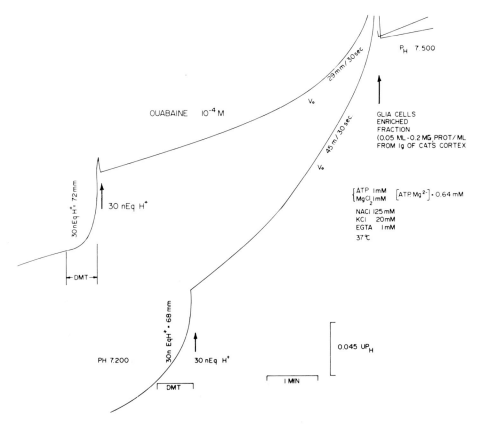

FIG. 3. Typical trace of the pH change during the hydrolysis of ATP by a glial-cell-enriched fraction isolated from 1 g of epileptogenic cortex of the cat exhibiting ECOG spike (F). Note the composition of the medium and the initial and final pH. The reaction was initiated by the addition of the sample. After about 3 min, 30 nEq H+ was added, causing a rapid fall in pH (68–72 mm), which was used to calibrate the system. Ouabain (10^{-4} M) caused an inhibition of about 39% of total activity. DMT: dead mixing time ($\sim$ 40 sec). See Glotzner (11) for details.

the technique was modified and adapted for the small amount of cerebral cortical tissue (usually 1 g) available using smaller filtration systems under slight vacuum and the 15-ml Spinco centrifugation tube for the ultracentrifugation step (Rotor Spinco SW 40). The relative purity of each fraction was tested by light and electron microscope as well as by determination of the specific glial fibrillary protein (GFA). The results are similar to those previously reported (13,14).

Determination of Na+ K+ -ATPase Activities

Na+ K+ -ATPase activities were measured as previously reported (15,16). Briefly, the rate of ATP hydrolysis was measured by the rate of liberation of ions using the hysteretic model (12). The incubation medium in a specially devised reaction vessel equilibrated at 37°C and stirred by means of a magnetic bar consisted of the following: ATP·Na$_2$ (vanadate-free disodium salt) 1 mM; MgCl$_2$ 1 mM; final concentration of NaCl 120 mM; KCl, as indicated; EGTA 0.1 mM at pH 7.420 in a final volume of 2 ml. Ouabain (10^{-4} M) was added in order to determine the Mg^{2+}-dependent ATPase activity. Mg^{2+} ATPase activity was subtracted from total enzyme activity, and the difference was considered to be the Na+K+ -ATPase activity expressed in nEq H+·mg prot^{-1}·sec^{-1}.

To eliminate variabilities in absolute values of enzyme-specific activities from one experiment to another, data were expressed in percent of activation by comparison with results obtained in 3-mM K+. Activities measured at these K+ concentrations, which corresponded to the baseline level of [K+]$_0$ in the CNS (4), were considered equivalent to 100% for each sample tested. A K+-induced 50% increase in activity was then equivalent to 150%. Proteins were determined as previously reported (13,15,16).

RESULTS

Kinetic Determination of Na$^+$K$^+$-ATPase Activity

A typical trace of the rate of H$^+$ ion production during ATP hydrolysis catalyzed by the glial fraction isolated from primary focus of the cat is shown in Fig. 3. As can be seen, 10 μg of glial protein produced ouabain-sensitive nonlinear progressive curves in the presence of 0.64-mM ATP·Mg^{2-} and 20-mM K$^+$. Initial velocities (V_0) were easily calculated according to a previously described hysteretic model (15). The results were expressed in nEq H$^+$·mg prot^{-1}·sec^{-1}. Inactivation rates were not significantly different from one sample to another and were the same in glial and synaptosomal fractions. Na$^+$K$^+$-ATPase activities were calculated by the difference between the activities in the absence (total ATPase) and the presence of 10^{-4}-M ouabain (Mg^{2+}-ATPase), respectively.

Na$^+$K$^+$-ATPase levels in Glia and Nerve Endings Isolated from Control and Epileptic Brains

Mg^{2+}-ATPase activities were not significantly different in most of the samples tested and reached 6 to 10 nEq H$^+$·mg prot^{-1}·sec^{-1}. However, synaptosomal fractions isolated from the primary focus (F) Mg^{2+}-ATPase enzyme activities were elevated threefold (21.1 ± 6.1 nEq H$^+$·mg prot^{-1}·sec^{-1}) when compared with control animals ($p < 0.001$) and brain samples (glia and synapses) from mirror foci and perifocal brain areas ($p < 0.01$). Table 1 shows the levels of Na$^+$K$^+$-ATPase activities measured in an incubation medium containing potassium concentrations close to those observed in brain extracellular fluid during resting states (~ 3 mM). As shown by the SD values, some variability in enzyme activities was observed that probably was a reflection of the impurity and the differences in protein yield of the Na$^+$K$^+$-ATP ase preparation; see Glotzner (11) for a discussion.

Total Na$^+$K$^+$-ATPase activity did not appear to change in the glial fractions of the primary focus. However, Na$^+$K$^+$-ATPase enzyme activity was significantly higher in glial cell fractions (and, to a lesser extent, in synaptosomes) isolated from the secondary focus (M) as compared with control animals. Some increase in the perifocal tissue was also present.

Synaptic Na$^+$K$^+$-ATPase increased activities in the primary and mirror foci, whereas they decreased within the perifocal area.

K$^+$ Activation of Na$^+$K$^+$-ATPase of Glia and Nerve Endings Isolated from Control and Epileptogenic Brain

Because the absolute activity of Na$^+$K$^+$-ATPase enzymes varied from one day's preparation to the next, initial velocities of enzyme reactions (Fig. 3) were expressed relative to the Na$^+$K$^+$-ATPase activity of a concurrent control incubation in the "standard medium," i.e., at 3-mM K$^+$ defined as 100%. K$^+$-dependent activities were then expressed in percent of activation (Fig. 4).

Synaptosomes

As shown in Fig. 4 (right), K$^+$ activation of the synaptosomal Na$^+$K$^+$-ATPase was, in a first approximation, the same in control and epileptogenic brain regions (F, M, PF). Indeed, Table 2 indicates that the maximum velocities were not significantly different from one sample to another. However, the activation constant for K$^+$ (the K$^+$ concentration corresponding to the half-maximum velocity) was significantly decreased within synaptosomal fractions from actively firing epileptogenic tissue, i.e., primary and secondary foci. The apparent affinity of the synaptosomal enzyme for K$^+$ therefore appeared to be increased within the firing tissue.

Glia

In glial fractions, significant differences in K$^+$ activation of the Na$^+$K$^+$-ATPase were observed between control and epileptogenic brains. In sham-operated (control) animals, curves relating rate reactions to external K$^+$ were indistinguishable from those of adult rabbit brains, newborn rat cultured astrocytes (25), and human brain astrocytes (14); the rate reaction is hyperbolic, with maximal activation at 18-mM K$^+$. This rate characteristic appeared more clearly in glial fractions isolated from the perifocal brain area devoid of ECOG epileptiform spikes (PF). In this surround region, maximum velocities and the activation constant for K$^+$ ($K_a$$^{K+}$) were significantly higher than those in control animals (Table 2).

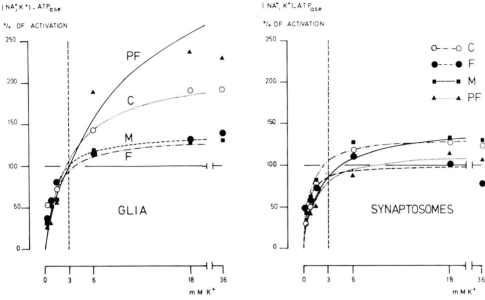

FIG. 4. Influence of K+ ions on the Na+K+-ATPase activities of glial (*left*) and synaptosomal (*right*) fractions isolated from control (C) and epileptogenic brain tissues exhibiting ECOG discharges (F, M) or not (PF). ATPase activities were determined as previously described (11,12) and summarized in Fig. 3. Data are expressed as percent of activation of activities measured in presence of 3-mM K+ (shown in Table 1) and considered equal to 100. Hyperbolic regression was calculated for each experience, and the mean curves are shown. In order to clarify the figure, the SD are not shown, but the significances of the kinetic parameters calculated from these curves (V_{max}, K_a^{K+}) are shown in Table 2.

TABLE 1. *Na+K+-ATPase activities of glial cells and synaptosomal fractions isolated from control and epileptogenic brain tissue*

K+ (3 mM)	Control (C)	Primary focus (F)	Perifocus (PF)	Secondary focus (M)
Glial cells enriched fractions	3.3 ± 1.3[a] (N = 6)	3.2 ± 1.0 (N = 8)	4.4 ± 3.4 (N = 8)	8.2 ± 4.8[b] (N = 8)
Synaptosomal fractions	4.1 ± 1.6 (N = 6)	6.5 ± 5.0 (N = 8)	2.9 ± 1.4[b] (N = 8)	6.0 ± 3.9 (N = 8)

[a]Values are expressed in nEq H+·mg prot^{-1}·sec^{-1} (see Fig. 3 for experimental conditions).
[b]$p < 0.01$ compared with C (t_1); $p < 0.001$ compared with F (t_2 or t test for matched sample).

The converse phenomenon was observed within actively firing epileptogenic tissue (F and M). The most striking feature of Fig. 4 is the appearance of a large difference in the activation curves for glial fractions isolated from the primary and mirror foci. Activation of glial enzyme between 3- and 18-mM K+ was no longer present (Fig. 4). Accordingly, both V_{max} and K_a^{K+} were significantly decreased as compared with both control animals and the PF area. In other words, within actively firing epileptogenic tissue, glial and synaptosomal enzymes exhibit the same response to K_0 saturation occurring between 3- and 6-mM K+. In the peri-focal tissue, however, the glial and synaptosomal K+ responses appeared in sharp contrast, the former remaining unsaturated in 18-mM K+ medium, the latter being saturated in 6-mM K+ medium.

DISCUSSION

Freezing a focal area of the cerebral cortex has proved to be an effective way of producing actively discharging chronic epileptogenic lesions in the cat (4–7). Epileptiform spikes and sharp waves can be observed 15 to 40 days after lesion production, and contralateral secondary spikes and sharp waves generally develop in more than half of experimen-

TABLE 2. Kinetic parameters (V_{max}, K_a^{K+}) of K^+ activation of glial and synaptosomal Na^+-K^+-ATPase isolated from control and epileptogenic brain tissue[a]

	Glia				Synaptosomes			
	C	F	PF	M	C	F	PF	M
V_{max} (% of activation)	215 ± 47 (N = 6)	140 ± 41[b] (N = 8)	386 ± 62[b,c] (N = 8)	134 ± 40[b] (N = 8)	146 ± 51[b] (N = 6)	99 ± 47 (N = 8)	116 ± 52 (N = 8)	133 ± 48 (N = 8)
K_a^{K+} (mM K^+)	3.1 ± 1.0 (N = 6)	1.1 ± 0.8[b] (N = 8)	8.5 ± 3.1[c] (N = 8)	1.3 ± 1.2[b] (N = 8)	2.1 ± 1.2 (N = 6)	0.4 ± 0.1[b] (N = 8)	1.4 ± 0.7[c] (N = 8)	0.7 ± 0.6[b] (N = 8)

[a]For experimental conditions and symbols, see Figs. 2 and 3 and Table 1.
[b]$p \leq 0.01$ compared with C (t_1).
[c]$p < 0.001$ compared with F (t_2).

tal animals (Fig. 2). Within the 10-mm freeze lesion, histological examination shows loss of nerve cells and dense gliosis. In this study we used bulk-isolation tissue-fractionation techniques to investigate the kinetic characteristics of Na^+K^+-ATPase isolated from different epileptogenic brain regions. Glial and synaptosomal fractions were isolated, and their purities were monitored by morphological and biochemical means, indicating a purity level of about 75%. A modified technique of Blomstrand and Hamberger (1) was adapted to the small amounts of tissue ($\sim$ 1 g) available. Glial-cell-enriched fractions (in milligrams of glial protein per gram of initial wet weight of brain tissue) harvested from the primary focus (F) yielded two to three times more protein than glial fractions isolated from other brain areas (C, M, PF). This result is consistent with the presence of extensive gliosis in the lesion site. The rationale for using bulk-isolated cellular and subcellular fractions for Na^+K^+-ATPase determination has been extensively discussed (13,15,16).

Absolute Level of Na⁺K⁺-ATPase Activity in Epileptogenic Brain Tissue

Table 1 shows that in the presence of 3-mM K^+, absolute levels of Na^+K^+-ATPase activities in brain fractions from chronic epileptogenic lesions varied greatly from one experimental preparation to another. Previous publications have discussed possible factors that influence levels of brain Na^+K^+-ATPase enzyme activities (13). Our results also demonstrated an increase in enzyme activity within the chronic secondary focus in both glial and synaptosomal fractions when compared with control animals (C), the primary focus (F), and its surrounding area (PF). Interestingly, some increases in enzyme activities were also observed in the area surrounding the focus (PF) when these regions were compared with controls. These results are clearly different from previous results published by other investigators. Indeed, Lewin and McCrimmon (22) showed that Na^+K^+-ATPase activities of homogenized brain tissue excised from acute epileptogenic freeze lesions increased 8 hr after lesion production, whereas it decreased 24 hr later. A slight reduction in enzyme level was also observed in 23-day-old cobalt-induced epileptogenic lesions (23). Using synaptosomes isolated from both primary and secondary foci, Delgado-Escueta and Horan (7) also showed increases in enzyme activity 18 hr and, to a lesser extent, 3 days after production of freeze lesions. Seven to 352 days later, Na^+K^+-ATPase activities stayed lower than control levels. Increased enzyme activities were often attributed to the presence of actively firing lesions or cerebral edema (7,22), whereas decreased enzyme levels were explained by cellular destruction during lesion production (23). Unilateral brain injury induced by freezing also has been shown to alter the response of the ATPase enzyme to K^+/Na^+ ratios and presumably has induced a loss of the total Na^+K^+-ATPase activity (29). Intravenous injection of CDP-choline partially restored the sensitivity of the enzyme to the Na/K ratio, indicating that cell damage induced by cold could be due to a disorder of protein-lipid interaction (25,29). Cultured astrocytes prepared from epileptogenic DBA mice also exhibit a decrease in ecto-ATPase activity compared with normal C57 mice (32). In some reports, alterations in membrane Na^+K^+-ATPase activities were used to explain the origin of seizures (4,20,33).

Although the Na^+K^+-ATPase is involved in the transport of Na^+ and K^+ across the cell membrane, its level of absolute activity might have no significance with regard to the physiological efficiency of the Na^+K^+ pump in vivo. In preceding sections we showed that absolute values of enzyme activity extensively varied from one preparation to another according to the technical procedures used for Na^+K^+-ATPase measurement. Moreover, embryonic structures like cultured astrocytes, neuroblastoma cells, and dorsal root ganglia very often exhibited low levels of enzymic activity while they actively pumped Na^+ against K^+ at high capacities; see Grisar et al. (13) for a review. In the case of synaptosomes isolated from cat brain with freeze lesions, however, reduction in Na^+K^+-ATPase activity was shown to exist, with a parallel impairment of the K^+-uptake mechanism within synaptosomes of chronic epileptogenic foci (4–7). In the absence of experiments determining the cationic fluxes across the membrane, it is difficult to draw conclusions from these studies, which measured the absolute levels of enzyme activities. It is possible that both the highly active nature of our mirror epileptogenic areas, which fired consistently with epileptiform spikes and sharp waves, and the associated influx of Na^+ inward contributed to the enhanced activities of Na^+K^+-ATPase. Delgado-Escueta (4) recently showed that ictal epileptiform paroxysms enhanced the activities of

Na+K+-ATPase that had chronically been decreased in the interictal state.

K+ Activation of Na+K+-ATPase Activity in Epileptogenic Brain Tissue

Understanding the K+-activation mechanisms of the Na+K+-ATPase enzyme within neuronal, synaptic, and glial fractions might reveal more important information in the clearance of extracellular K+ during neuronal firing and epilepsy. A reliable technique was devised for measurment of the initial velocity of the enzyme (Fig. 3), taking into account the well-demonstrated inactivation process of enzyme catalysis; see Grisar et al. (15) for detailed discussion. Our results indicated that within firing epileptogenic tissue, i.e., primary (F) and secondary (M) foci, glial Na+K+-ATPase enzyme increased sensitivity to external K+. The enzyme practically lost its response over the range of K concentrations previously shown to activate, i.e., between 3- and 18-mM K+ (10,12,19) (Fig. 4). Because the activation constant for K+ (K_a^{K+}) was reduced, it is reasonable to conclude that the enzyme increased its apparent affinity for K+ (Table 2). Interestingly, when epileptiform paroxysms increased frequency, glial Na+K+-ATPase exhibitied kinetic characteristics similar to those of the synaptosomal enzyme (Fig. 4, Table 2). According to our previous model, which explained increased physiological efficiency (V_{max}/K_{mapp}) of glial enzyme in the presence of high K+ concentrations, our present findings suggest that glial membranes have reduced their capacities in actively controlling elevated concentrations of external potassium ($[K+]_0$) during epileptiform paroxysms.

The converse phenomenon and, as a result, the converse interpretation could be proposed for the glial enzyme isolated from brain areas surrounding the primary focus (PF). Few earlier reports indicated modifications of glial metabolism within the epileptogenic brain tissue. Reactive astrocytes with histoenzymological abnormalities were described in human and experimental seizure (3). Cobalt-induced focal epileptogenic lesions in the frontal cortex of rats were associated with an increase in glial carbonic anhydrase (CA) activity in regions of epileptiform spikes (33,34). These results were interpreted to mean that glial cells increased CA activities and thus handled the increased metabolic production of CO_2 that was induced by the enhanced neuronal activities of epilepsy. Hence, the glial CA response was considered to be protective

rather than a cause of seizure. By maintaining acid-base homeostasis, glial cells helped limit the spread of seizure activity (33,34). From our results, a similar interpretation could be proposed. However, a protective role for glial cells in $[K+]_0$ homeostasis can be proposed only for the surround or perifocal area, where its physiological efficiency remains maintained even at high K+ concentrations. Within the primary and mirror foci, however, our data indicated a reduction rather than an increase in the protective ability of glial membranes. These abnormalities probably are not totally responsible for the development of PDSs in neurons of the seizure focus, because electrophysiological studies have shown that the baseline levels of $[K+]_0$ are not modified within the gliotic cortex (~ 3-mM K+). Inefficient Na+ and K+ pumping mechanisms within synaptic terminals and an enhanced Ca^{2+} influx process might all contribute to the generation of PDSs (6). However, the impairment in glial control of elevated $[K+]_0$ could be mainly responsible for the transition of discharges to ictal episodes (8) within the primary and the secondary foci. Recent experiments by Delgado-Escueta (4) on interictal and ictal states have shown that sustained epileptiform discharges increase synaptic Na+K+-ATPase activity. Our present results show that a continuously firing focal lesion and in its mirror focus, glial membranes decrease their ability to respond to high concentrations of extracellular K. Indeed, others reported that the transition from interictal to ictal episodes seemed to be due to an impaired faculty of silent cells to buffer $[K+]_0$ within the epileptogenic scar tissue (8,23). Although these results were questioned by Pedley et al. (26) and by Somjen (30), we believe that these contradictions in electrophysiological data may be more a reflection of the limitations of the technical methods used. Specific K+ microelectrodes are unable to measure the fine kinetic characteristics of cations *in vivo*. Our results also show that for adequate studies, brain areas should be explored separately, and the primary lesion and the mirror focus should be contrasted not only against control tissues but also against the surround.

In conclusion, our results present membrane biochemical data suggesting that a deficit in the glial capacity to actively control elevated $[K+]_0$ during sustained epileptiform paroxysms is present in focal seizures. In brain tissue surrounding the focus, the physiological efficiencies of glial cells are maintained at optimal levels. Further experiments are necessary in order to determine if these observations hold true as well for the genetic epilepsies.

ACKNOWLEDGMENTS

This work was supported by grants from the Belgium Rotary Foundation and the Epilepsy Foundation of America (T.G.) and by Department of Health and Human Services contract NO1-NS-0-2332. We thank A. Minet and M. Burette for their excellent technical assistance. We are grateful to M. Fodor for secretarial assistance and to Bob Mitchell for text processing.

REFERENCES

1. Blomstrand, C., and Hamberger, A. (1969): Protein turnover in cell-enriched fractions from rabbit brain. *J. Neurochem.*, 16:1401–1408.
2. Bowler, K., and Ducan, C. J. (1968): The temperature characteristics of the ATPase from a frog brain microsomal preparation. *Comp. Biochem. Physiol.*, 24:223–227.
3. Brotchi, J. (1972): Astrocytes reactionnels et epilepsie. *Acta Neurol. Belg.*, 72:137–142.
4. Delgado-Escueta, A. V. (1982): Na+K+ATPase activity during interictal and ictal states of the freezing lesion. *Brain Res (in press)*.
5. Delgado-Escueta, A. V., Davidson, G. H., and Reilly, E. (1974): The freezing lesion. II. Potassium transport within nerve terminals isolated from epileptogenic foci. *Brain Res.*, 78:223–237.
6. Delgado-Escueta, A. V., Davidson, G. H., and Reilly, E. (1974): The freezing lesion. III. The effect of diphenylhydantoin on potassium transport within nerve terminals from the primary foci. *Brain Res.*, 86:85–96.
7. Delgado-Escueta, A. V., and Horan, M. P. (1980): Brain synaptosomes in epilepsy: Organization of ionic channels and the Na+K+ pump. In: *Advances in Neurology, Vol. 27*, edited by G. H. Glaser, J. K. Penry, and D. M. Woodbury, pp. 85–126. Raven Press, New York.
8. Dichter, M. A., Herman, C. I., and Selzer, M. (1972): Silent cells during interictal discharges and seizures in hippocampal penicillin foci. Evidence for the role of extracellular K+ in the transition from the interictal state to seizures. *Brain Res.*, 48:173–183.
9. Franck, G. (1970): Exchanges cationiques au niveau des neurones et des cellules gliales du cerveau. *Arch. Int. Physiol. Biochim.*, 78:613.
10. Franck, G., Grisar, T., Moonen, G., and Schoffeniels, E. (1978): Potassium transport in mammalian astroglia. In: *Dynamic Properties of Glia Cells*, edited by E. Schoffeniels, G. Franck, D. B. Tower, and L. Hertz, pp. 315–325. Pergamon Press, Oxford.
11. Glotzner, F. L. (1973): Membrane properties of neuroglia in epileptogenic gliosis. *Brain Res.*, 55:159–171.
12. Grisar, T., and Franck, G. (1975): Glial cell control of extracellular K+ content in the CNS. In: *Abstracts of the Fifth Meeting of the International Society for Neurochemistry*, 160:228, Barcelona.
13. Grisar, T., Franck, G., and Schoffeniels, E. (1978): K+ activation mechanisms of the Na+K+ATPase of bulk isolated glia cells and neurons. In: *Dynamic Properties of Glia Cells*, edited by E. Schoffeniels, G. Franck, D. B. Tower, and L. Hertz, pp. 359–369. Pergamon Press, Oxford.
14. Grisar, T., Franck, G., and Schoffeniels, E. (1980): Glial control of neuronal excitability in mammals. II. Enzymatic evidence: Two molecular forms of the Na+K+ATPase in brain. *Neurochemistry International*, 2:311–320.
15. Grisar, T., Frere, J. M., Charlier-Grisar, J., and Schoffeniels, E. (1978): Synaptosomal Na+K+ATPase in a hysteretic enzyme. *F.E.B.S. Lett.*, 89:173–176.
16. Grisar, T., Frere, J. M., and Franck, G. (1979): Effect of K+ ions on kinetic properties of the Na+K+ATPase (E.C. 3.6.1.3) of bulk isolated glial cells, perikaria and synaptosomes from rabbit brain cortex. *Brain Res.*, 165:87–103.
17. Grossman, R. G., and Rosman, L. J. (1971): Intracellular potentials of inexcitable cells in epileptogenic cortex undergoing fibrillary gliosis after local injury. *Brain Res.*, 28:181–201.
18. Hamberger, A., Eriksson, O., and Norrby, K. (1971): Cell size distribution in brain suspensions and in fractions enriched with neuronal and glial cells. *Exp. Cell Res.*, 67:380–388.
19. Henn, F. A., Haljamae, H., and Hamberger, A. (1972): Glial cell function: Active control of extracellular K concentration. *Brain Res.*, 43:437–448.
20. Hunt, W. A., and Craig, C. R. (1973): Alterations in cation levels and Na+K+ATPase activity in rat cerebral cortex during the development of cobalt-induced epilepsy. *J. Neurochem.*, 20:559–567.
21. Kimmelberg, H. K., Biddlecome, S., Narumi, S., and Bourke, R. S. (1978): ATPase and carbonic anhydrase activities of bulk isolated neuron, glia and synaptosome fractions from rat brain. *Brain Res.*, 141:305–323.
22. Lewin, E., and McCrimmon, A. (1967): ATPase activity in discharging cortical lesions induced by freezing. *Arch. Neurol.*, 16:321–325.
23. Lewis, D. V., Mutsuga, N., Schuette, W. H., and Van Buren, J. (1977): Potassium clearance and reactive gliosis in the alumina gel lesion. *Epilepsia*, 18:132–136.
24. Lux, H. D. (1974): The kinetics of extracellular potassium: Relation to epileptogenesis. *Epilepsia*, 15:375–393.
25. Moonen, G., and Franck, G. (1977): Potassium effect on Na+K+ATPase activity of cultured newborn rat astroblasts during differenciation. *Neurosci. Letters*, 4:263–267.
26. Pedley, A. T., Fisher, R. S., Futamachi, K. J., and Prince, D. A. (1976): Regulation of extracellular potassium concentration in epileptogenesis. *Fed. Proc.*, 35:1254–1259.
27. Peter, H. W., and Wolf, H. V. (1976): Kinetics of Na+K+ATPase of human erythrocyte membranes. I.

Activation by Na⁺ and K⁺. *Biochim. Biophys. Acta*, 290:300–309.

28. Pollen, D. A., and Trachtenberg, M. C. (1970): Neuroglia: Gliosis and focal epilepsy. *Science*, 167:1252–1253.

29. Rigoulet, M., Guerin, B., Cohadon, F., and Vandendreissche, M. (1979): Unilateral brain injury in the rabbit: Reversible and irreversible damage of the membranal ATPases. *J. Neurochem.*, 32:535–541.

30. Somjen, G. G. (1980): Influence of potassium and neuroglia in the generation of seizures and their treatment. In: *Advances in Neurology, Vol. 27*, edited by G. H. Glaser, J. K. Penry, and D. M. Woodbury, pp. 155–167. Raven Press, New York.

31. Sweadner, K. J. (1979): Two molecular forms of Na⁺K⁺-stimulated ATPase in brain: Separation and difference in affinity for strophanthidin. *J. Biol. Chem.*, 254:6060–6067.

32. Trams, E. G., and Lauter, C. J. (1978): Ecto-ATPase in DBA mice. *Nature*, 271–270.

33. Woodbury, D. M., and Kemp, J. W. (1977): Basic mechanisms of seizures: Neurophysiological and biochemical etiology. In: *Psychopathology and Brain Dysfunction*, edited by C. Shagass, S. Gershon, and A. J. Friedhoff, pp. 149–182. Raven Press, New York.

34. Woodbury, D. M., and Kemp, J. W. (1979): Initiation, propagation and arrest of seizures. In: *Pathophysiology of Cerebral Energy Metabolism*, edited by B. B. Mrsulja, L. M. Rakic, I. Klatzo, and M. Spatz, pp. 313–351. Plenum Press, New York.

Advances in Neurology, Vol. 34: Status Epilepticus, edited by A.V. Delgado-Escueta, C.G. Wasterlain, D.M. Treiman, and R.J. Porter. Raven Press, New York © 1983.

20

Cerebral Energy Metabolism During Experimental Status Epilepticus

David C. Howse

Status epilepticus, occurring as either intermittent or continuous prolonged seizure activity, has long been recognized by physicians as a cause of permanent brain damage (1,15,18). When it occurs, it is often an ominous clinical development. The infantile brain is particularly susceptible to its destructive effects, with the tragic sequelae of cerebral palsy and mental retardation and the development in later life of a disabling seizure disorder. This reality of clinical practice has never surprised clinicians, who have repeatedly witnessed the intense muscle contractions, the subsequent respiratory insufficiency, and the profound disturbances in brain function that occur during a convulsion. These clinical observations led to the notion that the brain damage occurred as a result of tissue anoxia, with increased metabolic needs of cerebral tissue occurring at a time of systemic asphyxia, creating a relative cerebral hypoxia in which the metabolic demands of the seizure could not be met by adequate delivery of substrate. Brain damage then resulted for the same (unknown) reason that hypoxia-ischemia damages the brain, an organ notoriously sensitive to such insults.

This suspected relationship between energy metabolism and brain damage was supported by neuropathological studies in patients following severe status epilepticus (7). A distinctive pattern is commonly observed, with the prominent findings of neuronal degeneration and loss in the h1 and h3 fields of the hippocampus, with sparing of the h2 sector and often of the dentate gyrus. Extensive neuronal loss may be seen in the deeper layers of the neocortex. Lesser degrees of neuronal degeneration are seen in the cerebellum, amygdala, and other nuclei. Because these findings are also characteristic of the encephalopathy following anoxic-ischemic insults or hypoglycemia, the suspicion that the common denominator was that of energy metabolism inadequate to support cell survival appeared reasonable.

This hypothesis has practical implications for clinical medicine. If it is correct, then treatment of status epilepticus should be directed primarily toward correction of the secondary systemic defects of the seizure. Ensuring the delivery of adequate substrate of the brain should prevent brain damage. Suppression of seizure activity by anticonvulsants would not be essential and would be of secondary importance. Because suppression of seizure activity in status often can be difficult, requiring at times general anesthesia for prolonged periods (a treatment that carries risks of its own), the question is of critical clinical importance. Thus, there is a central question relating to management of status epilepticus: In the absence of hypoxemia, hyperthermia, hypoglycemia, and other systemic disturbances, is prolonged seizure activity destructive to the brain? Answers to this question have been sought in studies of cerebral energy metabolism in experimental animals.

CEREBRAL ENERGY METABOLISM IN THE SINGLE SEIZURE

Most investigators have studied this problem by measuring brain tissue concentration of substrates of energy metabolism at various stages during the progression of seizures (6,8,10,16,17). Taking into account differences in the models used, the species of animals, the epileptogens, and differing efficiencies and techniques used to preserve *in vivo* substrate levels, a fairly characteristic response has been observed in freely convulsing animals. There is rapid and abrupt depletion in the high-energy phosphates, adenosine triphosphate (ATP) and phosphocreatine (PCr), the ultimate sources of energy used by virtually all metabolic processes in the brain. Corresponding rises in the breakdown products adenosine diphosphate (ADP), adenosine monophosphate (AMP), and creatine occur, along with marked elevations in lactate and the lactate/pyruvate ratio. If the convulsion is severe, the high-energy phosphates can be almost depleted. Following termination of the seizure, these values tend to revert to normal promptly and correspond with clinical recovery. The magnitudes of these changes tend to reflect the intensity of the electrophysiological seizure rather than the nature of the epileptogen. Because these are the chemical changes also seen in acute ischemia, these studies have all supported the view that in freely convulsing animals the synthesis of metabolic energy by normal oxidative mechanisms or by anaerobic mechanisms is inadequate to meet the demands for its use.

In these studies it was evident that the effects of the secondary systemic responses associated with the asphyxia could not be separated from the primary responses of the brain metabolic processes to increased metabolic demands. Thus animal models were developed, using paralysis and ventilation, in which the effects of these systemic responses could be eliminated or minimized and physiological variables such as blood pressure, blood gases, and temperature could be carefully monitored.

In using these models, it was found that the profound depletion of high-energy phosphates and

related changes observed in the brains of the freely convulsing animals could be substantially modified (4,5,9,12–14,23). Nevertheless, changes did occur. There were small but highly significant decreases in ATP and PCr, with corresponding increases in ADP, AMP, and creatine. In addition, there were fivefold to sevenfold increases in lactate, lactate/pyruvate ratio, and tissue acidosis. These occurred in the mouse, rat, and cat and were similar for the convulsant drugs flurothyl and pentylenetetrazol (PTZ) and for electroshock. However, the studies of oxygen availability all indicated that as a consequence of the marked increase in cerebral blood flow, the sagittal sinus Po_2 actually rose, indicating that the blood flow increase exceeded the requirements of the metabolizing tissue. Thus, the energy changes observed represented the responses of the brain metabolic processes to a condition of markedly increased energy use in which substrate availability was not limiting. The increased use of ATP was presumably to support ion pumping and neurotransmitter metabolism. These changes promptly reversed on termination of the seizure. Thus, these studies on the single seizure emphasized the importance of the asphyxial response in perturbing the metabolic state of the brain, but they further identified changes in the energy state that occurred in response to increased energy use and provided a useful background for consideration of status epilepticus.

CEREBRAL ENERGY METABOLISM IN MULTIPLE OR PROLONGED SEIZURES (STATUS)

The transient perturbations of the energy state in the single seizure proved remarkably reproducible when multiple seizures were induced as a model of status epilepticus (9). Thus, when seizures lasting 15 to 30 sec were induced every 2 min in paralyzed ventilated mice by flurothyl or electroshock, the pattern of changes evident in the first seizure was seen after 20 seizures, providing evidence that even with frequent seizures, metabolic responses were unimpaired when ventilation was maintained. However, after 20 such seizures, some deterioration in the energy state occurred, accompanied by a tendency for spontaneous recurrent seizures to develop, indicating that deleterious effects had occurred.

In order to further study the problem, it seemed reasonable to create an intense seizure and follow

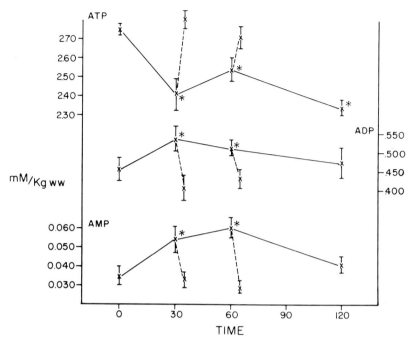

FIG. 1. Adenine nucleotide levels in the rat cortex during status epilepticus induced by PTZ. Animals were paralyzed, ventilated, and maintained under close physiological control. Values connected by dash lines represent concentrations 5 min after administration of diazepam and nitrous oxide:oxygen (70:30). Values are micromoles per gram. Asterisk indicates statistically significant change ($p < 0.05$ compared with controls).

it for a prolonged period. This was done using PTZ (120–150 mg/kg) as the epileptogen in paralyzed ventilated cats and rats under careful physiological control (12). Assays of brain substrates were done after 1, 10, 30, 60, and 120 min of seizure activity. The results in the cats and rats were similar in most respects. There were changes in the levels of high-energy phosphates and hence the metabolic energy state of the tissue. This occurred abruptly within 1 min and, once established, persisted for the duration of the seizure (Fig. 1). Lactic acidosis and elevation of the lactate/pyruvate ratio indicating an altered redox state occurred; this could not be ascribed to hypoxia, because brain tissue oxygen tension actually rose. These experiments could not be continued beyond 2 hr because of problems in maintaining blood pressure, which tended to fall after an initial marked rise. However, after 120 min of seizure activity in the rat, a modest deterioration in the energy state occurred. Also notable was a decline in brain glucose, with an increasing blood/brain glucose ratio (Fig. 2).

Furthermore, the changes at both 30 and 60 min could be rapidly reversed within 5 min of admin-

istration of the anticonvulsant diazepam, combined with reintroduction of nitrous oxide/oxygen anesthesia (70/30), suggesting that the metabolic changes in brain tissue were reflections of the increased metabolic needs created by the seizure and were not intrinsic to the epileptogen nor the consequences of secondary changes in the tissue.

These results demonstrated a remarkable ability of brain metabolic mechanisms to respond promptly to increased metabolic requirements to provide ATP to support cellular energy-requiring processes, particularly ion pumping and the metabolic mechanisms for synthesis and reuptake of neurotransmitters. This stability did not suggest serious failure of oxidative metabolic capacity exerted, despite 2 hr of intense seizure activity. This was not, however, interpreted as evidence that cellular damage had not occurred, because studies of anoxia-ischemia had established that a normal energy state could exist at a time of significant cellular damage (20) but rather if it did so it seemed unlikely to have occurred from inadequacies of energy metabolism. This stability of the energy state has also been demonstrated in status epilepticus induced by bicuculline and allylglycine (4).

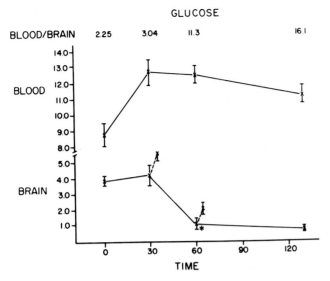

FIG. 2. Blood and brain tissue concentrations of glucose after 30, 60, and 120 min of status epilepticus induced by PTZ in rats. Values are means ± SD expressed as micromoles per gram (brain) and micromoles per milliliter (blood). Dash lines indicate concentrations 5 min after administration of diazepam and nitrous oxide:oxygen (70:30). Note the progressive increase in the blood/brain ratio. Asterisk indicates statistically significant change ($p < 0.05$ compared with controls).

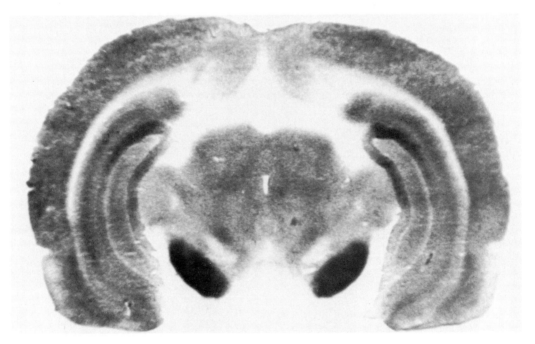

FIG. 3. Autoradiograph of rat brain showing glucose utilization. ^{14}C-2-DG was administered 1 min after seizure induction by PTZ, and the animal was killed 45 min later. Note the marked increase in glucose use in the substantia nigra and the molecular layer of the dentate gyrus.

STUDIES OF REGIONAL GLUCOSE METABOLISM IN PTZ-INDUCED STATUS EPILEPTICUS

The measurement of regional glucose metabolism using the technique of autoradiography with [^{14}C]2-deoxy-D-glucose (^{14}C-2-DG) (22) provided a means to further study energy metabolism during seizure activity. Electrophysiological studies and studies of regional glucose metabolism in both focal epilepsy and generalized epilepsy have all indicated marked differences in the involvement of different brain regions (3,5). Thus, studies of re-

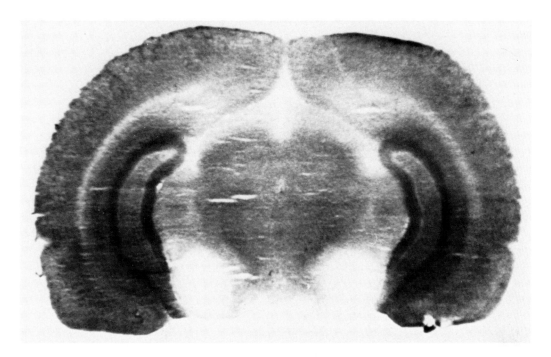

FIG. 4. Autoradiograph of a rat brain showing glucose utilization. ^{14}C-2-DG was administered 90 min after seizure induction by PTZ. Note the marked lack of activity in the region of the substantia nigra, as compared with Fig. 3.

gional glucose utilization were carried out in order to identify regional differences as they might affect seizure function and the development of brain damage.

The paralyzed ventilated rat model used for biochemical studies was adapted for ^{14}C-2-DG autoradiography. Following surgical preparation and assessment of physiological stability, status was induced by PTZ (120–150 mg/kg intraarterially). After 1, 5, 15, 20, 60, and 90 min of seizure activity, a pulse dose of 25 μCi of ^{14}C-2-DG was administered. After a time sufficient to allow uptake and phosphorylation of the glucose analogue in the brain and for elimination of the tracer from the blood (35–45 min), the animal was killed and the brain processed for quantitative autoradiography.

The autoradiographs taken at all times during the seizure differed markedly from those of controls. In general, they showed the expected increase in glucose metabolic rate. Certain areas showed marked increases. These included the substantia nigra, hippocampus, most areas of the cerebral cortex, the striatum, and the reticular formation of the brainstem. The regions most active in the

normal brain, the inferior colliculus, the interpeduncular nucleus, the olivary complex, and dorsal layers of the superior colliculus, were relatively inactive. This variation in the participation of different regions is of particular interest, with implications for interpretation of the patterns of energy metabolism. Furthermore, the pattern of activation, once established, tended to persist for the duration of the seizure. The striking exception was the substantia nigra (Fig. 3).

This nucleus initially showed a 6- to 10-fold increase in glucose utilization. Patterns of glucose uptake begun after 1, 5, and 15 min of seizure activity (thus measuring glucose uptake over the subsequent 45 min) all showed calculated metabolic rates ranging from 4 to 7 μmole/g/min. However, when the ^{14}C-2-DG was administered after 30 min of seizure activity, measured metabolic activity had fallen substantially to normal levels. After 60 to 90 min of seizure activity, glucose metabolism was markedly depressed (0.23 μmole/g/min), which represents more than a 15-fold change (Fig. 4). This was present both in the pars reticulata and, to a lesser degree, the pars compacta. The active participation of the substan-

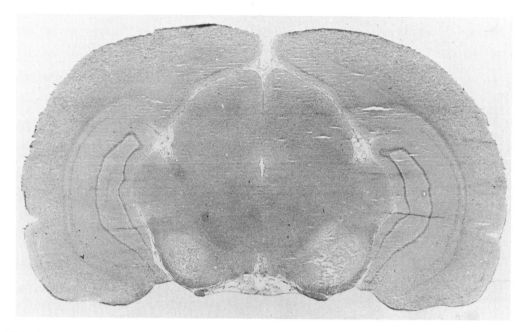

FIG. 5. Hematoxylin-eosin stain of rat brain section used for autoradiography after 90 min of continuous seizure activity induced by PTZ. This section taken from the same rat as in Fig. 4. Note the loosening and disruption of the substantia nigra.

tia nigra in various seizure processes has been recognized electrophysiologically and metabolically (3–6). However, the intensity of this response is particularly striking. It is also notable that the calculated glucose metabolic rate is substantially higher than the estimated V_{max} for glucose transport into whole brain (21). This implies that the maximal rate of transport of glucose by the glucose carrier into brain shows regional variations. The effect of increased blood flow may also be pertinent (19).

The dramatic decline in metabolic activity in the substantia nigra was also of particular interest. There is no obvious physiological explanation, because the metabolism in regions with known afferent and efferent connections to the substantia nigra remained relatively constant. Rather, the explanation appears to be that the most dramatic changes occur in the region most active metabolically because of cellular damage. This is suggested by hematoxylin-eosin staining of the autoradiograph, which shows altered staining of the substantia nigra and evidence of tissue disruption (Fig. 5). This was evident throughout both nuclei but was limited to them.

Microscopic examinations were carried out on the brains of 2 animals killed after 125 min of PTZ status epilepticus, thereby corresponding to the an-

imals given ^{14}C-2-DG after 90 min of seizure activity. These brains were perfuse-fixed with formalin:acetic acid:methanol (10:10:80). In the substantia nigra, particularly in the pars reticularis, many neurons with ischemic cell changes were identified; this was not seen in controls.

The second area of intense glucose utilization was that of the molecular layer of the dentate. The hippocampus is of particular interest because of its vulnerability in the human to status epilepticus. The hypermetabolism of glucose extended diffusely throughout the molecular layer. Interestingly, the layer of cell bodies of the granule cells appeared as a whitish line, suggesting relative inactivity during the seizure that was not apparent in controls. In contrast to the situation with the substantia nigra, the glucose hyperactivity persisted during the period of study, as did the pattern of activity in the hippocampus itself.

However, despite this evidence of metabolic activity, histological studies of the perfused fixed brains showed evidence of marked ischemic cell change and edema in the pyramidal cell layer. This was present throughout, but it appeared maximal in the h1 and h3 sections. In contrast, the majority of neurons in the granule cells of the dentate appeared normal.

The 2-DG technique, whether for qualitative or quantitative study, requires certain assumptions that may not be entirely valid when applied to the generalized seizure. The glucose level, which is assumed to be stable, may fluctuate during the seizure. It is also known that the blood-brain barrier breaks down during the convulsion, thereby disturbing the normal pattern of glucose transport into and out of the brain. In addition, the kinetic constants will change with increased glucose use and blood flow. Finally, the "lumped constant" may vary during the experimental conditions. Indeed, evidence exists that it is altered more than twofold in ischemic brain damage (11). Obviously, caution is required in interpreting density patterns in brains with other forms of damage. However, despite these cautions, the method appears to be a useful means of studying brain energy metabolism.

Two findings pertinent to the question posed initially were those in the substantia nigra and the hippocampus. The finding of failing glucose metabolism in the substantia nigra, combined with evidence of cell and tissue damage, provides evidence that seizure activity, particularly if intense, does indeed damage the brain. Similar conclusions can be drawn from the findings of pyramidal cell damage in the hippocampus. The extent of this damage is surprising in view of the much more modest changes reported in the bicuculline model of status (2). This may reflect greater intensity of seizure activity or possibly intrinsic toxic effects of the epileptogen. Studies to clarify this question appear highly desirable.

ACKNOWLEDGMENTS

This work was supported by the Medical Research Council of Canada (grant number MA5148). The author acknowledges the assistance of the Department of Pathology, Queen's University, in the preparation of histological sections. The author also is grateful for the excellent technical assistance of Dan Waiman.

REFERENCES

1. Aicardie, J., and Chevrie, J. J. (1971): Convulsive status epilepticus in infants and children: A study of 239 cases. *Epilepsia*, 11:187–197.
2. Blennow, C., Brierley, J. B., Meldrum, B. S., and Siesjö, B. K. (1978): Epileptic brain damage: The role of factors that modify cerebral energy metabolism. *Brain*, 101:687–700.
3. Caveness, W. F., Kato, M., Malamud, B. L., Hosokawa, S., Wakisaka, S., and O'Neill, R. P. (1980): Propagation of focal motor seizures in the pubescent monkey. *Ann. Neurol.*, 7:213–221.
4. Chapman, A. G., Meldrum, B. S., and Siesjö, B. K. (1977): Cerebral metabolic changes during prolonged epileptic seizures in rats. *J. Neurochem.*, 28:1025–1035.
5. Collins, R. C. (1978): Use of cortical circuits during focal penicillin seizure: An autoradiographic study with ^{14}C-deoxy-glucose. *Brain Res.*, 150:487–501.
6. Collins, R. C., Posner, J. B., and Plum, F. (1970): Cerebral energy metabolism during electroshock seizures in mice. *Am. J. Physiol.*, 218:943–950.
7. Corsellis, J. A. N., and Meldrum, B. S. (1976): Epilepsy. In: *Greenfield's Neuropathology*, edited by W. Blackwood and J. A. N. Corsellis, pp. 771–795. Year Book Medical Publishers, Chicago.
8. Dawson, R. M., and Richter, D. (1950): Effects of stimulation on the phosphate esters of the brain. *Am. J. Physiol.*, 160:203–211.
9. Duffy, T. E., Howse, D. C., and Plum, F. (1975): Cerebral energy metabolism during experimental status epilepticus. *J. Neurochem.*, 24:925–934.
10. Ferrendelli, J. A., and McDougall, D. B. (1971): The effect of electroshock on regional CNS energy reserves in mice. *J. Neurochem.*, 18:1197–1205.
11. Ginsberg, M., and Reivich, M. E. (1979): Use of the 2-deoxy-glucose method of local cerebral glucose utilization in the abnormal brain: Evaluation of the lumped constant during ischemia. *Acta Neurol. Scand. [Suppl. 72]*, 10:226–227.
12. Howse, D. C. (1978): Metabolic response to status epilepticus in the rat, cat, and mouse. *Can. J. Physiol. Pharmacol.*, 57:205–212.
13. Howse, D. C., Caronna, J. J., Duffy, T. E., and Plum, F. (1974): Cerebral energy metabolism, pH and blood flow during seizure in the cat. *Am. J. Physiol.*, 227:1444–1451.
14. Howse, D. C., and Duffy, T. E. (1975): Control of the redox state of the pyridine nucleotides in the rat cerebral cortex. *J. Neurochem.*, 24:935–940.
15. Hunter, R. A. (1959): Status epilepticus: History, incidence and problems. *Epilepsia*, 1:162–188.
16. King, L. K., Webb, O. L., and Carl, J. (1970): Effects of the duration of convulsions on energy reserves of the brain. *J. Neurochem.*, 17:13–18.
17. Klein, R. J., and Olsen, N. S. (1947): Effect of convulsive activity on the concentration of brain glucose, lactate and phosphate. *J. Biochem.*, 167:747–756.
18. Oxbury, J. M., and Whitty, C. W. (1971): Causes and consequences of status epilepticus in adults. *Brain*, 94:733–744.
19. Pardridge, W. M., and Oldendorf, W. H. (1975): Kinetics of blood/brain barrier transport of hexoses. *Biochim. Biophys. Acta*, 382:377–392.
20. Salford, L. G., Plum, F., and Siesjö, B. K. (1973): Graded hypoxia-oligemia in rat brain: I. Biochemical alterations and their implications. *Arch. Neurol.*, 29:227–233.
21. Siesjö, B. K. (1978): Brain Energy Metabolism, pp. 115–116. John Wiley & Sons, New York.
22. Sokoloff, L., Reivich, M., Kennedy, C., DesRossiers, M. H., Patlack, C., Pettigrew, K., Saku-

rada, O., and Shinohara, M. (1977): The ^{14}C-deoxy-glucose method for the measurement of local cerebral glucose utilization. *J. Neurochem.*, 28:897–916.

23. Whistler, K. E., Tews, J. K., and Stone, W. E. (1968): Cerebral amino acids and lipids in drug induced status epilepticus. *J. Neurochem.*, 15:215–220.

Advances in Neurology, Vol. 34: Status
Epilepticus, edited by A.V. Delgado-Escueta,
C.G. Wasterlain, D.M. Treiman, and R.J. Porter.
Raven Press, New York © 1983.

21

Local Cerebral Circulation and Metabolism in Bicuculline-Induced Status Epilepticus: Relevance for Development of Cell Damage

Bo K. Siesjö, Martin Ingvar, Jaroslava Folbergrová,
and Astrid G. Chapman

Among the clinical conditions that lead to brain dysfunction and/or irreversible neuronal cell damage in the brain, severe hypoxia, ischemia, and hypoglycemia have in common gross perturbation of the cerebral energy state, as evidenced by depletion of the high-energy phosphate compounds phosphocreatine and adenosine triphosphate (ATP) and accumulation of adenosine diphosphate (ADP) and adenosine monophosphate (AMP); a review of the literature is available (50). In two of these conditions (hypoxia and ischemia), anaerobic glycolysis is stimulated, with ensuing lactic acidosis, whereas the third (hypoglycemia) is characterized by energy failure at normal or increased intracellular pH. It is now known that excessive acidosis contributes to brain damage in hypoxia and ischemia (24,38,44). In hypoglycemia, this cannot be the case. It is therefore tempting to conclude that the mechanisms involved are related to energy failure. However, because deterioration of the tissue energy state during hypoglycemia is also observed in the cerebellum, a structure that shows virtually no histopathological alterations (1), other mechanisms must contribute. Results of this type, and the possibility that at least part of the final damage resulting from hypoxia-ischemia may be

incurred (or may mature) in the reoxygenation/recirculation period, have led to suggestions that "oxidative" mechanisms could be common to several adverse conditions (50,52). At present, such mechanisms are poorly defined, but suggestions have been made that they include lipid peroxidation and enzyme inactivation due to free-radical formation (2,19,34,53,59). Another possible cause of oxidative damage is that related to excessive accumulation of polyenoic fatty acids, chiefly arachidonic acid, which will trigger a burst of oxidative reactions along the fatty acid cyclo-oxygenase and lipoxygenase pathways, leading to formation of prostaglandins and leucotrienes, respectively (9,22). It is of interest that some of the potentially toxic compounds thus formed are free radicals.

Status epilepticus represents yet another condition in which neuronal cell damage may be incurred by mechanisms that are currently under debate. Neuropathological observations on human material have revealed cell injury localized to the classic selectively vulnerable regions, chiefly the cerebral cortex, limbic structures such as the hippocampus, and the cerebellum (17,39,). Because it could not be excluded that complicating hypoxia-ischemia contributed to the histopathological alterations, several groups have attempted to elucidate the pathophysiology of epileptic brain damage in animal experiments in which seizures were induced by electroshock or by drugs. Although some of these studies, especially those with seizure durations of 90 min or less, have failed to show the development of cell damage (42,48), others have demonstrated that such damage occurs. The latter studies fall into two categories. One series of experiments has been concerned with the adverse effects of repeated seizures on brain development in the immature animal (60) (see chapter 23). The other category, one that is of primary concern for the present discussion, includes experiments with drug-induced status epilepticus in mature animals. Because there is now relatively extensive information on seizures induced by the GABA receptor blocker bicuculline, we shall concentrate on the description of that model.

Working on baboons, Meldrum and Brierley (35) observed that prolonged seizures gave rise to "ischemic cell damage" in the selectively vulnerable regions (*vide supra*). When variables such as arterial oxygenation, blood pressure, and body temperature were controlled in ventilated animals, the damage was somewhat less pronounced, and the Purkinje cells of the cerebellum were spared (37). Such results make it tempting to conclude that vulnerable neurons succumb in spite of adequate oxygenation. Much information on this problem has been collected in artificially ventilated rats. First, it has been documented that bicuculline-induced seizures give rise to twofold to threefold increases in cerebral oxygen consumption (CMR_{O_2}) and glucose utilization (CMR_{gl}), with a corresponding increase in cerebral blood flow (10,36). Second, although biochemical results demonstrated an initial perturbation of the cerebral cortical energy state, a sustained reduction in phosphocreatine (PCr) concentration and sustained increases in creatine and lactate concentrations, with an associated rise in the lactate/pyruvate ratio, the phosphorylation state of the adenine nucleotide pool was upheld close to normal over a 2-hr seizure period (8,15). Third, in spite of this seemingly adequate energy state, neuronal lesions were observed in the cerebral cortex and hippocampus (6,55). In fact, because these experiments indicated that lesions were ameliorated, rather than accentuated, by restriction of the cerebral oxygen supply, with an accompanying exaggeration of tissue lactic acidosis, they lend further support to the possibility that the mechanisms involved are oxidative.

At present, interpretation of available information is hampered by lack of information on regional changes in blood flow, metabolic rate, and metabolic state. Specifically, it seems warranted to study such changes in "vulnerable" and "resistant" areas, i.e., to correlate changes in blood flow and metabolism to histopathological alterations. In pursuing this problem we adopted the following approach: First, we analyzed changes in local cerebral blood flow (CBF) and local CMR_{gl} using quantitative autoradiographic techniques (30). The objective of that study was to determine whether the localization of lesions to certain brain structures correlated to the increase in metabolic rate or to a mismatch between blood flow and metabolic rate. Second, in order to explore whether or not a correlation exists between histopathological findings and metabolic state, we analyzed two vulnerable regions (cerebral cortex and hippocampus) and a resistant one (cerebellum), measuring labile metabolites reflecting cellular energy balance (23). Third, in order to determine if conditions favoring oxidative damage were at hand, we measured phospholipid-bound fatty acids, free fatty acids, and glutathione redox ratios. In these studies we also found it of interest to explore changes occurring in cyclic nucleotides (cyclic AMP and cyclic GMP), because these may have a bearing on the balance between inhibition and excitation, as well as on the presence of adverse oxidative reactions (see Discussion).

MATERIALS AND METHODS

The material presented in this chapter is derived from four publications. Thus, data on cerebral cortical concentrations of fatty acids and cyclic nucleotides (as well as adenosine) for seizure periods of 1, 30, and 60 min are from Chapman et al. (14); results on regional metabolite concentrations (seizure periods of 20 and 120 min) are from Folbergrová et al. (23); results on l-CBF and l-CMR_{gl} are from Ingvar and Siesjö (30); results on free fatty acids at 20 and 120 min are from Siesjö et al. (51). Detailed accounts of methods and analytical techniques are given in these publications. The following is a brief summary of experimental procedures.

All experiments were performed on fed Wistar rats that were anesthetized with halothane-N_2O and maintained artificially ventilated on 70% N_2O and 30% O_2, with control of body temperature, blood pressure, arterial P_{O_2}, P_{CO_2}, and pH. Operative procedures included cannulation of one or both femoral arteries (for l-CBF measurements, a short brachial artery catheter was used) and one or both femoral veins, as well as insertion of EEG electrodes into the skull bone. After completion of the operative procedures, the animals were maintained at steady state for at least 30 min before seizures were induced. During that time, body temperature was kept at 37°C, Pa_{O_2} at about 100 mm Hg, and Pa_{CO_2} at 35 to 40 mm Hg.

Seizures were induced by intravenous injection of bicuculline (1.2 mg·kg^{-1}). To minimize the ictal increase in pressure, 3 to 5 ml of blood were slowly withdrawn just before the injection of bicuculline. When blood pressure subsequently fell, the shed blood was reinfused (or blood from a donor rat was given), so as to maintain mean arterial blood pressure at 110 to 120 mm Hg.

We measured local CBF after seizure periods of 20, 60, and 120 min using the autoradiographic ^{14}C technique described by Sakurada et al. (47). Local CMR_{gl} was measured with the autoradiographic ^{14}C-deoxyglucose technique of Sokoloff et al. (57). In these experiments the tracer was infused after 20, 45, and 105 min of seizure activity, and sampling of arterial blood was continued for 45 min. Because the l-CMR_{gl} values obtained can be assumed to be heavily weighted in favor of the first 5 to 15 min following isotope infusion (57), the values for blood flow and glucose utilization should pertain to seizure periods of similar duration. In both series of autoradiographic measurements the densities of 21 different brain structures and of a set of calibrated ^{14}C standards were evaluated with a densitometer with an aperture of 1 mm. Whole blood (^{14}C-iodoantipyrine) and plasma (^{14}C-deoxyglucose) tracer activities were measured by liquid scintillation techniques, and plasma glucose concentrations were measured with a fluorometric hexokinase method. Local CBF and CMR_{gl} were calculated as described in the references cited. Because the lumped constant used for calculating l-CMR_{gl} varies with the blood glucose concentration, we initially used corrected values, as determined by Sokoloff and associates (56). However, in spite of this, l-CMR_{gl} values obtained in cerebral cortical (and limbic) structures after 2 hr of status epilepticus greatly exceeded those expected from CMR_{O_2} data. We therefore made no attempts to interpret the results obtained quantitatively.

For measurements of tissue metabolites, the tissue was frozen *in situ* with liquid nitrogen (41). Samples of cerebral cortex (parietal-sensorimotor), hippocampal formation, and cerebellum (vermis excluded) were separated at -22°C. For the measurement of concentrations of PCr, ATP, ADP, AMP, glycogen, glucose, lactate, pyruvate, reduced gluthathione (GSH), and cyclic nucleotides, we extracted the tissues with HCl-methanol (-22°C) and perchloric acid (0°C). Oxidized glutathione (GSSG) was measured after extraction with trichloroacetic acid, and alkylation of SH groups was measured with *N*-ethylmaleimide (NEM) (43). Cyclic AMP was measured by a protein-binding technique, and cyclic GMP was measured by radioimmunoassay. All other metabolites were measured with enzymatic-fluorometric techniques.

For measurements of fatty acids, the tissues were extracted with chloroform-methanol. Phospholipid concentrations were estimated by fatty acid analyses and by phosphorous determinations. For measuring free fatty acids (FFA), these were first isolated by thin-layer chromatography; following esterification, the individual fatty acids were measured by gas-liquid chromatography.

RESULTS

In all the experiments the EEG seizure patterns were similar to those described previously (15,36), and a continuous burst-suppression pattern was upheld during the seizure periods. Arterial P_{O_2} was around 100 mm Hg, P_{CO_2} was in the range 30 to 40 mm Hg, and mean arterial blood pressure was 110 to 120 mm Hg.

Local CBF and CMR_{gl}

Absolute values for l-CBF and l-CMR_{gl} after 20, 60, and 120 min of seizure activity will be described in a forthcoming publication (30). In this chapter we shall exemplify changes observed by depicting percentage changes from control after 20 min of seizure activity in all structures analyzed and confine the description of time-related changes to those structures that were analyzed with respect to labile metabolites (cerebral cortex, hippocampus, and cerebellum).

Figure 1 shows changes in l-CBF and l-CMR_{gl} after 20 min of continuous seizure activity. The increase of CBF was fairly heterogeneous, with

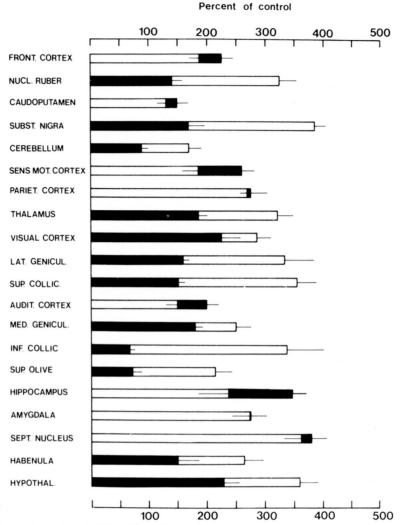

FIG. 1. Changes in local cerebral blood flow (CBF) and glucose consumption (CMR$_{gl}$) after 20 min of continuous bicuculline-induced seizures. All values are expressed as percent of control ($\pm$ SEM). The lengths of the unfilled bars denote CBF, and the filled bars indicate CMR$_{gl}$.

flow rates varying between 130% (caudate-putamen) and 380% (substantia nigra) of control. Cortical structures had CBF values varying between 150% (auditory) and 280% (parietal and visual) of control; hippocampus and amygdala had values about 2.5 times control; the cerebellum l-CBF value was 170% of control.

In this initial period of continuous seizure activity, the l-CMR$_{gl}$ values for parietal and sensorimotor cortex (260%–270% of control) were in excellent agreement with previous data for regional (cortical) CMR$_{O_2}$ and CMR$_{gl}$ (10,36). We can therefore confidently use these data to illustrate the

ratio between blood flow and metabolic rate. Figure 1 illustrates two main points: First, there was a marked heterogeneity in seizure-induced alterations in metabolic rate. Thus, two limbic structures (hippocampus and septal nucleus) showed increases in l-CMR$_{gl}$ (340% and 380% of control, respectively) that were even more pronounced than those observed in cerebral cortical areas. Furthermore, many other structures showed only moderate increases in metabolic rate, and in three of them (inferior colliculus, superior oliva, and cerebellum) the mean l-CMR$_{gl}$ values were below control. Second, although many structures showed similar relative changes in l-CBF and l-CMR$_{gl}$, others had flow rates that clearly exceeded any increase in metabolic rate. In other words, the increase in blood flow did not correlate with the enhancement in metabolic rate. We note that a "relative hyperperfusion" did not occur in cerebral cortical areas or in limbic structures (except habenula).

Prolongation of the seizure period from 20 to 60 min was associated with further increases in CBF in more than half the structures analyzed. This increase may, at least in part, reflect a corresponding augmentation of local glucose consumption (*vide infra*). However, the most striking time-related change was the pronounced reduction in flow that occurred with prolongation of the seizure period from 60 to 120 min. These changes in local blood flow were unrelated to differences in blood pressure, because the 60- and 120-min groups had mean arterial blood pressures of 114 ± 2 and 113 ± 3 mm Hg, respectively. Figure 2 demonstrates time-dependent changes in CBF in five cortical structures, two limbic areas, and cerebellar cortex. We observed that in all these structures, prolongation of status epilepticus was associated with secondary reduction in CBF, and in some the 2-hr CBF values were lower than those measured at 20 min.

After 1 hr, the l-CMR$_{gl}$ values calculated increased in all structures shown in Fig. 2, and be-

cause the percentage increases were similar, the relative changes in CBF and CMR$_{gl}$ were about the same as those illustrated in Fig. 1. However, after 2 hr a further increase in calculated l-CMR$_{gl}$ was observed, indicating that a pronounced mismatch between blood flow and metabolic rate had developed. In the cerebral cortical structures and in the limbic structures the l-CMR$_{gl}$ values ranged between 400% and 470% of control, whereas cerebellum showed a value that was only 175% of control. Because the value for frontal, parietal, and sensorimotor structures corresponded to a glucose utilization rate of about 3 $\mu mole \cdot g^{-1} \cdot min^{-1}$, we suspected that the deoxyglucose method, with the lumped constant applied, grossly overestimated glucose consumption in cerebral cortical and limbic structures. Measurements of oxygen consumption with a ^{133}Xe modification of the Kety-Schmidt technique (with sampling of venous blood from the superior sagittal sinus) corroborated this suspicion. Thus, 4 animals studied after 2 hr of status epilepticus had a CMR$_{O_2}$ of 9.31 ± 0.19 $\mu mole \cdot g^{-1}$, corresponding to a glucose consumption of 1.6 $\mu mole \cdot g^{-1}$, i.e., about 225% of control. If we assume that the superior sagittal sinus drains predominantly frontal, parietal, and sensorimotor cortex, the results reveal that a mismatch between blood flow and metabolic rate still must have existed, albeit less pronounced than that indicated by the obviously erroneous l-CMR$_{gl}$ values (see Discussion).

Cerebral Metabolic State

On the basis of the autoradiographic results described and previous histopathological findings (*vide supra*) we chose to analyze labile metabolites in the cerebral cortex, hippocampus, and cerebellum. We shall discuss two series of results. In one series, which was devoted to analyses of changes in free fatty acids (14), the brain was frozen *in situ* after 1, 30, and 60 min of seizure activity, and cerebral cortex only was sampled for measurements of labile metabolites. The data are shown to facilitate discussion of changes in fatty acids and cyclic nucleotides (*vide infra*). In the second series, metabolites were analyzed in cerebral cortex, hippocampus, and cerebellum after 20 and 120 min of status epilepticus.

The data in Fig. 3, which confirm those previously published (15), illustrate that the cerebral cortical energy state was perturbed at seizure onset (1 min). At that time we also observed a fivefold

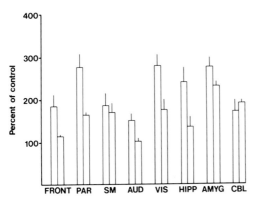

FIG. 2. Time-dependent changes in local CBF during bicuculline-induced seizures in eight cerebral structures (20 and 120 min). The values, which are in percent of control, pertain to (from left to right) frontal, parietal, sensorimotor, auditory, and visual cortex, hippocampus, amygdala, and cerebellum. After 120 min, clear reductions in CBF were noted in frontal, parietal, auditory, and visual cortex and in the hippocampus. These changes were even more pronounced (and also involved sensorimotor cortex and habenula) when the comparison was made to the 60-min values (data not shown).

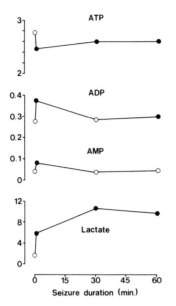

FIG. 3. Time-dependent changes in cerebral cortical concentrations of adenine nucleotides and lactate during bicuculline-induced seizures. The values (μmole·g^{-1} wet weight) are means for groups of 6 animals (SEM values smaller than the sizes of the symbols). Filled symbols denote significant changes from control ($p < 0.05$).

increase in tissue adenosine content (data not shown). Although the ATP concentration remained reduced during the subsequent 60-min period, the adenylate energy charge was close to normal at 30 and 60 min, and the adenosine content normalized. Thus, the remaining metabolic perturbation was dominated by an elevated lactate concentration and by a decrease in PCr concentration from a control value of 4.4 to about 2.75 μmole · g^{-1} (not shown).

Table 1 shows key metabolites in the cerebral cortex, hippocampus, and cerebellum after 20 and 120 min of status epilepticus (23). After 20 min, changes observed in the cerebral cortex were very similar to those illustrated in Fig. 1 for seizure durations of 30 and 60 min. Thus, PCr and ATP concentrations were reduced, but the energy charge did not deviate from control, and the lactate concentration was about 10 μmole·g^{-1}. The results further demonstrate a decrease in glucose concentration and extensive breakdown of glycogen. Metabolic changes in the hippocampus were virtually identical. Somewhat unexpectedly, signs of metabolic perturbation were observed in cerebellum as well, albeit somewhat less pronounced than in the two "vulnerable" structures.

Results obtained after 2 hr of status epilepticus allow two main conclusions. First, in contrast to previous findings (15), the cerebral cortex showed signs of a further perturbation of the cerebral energy state, with little evidence of resynthesis of glycogen and strikingly low glucose concentrations. Changes observed in the hippocampus were relatively similar, although lactate concentrations were lower and resynthesis of glycogen had occurred. For both structures, one can note the paradoxical finding that a reduction in energy charge was unassociated with a further increase in lactate concentration. Second, in the cerebellum the energy state was virtually normalized, extensive resynthesis of glycogen had occurred, and the slight increase in lactate concentration was associated with a normal lactate/pyruvate ratio (not shown).

The low tissue glucose concentrations in cortex and hippocampus suggested that the substrate supply had become limiting for cellular energy production. This suggestion was corroborated when the energy charge values of individual animals were related to the corresponding tissue glucose concentrations (Fig. 4). Thus, relatively marked reductions in energy charge were observed when tissue glucose concentrations fell well below 1 μmole·g^{-1}. In these animals, glycogen and lactate concentrations were low as well, suggesting that cellular glucose supply had become limiting, not only for energy production but also for lactate production and glycogen synthesis.

The data presented in Fig. 4 give the impression that in animals with "adequate" substrate supply, the phosphorylation state of the hippocampus may be upheld at control values. However, results obtained in a series of animals that were infused with glucose during the second hour of status epilepticus demonstrate that even if tissue glucose concentrations are upheld above 1 μmole·g^{-1} there is a small but highly significant reduction in adenylate energy charge. These results further demonstrate that the perturbations of the cerebral energy state are similar in the cerebral cortex and the hippocampus (23). Therefore, these "vulnerable" and hypermetabolic structures display perturbations of cerebral energy metabolism that are not observed in the "resistant" structure, the cerebellum.

Cyclic Nucleotides

Cyclic AMP (cAMP) and cyclic GMP (cGMP) concentrations were measured in the same series of experiments that were used for studying other

TABLE 1. *Metabolic changes in cerebral cortex, hippocampus, and cerebellum in bicuculline-induced status epilepticus*

Metabolite	Control	Seizure (20 min)	Seizure (120 min)
Cerebral cortex			
PCr	4.95 ± 0.09[a]	3.50 ± 0.19***	2.85 ± 0.20***
ATP	2.80 ± 0.09	2.60 ± 0.05*	2.50 ± 0.08**
EC[b]	0.938 ± 0.002	0.932 ± 0.003	0.895 ± 0.012**
Glycogen	2.68 ± 0.26	0.48 ± 0.08***	0.78 ± 0.23***
Glucose	3.43 ± 0.27	2.07 ± 0.22**	0.92 ± 0.16***
Lactate	2.58 ± 0.37	10.28 ± 0.46***	7.35 ± 1.71*
Hippocampus			
PCr	5.25 ± 0.10	3.99 ± 0.25***	4.04 ± 0.24***
ATP	2.93 ± 0.02	2.65 ± 0.08**	2.61 ± 0.05***
EC	0.941 ± 0.002	0.925 ± 0.005*	0.909 ± 0.012*
Glycogen	3.30 ± 0.31	0.48 ± 0.08***	1.78 ± 0.48*
Glucose	3.14 ± 0.29	1.60 ± 0.24**	0.84 ± 0.20***
Lactate	1.85 ± 0.06	8.96 ± 0.54***	4.63 ± 0.70**
Cerebellum			
PCr	7.02 ± 0.16	5.98 ± 0.07***	7.10 ± 0.20
ATP	2.61 ± 0.03	2.47 ± 0.03*	2.61 ± 0.06
EC	0.945 ± 0.002	0.941 ± 0.001	0.943 ± 0.002
Glycogen	3.82 ± 0.23	0.67 ± 0.11***	2.86 ± 0.12**
Glucose	4.37 ± 0.33	4.35 ± 0.53	2.45 ± 0.39**
Lactate	1.49 ± 0.21	6.67 ± 0.69***	2.31 ± 0.21*

[a] Values are means ± SEM for groups of 6 animals.
[b] EC = adenylate energy charge (ADP and AMP values not shown).
*$p < 0.05$.
**$p < 0.01$.
***$p < 0.001$.

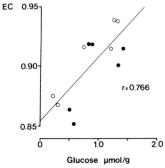

FIG. 4. Relationship between tissue glucose concentrations and energy charge values (EC) at the end of 2-hr seizure periods. Open symbols: hippocampus. Filled symbols: cerebral cortex. The correlation between glucose concentration and energy charge was significant ($p < 0.01$).

metabolites. Pooled data for the cerebral cortex are shown in Fig. 5 for seizure periods of 1 to 120 min. Concurrent with the initial perturbation of the cerebral energy state at 1 min and with the rise in adenosine content (Fig. 3), cAMP concentration increased 3.5-fold. Thereafter the values decreased, and after 60 min the values had normalized. After 120 min, a significant secondary increase was observed ($p < 0.05$). However, this increase was due to three values (2.21, 2.72, and 2.85 μmole·g⁻¹) obtained in those animals having the lowest energy charge values (0.901, 0.864, and 0.852, respectively). In the remaining 3 animals the cAMP values were within the normal range. The secondary rise in cAMP could well be related to energy failure, e.g., due to accumulation of adenosine.

Although the cGMP concentration also increased threefold at seizure onset, the values were upheld at about 300% of control throughout the seizure period. The individual values in the 2-hr group did not correlate with energy charge, and marked increases in cGMP were also noted in those 2 animals having energy charge values below 0.87.

In the hippocampus and cerebellum, cyclic nucleotides were measured only after 20 and 120 min

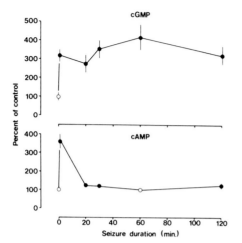

FIG. 5. Cerebral cortical concentrations of cyclic nucleotides during bicuculline-induced seizures (maximal 120 min duration). The values (percent of control) are means ± SEM (not shown if smaller than the sizes of the symbols). Filled symbols denote significant differences from controls ($p < 0.05$).

(23). At those times, the cAMP values in the hippocampus did not differ from control, but because the cGMP values at 20 and 120 min were 380% and 360% of control, respectively, the changes were similar to those observed in the cortex. In the cerebellum, cAMP concentrations did not differ from control. However, at 20 min, cGMP was 1,400% of control, and at 2 hr the values remained markedly elevated (450% of control).

Metabolic Changes Reflecting Oxidative Damage

Previous experiments have shown that when free-radical formation is induced in brain homogenates *in vitro*, the peroxidative reactions elicited are reflected in decreases in the concentrations of phospholipid-bound polyenoic fatty acids (20:4 and 22:6) and an oxidation of GHS to GSSG (43,45). In theory, therefore, measurements of phospholipids or phospholipid-bound fatty acids could yield information on peroxidative reactions operating *in vivo*. Furthermore, provided that the glutathione reductase reaction and the phosphogluconate pathway ("hexose monophosphate shunt") do not achieve instantaneous re-reduction of any GSSG formed, an increased GSSG/GSH ratio should be found.

Table 2 shows values for total phospholipid-bound fatty acid and percentage fatty acid composition in the cerebral cortex in animals exposed to seizure periods of 1, 30, and 60 min. As observed, seizures did not significantly alter total fatty acid content. In all seizure groups the mean values for arachidonic acid (20:4) were slightly below control. However, the change was not significant, and because the concentration of docosahexanoic acid (22:6) remained constant, the data fail to indicate that lipid peroxidation occurred.

Measurements of reduced (GSH) and oxidized (GSSG) glutathione concentrations gave equally negative results. Thus, after 2 hr of sustained seizure activity, cerebral cortex concentrations of GSH and GSSG did not deviate from control, and the GSSG concentration remained below 0.4% of the glutathione pool (in controls, GSH and GSSG concentrations were 2.27 ± 0.02 and 0.0080 ± 0.004 μmole · g^{-1}, respectively, and after 2 hr of seizures 2.29 ± 0.06 and 0.0086 ± 0.0003 μmole·g^{-1}, respectively).

We have previously reported that bicuculline-induced seizures are accompanied by a pronounced accumulation of FFA, the largest relative change occurring in arachidonic acid concentration (14). As was mentioned earlier, accumulation of polyenoic fatty acids may trigger potentially harmful reactions. We therefore analyzed FFA in cerebral cortex, hippocampus, and cerebellum. Data for cerebral cortex are available for seizure periods of 1, 20, 30, 60, and 120 min. Figure 6 shows changes in total FFA content and those affecting arachidonic acid. Total FFA content increased 2.3 times after 1 min, and the values were upheld at 250% to 300% of control during the first 30 min. Subsequently the values were reduced, but even after 2 hr the FFA content remained significantly increased (by about 30%). The peak arachidonic acid concentration occurred after 1 min, and the values were then gradually reduced. However, the value was twice control even after 2 hr.

In the hippocampus, total FFA content after 20 min had increased to 230% of control, with a five-fold increase in arachidonic acid concentration. At 2 hr the total FFA content was still increased 44% above control, but the differences did not reach statistical significance. However, because one control brain had an unusually high total FFA content and an arachidonic acid concentration more than twice the mean of the rest, we concluded that FFA changes in the hippocampus were similar to those observed in the cerebral cortex. However, the cerebellum provided an exception. Thus, although arachidonic acid concentration increased sevenfold after 20 min, the control value was much

TABLE 2. *Influences of bicuculline-induced seizures on major phospholipid-bound fatty acids in rat cerebral cortex*

Group	Total FA	16:0	18:0	18:1	20:4	22:6
Control	129 ± 3	32.6 ± 0.8	28.3 ± 0.6	24.2 ± 0.5	14.2 ± 0.8	21.6 ± 0.6
Seizures						
1 min	127 ± 2	33.5 ± 0.6	28.5 ± 0.7	23.9 ± 1.0	13.0 ± 0.3	21.1 ± 0.7
30 min	132 ± 2	33.9 ± 0.7	29.8 ± 0.4	25.6 ± 0.6	13.0 ± 0.2	22.2 ± 0.4
60 min	132 ± 3	33.5 ± 0.8	29.7 ± 0.6	25.5 ± 0.5	13.2 ± 0.4	21.9 ± 0.7

[a] Values are means ± SEM (μmole·g^{-1} wet weight; $N = 6$).

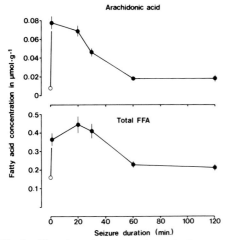

FIG. 6. Time-dependent changes in cerebral cortex concentrations of total FFA and arachidonic acid during bicuculline-induced seizures (maximal 120 min duration). Values are means ± SEM. Filled symbols denote values significantly different from controls ($p < 0.05$).

lower than those in the cortex and hippocampus. As a result, the value at 20 min of seizure activity was similar to the control values measured in the other structures. Furthermore, the total FFA content did not increase significantly. Finally, all individual acids were at control concentrations after 2 hr.

DISCUSSION

Our results can be summarized as follows: (a) Measurements of local CBF have confirmed previous results (36) in showing that bicuculline-induced status epilepticus is accompanied by an increase in CBF that is initially very marked but is attenuated in the later stages. In addition, the data demonstrate a marked heterogeneity in cir-

culatory response. Most important, structures considered vulnerable (neocortical and limbic areas), which have greatly increased perfusion rates in the initial phases, display pronounced reductions in CBF after 2 hr of status epilepticus. (b) The increase in local CMR$_{gl}$ is equally heterogeneous, the most pronounced changes being observed in these "vulnerable" areas. However, whereas CBF is reduced in these areas, metabolic rate is not, demonstrating that a mismatch between blood flow and metabolic rate develops. (c) The changes in metabolic rate and/or in the ratio between blood flow and glucose utilization correlate with the cerebral energy state. Thus, whereas sustained status epilepticus is accompanied by signs of moderate energy failure in neocortex and hippocampus, it leaves the metabolic state of a "resistant" area (the cerebellum) virtually unchanged. At least partly, the deterioration of the cerebral energy state in neocortex and hippocampus reflects curtailment of glucose supply that probably is secondary to the excessively increased metabolic demands. (d) During seizures, an initial increase in cAMP concentration is followed by a later return toward control values, whereas cGMP concentration remains elevated throughout the seizure period, the most pronounced changes being observed in the cerebellum. (e) Analyses of phospholipid-bound fatty acids or of glutathione redox ratios fail to reveal signs of peroxidative damage. However, seizures are accompanied by accumulations of FFA that are equally pronounced in cortex and hippocampus but strikingly moderate in the cerebellum. We shall discuss how these results relate to the known localization of neuronal lesions. However, it seems warranted to begin by briefly discussing the validity of the deoxyglucose technique for assessment of cerebral metabolic rate in seizures.

^{14}C-Deoxyglucose Technique during Seizures

The deoxyglucose technique of Sokoloff et al. (57) has been extensively used for measurements of local glucose utilization in seizures, particularly those elicited by topical application of convulsant drugs (12,16) and for limbic seizures induced by lidocaine (29) or kainic acid (see Chapter 25). In these studies it has been tacitly assumed that the "lumped constant" used for calculation of l-CMR$_{gl}$ is not influenced by the pathologically enhanced glucose utilization.

We have previously shown that under normal conditions (ventilated rats under 70% N$_2$O) the deoxyglucose technique yields values for glucose utilization in frontal, parietal, and sensorimotor cortex that fit well with previous measurements of *regional* CMR$_{O_2}$ and CMR$_{gl}$ (28). A corresponding agreement was obtained in the present material for the 20-min seizure group, but after 120 min of seizures the l-CMR$_{gl}$ values greatly exceeded those expected from CMR$_{O_2}$ measurements. In view of the low V_{max} values for transport of lactate between blood and tissue (40) and the small tissue-to-blood transport gradient, the discrepancy between l-CMR$_{gl}$ and CMR$_{O_2}$ cannot be explained by aerobic lactic acid production, nor can it be explained by glycogen synthesis (*vide supra*).

It is tempting to conclude that the lumped constant is changed at a time when cell damage and astrocytic swelling develop (see Chapter 16). However, it seems necessary to explore another possibility, i.e., that the lumped constant increases when glucose supply becomes limiting for the hexokinase reaction. Thus, when tissue glucose concentrations are reduced to very low values, the lumped constant increases (18,25). If this is so, a single lumped constant cannot be used for different structures, because such limiting glucose concentrations are observed only in areas with marked increases in metabolic rate. We are currently redetermining l-CMR$_{gl}$ in animals in which enough glucose is infused to maintain tissue glucose concentrations above 1 μmole·g^{-1} also in neocortex and hippocampus.

The Metabolic-Rate/CBF Couple and Localization of Neuronal Cell Damage

As remarked earlier, bicuculline-induced status epilepticus in artificially ventilated rats is accompanied by signs of neuronal cell damage, mainly localized to the neocortex and hippocampus, with sparing of most other structures, including the cerebellum. Clearly, this localization correlates both with the relative increases in local metabolic rate and with the reduced ratio between blood flow and metabolic rate. In view of the relative underperfusion of selectively vulnerable areas (at 2 hr), it is tempting to conclude that a deficient supply of oxygen and/or substrate contributes. At first sight, the results reported by Blennow et al. (7) would seem to provide direct evidence against this possibility. However, because curtailment of oxygen or glucose supply may reduce the firing rates of vulnerable neurons (*vide infra*), thereby reducing their metabolic demands, we put more confidence in two other findings. First, histopathological results reveal pronounced alterations already after 1 hr of status epilepticus (see Chapter 16), i.e., at a time when a mismatch between metabolic rate and blood flow has not yet developed. Second, ventilation of animals with 100% O$_2$ does not ameliorate the lesions (54).

In view of these results, we tentatively conclude that the excessive enhancement of local metabolic rate is what causes neuronal damage and that this, together with the associated swelling of astrocytic elements, gives rise to the delayed reduction in CBF.

Regional Metabolic Changes

The extent of metabolic perturbation observed in cerebral cortex, hippocampus, and cerebellum obviously correlates with the alterations in metabolic rate. At least at first sight, it is tempting to conclude that deterioration of the tissue energy state contributes to the development of cell damage. However, in analogy with what has been argued earlier, we must raise the question whether or not the dissociation in metabolic state after 2 hr of status epilepticus (cortex-hippocampus versus cerebellum) is merely the result of the differences in metabolic rates. Thus, because histopathological alterations in cerebral cortex appear marked already after 1 hr, when the adenylate energy charge is close to control (see Results), it is difficult to argue that the further metabolic deterioration observed after 2 hr is pathogenetically important. It is tempting to conclude, therefore, that structures that exhibit excessive enhancement of cellular metabolism develop signs of metabolic imbalance because their energy demands outstrip oxygen supply and that this imbalance, which is exaggerated when glucose supply becomes limiting, has little to do with the development of cell damage. However, this must remain a tentative conclusion until information is available on metabolic alterations, not of tissue in bulk, but of those cell populations that show signs of damage. Until such information is available, we can only note that "vulnerable" areas (cerebral cortex and hippocampus) show more pronounced metabolic changes than a "resistant" one (the cerebellum).

The analyses of cyclic nucleotides provided no clues to the mechanisms of damage. It has been suggested that the cAMP concentration, with its assumed relationship to catecholaminergic (chiefly noradrenergic) systems, reflects inhibitory influences, whereas cGMP bears some relationship to excitatory events, e.g., those associated with cholinergic pathways; discussions and reviews are available (20,21,26,31,32,58). In this context, it should also be recalled that the cGMP concentration has been claimed to reflect oxidative breakdown of polyenoic FFA (26). If we set aside the complexity of regulation of adenylate and guanylate cyclases, we can ask the simplifying question whether or not the cAMP/cGMP couple reflects the balance between inhibition and excitation during seizures. The results obtained in the cerebral cortex (a transient rise in cAMP and a sustained increase in cGMP concentration) are seemingly in accordance with such a view ("unbalanced excitation"). However, because similar changes occurred in the cerebellum, it is difficult to attach any pathogenetic importance to the alterations in the cAMP/cGMP couple.

In all probability, changes observed in FFA concentrations, particularly in arachidonic acid concentration, may be more relevant to a discussion of pathogenetic factors underlying cell damage. Many previous studies have shown that seizures induced by a variety of means raise tissue FFA concentrations (3,4,33). In this study we demonstrated that the FFA concentration increased in spite of maintained oxygenation of arterial blood and that, albeit reduced, this accumulation persisted throughout the seizure period. Furthermore, whereas FFA concentration increased threefold in the cerebral cortex (and hippocampus), the changes observed in the cerebellum were clearly less pronounced. The possible implication of this finding will be discussed later.

Is Oxidative Damage Occurring?

In view of what has been discussed, it is tempting to assume that damage is incurred in cell populations showing an excessive increase in metabolic turnover, by mechanisms that require oxygen to be present. Admittedly, analyses of phospholipid-bound fatty acids and of glutathione redox ratios failed to reveal the occurrence of peroxidative damage. However, as remarked earlier, the accumulation of polyenoic fatty acids, particularly of arachidonic acid, may trigger a burst of reactions along the cyclo-oxygenase and lipoxygenase pathways, leading to production of potentially toxic compounds. In this context, it suffices to recall the fact that polyenoic fatty acids may induce brain edema both *in vitro* (13) and *in vivo* (34). At present, we can only speculate on the pathogenetic importance of the accumulation of fatty acids. However, because the accumulations of FFA were regionally different and because they seem to correlate with pathological findings, the oxidative metabolism of polyenoic fatty acids seems worth pursuing.

Mechanisms of Epileptic Brain Damage: A Speculative Synthesis

Two pertinent questions remain to be answered: First, why is cell damage incurred in a tissue whose energy state is minimally perturbed? Second, why are certain cells selectively vulnerable? A tentative explanation is as follows (50): When seizures lead to enhanced neuronal firing, the intracellular Ca^{2+} concentration is raised by at least two mechanisms: influx from extracellular to intracellular fluids (27) and release from synaptic vesicles; see Calderini et al. (11) for changes in monoamine metabolism during bicuculline-induced seizures. Possibly, metabolically "strained" mitochondria may have a reduced Ca^{2+} transport capacity and thereby contribute to Ca^{2+} accumulation. Once the Ca^{2+} concentration rises, various hydrolyses, including phospholipase A_2, are activated, leading, among other things, to accumulation of FFA. This accumulation can then inhibit or uncouple mitochondria (5,61) and, because oxygen is present, activate cyclo-oxygenase and lipoxygenase, with resulting production of hydroperoxides and related free-radical compounds.

It is clear that if these events occur in circumscribed tissue loci, evidence of peroxidative damage is difficult to obtain by whole tissue analysis. The mere concept of selective neuronal vulnerability attests to the fact that the alterations are indeed circumscribed. Possibly this selective vulnerability resides in the electrophysiological (and metabolic) characteristics of such cells. Thus, pyramidal cells in the neocortex and hippocampus have been considered to have an innate capacity for spontaneous firing (46,49) and are supposed to have large (dendritic) Ca^{2+} conductances. In these cells, therefore, the proposed Ca^{2+}-triggered events could be grossly exaggerated.

We submit that the mechanisms proposed are speculative. However, there seems to be enough suggestive evidence to adopt this as a working hypothesis.

ACKNOWLEDGMENTS

This study was supported by a grant from the Swedish Medical Research Council (project B79-14X-263) and by U.S. Public Health Service grant R01 NS-07838. The excellent technical assistance of Kerstin Beirup, Barbro Asplund, Gertie Johansson, Karin Hansson, Gunilla Gidö, and Lena Sjöberg is gratefully acknowledged.

REFERENCES

1. Agardh, C.-D., Kalimo, H., Olsson, Y., and Siesjö, B. K. (1981): Hypoglycemic brain injury. Metabolic and structural findings in rat cerebellar cortex during profound insulin-induced hypoglycemia and in the recovery period following glucose administration. *J. Cerebral Blood Flow and Metabolism*, 1:71–84.
2. Barber, A. A., and Bernheim, F. (1967): Lipid peroxidation: Its measurement, occurrence and significance in animal tissues. *Adv. Gerontol. Res.*, 2:355–386.
3. Bazán, N. G. (1970): Effects of ischemia and electroconvulsive shock on free fatty acid pool in the brain. *Biochim. Biophys. Acta*, 218:1–10.
4. Bazán, N. G. (1976): Free arachidonic acid and other lipids in the nervous system during early ischemia and after electroshock. *Adv. Exp. Med. Biol.*, 72:317–335.
5. Björntorp, P., Ellis, H. A., and Bradford, R. H. (1964): Albumin antagonism of fatty acid effects on oxidation and phosphorylation reactions in rat liver mitochondria. *J. Biol. Chem.*, 239:339–344.
6. Blennow, G., Brierley, J. B., Meldrum, B. S., and Siesjö, B. K. (1978): Epileptic brain damage. The role of systemic factors that modify cerebral energy metabolism. *Brain*, 101:687–700.
7. Blennow, G., Folbergrová, J., Nilsson, B., and Siesjö, B. K. (1979): Effects of bicuculline-induced seizures on cerebral metabolism and circulation of rats rendered hypoglycemic by starvation. *Ann. Neurol.*, 5:139–151.
8. Blennow, G., Nilsson, B., and Siesjö, B. K. (1977): Sustained epileptic seizures complicated by hypoxia, arterial hypotension or hyperthermia: Effects on cerebral energy state. *Acta Physiol. Scand.*, 100:126–128.
9. Borgeat, P., and Samuelsson, B. (1979): Arachidonic acid metabolism in polymorphonuclear leukocytes: Effects of ionophore A23187. *Proc. Natl. Acad. Sci. U.S.A.*, 76:2148–2152.
10. Borgström, L., Chapman, A. G., and Siesjö, B. K. (1976): Glucose consumption in the cerebral cortex of rat during bicuculline-induced status epilepticus. *J. Neurochem.*, 27:971–973.
11. Calderini, G., Carlsson, A., and Nordström, C.-H. (1978): Monoamine metabolism during bicuculline-induced epileptic seizures in the rat. *Brain Res.*, 157:295–302.
12. Caveness, W. F., Kato, M., Malamut, B. L., Hosokawa, S., Wakisaka, S., and O'Neill, R. R. (1980): Propagation of focal motor seizures in the pubescent monkey. *Ann. Neurol.*, 7:213–221.
13. Chan, P. H., and Fishman, R. A. (1978): Brain edema: Induction in cortical slices by polyunsaturated fatty acids. *Science*, 201:358–360.
14. Chapman, A., Ingvar, M., and Siesjö, B. K. (1980): Free fatty acids in the brain in bicuculline-induced status epilepticus. *Acta Physiol. Scand.*, 110:335–336.
15. Chapman, A., Meldrum, B. S., and Siesjö, B. K. (1977): Cerebral metabolic changes during prolonged epileptic seizures in rats. *J. Neurochem.*, 28:1025–1035.
16. Collins, R. C., Kennedy, C., Sokoloff, L., and Plum, F. (1976): Metabolic anatomy of focal motor seizures. *Arch. Neurol.*, 33:536–542.
17. Corsellis, J. A. N., and Meldrum, B. S. (1976): Epilepsy. In: *Greenfield's Neuropathology*, edited by W. Blackwood and J. A. N. Corsellis, pp. 771–795. Edward Arnold, London.
18. Crane, P. D., Pardridge, W. M., Braun, L. D., Nyerges, A. M., and Oldendorf, W. H. (1981): The interaction of transport and metabolism on brain glucose utilization: A reevaluation of the lumped constant. *J. Neurochem.*, 36:1601–1604.
19. Demopoulos, H. B., Flamm, E., Seligman, M., Power, R., Pietronigro, D., and Ransohoff, J. (1977): Molecular pathology of lipids in CNS membranes. In: *Oxygen and Physiological Function*, edited by F. F. Jöbsis, pp. 491–508. Professional Information Library, Dallas.
20. Ferrendelli, J. A., Rubin, E. H., and Kinscherf, D. A. (1976): Influence of divalent cations on regulation of cyclic GMP and cyclic AMP levels in brain tissue. *J. Neurochem.*, 26:741–748.
21. Ferrendelli, J. A., Steiner, A. L., McDougal, D. B., and Kipnis, D. M. (1970): The effect of oxytremorine and atropine on cGMP and cAMP levels in the mouse cerebral cortex and cerebellum. *Biochem. Biophys. Res. Commun.*, 41:1061–1067
22. Flower, R. J. (1979): Biosynthesis of prostaglandins. In: *Oxygen Free Radicals and Tissue Damage. Ciba Foundation Symposium 65*, pp. 120–142. Excerpta Medica, Amsterdam.
23. Folbergrová, J., Ingvar, M., and Siesjö, B. K. (1981): Metabolic changes in cerebral cortex, hippocampus,

and cerebellum during sustained bicuculline-induced seizures. *J. Neurochem.*, 35:1228–1238.

24. Ginsberg, M. D., Graham, D. I., and Welsh, F. A. (1979): Neuropathological sequelae of severe diffuse cerebral ischemia in the cat: Relationship to postischemic impairments of perfusion and metabolism. *Acta Neurol. Scand. [Suppl. 72]*, 60:290–291.

25. Gjedde, A. (1982): Calculation of cerebral glucose phosphorylation from brain uptake of glucose analogs *in vivo*: A re-examination. *Brain Res., (in press).*

26. Goldberg, N. D., and Haddox, M. K. (1977): Cyclic GMP metabolism and involvement in biological regulation. *Annu. Rev. Biochem.*, 46:823–896.

27. Heinemann, U., and Gutnick, M. J. (1979): Relation between extracellular potassium concentration and neuronal activities in cat thalamus (VPL) during projection of cortical epileptiform discharge. *Electroencephalogr. Clin. Neurophysiol.*, 47:345–357.

28. Ingvar, M., Abdul-Rahman, A., and Siesjö, B. K. (1980): Local cerebral glucose consumption in the artifically ventilated rat: Influence of nitrous oxide analgesia and of phenobarbital anesthesia. *Acta Physiol. Scand.*, 109:177–185.

29. Ingvar, M., and Shapiro, H. M. (1981): Selective metabolic activation of the hippocampus during lidocaine induced pre-seizure activity. *Anesthesiology*, 54:27–31.

30. Ingvar, M., and Siesjö, B. K. (1982): Article in preparation.

31. Iversen, L. L. (1977): Catecholamine-selective adenylate cyclases in nervous tissues. *J. Neurochem.*, 29:5–12.

32. Lee, T. P., Kuo, J. F., and Greengard, P. (1972): Role of muscarinic cholineric receptors in regulation of guanosine 3′,5′-cyclic monophosphate content in mammalian brain, heart, muscle, and intestinal smooth muscle. *Proc. Natl. Acad. Sci. U.S.A.*, 69:3287–3291.

33. Marion, J., and Wolfe, L. S. (1978): Increase in vivo of unesterified fatty acids, prostaglandin F_2, but not thromboxane B_2 in rat brain during drug induced convulsions. *Prostaglandins*, 16:99–110.

34. Mead, J. F. (1976): Free radical mechanisms of lipid damage and consequences for cellular membranes. In: *Free Radicals in Biology*, edited by W. A. Pryor, pp. 51–68. Academic Press, New York.

35. Meldrum, B. S., and Brierley, J. B. (1973): Prolonged epileptic seizures in primates: Ischaemic cell change and its relation to ictal physiological events. *Arch. Neurol.*, 28:10–17.

36. Meldrum, B. S., and Nilsson, B. (1976): Cerebral blood flow and metabolic rate early and late in prolonged epileptic seizures induced in rats by bicuculline. *Brain*, 99:523–542.

37. Meldrum, B. S., Vigoroux, R. A., and Brierley, J. B. (1973): Systemic factors and epileptic brain damage. Prolonged seizures in paralysed artifically ventilated baboons. *Arch. Neurol.*, 29:82–87.

38. Myers, R. E. (1979): A unitary theory of causation of anoxic and hypoxic brain pathology. In: *Cerebral Hypoxia and Its Consequences, Advances in Neurology, Vo. 26*, edited by S. Fahn, J. N. Davis, and L. P. Rowland, pp. 195–213. Raven Press, New York.

39. Norman, R. M. (1964): The neuropathology of status epilepticus. *Med. Sci. Law*, 4:46–51.

40. Pardridge, W. M., Connor, J. D., and Crawford, L. L. (1975): Permeability changes in the blood-brain barrier: Causes and consequences. *C.R.C. Crit. Rev. Toxicol.*, 3:159–199.

41. Pontén, U., Ratcheson, R. A., Salford, L. G., and Siesjö, B. K. (1973): Optimal freezing conditions for cerebral metabolites in the rat. *J. Neurochem.*, 21:1127–1138.

42. Purpura, D. P., and Gonzalez-Monteagudo, O. (1960): Acute effects of methoxypyridine on hippocampal endblad neurons: An experimental study of "special pathoclisis" in the cerebral cortex. *J. Neuropathol. Exp. Neurol.*, 19:421–432.

43. Rehncrona, S., Folbergrová, J., Smith, D. S., and Siesjö, B. K. (1980): Influence of complete and pronounced incomplete cerebral ischemia and subsequent recirculation on cortical concentrations of oxidized and reduced glutathione in the rat. *J. Neurochem.*, 34:477–486.

44. Rehncrona, S., Rosén, I., and Siesjö, B. K. (1980): Excessive cellular acidosis: An important mechanism of neuronal damage in the brain? *Acta Physiol. Scand.*, 110:435–437.

45. Rehncrona, S., Smith, D. S., Åkesson, B., Westerberg, E., and Siesjö, B. K. (1980): Peroxidative changes in brain cortical fatty acids and phospholipids, as characterized during Fe^{2+}- and ascorbic acid-stimulated lipid peroxidation in vitro. *J. Neurochem.*, 34:1630–1638.

46. Roberts, E. (1980): Epilepsy and antiepileptic drugs: A speculative synthesis. In: *Antiepileptic Drugs: Mechanisms of Action*, edited by G. H. Glaser, J. K. Penry, and D. M. Woodbury, pp. 667–713. Raven Press, New York.

47. Sakurada, O., Kennedy, C., Jehle, J., Brown, J. D., Carbin, G. L., and Sokoloff, L. (1978): Measurement of local cerebral blood flow with ^{14}C iodoantipyrine. *Am. J. Physiol.*, 234:H59–H66.

48. Schwartz, J. R., Broggi, G., and Pappas, G. D. (1970): Fine structure of cat hippocampus during sustained seizures. *Brain Res.*, 18:176–180.

49. Schwartzkroin, P. A., and Wyler, A. R. (1980): Mechanisms underlying epileptiform burst discharge. *Ann. Neurol.*, 7:95–107.

50. Siesjö, B. K. (1981): Cell damage in the brain: A speculative synthesis. *J. Cerebral Blood Flow and Metabolism*, 1:155–185.

51. Siesjö, B. K., Ingvar, M., and Westerberg, E. (1982): The influence of bicuculline-induced seizures on free fatty acid concentrations in cerebral cortex, hippocampus, and cerebellum. *J. Neurochem. (in press)*.

52. Siesjö, B. K., and Rehncrona, S. (1980): Adverse factors affecting neuronal metabolism: Relevance to the dementias. In: *Biochemistry of Dementia*, edited by P. J. Roberts, pp. 91–120. John Wiley & Sons, New York.

53. Slater, J. F. (1972): *Free Radical Mechanisms in Tissue Injury*. Pion, London.

54. Söderfeldt, B. (1982): article in preparation.

55. Söderfeldt, B., Kalimo, H., Olsson, Y., and Siesjö, B. K. (1981): Pathogenesis of brain lesions caused by experimental epilepsy. Light- and electron-microscopic changes in the rat cerebral cortex following

bicuculline-induced status epilepticus. *Acta Neuropathol. (Berl.)*, 54:219–231.

56. Sokoloff, L. (1981): personal communication.
57. Sokoloff, L., Reivich, M., Kennedy, C., Des Rosiers, M. H., Patlak, C. S., Pettigrew, K. D., Sakurada, O., and Shinohara, M. (1977): The ^{14}C-deoxyglucose method for the measurement of local cerebral glucose utilization: Theory, procedure, and normal values in the conscious and anaesthetized albino rat. *J. Neurochem.*, 28:897–916.
58. Stone, T. W., Taylor, D. A., and Bloom, F. E. (1975): Cyclic AMP and cyclic GMP may mediate opposite neuronal responses in the rat cerebral cortex. *Science*, 187:845–847.
59. Tappel, A. L. (1973): Lipid peroxidation damage to cell components. *Fed. Proc.*, 32:1870–1874.
60. Wasterlain, C. G., and Duffy, T. E. (1976): Status epilepticus in immature rats. Protective effects of glucose on survival and brain development. *Arch. Neurol.*, 33:821–827.
61. Wojtczak, L. (1976): Effect of long-chain fatty acids and acyl-CoA on mitochondrial permeability, transport, and energy-coupling processes. *J. Bioenerget. Biomembr.*, 8:293–311.

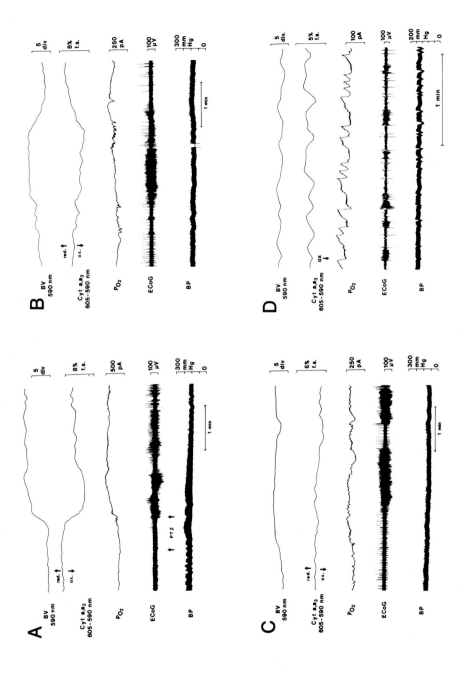

TABLE 2. *Metabolic and vascular changes associated with pentylenetetrazol seizures in the rat*

	Systemic blood pressure	Cerebral cytochrome a,a₃	Cerebral blood volume	Cerebral Po₂
Initial seizures	Increase	Oxidation	Increase	Increase
Later seizures	No increase	Reduction or no oxidation	No increase	Decrease or no change

There are several possible causes of oxygen insufficiency during seizures subsequent to the transition: (a) arterial blood Po_2 is decreased, (b) oxygen transport from blood to the mitochondria is limited or (c) utilization of oxygen by the mitochondria is lowered. The close correspondence between the amplitude of cytochrome a,a₃ reduction and the magnitude of the decrease in tissue oxygen tension after transition (25) suggests that oxygen supply to the tissue is the limiting factor and that mitochondrial function remains intact during recurrent seizures. If this hypothesis is correct, then failure to maintain adequate cerebral oxygenation during recurrent seizures probably is the result of derangements in cardiovascular or pulmonary physiology.

We then assessed the roles of various physiological changes in transition. During the initial seizure after transition in 15 rats, arterial blood pressure failed to increase (or incremented only slightly) in 9 animals; cerebral blood volume failed to increase in another 9 animals (not necessarily the same 9 animals); 7 animals developed systemic hypotension; and 8 animals exhibited the onset of sustained repetitive seizures. There were different combinations of these events associated with transition in different animals, suggesting that none of these events was necessary to bring about transition. One common finding, however, was that two or more of the measured cardiovascular changes accompanied transition. Any combination of these cardiovascular changes could produce decreases in cerebral blood flow and oxygen delivery, emphasizing their importance in contributing to transition. I 12 of 15 rats, however, transition was preceded by one or more seizures accompanied by a prolonged elevation of blood pressure that outlasted the ictal burst by several minutes. It is difficult to see how such a prolonged increase in blood pressure could contribute directly to transition. More likely, the prolonged blood pressure increase is a compensatory response to other physiological changes such as arterial hypoxemia. This possi-

bility is supported by some of our preliminary data, which suggest that pulmonary problems can cause arterial hypoxemia in conjunction with the prolonged blood pressure increases.

OXYGEN INSUFFICIENCY IN SEIZURES

The transition from oxygen sufficiency to insufficiency in recurrent seizures may explain the lack of consensus about cerebral oxygenation in other reports (5,8,13,41,44). The numbers of seizures in the series studied could have influenced conclusions regarding oxygen sufficiency. Plum et al. (45) concluded that oxygen supply was more than adequate to meet demand during seizures because of an associated rise in venous Po_2. However, only the first few seizures of a series were studied, and the animals were respired on 100% O_2. Also, there is some question about the validity of venous Po_2 as a measure of adequacy of tissue oxygenation (51). Caspers and Speckmann (5) reported that cerebral Po_2 increased during the first several seizures but then fell during each subsequent seizure. These data provided the first suggestion that a transition to oxygen insufficiency might occur during serial seizures. They proposed that failure of either blood pressure or cerebral blood flow to increase adequately was responsible for the decreases in cerebral oxygenation during later seizures. This hypothesis has been supported by results obtained in the investigation reported here and preceding investigations. For example, Plum et al. (45) were the first to demonstrate that cerebral venous Po_2 rose during each seizure only when blood pressure and cerebral blood flow increased. Spinal transection or ganglionic blockade, which prevented seizure-associated blood pressure increases, led to a fall rather than a rise in venous Po_2 during seizures. Blood pressure decreases during seizures also have been shown to reverse the direction of mitochondrial respiratory chain redox shifts (16,52) and produce metabolic and functional changes indicative of ischemia (2). These observations emphasize the importance of the blood pressure increase in providing adequate blood flow and oxygen supply to the brain during seizures.

A fall in cerebrovascular resistance also plays an important role in elevating cerebral blood flow during seizures (32,42,44). Dilation of pial arteries accompanies individual seizures (24,41–43), but cerebral vessels fail to recover tone completely after termination of each successive seizure in a series (24,32). Also, cerebral blood flow has been observed to increase progressively in smaller increments until a plateau is reached after several successive ictal episodes (5,21,49). Such cerebrovascular changes probably underlie the progressive increase in basal blood volume and eventual failure of blood volume to increase transiently that we observed during seizures following transition. Collectively, these data suggest that progressive dilation of the cerebral vasculature reaches a limit beyond which this mechanism can no longer respond to increases in metabolic rate. Thus, local chemical autoregulation of the cerebral vasculature would be suspended along with the more well known suspension of pressure autoregulation (44). In support of this suggestion, uncoupling of local cerebral blood flow and neuronal activity has been observed in experimental status epilepticus (15). The resultant loss of ability to increase blood flow to match any additional local increases in metabolic rate could be responsible for local oxygen insufficiency. The progressive loss of cerebrovascular tone could be caused by either decreased arterial oxygen tension or excessive release of vasodilator substances. Local oxygen insufficiency could also be caused by arteriovenous shunting of oxygen or cellular swelling and impairment of oxygen diffusion to mitochondria.

NEURONAL DAMAGE AND FOCAL OXYGEN INSUFFICIENCY DURING RECURRENT SEIZURES

Neuronal damage is commonly observed in adults and children who die shortly after prolonged episodes of status epilepticus (9). Injury is confined primarily to brain structures known to be most vulnerable to lack of oxygen; cerebral cortex, thalamus, and hippocampus. Such a pattern of neuronal damage also has been observed in awake animals (36) and in paralyzed artificially ventilated animals after prolonged seizures (39). Individual seizures, however, seldom harm nerve cells. The occurrence of vascular or pulmonary problems and the resultant oxygen insufficiency during recurrent seizures suggest that hypoxia is a mechanism underlying neuronal damage. Such abnormal physiological responses to seizures have already been implicated in the production of neuronal damage (4,36–39), other morbidity (35), and mortality (35,53) in prolonged status epilepticus. It remains unclear, however, whether or not oxygen lack is the primary factor responsible for neuronal injury in seizures, because lesions similar in appearance to those labeled hypoxic/ischemic can result from a number of abnormalities other than hypoxia or ischemia (9).

If hypoxia is a causative factor in brain damage with seizures, as our study suggests, then some discrepancies remain to be resolved. For example, it was reported recently that recurrent seizures in mildly hypoxic animals resulted, paradoxically, in less severe neuronal damage than in normoxic animals (4). However, the decreased severity of neuronal damage in mildly hypoxic animals may have resulted from decreased neuronal activity and therefore decreased energy demand. Horton et al. (17) reported that local blood flow during prolonged seizures in regions vulnerable to neuronal damage was higher than in regions not showing brain damage. They concluded that maintained intense seizure discharge was the primary requirement for the production of brain damage, not local vascular factors. Others have reported, however, that the local glucose consumption rate is elevated nonuniformly during prolonged seizures and that increases in local blood flow do not match energy demands in many regions (50). It remains to be determined if the mismatch between blood flow and metabolic rate in these vulnerable brain regions is the primary factor in the production of neuronal abnormalities or if other factors are involved. Nevertheless, the recurrent episodes of transient oxygen insufficiency reported here indicate serious pathophysiological consequences, whether or not they are sufficiently injurious to produce histologically evident neuronal changes.

CONCLUSIONS

Our findings place the previous and sometimes conflicting reports concerning O_2 sufficiency in status epilepticus into a new perspective. It is clear that oxygen insufficiency, to a degree that conceivably could be responsible for neuronal damage, develops during recurrent seizures in several animal models. This transition from oxygen sufficiency to insufficiency is probably related to deteriorating or inappropriate vascular reactivity that results in decreased ability to deliver oxygen to focal areas of metabolically hyperactive cerebral tissue. Neuronal damage could ensue directly as a result of the episodes of transient local hypoxia that occur during seizures following the transition. By amelioration of the deteriorating systemic factors, it should be possible to retard the development of local cerebral hypoxia and prevent or lessen the extent of permanent neuronal dysfunction.

ACKNOWLEDGMENTS

These studies were supported by grants from the Epilepsy Foundation of America and the American Heart Association of Louisiana (to N.R.K.), NIH grants NS-14319 and NS-14325 (to M.R.), research career development award NS-00399 (to J.C.L.), and postdoctoral fellowship NS-06300 (to T.J.S.).

REFERENCES

1. Aizawa, T., Muramatsu, F., Hamaguchi, K., Tomita, M., Kakimi, R., and Toyoda, M. (1965): Cerebral circulation, metabolism, and electrical activity during convulsion induced by megimide. *Jpn. Circ. J.*, 29:449–453.
2. Astrup, J., Blennow, G., and Nilsson, B. (1979): Effects of reduced cerebral blood flow upon EEG pattern, cerebral extracellular potassium, and energy metabolism in the rat cortex during bicuculline-induced seizures. *Brain Res.*, 177:115–126.
3. Beresford, H. R., Posner, J. B., and Plum, F. (1969): Changes in brain lactate during induced cerebral seizures. *Arch. Neurol.*, 20:243–248.
4. Blennow, G., Brierley, J. B., Meldrum, B. S., and Siesjö, B. K. (1978): Epileptic brain damage: The role of systemic factors that modify cerebral energy metabolism. *Brain*, 101:687–700.
5. Caspers, H., and Speckmann, E. J. (1972): Cerebral pO_2, pCO_2 and pH: Changes during convulsive activity and their significance for spontaneous arrest of seizures. *Epilepsia*, 13:699–725.
6. Chance, B., and Williams, G. R. (1956): The respiratory chain and oxidative phosphorylation. *Adv. Enzymol.*, 17:65–134.
7. Chapman, A. G., Meldrum, B. S., and Siesjö, B. K. (1977): Cerebral metabolic changes during prolonged epileptic seizures in rats. *J. Neurochem.*, 28:1025–1035.
8. Cooper, R. H., Crow, J., Walter, W. G., and Winter, A. L. (1966): Regional control of cerebral vascular reactivity and oxygen supply in man. *Brain Res.*, 3:174–191.
9. Corsellis, J. A. N., and Meldrum, B. S. (1976): Epilepsy. In: *Greenfield's Neuropathology*, ed. 3, edited by W. Blackwood and J. A. N. Corsellis, pp. 771–795. Edward Arnold, London.
10. Davies, P. W., Remond, A. (1947): Oxygen consumption of the cerebral cortex of the cat during metrazol convulsions. *Res. Publ. Assoc. Res. Nerv. Ment. Dis.* 26:205–217.
11. Davis, E. W., McCulloch, W. S., and Roseman, E. (1943): Rapid changes in the O_2 tension of cerebral cortex during induced convulsions. *Am. J. Psychiatry*, 100:825–829.
12. Duffy, T. E., Howse, D. C., and Plum, F. (1975): Cerebral energy metabolism during experimental status epilepticus. *J. Neurochem.*, 24:925–934.
13. Dymond, A. M., and Crandall, P. H. (1976): Oxygen availability and blood flow in the temporal lobes during spontaneous epileptic seizures in man. *Brain Res.*, 102:191–196.
14. Gurdjian, E. S., Webster, J. E., and Stone, W. E. (1947): Cerebral metabolism in metrazol convulsions in the dog. *Res. Publ. Assoc. Res. Nerv. Ment. Dis.*, 26:184–204.
15. Heiss, W.-D., Turnheim, M., Vollmer, R., and Rappelsberger, P. (1979): Coupling between neuronal activity and focal blood flow in experimental seizures. *Electroencephalogr. Clin. Neurophysiol.*, 27:396–403.
16. Hempel, F. G., Kariman, K., and Saltzman, H. A. (1980): Redox transitions in mitochondria of cat cerebral cortex with seizures and hemorrhagic hypotension. *Am. J. Physiol.*, 238:H249–H256.
17. Horton, R. W., Meldrum, B. S., Pedley, T. A., and McWilliam, J. R. (1980): Regional cerebral blood flow in the rat during prolonged seizure activity. *Brain Res.*, 192:399–412.
18. Howse, D. C. N. (1978): Metabolic responses to status epilepticus in the rat, cat and mouse. *Can. J. Physiol. Pharmacol.*, 57:205–212.
19. Howse, D. C., Caronna, J. J., Duffy, T. E., and Plum, F. (1974): Cerebral energy metabolism, pH, and blood flow during seizures in the cat. *Am. J. Physiol.*, 227:1444–1451.
20. Ingvar, D. H., Lübbers, D. W., and Siesjö, B. K. (1962): Normal and epileptic EEG patterns related to cortical oxygen tension in the cat. *Acta Physiol. Scand.*, 55:210–224.
21. Jasper, H., and Erickson, T. C. (1941): Cerebral blood flow and pH in excessive cortical discharge induced by metrazol and electrical stimulation. *J. Neurophysiol.*, 4:333–347.
22. Jöbsis, F. F., O'Connor, M., Vitale, A., and Vreman, H. (1971): Intracellular redox changes in functioning cerebral cortex. I. Metabolic effects of epileptiform activity. *J. Neurophysiol.*, 34:735–749.
23. Jöbsis, F. F., Rosenthal, M., LaManna, J. C., Lothman, E., Cordingley, G., and Somjen, G. (1975): Metabolic activity in epileptic seizures. In: *Brain Work, Alfred Benzon Symposium VIII*, edited by D. H. Ingvar and N. A. Lassen, pp. 185–196. Munksgaard, Copenhagen.
24. Kontos, H. A., Wei, E. P., Raper, A. J., Rosenblum, W. I., Navari, R. M., and Patterson, J. L. Jr.(1978): Role of tissue hypoxia in local regulation of cerebral microcirculation. *Am. J. Physiol.*, 234:H582–H591.
25. Kreisman, N. R., LaManna, J. C., Rosenthal, M., and Sick, T. J. (1981): Oxidative metabolic responses

with recurrent seizures in rat cerebral cortex: Role of systemic factors. *Brain Res.*, 218:175–188.

26. Kreisman, N. R., Sick, T. J., and Bruley, D. F. (1979): Local oxygen tension and its relationship to unit activity during penicillin interictal discharges in the bullfrog hippocampus. *Electroencephalogr. Clin. Neurophysiol.*, 46:619–633.

27. Kreisman, N. R., Sick, T. J., LaManna, J. C., and Rosenthal, M. (1981): Local tissue oxygen tension–cytochrome a,a₃ redox relationships in rat cerebral cortex *in vivo*. *Brain Res.*, 218:161–174.

28. LaManna, J. C., Peretsman, S. J., Light, A. I., and Rosenthal, M. (1981): Oxygen sufficiency in the "working" brain. In: *Advances in Physiological Sciences, Vol. 25, Oxygen Transport to Tissue*, edited by A. G. B. Kovách, E. Dóra, M. Kessler,and I. A. Silver, pp. 95–96. Akadémiai Kiadó, Budapest.

29. Leninger-Follert, E., and Lübbers, D. W. (1976): Behavior of microflow and local PO₂ of the brain cortex during and after direct electrical stimulation. *Pfluegers Arch.*, 366:39–44.

30. Lewis, D. V., O'Connor, M. J., and Schuette, W. H. (1974): Oxidative metabolism during recurrent seizures in the penicillin treated hippocampus. *Electroencephalogr. Clin. Neurophysiol.*, 36:347–356.

31. Lothman, E., LaManna, J., Cordingley, G., Rosenthal, M., and Somjen, G. (1975): Responses of electrical potential, potassium levels, and oxidative metabolic activity of the cerebral neocortex of rats. *Brain Res.*, 88:15–36.

32. Magnaes, B., and Nornes, H. (1974): Circulatory and respiratory changes in spontaneous epileptic seizures in man. *Eur. Neurol.*, 12:104–115.

33. Mayevsky, A., and Chance, B. (1975): Metabolic responses of the awake cerebral cortex to anoxia, hypoxia, spreading depression and epileptiform activity. *Brain Res.*, 98:149–165.

34. Mayevsky, A., Zarchin, N., and Rosenshein, U. (1980): The effects of anesthesia on the metabolic response to cortical spreading depression in the gerbil. *Neurosci. Abstr.*, 6:768.

35. McNamara, J. O. (1980): Human hypoxia and seizures: Effects and interactions. In: *Cerebral Hypoxia and Its Consequences, Vol. 26, Advances in Neurology*, edited by S. Fahn, J. N. Davis, and L. P. Rowland, pp. 137–143. Raven Press, New York.

36. Meldrum, B. S., and Brierley, J. B. (1973): Prolonged epileptic seizures in primates: Ischemic cell change and its relation to ictal physiological events. *Arch. Neurol.*, 28:10–17.

37. Meldrum, B. S., and Horton, R. W. (1973): Physiology of status epilepticus in primates. *Arch. Neurol.*, 28:1–9.

38. Meldrum, B. S., and Nilsson, B. (1976): Cerebral blood flow and metabolic rate early and late in prolonged epileptic seizures induced in rats by bicuculline. *Brain*, 99:523–542.

39. Meldrum, B. S., Vigouroux, R. A., and Brierley, J. B. (1973): Systemic factors and epileptic brain damage: Prolonged seizures in paralyzed, artificially ventilated baboons. *Arch. Neurol.*, 29:82–87.

40. Meyer, J. S., Gotoh, F., and Favale, E. (1966): Cerebral metabolism during epileptic seizures in man. *Electrocephalogr. Clin. Neurophysiol.*, 21:10–22.

41. Meyer, J. S., and Portnoy, H. D. (1959): Post-epileptic paralysis: A clinical and experimental study. *Brain*, 82:162–185.

42. Myers, R. R., and Intaglietta, M. (1976): Brain microvascular hemodynamic responses to induced seizures. *Stroke*, 7:83–88.

43. Penfield, W. K., von Santha, K., and Cipriani, A. (1939): Cerebral blood flow during induced epileptiform seizures in animals and man. *J. Neurophysiol.*, 2:257–267.

44. Plum, F., Howse, D. C., and Duffy, T. E. (1974): Metabolic effects of seizures. In: *Brain Dysfunction in Metabolic Disorders*, edited by F. Plum, pp. 141–157. Raven Press, New York.

45. Plum, F., Posner, J. B., and Troy, B. (1968): Cerebral metabolic and circulatory responses to induced convulsions in animals. *Arch. Neurol.*, 18:1–13.

46. Rosenthal, M., and Jöbsis, F. F. (1971): Intracellular redox changes in functioning cerebral cortex. II. Effects of direct cortical stimulation. *J. Neurophysiol.*, 34:750–761.

47. Rosenthal, M., LaManna, J. C., Jöbsis, F. F., and LeVasseur, J. E., Kontos, H. A., and Patterson, J. L. (1976): Effects of respiratory gases on cytochrome A in intact cerebral cortex: Is there a critical PO₂? *Brain Res.*, 108:143–154.

48. Rosenthal, M., LaManna, J. C., Yamada, S., Younts, B. W., and Somjen, G. (1979): Oxidative metabolism, extracellular potassium and sustained potential shifts in cat spinal cord in situ. *Brain Res.*, 162:113–127.

49. Shalit, M. N. (1965): The effect of Metrazol on the hemodynamics and impedance of the cat's brain cortex. *J. Neuropathol. Exp. Neurol.*, 24:75–84.

50. Siesjö, B. K., Ingvar, M., Folbergrová, J., and Chapman, A. G. (1982): Chapter 21, this volume.

51. Siesjö, B. K., and Plum, F. (1973): Pathophysiology of anoxic brain damage. In: *Biology of Brain Dysfunction, Vol. 1*, edited by G. E. Gaull, pp. 319–372. Plenum Press, New York

52. Vern, B., Schuette, W. H., Whitehouse, W. C., and Mutsuga, N. (1976): Cortical oxygen consumption and NADH fluorescence during Metrazol seizures in normotensive and hypotensive cats. *Exp. Neurol.*, 52:83–98.

53. Wasterlain, C. G. (1974): Mortality and morbidity from serial seizures. *Epilepsia*, 15:155–176.

Advances in Neurology, Vol. 34: Status Epilepticus, edited by A.V. Delgado-Escueta, C.G. Wasterlain, D.M. Treiman, and R.J. Porter. Raven Press, New York © 1983.

23

Brain Metabolism During Prolonged Seizures in Neonates

Claude G. Wasterlain and Barney E. Dwyer

This chapter deals exclusively with the consequences of seizures for the brain of the neonate. It has been shown that the most important factor in the prognosis in neonatal seizures is their cause (60), and indeed it is intuitively obvious that there must be an enormous difference in outcome between sustained seizures associated with an incurable brain disease, such as many inborn errors of metabolism, and brief seizures associated with a transient, treatable metabolic abnormality, such as hypocalcemia (see Chapter 10). However, regardless of their cause, sustained seizures can trigger in brain and body a number of physiological and biochemical changes that can cause brain damage or add to it (1–3,10,75,76,78). Many of these changes are preventable or treatable and therefore important to the clinician.

In species that are moderately to markedly immature at birth, such as the dog, pig, cat, rat, rabbit, mouse, and human, the neonatal brain is physiologically quite different from the adult brain. The neonatal brain's physiological and biochemical adaptation to sustained seizures is entirely different from that in the adult. Current evidence indicates that the neonatal brain is much more efficiently protected against some deleterious biochemical consequences of seizures, such as lactate accumulation, but is much more vulnerable to others, such as an inadequate supply of carbohydrates.

Brain development follows a relatively inflexible chronology, different nerve cell populations being generated in different regions at specific times. For example, in the rat, the basket cells of the cerebellar cortex are produced only during the first week after birth (26). Metabolic insults, such as sustained seizures, that occur during the process of generation of a particular neuronal type could result in its irreversible loss or abnormal development, with consequent alteration in cell populations and possibly in behavior. This is one of the reasons why developmental steps that have been bypassed frequently cannot be retraced. On the other hand, the tremendous regenerative potential of the neonatal brain makes possible recovery from insults that would irreversibly damage the adult brain.

In recent years we have begun to understand the developing brain's reactions to metabolic insults, including seizures. An account of the changes they induce will highlight their importance in the medical management of epilepsy and in the prevention of mental retardation.

ENERGY METABOLISM OF THE DEVELOPING BRAIN

The low oxygen consumption of the immature brain (32,33,36) is part of an overall much lower metabolic rate, as compared with the adult. The

TABLE 1. *Brain energy substrates during seizures in 4-day old rats*

	Controls		Flurothyl seizures	
	Frozen	Decapitated	Frozen	Decapitated
ATP	2.34 ± 0.04^a	2.29 ± 0.03	$1.98 \pm 0.06^*$	$1.80 \pm 0.04^*$
Phosphocreatine	2.03 ± 0.07	1.35 ± 0.07	$1.14 \pm 0.04^*$	$0.53 \pm 0.03^*$
Glucose	1.36 ± 0.05	1.26 ± 0.17	1.50 ± 0.14	$0.59 \pm 0.08^*$
Glycogen	2.76 ± 0.18	2.74 ± 0.32	3.09 ± 0.20	2.70 ± 0.36
Metabolic rates (mmole ~P/kg/min)	1.04		3.92*	

^{a}Values represent means $\pm$ SE in mmole/kg. Metabolic rate = $(2\Delta ATP + \Delta phosphocreatine + 2\Delta glucose + 2.9\Delta glucogen)/\Delta time$.
*Significant difference from appropriate controls ($p < 0.05$).

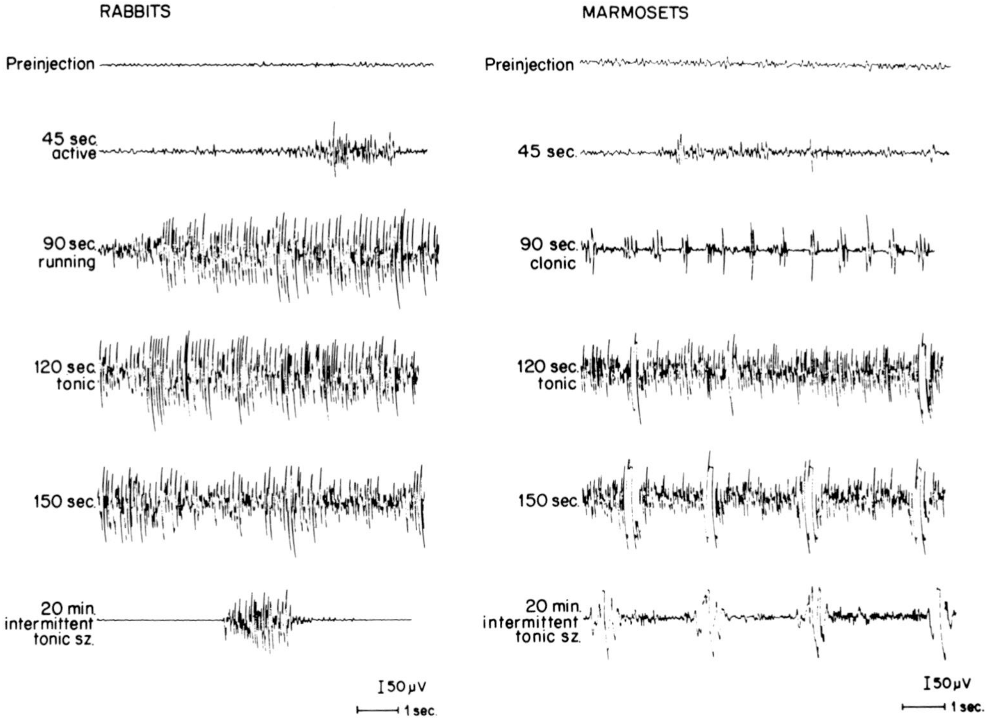

FIG. 1. Scalp EEGs during sustained seizures in 1-day-old rabbits and 1- to 7-day-old marmosets.

relative proportions of glycolysis and respiration, however, do not change drastically with age (23). It is this slow metabolic rate that permits the brain of the neonate to tolerate much longer periods of hypoxia than that of the adult, a property that is progressively lost during maturation as the cerebral metabolic rate increases.

The brain's endogenous stores of substrates for energy metabolism are quite low compared with their rates of utilization; therefore the brain is de-pendent on continued replenishment of its sub-strates through the cerebral circulation and the blood-brain barrier.

The immature brain produces its energy in the form of ATP by four major pathways: in the cell's cytoplasm, anaerobic glycolysis transforms one molecule of glucose into two of pyruvate then lac-tate, and in the process generates two molecules of ATP. Respiration, a predominantly mitochon-drial process, requires molecular oxygen and produces 36 molecules of ATP per molecule of glucose, which is oxidized to CO_2 and water. The oxidation of ketone bodies (acetoacetate and β-hydroxybutyrate) also requires molecular oxygen, as does the hexosemonophosphate shunt, which generates NADPH (required for lipid synthesis) and ribosephosphate (a building block of nucleic acids). Those two pathways are of little importance in adult animals (5,45,46,54,57,61,66) but may provide a significant portion of the energy requirements of the immature brain (38,53,55).

Rates of respiration (CMR_{O_2}, cerebral metabolic rate for oxygen) have been measured in fetal and newborn lambs (37,43,45,59) and have been calculated in rodents from the ratio of synthesized high-energy phosphate bonds per molecule of oxygen consumed. This P/O ratio (34) is lower in neonates, suggesting a lower rate of respiration (approximately 1 mmole/100 g/min versus 2.5 mmole/100 g/min measured in lambs). In any case, the cerebral metabolic rate is much lower in neonates (1.33 mmole P/kg/min) than in adults (26.8 mmole P/kg/min). In rats, CMR_{O2} is between 0.96 and 2.5 mmole/100 g/min in neonates and 10.3 mmole/100 g/min in adults.

Glycolysis transforms one molecule of glucose into two molecules of pyruvic acid. When oxygen is available, 85% of this pyruvic acid enters the tricarboxylic acid cycle and is converted to CO_2 and water. When it is not, pyruvic acid is reduced to lactic acid (46). The rate of glycolysis is controlled by several regulatory enzymes, the main control point being phosphofructokinase (PFK), with hexokinase and possibly pyruvate kinase playing secondary roles (42). ATP, citric acid, and H^+ ions inhibit PFK, whereas ADP, AMP, and P_i stimulate its activity (4). During seizures, the decrease in ATP and the marked increases in ADP, AMP, and P_i stimulate PFK. However, in status epilepticus, a marked increase in intracellular H^+ ion concentration can reduce that stimulation.

Duffy et al. (22) measured the glycolytic rate in rats using the Lowry decapitation technique. Lactate accumulation averaged 0.69 mmole/kg/min in neonates, 1.4 mmole/kg/min in 7-day-old rats, and nine times the neonatal rate in adult rats (67). A similar curve was observed in mice (70).

We measured energy reserves in 4-day-old rats subjected to flurothyl-induced seizures (76). Animals were matched by litter, sex, and body weight and were maintained in a 1-liter jar at 33°C, which is close to their natural core temperature, by means

of a water bath. Previous experiments showed that the oxygen content in the jar did not vary during the course of the experiment.

At the onset of the experiment, 50 μl of flurothyl was injected into the jar. This was followed by hyperactivity, then by tonic seizures. At the time of onset of clinical seizures, half the animals were frozen in liquid nitrogen. The other half were decapitated and their heads frozen 60 sec later. Controls were similarly processed. In this fashion, the metabolic rate for experimental animals reflected the first 30 sec of tonic seizure activity and was presumably close to the highest metabolic rate obtainable at that age. It increased nearly fourfold during seizures, demonstrating that the immature rat brain is able to markedly elevate its metabolic rate at times of maximal seizure activity (Table 1).

It is obvious that glycogen mobilization was not sufficiently rapid to prevent marked decreases in brain glucose, phosphocreatine, and ATP in the decapitated heads of seizing rats and that relative changes in those substrates were remarkably similar to those observed in adults (21).

BRAIN GLUCOSE DURING SUSTAINED SEIZURES

Blood and brain glucose concentrations were measured in immature rats, rabbits, and monkeys during sustained seizures (25,76). In 1-day-old rabbit experiments, experimental animals were injected with bicuculline (2.5 mg/kg i.m.) (Fig. 1). One-half received 10% of their body weight of isotonic glucose solution subcutaneously 30 min before receiving bicuculline. Matched animals received isotonic saline solution instead of glucose.

Four-day-old Wistar rats matched for sex, body weight, and litter received similar loads (10% of body weight) of isotonic glucose, isotonic saline, or a sham injection intraperitoneally, followed 30 min later by flurothyl seizures, as previously described (76).

Newborn marmoset monkeys were subjected to bicuculline seizures (5 mg/kg i.m.) during the first week of life. Because most births are twin pairs, each control was matched with its experimental sibling. Temperature was maintained at 36°C to 37°C, and arterialized venous blood was sampled from the tail while vasodilation was induced by local application of hot compresses.

In all three species, blood glucose concentrations remained normal or slightly elevated during a considerable span of seizure activity (Fig. 2). In

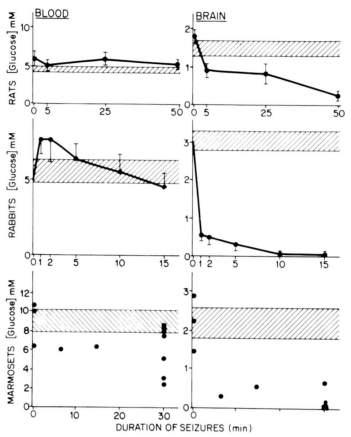

FIG. 2. Blood and brain glucose concentrations during neonatal seizures. The hatched areas represent means ± SE of untreated controls.

rabbits, a mild elevation at the onset of seizure activity was followed by normoglycemia at 10 to 15 min and by mild hypoglycemia at 30 min (mean 47 mg/dl). Rats remained normoglycemic or mildly hyperglycemic throughout 50 min of seizure activity. Control and experimental monkeys were quite hyperglycemic at the beginning of the experiment, presumably because they are relatively more mature at birth than rodents and were stressed by handling and separation from their parents. Seizing animals became less hyperglycemic, but mean blood glucose concentration at 30 min was above normoglycemic values for humans, and the lowest glucose concentration measured in one animal was 42 mg/dl.

Brain glucose concentrations (calculated after subtraction of glucose in brain blood, which was assumed to represent 3% of brain volume, a probable underestimation in experimental animals) fell markedly in all three species. In rabbits, which

TABLE 2. *Blood glucose concentration and transport across blood-brain barrier*

$V = \dfrac{V_{max} \times (S)}{K_m + (S)}$ Blood (glucose)	$K_m = 7$ mM Transport rate
27 mg/dl = 1.8 mM	18% V_{max} = 0.07 mmole/kg/min
90 mg/dl = 5 mM	42% V_{max} = 0.17 mmole/kg/min
200 mg/dl = 11 mM	61% V_{max} = 0.24 mmole/kg/min

were sacrificed by focused-beam microwave irradiation in a high-power oven, the decrease in brain glucose concentration induced by seizures was rapid and severe, and after 10 min of seizures it is likely that brain glucose concentrations were rate-limiting for hexokinase activity, a situation similar to that observed in severe hypoglycemia and anoxia (68,69,70), but here associated with normoglycemia. In rats that were sacrificed by freezing in liquid nitrogen, brain glucose concen-

TABLE 3. *Cerebral energy balance during neonatal seizures*

Blood (glucose)	27 mg/dl	90 mg/dl	200 mg/dl
Maximum rate of glycolysis (nmole ~P/kg/min)	0.69	0.69	0.69
Maximum rate of glucose transport (nmole /kg/min)	0.072	0.168	0.24
Maximum rate of glycolysis from glucose transported across BBB (nmole ~P/kg)	0.144	0.336	0.48
Energy reserves (nmole ~P/kg)	24	24	24
Maximum rate of reserve mobilization (nmole ~P/kg/min)	0.37	0.37	0.37
Energy balance (nmole ~P/kg/min)			
Calculated	-0.176	$+0.016$	$+0.160$
Measured	negative	-0.028	positive

tration decreased rapidly with the first seizure, then more slowly for the next 20 min, possibly because of glycogen mobilization. This was followed by a more profound depletion, with a precipitous decrease in the ratio of brain glucose to blood glucose. Monkeys were also sacrificed by freezing in liquid nitrogen. Initial brain glucose concentrations were quite high, but they decreased precipitously to reach very low levels in 3 animals at 30 min and moderate depletion in another 5 animals. These data demonstrate that a decrease in brain glucose concentration during seizures in normoglycemic neonates is not restricted to rodents but can occur in primates as well. Because abundant supplies of glucose were available in blood, this implies that transport from blood to brain was unable to keep up with the rate of glucose utilization in all three species.

GLUCOSE TRANSPORT ACROSS THE BLOOD-BRAIN BARRIER

The devastating effects of hypoglycemia on the brain of the neonate highlight its dependence on a continuous supply of glucose. Based on the suggestion that the blood-brain barrier of the newborn is incomplete, it has been assumed that glucose enters the cerebral extracellular space by simple diffusion. However, more rigorous investigations (7,13,14,49) have shown that only negligible amounts of hexoses penetrate the immature rat brain by simple diffusion. Preliminary evidence from our laboratory suggests that a similar situation applies in rabbits and monkeys. In neonates (13,14,49), as in adults (9,16,27,29,52,56), glucose crosses the blood-brain barrier by carrier-me-

diated, non-energy-requiring facilitated transport, identified in the infant, as in the adult, by transport selectivity, competition, and counterflow. However, in infant rats up to 2 weeks of age, the flux of glucose into brain is only about 20% of the adult rate (49), mostly because of lower carrier concentration in the immature blood-brain barrier. The affinity of the carrier system for hexoses in neonates is very similar to that in adults, as well as across species, suggesting that the marked increase in transport capacity with age is due to an increase in brain concentration of carrier, not to a change in its molecular nature (49).

At physiological glucose concentrations, the carrier is never saturated (9,13,14). As a result, an increase in blood glucose concentration increases carrier saturation and the brain's supply of glucose; a decrease has the opposite effect. At a blood glucose concentration of 27 mg/dl, the blood-brain barrier is able to utilize only 18% of its maximum transport capacity for glucose. An increase in glucose concentration to 200 mg/dl in blood triples glucose flux into brain, permitting utilization of 61% of the maximal capacity of the system (Table 2).

The resting intracellular glucose concentration in brain is at least 20 times higher than the concentration necessary to saturate hexokinase, the first enzyme of the glycolytic pathway. In other words, under physiological conditions, glucose concentration is never rate-limiting. However, when glycolytic rates increase markedly, as they do during seizures or ischemia, or when hypoglycemia lowers the saturation of the glucose carrier, the lower transport capacity of the blood-brain barrier in the neonate may become the rate-limiting factor for the generation of energy.

In 1-day-old rats, the maximal transport capacity for glucose across the blood-brain barrier (T_{max}) is of the order of 0.4 mmole/kg/min (49). We can assume that transport is unidirectional, because sustained seizures deplete brain glucose. However, this will result in a slight lowering of T_{max} because the movement of free carrier across the membrane is slightly slower than that of the glucose-carrier complex (6). Even if this small slowing is neglected, T_{max} for glucose will be 0.072, 0.168, and 0.24 mmole/kg/min at blood glucose concentrations of 27, 90, and 200 mg/dl, respectively (Table 3). The maximal rate of energy utilization in 1-day-old rats is 1.33 mmole $\sim$P/min, and the maximal rate of lactate production through the glycolytic pathway is 0.69 mmole $\sim$P/kg/min (71). Because through glycolysis one molecule of glucose produces two molecules of lactate, the maximal rate of glucose utilization through the glycolytic pathway in 1-day-old rats is 0.35 mmole/kg/min. It will be obvious from the comparison of this value with T_{max} that in the neonate, glucose can be metabolized through the cerebral glycolytic pathway faster than it can be transported into brain from blood. If high glycolytic rates are sustained, a progressive deficit in brain glucose must follow. The extent of the deficit varies with the blood glucose concentration, from 0.55 mmole/kg/min at a blood glucose concentration of 27 mg/dl to 0.21 mmole/kg/min at a concentration of 200 mg/dl. This latter situation, however, permits the brain to sustain its metabolic rate as long as it can use its reserves of glycogen *(vide infra)*.

GLYCOGENOLYTIC CAPACITY

Glycogen constitutes the main storage form of oxidizable carbohydrates in brain. It is present in sizable quantities in the neonate (71). In fact, the total energy reserves of the brain for 1-day-old rats are as high as in the adult. Those reserves could sustain the maximal rate of brain metabolism for 18 min (against 0.85 min in the adult, where energy-use rates are much faster) if they could be mobilized rapidly enough and in totality. In fact, glycogen metabolism can sustain some brain metabolism in the neonate for much longer periods than in the adult, but several factors may slow its mobilization in response to energy demands even when brain glucose concentrations are rapidly depleted (23,68–70). The concentrations of two enzymes necessary for glycogen breakdown to glucose-6-phosphate or glucose-1-phosphate (which then enters the glycolytic pathway) are very low in newborn rat brain. Phosphorylase, probably the rate-limiting enzyme (71), is present at only 10% of the adult concentration, and phosphoglucomutase is very low (62). In addition, histochemical stains have revealed that phosphorylase activity in the neonate is detected only in ependymal and subependymal regions (63) and thus is located at some distance from neurons where most of the demand presumably occurs. Furthermore, the mechanism by which phosphorylase is activated in the adult is poorly developed at birth in most brain regions. The transformation of phosphorylase B to phosphorylase A requires a cyclic-AMP-stimulated protein kinase (Fig. 3). Cyclic AMP in glial cells is in turn generated by stimulation of β-adrenergic receptors, presumably by norepinephrine liberated from free terminals. However, in the neonate, glial cells are quite immature and contain few β-adrenergic receptors. The rate of generation of cyclic AMP in response to seizures in the neonate is considerably lower than in the adult (Fig. 4). As a result, the activation of phosphorylase is much slower, further reducing the ability of the immature brain to mobilize glycogen rapidly in situations such as seizures and anoxia. During the first 10 min of total anoxia, newborn rats metabolize glycogen at 1.29 mmole/kg, or 0.129 mmole/kg/min. This is presumably close to the maximal rate of glycogen mobilization in the neonate (71). Because breakdown of glycogen during anoxia produces 2.9 mole of $\sim$P per mole of glycogen as glucosyl equivalents (41), glycogen mobilization in neonates contributes $\sim$P at 0.129 × 2.9 = 0.374 mmole/kg/min to brain metabolism. This is 28% of the maximum rate of energy use in a newborn brain and 54% of the glucosyl equivalents needed to maintain its glycolytic rate (Table 3).

ALTERNATIVE FUELS

The immature brain has a high capacity for utilizing glucose by the hexosemonophosphate shunt, which produces NADPH and ribose phosphate (5,53,61). However, this pathway cannot generate ATP from glucose under anaerobic conditions, because NADP cannot be regenerated from NADPH. When convulsions or seizures are accompanied by signficant anoxemia and cerebral anoxia (11,72,73), this pathway is probably of little use in energy production.

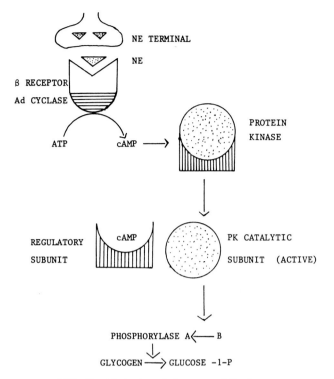

FIG. 3. Mechanism of glycogen mobilization.

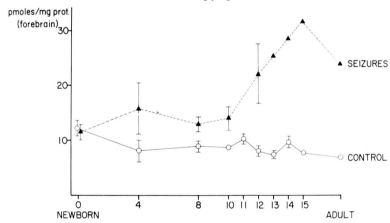

FIG. 4. Cyclic AMP concentrations in whole forebrains of rats microwave-fixed at the peak of tonic seizures induced by intraperitoneal bicuculline compared with paired littermates. The elevation of cyclic AMP in response to seizures is much lower in neonates than in juveniles or adults.

During the suckling period, both rats and humans show ketosis of nutritional origin that reflects the high fat content of maternal milk (8) and disappears after weaning. During this period, as much as one-third of the brain's energy may be derived from ketone bodies (14,15). Positive arteriovenous differences indicate cerebral uptake of ketone bodies (28,39) that are carried across the blood-brain barrier by facilitated, non-energy-requiring transport on the lactate carrier (56). Both the carrier (which appears inducible) and the enzymes of ketone metabolic pathways are considerably more active in early postnatal life than in adults. We have investigated the possibility that ketone bodies might be able to protect immature rats against mortality and inhibition of brain growth from repetitive seizures. Table 4 shows that whereas glucose was very effective in reducing mortality during a single bout of status epilepticus in 4-day-old rats, both ketone bodies and amino acids failed to provide any protection. This is not surprising, because utilization of β-hydroxybutyrate or acetoacetate requires molecular oxygen at several steps. The NADH generated by the first oxidation cannot be regenerated to NAD in the absence of oxidative phosphorylation, which is compromised during repetitive seizures when they are accompanied by cerebral hypoxia (Fig. 5).

ROLE OF HYPOXEMIA

In adult rats and mice, oxygen availability often is the key to survival during repetitive seizures (Fig. 6). When two groups of adult rats were given supramaximal electroconvulsive seizures every 30 sec and cerebral anoxia was prevented in one group by curarization (which prevents competition for

available oxygen among brain, heart, and muscle), artificial ventilation on a respirator, and a supply of 100% oxygen, we found that a treatment that killed all freely convulsing animals was survived by 100% of the oxygenated animals (72). Similarly, Posner et al. (58), in humans, Collins et al. (11), in mice, and Duffy et al. (21), in rats, showed that oxygenation drastically reduces both oxygen and energy debt during seizures. However, in 4-day-old rats subjected to repetitive flurothyl seizures, carrying out those seizures in an atmosphere of 100% oxygen instead of air had no effect on mortality or brain development (76). Because we did not measure blood oxygen concentrations in those animals, it is possible that the oxygen atmosphere failed to prevent anoxemia and cerebral anoxia. However, the dramatic decreases in brain glucose concentrations observed in these animals may reduce the effectiveness of oxygen in neonates as compared with adults. Two additional experiments suggested that some damage may be produced even if anoxemia is completely prevented. Seizures produced profound inhibition of brain protein synthesis. This inhibition was found even in animals that were paralyzed and mechanically ventilated with oxygen so that anoxemia was completely prevented (74). In a separate experiment, newborn rats were paralyzed and ventilated with oxygen at the time of delivery of electroshock seizures (100 mA, AC, 1 sec, twice per day). These animals were compared to respirator controls not subjected to seizures, to untreated controls, and to experimental animals that convulsed freely during

TABLE 4. *Failure of ketone bodies to protect young rats in status epilepticus*

Injection	Mortality	N
—	23	50
Glucose	2	50
Acetoacetate	31	50
β-hydroxybutyrate	28	50
Amino acids	21	50

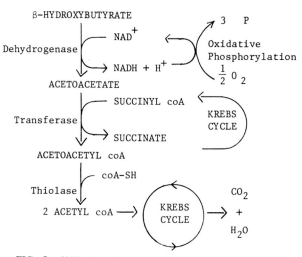

FIG. 5. Utilization of ketone bodies by the immature brain.

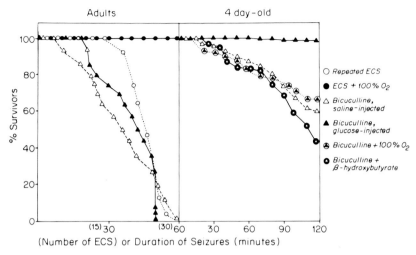

FIG. 6. Effects of O_2 or glucose on mortality from status epilepticus. Two groups (10 each) of 300- to 400-g Wistar rats were treated with electroconvulsive shock every 30 sec. One group was breathing room air and convulsed freely; the others were paralyzed and mechanically ventilated with 100% O_2. Two additional groups of 28 adult Wistar rats received bicuculline (10 mg/kg i.p.) following a load of isotonic glucose or saline solution i.p. (10% of body weight, 30 min before bicuculline). Four-day-old rats were treated with i.p. bicuculline and were allowed to convulse freely in an atmosphere of 100% O_2 or of room air; some received a load of isotonic glucose or saline solution i.p. 30 min before bicuculline.

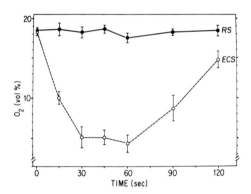

FIG. 7. Oxygen content of heart blood during electroconvulsive seizures (100 mA, AC, 2 sec) in 2-day-old rats paralyzed with succinylcholine and ventilated with O_2 (filled circles, RS) or without any other treatment (open circles, ECS). The time elapsed after the delivery of electroshock is indicated on the abscissa. Heart blood obtained by direct puncture of the left ventricle was analyzed for O_2 content using an oxygen-sensitive electrode.

seizures (73). These animals were littermates raised by the same dam and were paired four by four at 2 days of age. Ventilation with oxygen completely prevented the anoxemia observed during seizures (Fig. 7). However, the delay in brain growth was as great in paralyzed, O_2-ventilated animals as in their convulsing littermates. This suggests that part of the inhibition of brain growth by seizures, as well as the inhibition of protein synthesis, is in-

dependent of anoxemia. It is, of course, possible that some physiological variable that could not be monitored because of the small size of the animals was abnormal in the ventilated group and introduced an artifact, but the current data clearly argue that the deleterious effects of seizures on brain growth can occur in the absence of anoxemia. The problem is of great practical importance. If retardation of brain growth results from cerebral anoxia, one would expect that treatment aimed at stopping or preventing vigorous convulsive activity would be adequate to prevent or minimize it. On the other hand, if sustained cerebral seizure activity without convulsions or anoxemia inhibits brain growth, one might consider treating not only those with convulsions but also those with epileptiform EEGs. It is, of course, common to see epileptiform EEGs in the absence of clinical convulsions in premature infants, as well as in neonates paralyzed with pancuronium and maintained on the respirator, and the possibility of adverse effects of anticonvulsants themselves must be kept in mind.

ROLE OF LACTATE

Recent evidence suggests that lactate accumulation may play a critical role in the generation of ischemic cell necrosis in the adult brain. Lactate accumulation has been shown to play a critical role

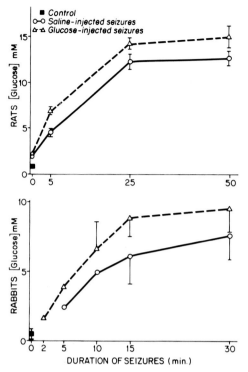

FIG. 8. Brain lactate concentrations during flurothyl seizures in 4-day-old rats and during bicuculline seizures in 1-day-old rabbits. Some animals were injected with isotonic glucose or saline solution (10% of body weight i.p.) 30 min before seizure induction.

in the vascular collapse that can result from status epilepticus in adult animals (77). Lactate accumulation in the adult brain during status epilepticus can also reach very high concentrations. Its precise role in the pathophysiology of brain damage from status is unknown, but it has been suggested to be an important factor in the production of ischemic cell changes, which are frequently found after status epilepticus in humans and animals alike (12,47).

We measured brain lactate concentrations during sustained seizures in 4-day-old rats, in 1-day-old rabbits, and in 1- to 7-day-old marmoset monkeys. Blood lactate concentrations were also measured in rabbits and monkeys. In rats, seizures were induced by inhalation of the volatile convulsant flurothyl (Indoklon®). Four-day-old pups were maintained at 37°C in 1-liter jars, and 50µl of flurothyl was injected into each jar every 5 min. After 3.5 min, the lid was removed, and air was circulated to purge the jar of convulsant. Every injection induced seizures that abated with ventilation. After 90 min, the amount of flurothyl in-

jected at 5-min intervals was increased to 100 µl in order to maintain an approximately even level of seizure activity throughout the 2 hr of the experiment. At appropriate times, animals were frozen in liquid nitrogen, and their cerebral cortices were processed in the frozen state according to the method of Lowry et al. (42). Some animals were injected with isotonic glucose or NaCl to elevate blood and brain glucose concentrations or to provide a similar osmotic load without changing carbohydrate supply.

Brain lactate concentrations increased severalfold with seizures (Fig. 8). Animals that received glucose supplements had slightly higher brain lactate concentrations, suggesting that when more glucose was available, more was utilized. Although no individual point showed a significant elevation of brain lactate in the glucose group, the curve as a whole was significantly higher than that for their saline-injected littermates. Concentrations never reached 15 mM in either group and therefore were well below the concentrations associated with ischemic cell necrosis in experimental models of ischemia in the rat. Other studies showed that the animals treated with glucose, in spite of their slightly higher brain lactate concentrations, had greatly reduced mortality when seizures were prolonged and that the brain was relatively protected against the effect of seizures on growth (Table 5). These data suggest clearly that the amounts of lactate accumulated in these brains had little if any adverse effect.

Rabbits were studied at the age of 1 day. Seizures were induced with intramuscular bicuculline (2.5 mg/kg). Animals were similarly injected with 10% of body weight of isotonic solution of glucose (Gl group) or NaCl (saline group). Sacrifice was by microwave irradiation with a focused beam in a high-power oven (Gehrling Moore). Bicuculline injection resulted in hyperactivity, followed within 2 min by clonic seizures, culminating in a generalized tonic seizure, followed by intermittent tonic-clonic activity that continued through the 30 min of the experiment. Blood and brain lactate concentrations increased severalfold with seizures but remained well below the concentrations associated with ischemic cell necrosis. Blood lactate concentration also remained well below those observed during status epilepticus in adult aimals.

In newborn monkeys, seizures were induced by intraperitoneal bicuculline (5 mg/kg), and sacrifice was by immersion in liquid nitrogen. Animals were

TABLE 5. *Brain development in immature rats after status epilepticus: protective effect of glucose*[a]

	Controls	Glucose-injected	Saline-injected
Brain weight (mg)	452 ± 24†	424 ± 18*	404 ± 18**†
Brain RNA (μg)	1,172 ± 42	1,141 ± 34	1,093 ± 39**
Brain DNA (μg)	819 ± 30	801 ± 18	753 ± 19**†
Brain protein (mg)	40.8 ± 2.2†	37.6 ± 1.9*	34.8 ± 1.8**††
Brain cholesterol (mg)	2.37 ± 0.13	2.26 ± 0.13	2.06 ± 0.14**†
RNA concentration (μg/g)	2,736 ± 92	2,763 ± 91	2,645 ± 110
DNA concentration (μg/g)	1,812 ± 64	1,889 ± 42	1,864 ± 44
Protein concentration (mg/g)	90.3 ± 4.5	88.7 ± 4.2	86.1 ± 4.1
Cholesterol concentration (mg/g)	5.24 ± 0.30	5.33 ± 0.29	5.10 ± 0.31
Protein-DNA ratio	49.8 ± 2.4	46.9 ± 2.1	46.2 ± 2.1
RNA-DNA ratio	1.43 ± 0.40	1.42 ± 0.40	1.45 ± 0.40
Cholesterol-DNA ratio	2.89 ± 0.20	2.82 ± 0.20	2.74 ± 0.20
Cell number ($\times 10^{-6}$)	132.1 ± 4.8	129.2 ± 2.9	121.4 ± 3.1**†
Mean weight per nucleus (ng)	3.31 ± 0.06	3.24 ± 0.09	3.28 ± 0.08

[a]Rats matched for sex, litter, and body weight (0.5 g) were treated at 4 days of age and killed at 7 days of age. Treatment consisted of injection of isotonic glucose (10% of body weight) followed by 2 hr of flurothyl-induced seizures (glucose group), injection of isotonic sodium chloride solution followed by 2 hr of seizures (saline group), or simple handling (control group). Different from controls: *$p < 0.05$; **$p \leq 0.01$. Different from glucose-injected: †$p < 0.05$; ††$p < 0.01$.

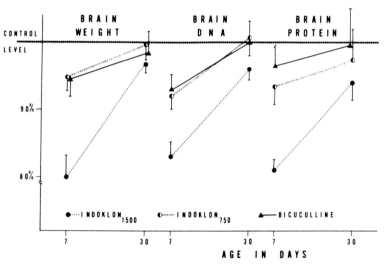

FIG. 9. Effects on brain growth of a single 2-hr episode of seizures in 4-day-old rats. Total forebrain contents of DNA and protein were depressed 3 days after seizures but recovered completely (bicuculline, flurothyl, 750 μl) or partially (flurothyl, 1,500 μl) by the age of 30 days.

not preinjected with either glucose or saline solutions. Measurements of blood glucose concentrations were carried out at infrequent intervals to avoid excessive volume depletion. The sequence of hyperactivity, followed by clonic-tonic-clonic seizures, was similar to that observed in rabbits. EEGs evolved from continued polyspike activity during the initial tonic manifestations to a burst-suppression pattern in which seizure activity alternated with electrical silence. In monkeys, as in rabbits and rats, most seizures were characterized by polyspike activity, but in contrast to the findings in rats and rabbits, in marmosets a small amount of slow-wave activity was observed in conjunction with the spikes (Fig. 1).

Lactate concentrations in blood and brain were elevated severalfold. However, they always stayed below the 10-mM range in spite of the associated

A,B

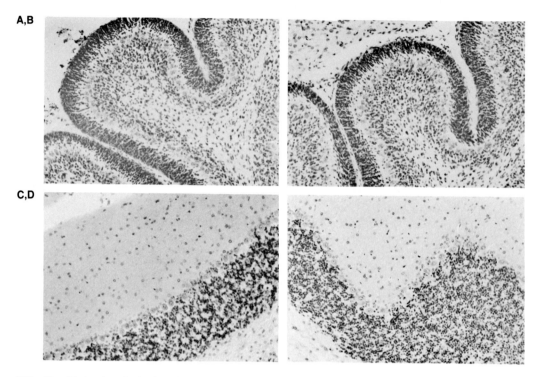

C,D

FIG. 10. Nissl stains of animals subjected to 2 hr of fluorthyl (1,500 μl) seizures at 4 days of age and paired littermate controls that were sacrificed at 7 or 30 days of age. Cerebellum in 7-day controls (**A**) and experimental animals (**B**) and in 30-day controls (**C**) and experimental animals (**D**). *(contd.)*

anoxia and cyanosis. Our preliminary and unpublished histological observations using routine light microscopy have revealed no histological changes.

All three species studied showed striking similarity, with severe status producing no ischemic cell necrosis in these immature animals, and with relatively modest elevations in brain lactate concentrations in spite of massive increases in metabolic rate. Glucose supplements in two species resulted in only modest elevations in brain lactate concentrations, but they were very effective in protecting the brain and in increasing survival. At first glance, these data appear to conflict with those of Myers (19,51) indicating an adverse effect of glucose with massive lactate accumulation in mixed anoxia-ischemia in neonates. However, these data are, in fact, compatible with those of Myers and can be integrated into a simple hypothesis: The integrity of the circulation in our model of status epilepticus differentiates the situation from that of anoxia plus hypotension. The high concentration of lactate carrier in the blood-brain barrier of immature and suckling animals is well known (56).

In fact, in older suckling rats (18 days) the maximal lactate flux from brain·to blood can exceed 2 mmole/kg/min (15). When circulation is intact, as was the case in our animals, brain lactate can escape from brain to blood. As a result, the role of lactate accumulation in neonates is probably of minor significance. Even a massive increase in glucose supplied to the brain in status epilepticus results in only a marginal increase in brain lactate that has no harmful effect. On the other hand, the correction by glucose supplements of the decrease in intracellular brain glucose concentration described elsewhere in this chapter protects the brain and increases survival. This would explain the relative paucity of cortical abnormalities in neonates and the lack of histological damage following most anoxic or hypermetabolic insults in experimental animals in the neonatal period (Fig. 9). In adults, both in experimental status epilepticus and in clinical status, and presumably in children past the suckling period, the small amounts of lactate carrier in the blood-brain barrier restrict escape of lactate from brain even when circulation is main-

E,F

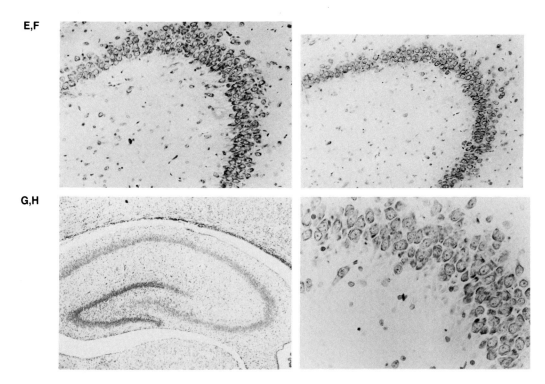

G,H

FIG. 10. *(contd.).* Hippocampus in 7-day controls **(E)** and experimental animals **(F)** and in 30-day controls **(G,H)** and experimental animals (see **I** and **J** on following page). *(contd.)*

tained; lactate reaches very high concentrations (>25 mM) and may contribute to the genesis of ischemic neuronal necrosis (77). If this hypothesis is correct, glucose supplements that protect the neonate when circulation is maintained might actually become harmful in case of circulatory collapse, because lactate might then be unable to escape from brain into blood and might reach toxic concentrations in brain. A similar reasoning might apply to anoxic states, so that in the neonate, glucose supplements might conceivably be helpful in anoxia and harmful in ischemia. The potential applications of these principles to the management of neonatal hypoxia, ischemia, and seizures are obvious, and considerably more work is needed in this area.

CARDIAC FACTORS

We do not know the respective roles of the heart and the brain in the reduction in mortality from status epilepticus brought about by a glucose load. However, in contrast to the brain, the immature heart has abundant stores of carbohydrates and can

mobilize them quickly in response to metabolic needs (17,18,50,64). Cardiac complications, which are frequent and serious during status epilepticus in adults (72), are rarely observed during experimental status epilepticus in newborn animals.

REGULATION OF CEREBRAL BLOOD FLOW

The limited studies involving newborn dogs (30,59) have suggested that the mechanisms that regulate cerebral blood flow are nearly fully mature at birth. Autoregulation of cerebral blood flow assures the brain of a constant supply of blood, despite wide variations in arterial blood pressure. In humans, fluctuations in blood pressure with each seizure have been noted in the neonatal intensive care unit. Autoregulation was abolished in human infants in respiratory distress (40,44). The effects of seizures on cerebral blood flow in neonates have never been studied directly, but in view of the maturity of the system at birth, they are presumed to be relatively similar to those observed in adults.

I,J

K,L

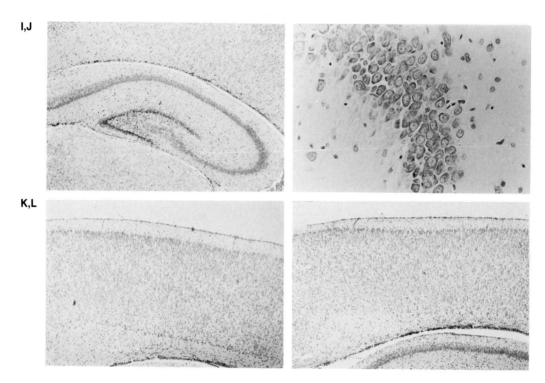

FIG. 10. *(contd.).* Hippocampus in 30-day experimental animals (**I,J**). Cortex in 7-day controls (**K**) and experimental animals (**L**).

TABLE 6. *Ontogeny of behavioral milestones after neonatal status epilepticus*

	Controls	Experimentals
Free-fall righting	16.5 ± 0.2[a]	18.2 ± 0.4*
Swimming ability	12.2 ± 0.3	13.3 ± 0.2*

[a]Values indicate the number of postnatal days required to reach the adult type of response (mean ± SEM).
*Different from controls (*p* < 0.01).

EFFECTS OF ANTICONVULSANTS ON THE IMMATURE BRAIN

The effects of phenobarbital and phenytoin on brain development have been studied in rats, mice, and rhesus monkeys. Long-term administration of phenobarbital has been shown to produce a reduction in brain growth that is dose-dependent (20). These effects were obtained at very high doses (60 mg/kg) and were not induced with lower amounts of anticonvulsants (30 mg/kg of phenobarbital) of the same order of magnitude as those that would be expected to be used to treat sustained seizures in the neonate. These effects on brain growth do not result from malnutrition because they have been observed in artificially reared, paired-fed animals. Other reports have indicated that the prenatally forming large neurons develop poorly after injection of phenobarbital in mice, but that granule cells that develop later are not altered (80). Similar studies in rats using phenytoin resulted in abnormalities such as anencephaly, growth retardation, and other dysmorphogenic features such as cleft palate (48). Such effects have not been produced in primates or in humans with therapeutic, nontoxic doses similar to those used in clinical practice. Other studies using smaller amounts of phenytoin showed no

TABLE 7. *Flurothyl seizure thresholds[a]*

	Controls	Experimentals
Seizure latency	599 ± 14 sec	529 ± 8 sec*
Quantity of flurothyl	199 ± 5 μl	176 ± 3 μl*

[a]Each rat was placed into a 1 gallon jar into which flurothyl was infused at the rate of 20 μl/min. Seizure threshold was defined as the amount of flurothyl infused into the jar at the time of onset of a full tonic seizure (mean ± SEM).
*Different from controls (*p* < 0.01).

microscopic abnormalities (79). Postnatal effects have not been demonstrated. In humans, most studies have shown little effect of maternal injection of anticonvulsants on a child's intellectual performance or head growth. However, a study demonstrating retardation at 2 years of age or above among such infants has been published (31). It is doubtful, however, that these studies are relevant to the acute treatment of seizures in human neonates, because no abnormalities have ever been demonstrated with short-term treatment, and therefore during neonatal seizures the risk of treatment, if any, appears much lower than the risk associated with the seizures.

NEONATAL SEIZURES IMPAIR BRAIN GROWTH

In infants and children, prolonged or repetitive seizures often are followed by learning difficulties in school, intellectual or motor deterioration, or even institutionalization (1,2). They can lead to cerebral atrophy, demonstrable by pneumoencephalography (3), or to death. We have studied the effects of repetitive seizures on brain development in the rat. Our findings indicate that a single bout of repetitive seizures too mild to cause neuronal necrosis can nevertheless inhibit brain DNA synthesis, permanently reduce brain size and the number of brain cells, and delay the appearance of some behavioral milestones (75). A considerable potential for recovery of cell number exists, and both the severity of the insult and the extent of recovery vary regionally within the brain. These studies reveal a new aspect of the vulnerability of developing at critical times. They suggest that even insults that stay short of inducing ischemic cell necrosis can permanently damage the immature brain.

Pregnant Wistar rats were housed individually and kept in a room with a 7 a.m. to 7 p.m. light–dark cycle. After delivery, each litter was kept with its natural mother. Littermates were paired by sex and body weight (± 0.5 g) at age 4 days. One member of each pair was subjected to seizures at 4 days of age; its companion was handled in similar fashion, but no seizures were induced. Animals were sacrificed at age 7 days to study the short-term effects of seizures on brain development, because cells injured during seizures would have lysed within 3 days. When we wanted to study the long-term effects of seizures, animals were sacrificed at the age of 30 days, because after that age very

little cell division takes place in the rat brain, and observed differences in brain DNA and brain cell number are likely to be permanent. Seizures were induced in a 33°C oven (bicuculline) or in a 33°C water bath (flurothyl). Periodic temperature checks in selected animals showed that their temperatures were close to that of the environment. All experiments and behavioral tests were carried out between 1 and 4 p.m. Seizures were induced by intraperitoneal bicuculline (10 mg/kg) or flurothyl vapor. For the latter, 1 to 4 rats were placed in a 1-liter cylindrical jar at 33°C in a water bath. Every 5 min, flurothyl was injected against the inner wall of the jar. The lid was kept on for 3.5 min and then removed for 1.5 min. The oxygen content of the jar did not vary during the experiment. Two dosages of flurothyl were used: "Mild" seizures were induced by injections of 25 μl for the initial 90 min and 50 μl for the last 30 min. For "severe" seizures, these amounts were doubled. Other groups of animals received two daily electroconvulsive seizures (1 sec, 100 mA, 60-Hz AC) and were also sacrificed at 30 days. For histological studies, animals were perfused-fixed with formalin/acetic acid/methanol. In selected animals we studied behavioral milestones such as the ability to swim and free-fall righting (ability of a rat dropped in the supine position from a height of 35 cm to turn over in midair and land on all fours). These milestones developed at highly predictable ages. Seizure threshold was tested at 28 days of age with flurothyl (75). For measurements of DNA synthesis, rats were injected intraperitoneally with methyl-[³H]thymidine (5 μCi/g) and decapitated 20 or 30 min after injection. Our methods were specific for radioactivity incorporated into DNA (75). For measurements of DNA breakdown, rats were injected with methyl-[³H]thymidine at age 2 days, followed by seizures at 4 days and later sacrifice.

Flurothyl seizures resulted in dose-dependent reductions in brain and body growth. Bicuculline had similar effects. Three days after severe flurothyl seizures, the mean deficit in number of cells in forebrain in experimental rats was 30,000,000. Brain RNA, DNA, protein, cholesterol, and weight were reduced to approximately the same extent, suggesting a reduction in number of brain cells without much change in mean cell size. Twenty days after seizures, a small but significant reduction in forebrain weight persisted. Forebrain DNA, protein, and cholesterol were also reduced in the experimental group. In other words, a single 2-hr

weight and brain DNA content were significantly higher in glucose-treated rats than in saline-treated animals (but lower than in untreated controls) (Table 5). Because diploid cells of the rat contain 6.2 pg DNA per nucleus, the mean cell deficit per brain was calculated to be 10.7 million cells in the saline group and 2.9 million cells in the glucose group.

The lower DNA content of brain in immature rats subjected to repeated seizures, as compared with controls, was found previously to reflect inhibition of synthesis rather than enhanced breakdown (75). Pretreatment with glucose reduced the inhibitory effect of seizures on brain DNA synthesis.

CONCLUSIONS

We are beginning to understand how seizures damage the developing brain. The combination of increased utilization and decreased supply depletes energy stores and, perhaps by raising the GDP/GTP ratio, inhibits the initiation of protein synthesis, which in turn dissociates polysomes, slows growth, and profoundly inhibits DNA synthesis. Because of the brain's limited mitotic potential, inhibition of cell multiplication causes defects that cannot be made up after it ceases. The resulting imbalance between cell populations can be permanent.

During sustained seizures in the immature brain, glucose transport cannot keep up with glucose utilization because of the low concentration of glucose carrier in the blood-brain barrier and because of its relatively effective glycolytic pathway. Glycogen stores cannot be rapidly mobilized because of low phosphorylase and phosphoglucomutase concentrations and low phosphorylase activation by cyclic AMP in glia. Ketone bodies cannot be used efficiently as alternative fuels when the redox state of the tissue is compromised, as it usually is by sustained convulsive seizures. The net result is profound depletion of intracellular glucose in brain, whereas blood glucose may remain entirely normal, and brain damage by a mechanism similar to that seen in hypoglycemia. Because of the unusual characteristics of the hexose carrier in the blood-brain barrier, this intracellular glucose depletion can be corrected by raising blood glucose concentration above normal, illustrating the therapeutic advantages of a better understanding of brain metabolism.

As long as cerebral circulation is maintained, brain lactate accumulation does not reach critical levels, even in the presence of hyperglycemia, pre-

sumably because the large amounts of lactate carrier present in the blood-brain barrier of suckling animals allow lactate to escape from brain. These results illustrate the large differences between the mechanisms of brain damage in the immature brain and the mature brain and the therapeutic importance of a better understanding of cerebral pathophysiology.

REFERENCES

1. Aicardi, J. (1977): Postnatal seizures. Clinical effects. In: *Brain, Fetal and Infant*, edited by S. R. Berenberg, p. 295. Martinus Nighoff, The Hague.
2. Aicardi, J., and Baraton, J. (1971): A pneumoencephalographic demonstration of brain atrophy following status. *Dev. Med. Child Neurol.*, 13:660.
3. Aicardi, J., and Chevrie, J. J. (1971): Convulsive status epilepticus in infants and children: A study of 239 cases. *Epilepsia*, 11:187.
4. Bachelard, H. S. (1970): Control of carbohydrate metabolism. In: *Handbook of Neurochemistry, Vol. IV*, edited by A. Lajtha, pp. 1–11. Plenum Press, New York.
5. Balazs, R. (1970): Carbohydrate metabolism. In: *Handbook of Neurochemistry, Vol. III*, edited by A. Lajtha, pp. 1–36. Plenum Press, New York.
6. Betz, A. L., Gilboe, D. D., and Drewes, L. R. (1975): Accelerative exchange diffusion, kinetics of glucose between blood and brain and its relation to transport during anoxia. *Biochim. Biophys. Acta*, 401:416–428.
7. Braun, L. D., Cornford, E. M., and Oldendorf, W. H. (1980): Newborn rabbit blood-brain barrier is selectively permeable and differs substantially from the adult. *J. Neurochem.*, 34:147–152.
8. Buckley, B. M., and Williamson, D. H. (1973): Acetoacetate and brain lipogenesis: Developmental pattern of acetoacetyl-coenzyme A synthetase in the soluble fraction of rat brain. *Biochem. J.*, 132:653–656.
9. Buschiazzo, P. M., Terrell, E. B., and Regen, D. M. (1970): Sugar transport across the blood-brain barrier. *Am. J. Physiol.*, 219:1505–1513.
10. Chevrie, J. J., and Aicardi, J. (1978): Convulsive disorders in the first year of life: Neurological and mental outcome and mortality. *Epilepsia*, 19:67.
11. Collins, R. C., Posner, J. B., and Plum, F. (1970): Cerebral energy metabolism during electroshock seizures in mice. *Am. J. Physiol.*, 218:943–950.
12. Corsellis, J. (1981): Neuropathology of status epilepticus (Chapter 12, *this volume*).
13. Cremer, J. E., Braun, L., and Oldendorf, W. H. (1976): Changes during development in transport processes of the blood brain barrier. *Biochim. Biophys. Acta*, 448:633–637.
14. Cremer, J. E., and Heath, D. F. (1974): The estimation of rates of utilization of glucose and ketone bodies in the brain of the suckling rat using compartmental analysis of isotopic data. *Biochem. J.*, 142:527–544.
15. Cremer, J. E., Teal, H. M., and Heath, D. F. (1975): Regulatory factors in glucose and ketone body utilization by the developing brain. In: *Normal and Path-*

ological Development of Energy Metabolism, edited by F. A. Hommes and C. J. Van den Berg, pp. 133–142. Academic Press, New York.

16. Crone, C. (1965): Facilitated transfer of glucose from blood into brain tissue. *J. Physiol.*, 181:103–113.

17. Dawes, G. S., Jacobson, H. N., Mott, J. C., and Shelley, H. J. (1960): Some observations on foetal and newborn rhesus monkeys. *J. Physiol.*, 152:271–298.

18. Dawes, G. S., Mott, J. C., and Shelley, H. J. (1959): The importance of cardiac glycogen for the maintenance of life in foetal lambs and newborn animals during anoxia. *J. Physiol.*, 146:516–538.

19. DeCourten, G. M., Myers, R. E., and Yamaguchi, S. (1981): Serum glucose concentration as determiner of brain pathologic response to marked hypoxia with hypotension. *Neurology (Minneap.)*, 31:41.

20. Diaz, J., and Schain, R. J. (1978): Phenobarbital: Effects of long-term administration on behavior and brain of artificially reared rats. *Science*, 199:90.

21. Duffy, T. E., Howse, D. E., and Plum, F. (1975): Cerebral energy metabolism during experimental status epilepticus. *J. Neurochem.*, 24:925–934.

22. Duffy, T. E., Kohle, S. J., and Vannucci, R. C. (1975): Carbohydrate and energy metabolism in perinatal rat brain: Relation to survival in anoxia. *J. Neurochem.*, 24:271–276.

23. Duffy, T. E., and Vannucci, R. C. (1977): Metabolic aspects of cerebral anoxia in the fetus and newborn. In: *Brain, Fetal and Infant*, edited by S. R. Berenberg, p. 316. Martinus Nijhoff, The Hague.

24. Dwyer, B. E., Racz, T., and Wasterlain, C. G. (1978): Effect of neonatal seizures on brain lipid accumulation. *Trans. Am. Soc. Neurochem.*, 9:140.

25. Dwyer, B. E., and Wasterlain, C. G. (1981): Prolonged seizures deplete brain glucose in normoglycemic neonates. *Neurology (Minneap.)*, 31:162.

26. Fish, I., and Winick, M. (1969): The effects of malnutrition on regional growth of the developing rat brain. *Exp. Neurol.*, 25:534.

27. Fishman, R. A. (1964): Carrier transport of glucose between blood and cerebrospinal fluid. *Am. J. Physiol.*, 206:836.

28. Gottstein, U., Muller, W., Berghoff, H., Gartner, H., and Held, K. (1971): Zur Utilisation von nicht-veresterten Feftsauren und Ketonkorpern im Gehirn des Menschen. *Klin. Wochenschr.*, 49:406–411.

29. Growdon, W. A., Bratton, T. S., Houston, M. C., Tarpley, H. L., and Regen, D. M. (1971): Brain glucose metabolism in the intact mouse. *Am. J. Physiol.*, 221:1738–1745.

30. Hernandez, M. J., Brennan, R. W., and Bowman, G. (1980): Autoregulation of cerebral blood flow in the newborn dog. *Brain Res.*, 184:199–202.

31. Hill, R. M., Verniaud, W. M., Horning, M. G., McCulley, L. V., and Morgan, N. F. (1974): Infants exposed in utero to antiepileptic drugs. A prospective study. *Am. J. Dis. Child.*, 127:645.

32. Himwich, H. E., Baker, Z., and Fazekas, J. F. (1939): The respiratory metabolism of infant brain. *Am. J. Physiol.*, 125:601–606.

33. Himwich, H. E., and Fazekas, J. F. (1941): Comparative studies of the metabolism of brain of infant and adult dogs. *Am. J. Physiol.*, 132:454–458.

34. Holtzman, D., and Moore, C. L. (1973): Oxidative phosphorylation in immature rat brain mitochondria. *Biol. Neonate*, 22:230–242.

35. Jorgensen, O. S., Dwyer, B. E., and Wasterlain, C. G. (1980): Synaptic proteins after electroconvulsive seizures in immature rats. *J. Neurochem.*, 35:1235–1237.

36. Kennedy, C., Grave, G. E., Jehle, J. W., and Sokoloff, L. (1972): Changes in blood flow in the component structures of the dog brain during postnatal maturation. *J. Neurochem.*, 19:2423–2433.

37. Kjellmer, I., Karlaaon, K., Olsson, T., and Rosen, K. G. (1974): Cerebral reactions during intrauterine asphyxia in the sheep. I. Circulation and oxygen consumption in the fetal brain. *Pediatr. Res.*, 8:50–57.

38. Klee, C. B., and Sokoloff, L. (1967): Changes in D(−)-β-hydroxybutyric acid-dehydrogenase activity during brain maturation in the rat. *J. Biol. Chem.*, 242:3880–3883.

39. Kraus, H., Schenker, S., and Schwedesky, D. (1974): Developmental changes of cerebral ketone body utilization in human infants. *Hoppe Seylers Z. Physiol. Chem.*, 355:164–170.

40. Lou, H. C., Lassen, N. A., and Friss-Hansen, B. (1979): Impaired autoregulation of cerebral blood flow in the distressed newborn infant. *J. Pediatr.*, 94:118–121.

41. Lowry, O. H., and Passonneau, J. V. (1972): *A Flexible System of Enzymatic Analysis.* Academic Press, New York.

42. Lowry, O. H., Passonneau, J. V., Hasselberger, F. X., and Schulz, D. W. (1964): Effect of ischemia on known substrates and cofactors of the glycolytic pathway in brain. *J. Biol. Chem.*, 239:18–30.

43. Lucas, W., Kirschbaum, T., and Assali, N. S. (1966): Cephalic circulation and oxygen consumption before and after birth. *Am. J. Physiol.*, 210:287–292.

44. Mann, L. I. (1970): Developmental aspects and the effect of carbon dioxide tension on fetal cephalic blood flow. *Exp. Neurol.*, 26:136–147.

45. Mann, L. I. (1970): Fetal brain metabolism and function. *Clin. Obstet. Gynecol.*, 13:638–651.

46. McIlwain, M., and Bachelard, H. S. (1971): *Biochemistry and the Central Nervous System.* Williams & Wilkins, Baltimore.

47. Meldrum, B. S., and Brierley, J. B. (1973): Prolonged epileptic seizures in primates: Ischaemic cell change and its relation to ictal physiological events. *Arch. Neurol.*, 28:10–17.

48. Mercier-Parot, L., and Tuchmann-Duplessis, H. (1974): The dysmorphogenic potential of phenytoin: Experimental observations. *Drugs*, 8:340.

49. Moore, T. J., Lione, A. P., Regen, D. M., Tarpley, H. L., and Raines, P. L. (1971): Brain glucose metabolism in the newborn rat. *Am. J. Physiol.*, 221:1746–1753.

50. Mott, J. C. (1961): The ability of young mammals to withstand total oxygen lack. *Br. Med. Bull.*, 17:144–148.

51. Myers, R. (1977): Experimental models of perinatal brain damage: Relevance to human pathology. In: *Intrauterine Asphyxia and the Developing Fetal Brain*, edited by L. Gluck, Yearbook Medical Publishers, Chicago.

52. Oldendorf, W. H. (1971): Brain uptake of radiola-beled amino acids, amines, and hexoses after arterial injection. *Am. J. Physiol.*, 221:1629–1639.

53. O'Neill, J. J., and Duffy, T. E. (1966): Alternate metabolic pathways in newborn brain. *Life Sci.*, 5:1849–1857.

54. Owen, O. E., Morgan, A. P., Kemp, H. G., Sullivan, J. M., Herrera, M. G., and Cahill, G. F. (1967): Brain metabolism during fasting. *J. Clin. Invest.*, 46:1589–1593.

55. Page, M. A., Krebs, H. A., Williamson, D. H. (1971): Activities of enzymes of ketone-body utilization in brain and other tissues of suckling rats. *Biochem. J.*, 121:49–53.

56. Pardrige, W. M., and Oldendorf, W. H. (1977): Transport of metabolic substrates through the blood-brain barrier. *J. Neurochem.*, 28:5–12.

57. Persson, B., Settergren, G., and Dahlquist, G. (1972): Cerebral arteriovenous difference of acetoacetate and D-β-hydroxybutyrate in children. *Acta Paediatr. Scand.*, 61:272–278.

58. Posner, J. B., Plum, F., and Van Poznak, A. (1969): Cerebral mechanism during electrically induced seizures in man. *Arch. Neurol.*, 20:388–395.

59. Purves, M. J., and James, F. M. (1969): Observations on the control of cerebral blood flow in the sheep fetus and newborn lamb. *Circ. Res.*, 25:651–667.

60. Rose, A. L., and Lombroso, C. T. (1976): A study of clinical, pathological, and electroencephalographic features in 137 full term babies with a long-term follow-up. *Pediatrics*, 45:404.

61. Sacks, W. (1969): Cerebral metabolism *in vivo*. In: *Handbook of Neurochemistry, Vol. I*, edited by A. Lajtha, pp. 301–324. Plenum Press, New York.

62. Shapiro, B., and Wertheimer, E. (1943): Phosphorolysis and synthesis of glycogen in animal tissues. *Biochem. J.*, 37:397–403.

63. Shimizu, N., and Okada, M. (1957): Histochemical distribution of phosphorylase in rodent brain from newborn to adults. *J. Histochem. Cytochem.*, 5:459–471.

64. Stafford, A., and Weatherall, J. A. C. (1960): The survival of young rats in nitrogen. *J. Physiol.*, 153:457–472.

65. Suga, S., and Wasterlain, C. G. (1980): Effects of neonatal seizures or anoxia on cerebellar mitotic activity in the rat. *Exp. Neurol.*, 67:573–580.

66. Swaab, D. F., and Boer, K. (1972): The presence of biologically labile compounds during ischemia and their relationship to the EEG in rat cerebral cortex and hypothalamus. *J. Neurochem.*, 19:2843–2853.

67. Swaab, D. F., and Boer, K. (1972): The presence of biologically active compounds during ischemia and their relationship to the EEG in rat cerebral cortex and hypothalamus. *J. Neurochem.*, 19:2843–2853.

68. Thurston, J. H., Hauhart, R. E., and Jones, E. M. (1974): Anoxia in mice: Reduced glucose in brain with normal or elevated glucose in plasma and increased survival after glucose treatment. *Pediatr. Res.*, 8:238–243.

69. Thurston, J. H., Hauhart, R. E., Jones, E. M., Ikossi, M. G., and Pierce, R. W. (1973): Decrease in brain glucose in anoxia despite elevated plasma glucose levels. *Pediatr. Res.*, 7: 691–695.

70. Thurston, J. H., and McDougal, D. B. (1969): Effect of ischemia on metabolism of the brain of the newborn mouse. *Am. J. Physiol.*, 216:348–352.

71. Vannucci, S. J., and Vannucci, R. C. (1980): Glycogen metabolism in neonatal rat brain during anoxia and recovery. *J. Neurochem.*, 34:1100–1105.

72. Wasterlain, C. G. (1974): Morbidity and mortality from serial seizures. *Epilepsia*, 15:155–176.

73. Wasterlain, C. G. (1980): Does anoxemia play a role in the effects of neonatal seizures on brain growth? An experimental study in the rat. *Eur. Neurol.*, 18:222–229.

74. Wasterlain, C. G. (1974): Inhibition of cerebral protein synthesis by epileptic seizures without motor manifestations. *Neurology (Minneap.)*, 24:175–180.

75. Wasterlain, C. G. (1976): Effects of neonatal status epilepticus on rat brain development. *Neurology (Minneap.)*, 76:975.

76. Wasterlain, C. G., and Duffy, T. E. (1976): Status epilepticus in immature rats. *Arch. Neurol.*, 33:821–827.

77. Wasterlain, C. G., and Graham, S. (1980): Autoregulation of cerebral blood flow: An asset during single seizures, a liability during status epilepticus. *Ann. Neurol.*, 8:94.

78. Wasterlain, C.G., and Plum, F. (1973): Vulnerability of developing rat brain to electroconvulsive seizures. *Arch. Neurol.*, 29:38.

79. Westmoreland, B., and Bass, N. H. (1971): Diphenylhydantoin intoxication during pregnancy. A chemical study of drug distribution in the albino rat. *Arch. Neurol.*, 24:158.

80. Yanai, J., Rosselli-Austin, L., and Tabakoff, B. (1979): Neuronal deficits in mice following prenatal exposure to phenobarbital. *Exp. Neurol.*, 64:237.

Advances in Neurology, Vol. 34: Status Epilepticus, edited by A.V. Delgado-Escueta, C.G. Wasterlain, D.M. Treiman, and R.J. Porter. Raven Press, New York © 1983.

24

Metabolic Factors During Prolonged Seizures and Their Relation to Nerve Cell Death

Brian S. Meldrum

In 1980, students of epileptic brain damage celebrated the centenary of two seminal observations. In 1880, Sommer (82) described regionally selective loss of pyramidal neurons within the hippocampus in chronic epilepsy. In that same year, Pfleger (66) noted hippocampal coloration indicative of recent pathological changes following seizures. He stated the hypothesis that impaired nutrition or blood flow during or after seizures could be responsible for the sclerosis.

One hundred years later we are still seeking to comprehend these observations. Many explanations have been offered, but none so far has proved adequate. Spielmeyer (84), on the basis of the similarity between hippocampal lesions in epilepsy and those in some cases of cerebral ischemia, proposed that cerebral vascular spasm ("angiospasmus"), which he believed to accompany seizures, was responsible for hippocampal sclerosis. Following demonstrations in humans and animals (65) that vascular dilatation, not constriction, accompanied seizures, German neuropathologists (64, 72,73) put forward various revised hypoxia/ischemia hypotheses to explain hippocampal damage in epilepsy. These included the following factors as possible contributory causes: (a) systemic hypoxia (due to apnea or muscular spasms); (b) increased cerebral metabolic rate ("consumptive hypoxia"); (c) bradycardia and a fall in arterial blood pressure; (d) increased permeability of the blood-brain barrier; (e) increased brain volume (vascular engorgement or cerebral edema) leading to compression of vessels, with the possibility of medial temporal herniation at the tentorial edge compressing branches of the posterior cerebral artery, described by Lindenberg (35) as a sequel of acute increases in supratentorial pressure. The nature of the clinical material did not permit firm conclusions about the relationship between physiological changes during seizures and epileptic brain damage. Indeed, it was widely believed that the sclerotic hippocampal lesions found in patients with chronic epilepsy were the results of trauma or asphyxia in the perinatal period and the causes of subsequent temporal lobe epilepsy (19).

Therefore, I began, 10 years ago, a series of experimental studies in primates and rodents intended to clarify the role of ictal and postictal events in the genesis of epileptic brain damage. Initially, sustained generalized seizures induced by systemic drug administration were studied in baboons and rodents (Table 1). More recently, focal limbic seizures induced by microinjections of kainic acid into the amygdala of marmosets, rats, and baboons have shown that purely focal seizures can be followed by hippocampal lesions. This chapter will summarize these studies and discuss possible mechanisms of selective neuronal loss.

TABLE 1. *Animal models of generalized seizures and pathological outcomes*

Convulsant	Animal	Duration (hr)	Paralysis	Neuronal loss			Gliosis	Reference
				Neocortex	Hippocampus	Cerebellum		
Sustained tonic-clonic seizure								
Bicuculline	Baboon	1.5–5.0	No	+ +	+ +	+ +		48
	Baboon	3.4–7.5	Yes	+	+ +	0		56
	Rat	2.0	Yes	+	+ +	0		6
PTZ	Baboon	1–2 (× 5–10)	Yes				+ +	54
Intermittent tonic-clonic seizures								
Allylglycine	Baboon	(28–62 seizures in 8–11 hr)	No	0	+ +	0	+	51

SUSTAINED GENERALIZED SEIZURES IN BABOONS

Preliminary tests using a variety of convulsant agents in rodents, rhesus monkeys, and baboons showed that bicuculline, an alkaloid that blocks the postsynaptic inhibitory action of GABA, is exceptional in inducing generalized seizures that are severe and sustained, but compatible with survival (49,50).

In the first experimental series, "unmodified" seizures (i.e., without peripheral paralysis, sedatives, or anesthetics) were induced with intravenous bicuculline, 0.2 to 0.6 mg/kg, in adolescent baboons chronically prepared to permit monitoring of the EEG and various critical physiological variables, including arterial and cerebral venous pressure and blood gases (50).

Seizure onset was associated with marked increases in systolic and diastolic arterial pressures and in cerebral venous pressure. There was severe plasma acidosis (arterial pH < 6.8; arterial lactate mean peak 11.6 mM/liter) in the first minutes of the seizure. Arterial glucose concentration was elevated after 15 to 65 min (mean peak 18.8 mM/liter). The sustained rhythmic myoclonus was associated with a progressive increase in rectal temperature, producing hyperpyrexia (40–42°C) after 60 to 90 min. Late in prolonged seizures there was mild to moderate arterial hypotension and, in some animals, hypoglycemia. However, cerebral venous oxygen tension remained above levels regarded as critical for hypoxic brain damage.

The brains were fixed by peroartic perfusion with a formalin/acetic acid/methanol mixture a few minutes to 4 hr after the end of seizure activity. Paraffin- and celloidin-embedded material was studied by light microscopy (48). The principal abnormality was "ischemic cell change" *(vide in-fra)*. This involved, selectively, the following: in the neocortex, small pyramidal neurons in the third, fifth, and sixth laminae; in the cerebellum, Purkinje and basket cells; in the hippocampus, pyramidal neurons in the Sommer sector and end folium; in the thalamus, neurons in the anterior and dorsomedial nuclei; in the amygdala, scattered neurons in the basolateral nuclei. In the neocortex, damage was diffuse, sometimes with accentuation occipitally and in the depths of sulci. In the hippocampus, asymmetrical lesions were observed in the Sommer sector. Cerebellar damage was in most cases accentuated in the boundary zone between the territories of the superior and posterior inferior cerebellar arteries, a pattern of damage found after severe arterial hypotension (10).

The presence and severity of brain damage did not correlate with the severity of any of the physiological changes observed early in seizures. It did correlate with the total duration of generalized seizures as assessed on the EEG and with the duration of hyperpyrexia (rectal temperature above 40°C). This was particularly true for cerebellar damage, which was not seen in the 2 brain-damaged animals without hyperpyrexia. There was also a tendency for the severity of brain damage to be related to arterial hypotension (all animals with mean pressure below 75 mm Hg during the last 30 min of seizure activity showed cerebellar "boundary zone" lesions, and 3 showed severe cortical lesions). Prolonged hypoglycemia (plasma glucose < 1.6 mM) was also associated with brain damage. This suggested that these secondary consequences of the generalized seizure might play a role in the initiation of ischemic cell change. In earlier experiments (10,11) we had observed the selective occurrence of ischemic neuronal changes following arterial hypotension and hypoglycemia in rhesus monkeys. However, it was possible that the cerebral seizure activity itself was the direct cause of the pathological changes, giving rise to a noncausal correlation between brain damage and secondary physiological events that would naturally vary with seizure severity and duration. A study was therefore undertaken in paralyzed, mechanically ventilated animals in which secondary physiological changes were minimized.

STATUS EPILEPTICUS IN PARALYZED VENTILATED BABOONS

Bicuculline was given intravenously in adolescent baboons with peripheral neuromuscular paralysis under mechanical ventilation (56). Generalized seizures, evaluated from EEG records, were sustained without interruption for up to 7.5 hr. Physiological monitoring showed early increases in arterial blood pressure, with minimal abnormalities in the later phase of the seizure. Arterial blood gases showed little variation. Acidosis was mild or absent. Cerebral blood flow was enhanced for the first 1 to 2 hr. Rectal temperature rose slightly but did not exceed 40°C.

Perfusion fixation of the brain after seizures lasting 3.4 to 7.5 hr revealed ischemic cell changes in the neocortex (diffusely involving small pyramidal neurons in the third, fifth, and sixth laminae, with some occipital accentuation), in the hippocampus (Sommer sector, end folium), and in the thalamus (scattered neurons in anterior and dorsomedial nuclei). The amygdala and cerebellum were not affected, except for a few Purkinje cells at the arterial boundary zone in the cerebellum of 1 baboon having had a rectal temperature of 39.8°C for 3 hr.

These experiments, in conjunction with the experiments with unmodified seizures, strongly suggested that secondary systemic consequences of seizures contribute to the cerebellar damage induced by status epilepticus. The abnormal motor activity leads to a powerful excitatory input to the cerebellar cortex (70) (from muscle spindle and joint receptor afferents) that will enhance metabolic activity. Arterial hypotension and hyperpyrexia, in the absence of epileptic activity, can lead to cerebellar abnormalities (11,44). Thus a role for these systemic factors appears probable. However, it appears that neocortical and hippocampal damage can occur in the absence of major changes in the secondary physiological changes that we have evaluated. This does not exclude the possibility

that respiratory or cardiovascular factors play a significant pathogenic role when they impair cerebral metabolic function.

Indeed, more prolonged seizures were necessary to produce a given pathological change (in the cortex or hippocampus) in the paralyzed baboons. Pathological changes were reported to be absent in paralyzed cats with carefully maintained respiratory and cardiovascular status after bicuculline-induced seizures lasting up to 5 hr (13). Furthermore, other subtle peripheral factors such as endocrine changes cannot be excluded. However, these experiments led us to seek the causes of hippocampal damage in cellular changes that are direct local consequences of a seizure discharge.

STATUS EPILEPTICUS IN BABOONS AND HUMANS

Are the physiological and pathological features of status epilepticus in baboons also found in humans? A recent study of 98 adults with status epilepticus admitted consecutively to the San Francisco General Hospital (2) permits a partial answer to this question. Recovery with no neurological sequelae was observed in 70 patients; in 18 patients, morbidity was attributable to the primary illness. Status epilepticus appeared responsible for neurological sequelae in 10 patients, including 2 patients who died (postmortem examination in one revealed ischemic changes in the basal ganglia and posterior parietal region and bilateral arterial boundary zone infarction). Unfavorable outcome ·correlated with prolonged duration where this was known precisely. Seizures lasted more than 2 hr in 5 of 6 patients with neurological sequelae and in 9 of 49 patients without sequelae. Hyperthermia was a frequent finding; when severe, it was associated with an unfavorable outcome. Acidosis was common (arterial pH below 7.00 in 23 patients), but this showed no correlation with unfavorable outcome. Late hypoglycemia was not encountered, because dextrose was given prophylactically.

Thus, brain damage in humans and baboons is a possible outcome of generalized seizures lasting more than 2 hr. Hyperthermia is a consequence of severe prolonged seizures. It is associated with a less favorable outcome and is a known independent cause of cerebellar damage in humans (22).

The overall pattern of brain damage in the baboon with unmodified bicuculline seizures is closely similar to that in humans after generalized status epilepticus (17). The prominence of diffuse laminar cortical pathological changes, the tendency for hippocampal lesions to be symmetrical in the end folium and asymmetrical in the Sommer sector, and the symmetrical involvement of the cerebellum and of particular nuclear groups in the amygdala and thalamus are common features.

ISCHEMIC CELL CHANGES AND METABOLIC STRESS

Ischemic cell change was the name given by Spielmeyer (83) to the appearance of selectively vulnerable neurons in the human brain examined 6 to 48 hr after an episode of cerebral hypoxia or ischemia. It is characterized by a pyknotic triangular nucleus, staining darkly with eosin. The cytoplasm is also eosinophilic and shrunken, with a triangular outline, which may show scalloping or may be surrounded by incrustations. Ischemic cell change is followed by appearances (naked nuclei inside large vacuoles; neuronophagia) that precede selective cell loss. A prodromal stage can be identified as "microvacuolation" by light microscopy and as swelling of mitochondria with disruption of the cristae with the electron microscope (9). This alteration in mitochondria is identifiable in the soma and apical dendrites of selectively vulnerable neurons from 20 min to 2 hr after the onset of hypoxia-ischemia in rodents or experimental primates (11,12). It precedes the swelling of astrocytic end feet that gives rise to the scalloped appearance of some neurons. These neuronal appearances occur in experimental material regardless of whether the stress is hypoxia-ischemia (as in ventilation with nitrogen in an animal with one carotid artery occluded), profound arterial hypotension, or drug-induced status epilepticus. Prolonged profound hypoglycemia is also followed by ischemia cell change: Prodromal mitochondrial swelling is identifiable during a "recovery" period with glucose administration, but it may be less pronounced than after ischemia.

We concluded (43,44) that ischemic cell change was the common end point in selectively vulnerable neurons for any process that leads to a critical impairment of energy metabolism. We presumed that in status epilepticus this would be the consequence of a combination of impaired circulation and substrate supply and enhanced metabolic demand. We therefore sought to investigate this in a rodent model where it was possible to make accurate measurements of blood flow, oxygen and glucose consumption, and cerebral metabolic intermediates.

PROLONGED SEIZURES IN PARALYZED RATS

In the rat, a single injection of bicuculline, 1.2 mg/kg i.v., induces an electroencephalographic seizure that continues for 2 hr or more in the paralyzed mechanically ventilated animal (53). In this preparation it is possible to maintain blood pressure and blood gases and body temperature within specific limits, so that their influences on cerebral metabolism and pathological changes can be determined (7,14).

We measured cerebral blood flow (CBF) by an isotope-clearance method and by a venous-outflow method (53). In the first minute, CBF increased to nine times the control value. It was still four times control after 20 min and two to three times control after 60 to 120 min of seizure activity. The increase in oxygen consumption was less marked; CMR_{O2} was two to three times control throughout the seizure period. In a parallel study (8), cerebral glucose consumption was found to be four times normal at seizure onset. The excess over the increase in oxygen consumption is accounted for by lactate production. In the second hour of seizure activity the increase in glucose consumption matches stoichiometrically the increase in oxygen consumption. Thus, provided that arterial pressure, oxygenation, and blood glucose are adequately maintained, cerebral metabolic rate (for oxygen and glucose) is maintained at two to three times normal throughout 2 hr of seizure activity. Nevertheless, ischemic cell change is detectable in selectively vulnerable neurons in the neocortex and the hippocampus after 2 hr of seizure activity with physiological circumstances adequately maintained (7).

Impaired energy metabolism can be evaluated by direct measurement of substrates, metabolic intermediates, and phosphonucleotides in cerebral tissue using rapid freezing of the cortex at different times during sustained seizure activity (14). The data presented in Table 2 show that after 1 to 5 min a new relatively stable metabolic state is established with reduced glucose and phosphocreatine contents, elevated lactate, but a stable ATP concentration (and "energy charge") and a glycogen level that returns to normal.

TABLE 2. *Effects of systemic factors on changes in labile metabolites in rat cerebral cortex induced by status epilepticus[a]*

	Phosphocreatine	ATP	EC[b]	Lactate
Control (N = 5)	4.85 ± 0.13	2.99 ± 0.03	0.948 ± 0.001	1.56 ± 0.20
Standard (N = 5)	3.39 ± 0.27	2.94 ± 0.03	0.937 ± 0.002	9.14 ± 1.76
Hypotension (N = 6)	2.65 ± 0.10*	2.94 ± 0.04	0.933 ± 0.002	16.06 ± 1.05**
Hypoxia (N = 6)	2.61 ± 0.30	2.80 ± 0.06	0.931 ± 0.004	23.22 ± 2.03***
Hypoglycemia (N = 6)	3.38 ± 0.15	2.33 ± 0.02***	0.913 ± 0.008**	1.31 ± 0.23*
Hyperthermia (N = 5)	2.38 ± 0.13**	2.92 ± 0.03	0.933 ± 0.002	17.72 ± 1.55**

From Blennow et al. (7).

[a]Cortex frozen *in situ* after 2 hr of sustained bicuculline-induced epileptic seizures in "standard" animals (normoxic, normotensive, normothermic) and in animals with moderate hypotension, hypoxia, hypoglycemia, or hyperthermia; means ± SEM in $\mu mole \cdot g^{-1}$ wet tissue. For statistical evaluation, the hypotensive, hypoxic, and hyperthermic groups were compared with the standard group, not the control group.

[b]EC: adenylate"energy charge" = $(ATP + 0.5ADP)/(ATP + ADP + AMP)$.

*$p < 0.05$, ** $p < 0.01$, ***$p < 0.001$.

In this model it is possible to test the influence of systemic factors on cerebral metabolism and epileptic brain damage by varying one factor at a time (7) and comparing the outcome with a "standard" group (i.e., arterial pressure above 120 mm Hg, arterial P_{O_2} above 100 mm Hg, and rectal temperature at 37°C throughout 2 hr of seizure activity). Moderate arterial hypotension, hypoxia, and hypoglycemia all apparently protect against the development of ischemic cell change in the hippocampus and cortex. Only hyperthermia produces a clear exacerbation of the pathological changes, with an accelerated time course of ischemic cell change. The energy state of the brain is not improved by hypotension, hypoxia, or hypoglycemia (Table 2). However, these stresses tend to diminish the intensity of the seizure discharge, as indicated by the EEG. In these experiments there was no recovery or restitution phase (i.e., perfusion followed directly after the seizure). The impaired energy state might delay the evolution of ischemic cell change. An energy state adequate to permit an intense and sustained seizure discharge seems to be necessary for the rapid appearance of selective epileptic brain damage.

Reduced hippocampal blood flow during sustained seizures has frequently been proposed as a possible explanation for selective hippocampal damage. We have used a particle-distribution method and a diffusible-tracer method to determine regional blood flow in the rat brain at different times in the course of bicuculline seizures (28). The increases in neocortical blood flow match those for total cerebral blood flow at all times. In the thalamus, increases in blood flow exceed those for whole brain at all times. This correlates with the high tendency for the thalamus to show diffuse breakdown of the blood-brain barrier (as indicated by the entry of protein-bound dyes) during seizures (30). However, there is no correlation between the regional selectivity of blood-brain barrier breakdown and postictal pathological changes. Increases in CBF in the hindbrain (including the cerebellum) are less than average throughout the 2 hr. Initially, increases in CBF in the hippocampus are equal to those for neocortex and whole brain, but in the second hour the increases are relatively greater in the hippocampus. Thus a purely vascular explanation for hippocampal changes can be excluded.

OTHER PATTERNS OF PATHOLOGICAL CHANGES IN THE BABOON

Although sustained generalized seizures induced by bicuculline most clearly reproduce the pattern of damage found after status epilepticus, other experimental models more readily reproduce certain pathological features found in patients with chronic epilepsy.

Thus, in baboons given pentylenetetrazol (PTZ) intravenously while paralyzed and mechanically ventilated, at weekly intervals for 5 to 10 weeks, seizures lasted 1 to 2 hr (terminated by diazepam i.v.) (54). The predominant pathological change was gliosis, with marked proliferation of fibrous astrocytes in the end folium and marginal or subpial gliosis (15) diffusely in the neocortex and some proliferation of Bergman glia in the cerebellum. Neuronal loss could not be positively identified in any brain region.

Compounds that inhibit the cerebral enzyme glutamic acid decarboxylase, and thus decrease the rate of synthesis of GABA, induce generalized seizures (42). With a just-convulsant dose, these are brief, and they recur with intervening EEG recovery, but with a higher dose they become closely consecutive (47,51). D,L-allylglycine (350–550 mg/kg i.v.) in adolescent baboons is followed by brief tonic-clonic seizures (total 6 to 63 in 2–11 hr), which sometimes terminate with a period of status epilepticus. Brains examined after status epilepticus with short survivals show a pattern of damage similar to that seen after bicuculline in paralyzed baboons, i.e., selective ischemic cell change in neocortex and hippocampus but not in cerebellum. Hyperpyrexia occurred during status epilepticus but was of relatively short duration. After long sequences of brief seizures (34–63 in 8–11 hr) and longer-term recovery (1–3 weeks), the pathological changes are similar to those seen after repeated PTZ-induced seizures (i.e., astrocytic reaction in the neocortex, hippocampus, and cerebellum), except that neuronal loss is clearly identifiable in the hippocampus (Sommer sector and end folium) (51,54).

Using baboons 6 to 12 months old, longer survival periods (up to 5 years) following a sequence of seizures induced by D,L-allylglycine have now been studied. Marked astrocytic proliferation in the hippocampus is evident. However, cell loss is only mild, and spontaneous temporal lobe seizures have not been observed (46).

The pattern of brain damage seen after brief repetitive seizures induced by allylglycine is similar to that found in patients with chronic epilepsy, particularly that associated with a temporal lobe focus (psychomotor seizures, complex partial seizures) (39,41,85). This raises the possibility that hippocampal or mesial temporal sclerosis could be the consequence of seizures that are less generalized or less sustained than status epilepticus, which produces widespread neuronal loss. Observations in humans with, for example, a temporal lobe tumor, malformation, or other primary lesion coexisting with hippocampal sclerosis (17) are consistent with temporal lobe epilepsy as a cause of hippocampal sclerosis.

Injection of ouabain into the septal region in rabbits has been reported to induce limbic seizures and hippocampal changes (4). We therefore began early in 1978 a series of experiments in rodents and primates to test the pathological effects of focal limbic seizures.

LIMBIC SEIZURES DUE TO FOCAL INJECTION OF KAINIC ACID

Kainic acid is a structural analogue of glutamic acid that has potent excitatory and neurotoxic actions (63,79). The direct neurotoxic action of kainic acid shows selectivity for particular cell types. Thus, in the cerebellum, Purkinje and basket cells are more vulnerable than granule cells (26).

Hippocampal lesions involving pyramidal neurons of CA_3 and CA_4 follow the injection of small quantities of kainic acid into one lateral ventricle, striatum, or amygdala (6,59,93). With injections into the amygdala it is possible to study the spread and duration of local seizure activity by EEG recording from deep electrodes and by tracer methods indicating changes in local blood flow or glucose utilization (6,52). By these means we have attempted to differentiate between regional or cellular selectivity in the neurotoxic action of kainic acid and the neuropathological effects of local seizure activity.

In the rat, EEG recordings show bursts of seizure activity in the amygdala within a few minutes of focal injection of kainic acid (0.4–2.0 μg in 0.1–0.5 μl). This spreads to the ipsilateral hippocampus and, later, contralaterally. Behavioral signs accompanying this seizure activity show a progression from wet shakes to facial clonus, rearing, circling, barrel rotation, and generalized clonic seizures. The brief seizure discharges recur for 2 to 6 hr. Subsequently, isolated spikes occur in the injected amygdala and sometimes also in the ipsilateral hippocampus.

At the injection site the lesion is concentric, with total neuronal loss centrally but only selective neuronal loss peripherally. The earliest and most consistent pathological changes occur in the ipsilateral hippocampal end folium, CA_3 and CA_4, with ischemic cell changes after survivals of a few hours, and nerve cell loss subsequently. With longer survival times, neuronal necrosis involves also the contralateral hippocampus, midline thalamic nuclei, and variably the bed nucleus of the stria terminalis, the septum, the claustrum, contralateral amygdala, and patchily in the third, fifth, and sixth laminae of the cortex (6).

The administration of diazepam, 3 to 5 mg/kg i.p. at 30-min intervals starting at seizure onset and continuing for 6 hr, blocks clinical signs of

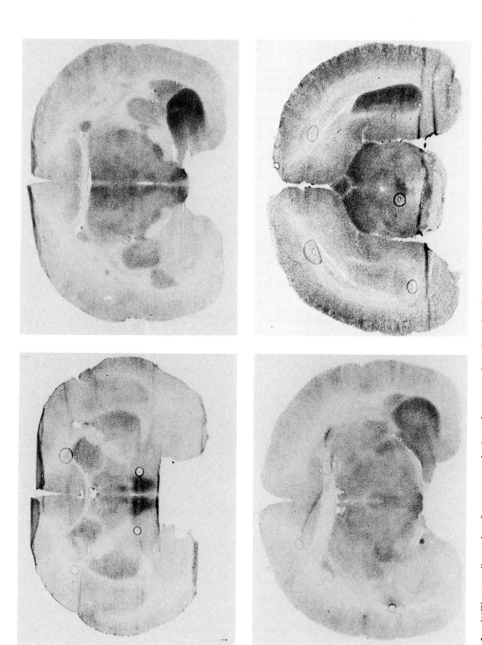

FIG. 1. [^{14}C] autoradiographs of a marmoset brain at four coronal sections showing the spread of seizure activity 10 min after the first discharges appeared in the right hippocampus, following the injection of 1 μg of kainic acid. Note the early bilateral and diffuse increase in metabolic activity in the hypothalamus.

seizure and EEG seizure activity remote from the injection site. It does not modify the lesion at the site of injection. This treatment prevents the occurrence of remote lesions, with the exception of the ipsilateral hippocampal CA_3 and CA_4 and the thalamic lesions, which are, however, reduced in severity (6).

In marmosets and baboons the behavioral and neuropathological consequences of intra-amygdaloid injection of kainic acid are more restricted. Deep electrodes show focal seizure discharges originate within the amygdala within a few minutes to an hour of the injection (57). Spread to the ipsilateral hippocampus usually occurs within a few minutes. Contralaterally, seizures appear in either or both amygdala and hippocampus with a much longer latency (1–3 hr). These brief recurrent focal limbic seizures are seen for 3 to 6 hr. Subsequently, irregular spikes are prominent in the ipsilateral amygdala, sometimes persisting for 3 to 7 days.

In both marmosets and baboons the clinical signs are very restricted. Arrest of movement, mouthing, and tongue protrusion variably accompany the focal seizures. At a later stage, facial myoclonus is sometimes present.

The only consistent secondary lesion is in the ipsilateral hippocampus, in which either or both the end folium and Sommer sector show initially ischemic cell changes and later nerve cell loss and gliosis. In some baboons, lesions occur also in restricted regions of the orbitofrontal and occipital cortex (57).

Physiological monitoring during seizures in marmosets reveals only slight increases in systolic pressure during seizures and slight increases in arterial blood glucose concentrations. Studies using [^{14}C]deoxyglucose autoradiography during the early stages of seizures in marmosets reveal clearly that the seizure spreads only to the hippocampus ipsilaterally and to the hypothalamus bilaterally (Fig. 1).

Thus the experiments in marmosets and baboons support the concept that focal limbic seizures can themselves induce hippocampal sclerosis of the kind classically associated with temporal lobe epilepsy.

VULNERABILITY TO KAINIC ACID AND SELECTIVE NEURONAL LOSS IN EPILEPSY

The similarity between the selective neuronal lesions following status epilepticus and those seen after kainic acid injection appears to be explicable in terms of regionally selective induction and spread of seizure activity following kainic acid. Thus in [^{14}C]deoxyglucose autoradiographs of rat brain after systemic kainic acid (16) there is a broad correspondence between the areas showing increased glucose utilization early in the period of seizure activity and those showing subsequent pathological changes. Systemic or focal amygdaloid injections of kainic acid are followed by mediodorsal thalamic lesions in the rat, in agreement with the focal activation of these nuclei on autoradiographs; in the marmoset, following intra-amygdaloid kainic acid, there is neither early activation (identifiable by autoradiography) nor subsequent focal abnormality in the thalamus (55).

Studies with focal injections of kainic acid into the ventricle, hippocampus, or amygdala in combination with prior chemical or surgical lesioning of afferent hippocampal pathways (commissural, perforant path, septohippocampal, or mossy fiber system) (6,58) show that a powerful excitatory input is required for lesions of CA_3 and CA_1 pyramidal neurons to occur. Using focal injections in various sites (6,77), remote pathological changes vary according to routes of axonal connection. Electron microscopic studies show that early dendritic swelling on hippocampal pyramidal neurons is localized to regions receiving powerful excitatory inputs (e.g., proximodendritic segment of CA_3 receiving mossy fiber input) (62,77).

Thus, many kinds of evidence support the conclusion that there is a very close linkage between an abnormal excitatory input and subsequent abnormalities and that remote lesions following kainic acid are due to spread of seizure activity, not diffusion of kainic acid. However, there is no evidence that permits definitive rejection of the additional hypothesis that kainic acid has selective neurotoxic properties that are not necessarily dependent on seizure activity. Kainic acid injected directly into the hippocampus at threshold doses spares pyramidal neurons (58). Kainic acid also exerts selective toxic actions on cerebellar neurons in culture that match its *in vivo* selectivity (78). It is also possible that neurons undergoing seizure activity are more susceptible to the toxic actions of kainic acid.

A REVISED METABOLIC HYPOTHESIS FOR EPILEPTIC BRAIN DAMAGE

A synthesis of the experimental studies in rodents and primates described earlier yields the conclusion that selective neuronal loss after focal or generalized status epilepticus is closely linked to the abnormal neuronal discharge itself. Evidence that increased oxygen and glucose consumption correlates closely in timing and regional distribution with seizure discharge, whereas regional blood flow can vary in a quantitatively different pattern (28), supports a revised metabolic hypothesis (44). This hypothesis stresses the primary role of enhanced energy demand (cf. "consumptive hypoxia") (64), with a possible secondary role for relative insufficiency of substrate delivery (due to local impairment of blood flow, arterial hypotension, or other systemic changes).

Superficially, this hypothesis appears to be consistent with a primary metabolic cell death as the explanation for the similar pattern of neuronal loss after cerebral hypoxia-ischemia (strangulation, cardiac arrest, atmospheric decompression) or hypoglycemia. However, complete ischemia without a recovery period is selective only in affecting neurons before glia, but not among types of neurons (29). Also, transient total ischemia or hypoxia can lead to severe depletion of cerebral substrate and high-energy compounds (i.e., glucose, ATP, and CrP), but it is compatible with complete restoration of function and absence of pathological changes (18,36,38). Depletion of energy reserves alone is an inadequate explanation for the selective appearances of ischemic cell changes after ischemia, hypoxia, or status epilepticus. Indeed, status epilepticus is associated with a relatively stable energy state in the cerebral cortex, with the "energy charge" well maintained (14) even after 2 hr of continuous seizure activity.

Because it is now clear that special features of vascular anatomy or vascular responses cannot explain the similar selective neuronal losses occurring in ischemia, hypoglycemia, and status epilepticus, a modern version of the pathoclisis hypothesis (89) is required. In seeking specific metabolic differences that characterize selectively vulnerable neurons, neurophysiological evidence from studies with seizures suggests that properties of the membranes relating to ionic conductances may be the relevant factors. One unifying hypothesis is that the selectively vulnerable neurons are those with a low seizure threshold, i.e., those particularly liable to show bursting responses or a "paroxysmal depolarizing shift" in membrane potential. Focal spike or seizure discharges are common features during the recovery period from hypoxia or ischemia, possibly because of differential rates of restoration of function in inhibitory and excitatory systems. Anticonvulsant drugs (barbiturates, benzodiazepines) given during the recovery phase protect against neuronal damage in some experimental models of cerebral ischemia (34,80).

CALCIUM MOVEMENTS AND NEURONAL ACTIVITY

The abnormal neuronal discharges associated with seizure activity are associated with increased efflux of potassium and influx of sodium. Restoration of the ionic gradients across the plasma membrane by ATPase-linked pumps is largely responsible for enhanced mitochondrial metabolism during seizures. An increased inward movement of calcium also accompanies seizure activity. If this calcium entry is sustained and exceeds the capacity of the neuron to sequester or transport Ca^{2+}, it could be a cause of ischemic cell change (45).

Extracellular calcium concentration in the brain is normally close to 1.2 to 1.3 mmoles/liter. Intraneuronal calcium activity (i.e., ionized calcium) is very much lower, around 5×10^{-8} mM (3). At least four mechanisms (87) operate to keep intracellular Ca^{2+} at this low level: (a) an energy-requiring uptake into mitochondria (that is osmotically active when phosphate is also being sequestered); (b) entrapment by other intracellular organelles, including endoplasmic reticulum and synaptic vesicles (this also requires ATP); (c) a membrane carrier that exchanges Ca^{2+} for extracellular Na^+; (d) binding to specific proteins, calmodulins.

The neuronal membrane shows a voltage-dependent increase in Ca^{2+} conductance during depolarization. The inward movement of Ca^{2+} is sufficient to give rise to a calcium spike in the dendrites of both hippocampal and neocortical pyramidal neurons and in cerebellar Purkinje cells (37,86).

During epileptic activity, neuronal membrane responses show a characteristic abnormality: bursts of spikes associated with a paroxysmal depolarizing shift in membrane potential (76). The initial spikes comprising a burst depend on a normal voltage-dependent increase in Na^+ conductance, but they may be followed by slower spikes that arise from increases in Ca^{2+} conductance (90). The paroxysmal depolarizing shift is associated with a substantial, prolonged inward movement of calcium.

TABLE 3. *Toxicity of intracellular Ca^{2+}*

Tissue	Cause	Change	Protection	References
Muscle (heart, vascular, skeletal)	Ischemia	Mitochondrial swelling and Ca^{2+} accumulation	Ca^{2+} antagonists	(21,23,60)
	A23187	Protein breakdown		(67)
	Dystrophy (Duchenne, chicks, hamsters)	Eosinophilia, degeneration	Penicillamine Ca^{2+} deficiency	(31,92) (20)
Liver	Various toxins	Cell death	Low extracellular Ca^{2+}	(71)
Nerve	Electrical stimuli	Mitochondrial swelling and Ca^{2+} accumulation; neuronal loss		(1)
	Spinal trauma	Axonal degeneration; Ca hydroxyapatite		(5)

Ion-sensitive microelectrodes in the cat cortex demonstrate a fall in extracellular Ca^{2+} activity (by 30%–40%) within a few seconds of initiation of a seizure discharge (25). A much larger fall (to 10% of control Ca^{2+} concentration) occurs during anoxia-ischemia (61).

CALCIUM TOXICITY

Several types of degeneration in skeletal, cardiac, and vascular smooth muscle are associated with an increase in intracellular Ca^{2+} concentration (Table 3). In dystrophic muscle, an increase in intracellular ionized calcium activates proteases that produce myofibrillar degeneration (20). Hypoxia or ischemia induces increases in intracellular calcium in arterial smooth muscle and in cardiac muscle. Mitochondria show accumulation of calcium and swelling, particularly during reoxygenation. These changes can be prevented by calcium antagonists that block the inward movement of calcium, e.g., verapamil (23,60). There is a wide range of cytotoxic agents that are lethal to cultured liver cells only in the presence of extracellular calcium (71). The toxins alter the plasma membrane permeability, and subsequent excessive calcium entry leads to cell death.

Evidence for an increase in intracellular calcium as the mechanism of nerve cell degeneration is thus far only indirect. After experimental spinal cord trauma, calcium hydroxyapatite appears intra-axonally and is associated with degenerative changes (5). Prolonged electrical stimulation of the cat cerebral cortex with high charge densities leads to the appearance of calcium hydroxyapatite in the superficial 2 mm of the cortex (1). Deposits are prominent in postsynaptic dendrites and are associated with neuronal degeneration and loss. Intraneuronal proteases are activated by an intracellular calcium concentration (1 mM) that approaches the extracellular concentration (69).

SELECTIVE VULNERABILITY AND CALCIUM TOXICITY

An attractive hypothesis is that selectively vulnerable neurons are those in which an abnormally large entry of Ca^{2+} during seizures overwhelms the capacity of the neurons to extrude or sequester Ca^{2+} (Table 4). The high entry of Ca^{2+} is directly related to burst firing and the associated paroxysmal depolarization shift. Neurons that show these phenomena probably have a high ratio of Ca^{2+} channels to Na^+ channels in the plasma membrane.

Activation of a powerful excitatory input is important in the induction of bursting behavior, in kainic acid toxicity, and in epileptic neuronal loss. Thus, bursting behavior is not seen in hippocampal CA_1 neurons during penicillin application in the absence of the excitatory input from hippocampal CA_3 (74). The CA_3 neurons can exhibit sponta-

TABLE 4. *Proposed sequence of changes in selectively vulnerable neurons in status epilepticus*

1. Burst firing, paroxysmal depolarization
   Sustained Ca^{2+} entry
   Enhanced ATP turnover and mitochondrial metabolism
2. a. Ca^{2+} calmodulin enzyme activations (protein kinases, phospholiase A, etc.)
   b. Ca^{2+} accumulation in mitochondria (requires ATP) displaces H^+ or, with PO_4^{2-}, is osmotically active
3. Mitochondrial failure ("microvacuolation")
   Cytoplasmic release of accumulated Ca^{2+}
   Activation of proteases and phospholipases
4. Ischemic cell change, neuronal loss

TABLE 5. *Selectively vulnerable neurons*

Type	Common features
Type I (general)	
Cerebellar Purkinje cells	1. Golgi type I morphology, with complex dendritic tree
Hippocampal pyramidal neurons	2. Symmetric GABAergic endings around soma
Neocortical small pyramidal neurons	3. Excitatory endings (glutamate or aspartate?) to dendrites
	4. Noradrenergic input to dendrites
	5. Ca^{2+} spikes in dendrites
	6. Bursting patterns can be induced
Type II (hypoxia)	
Cerebellar basket cells	1. Golgi type II morphology
Neocortical aspinous stellate cells	2. Inhibitory (GABAergic) in function
?Hippocampal basket cells	3. High density of mitochondria

neous bursting patterns of firing and paroxysmal depolarization (32). Burst firing can be induced by appropriate excitatory afferent (climbing fiber) stimulation in cerebellar Purkinje cells (70). This observation could thus explain the necessity for peripheral motor activity, during seizures, in order to produce Purkinje cell damage.

Glutamate or other excitatory amino acids act to increase sodium conductance, the resulting depolarization leading to enhancement of the voltage-dependent Ca^{2+} conductance. This increased Ca^{2+} conductance is not normally sustained in the presence of maintained depolarization. However, there is evidence that the continued presence of glutamate or aspartate may prolong the increased Ca^{2+} conductance (33). This phenomenon may be related to the importance of excitatory inputs for the paroxysmal depolarizing shift and the role of glutamate in kainic acid toxicity. Removal of glutamergic afferents protects against primary kainic acid lesions (40), and coadministration of glutamate with kainic acid restores the toxicity (86).

METABOLIC FAILURE AND CALCIUM ACCUMULATION

Various sequential interactions between failure of energy metabolism and increases in intracellular Ca^{2+} are possible. During seizures, a new metabolic state exists (14), with mitochondrial metabolism increased about threefold (largely in response to ionic movements and increased utilization of high-energy phosphate). Mitochondrial accumulation of Ca^{2+} is osmotically active when both ATP and inorganic phosphate are available (24).

This is the circumstance in the neocortex during seizures: ATP concentration is maintained, but PO_4^{2-} is increased through the hydrolysis of crea-

tine phosphate (14). This could thus explain the nonhypoxic mitochondrial swelling ("microvacuolation") observed during status epilepticus following bicuculline or kainic acid (48,62). Eventually the swollen mitochondria release the sequestered calcium, with pathological consequences comparable to those of calcium overload of mitochondria in muscle ("eosinophilic degeneration") (92).

This hypothesis can be extended to cover selective neuronal loss in hypoxia, ischemia, and hypoglycemia, with events occurring in a slightly different sequence. Selectively vulnerable neurons are those in which Ca^{2+} entry is favored by neuronal depolarization or by bursting behavior during a restitution phase in hypoxia or ischemia (Table 5).

INHIBITORY INTERNEURONS

The vulnerable neurons in neocortex, hippocampus, and cerebellum receive inhibitory inputs to the neuronal soma from GABAergic interneurons (basket cells or aspinous stellate cells) (68). There is evidence that these neurons are particularly vulnerable to hypoxia. In infant monkey cortex, the aspinous stellate neurons degenerate after 30 min of moderate hypoxia (81). Bicuculline and allylglycine both impair GABA-mediated inhibition as their primary action (27,75), secondarily producing seizures and selective neuronal loss. Thus, impairment of GABA-mediated inhibition could be an intermediate step in hypoxic-ischemic neuronal damage, leading to selective neuronal damage matching that after status epilepticus.

SUMMARY

Convulsant drugs (bicuculline, allylglycine, kainic acid) given systemically or intracerebrally to rodents or primates so as to produce focal or generalized seizures induce a wide range of patterns of brain damage. These patterns correspond closely in distribution and cellular characteristics not only to the patterns seen acutely after status epilepticus in humans but also to patterns identified in patients with chronic generalized seizures and complex partial seizures (temporal lobe epilepsy).

A temporal sequence of mitochondrial swelling, ischemic cell change, and selective neuronal loss and glial proliferation is consistently identifiable.

The selective neuronal changes are directly related to enhanced neuronal firing during seizures and the accompanying increase in metabolic rate (for oxygen and glucose) and the increased ionic exchanges.

Explanations of neuronal loss that depend on regional abnormalities of vascular responses or on cellular energy failure do not provide an adequate explanation of the similar selectivities of neuronal loss under diverse circumstances.

A hypothesis has been outlined that seeks to explain ischemic cell change as a result of the toxicity of excess intracellular Ca^{2+}. Selective vulnerability, it is proposed, arises from the greater tendency of certain neurons to show bursting behavior and a paroxysmal depolarizing shift associated with enhanced Ca^{2+} entry. When seizure activity is sustained, the capacity of the cell to sequester or extrude Ca^{2+} is exceeded. Mitochondrial swelling and failure release Ca^{2+} into the cytoplasm and initiate ischemic cell change.

ACKNOWLEDGMENTS

The financial support of The Wellcome Trust, the Medical Research Council, and the National Fund for Research into Crippling Diseases is gratefully acknowledged.

REFERENCES

1. Agnew, W. F., Yuen, T. G. H., Bullara, L. A., Jacques, D., and Pudenz, R. H. (1979): Intracellular calcium deposition in brain following electrical stimulation. *Neurol. Res.*, 1:187–202.
2. Aminoff, M. J., and Simon, R. P. (1980): Status epilepticus. Causes, clinical features and consequences in 98 patients. *Am. J. Med.*, 69:15.
3. Baker, P. F. (1976): Regulation of intracellular Ca and Mg in squid axons. *Fed. Proc.*, 35:2589–2595.
4. Baldy-Moulinier, M., Arias, L. P., and Passouant, P. (1973): Hippocampal epilepsy produced by ouabain. *Eur. Neurol.*, 9:333–348.
5. Balentine, J. D., and Spector, M. (1977): Calcification of axons in experimental spinal cord trauma. *Ann. Neurol.*, 2:520–523.
6. Ben-Ari, Y., Tremblay, E., Ottersen, O. P., and Meldrum, B. S. (1980): The role of epileptic activity in hippocampal and 'remote' cerebral lesions induced by kainic acid. *Brain Res.*, 191:79–97.
7. Blennow, G., Brierley, J. B., Meldrum, B. S., and Siesjö, B. K. (1978): Epileptic brain damage. The role of systemic factors that modify cerebral energy metabolism. *Brain*, 101:687–700.
8. Borgström, L., Chapman, A. G., and Siesjö, B. K. (1976): Glucose consumption in the cerebral cortex of rat during bicuculline-induced status epilepticus. *J. Neurochem.*, 27:971–973.
9. Brierley, J. B. (1976): Cerebral hypoxia. In: *Greenfield's Neuropathology*, edited by W. Blackwood and J. A. N. Corsellis, pp. 43–85. Edward Arnold, London.
10. Brierley, J. B., Brown, A. W., Excell, B. J., and Meldrum, B. S. (1969): Brain damage in the rhesus monkey resulting from profound arterial hypotension. I. Its nature, distribution and general physiological correlates. *Brain Res.*, 13:68–100.
11. Brierley, J. B., Brown, A. W., and Meldrum, B. S. (1971): The nature and time course of the neuronal alterations resulting from oligaemia and hypoglycaemia in the brain of *Macaca mulatta*. *Brain Res.*, 25:483–499.
12. Brown, A. W., and Brierley, J. B. (1973): The earliest alterations in rat neurones after anoxia-ischaemia. *Acta Neuropathol. (Berl.)*, 23:9–22.
13. Brown, W. J., Mitchell, A. G., Babb, T. L., and Crandall, P. H. (1980): Structural and physiologic studies in experimentally induced epilepsy. *Exp. Neurol.*, 69:543–562.
14. Chapman, A. G., Meldrum, B. S., Siesjö, B. K. (1977): Cerebral metabolic changes during prolonged epileptic seizures in rats. *J. Neurochem.*, 28:1025–1035.
15. Chaslin, P. (1889): Note sur l'anatomie pathologique de l'épilepsie dite essentielle—La sclerose nevroglique. *C. R. Soc. Biol. (Paris)*, 1:169–171.
16. Collins, R. C., McLean, M., and Olney, J. (1980): Cerebral metabolic response to systemic kainic acid: ^{14}C-deoxyglucose studies. *Life Sci.*, 27:855–862.
17. Corsellis, J. A. N., and Meldrum, B. S. (1976): Epilepsy. In: *Greenfield's Neuropathology*, edited by W. Blackwood and J. A. N. Corsellis, pp. 771–795. Edward Arnold, London.
18. Duffy, T. E., Nelson, S. R., and Lowry, O. H. (1972): Cerebral carbohydrate metabolism during acute hypoxia and recovery. *J. Neurochem.*, 19:959–977.
19. Earle, K. M., Baldwin, M., and Penfield, W. (1953): Incisural sclerosis and temporal lobe seizures produced by hippocampal herniation at birth. *Arch. Neurol. Psychiatry*, 69:27–42.
20. Emery, A. E. H., and Burt, D. (1980): Intracellular calcium and pathogenesis and antenatal diagnosis of Duchenne muscular dystrophy. *Br. Med. J.*, 280:355–357.
21. Flameng, W., Daenen, W., Xhonneux, Van de Water, A., Thone, F., and Borgers, M. (1980): Lidoflazine protects against normothermic myocardial ischemia in the dog. *Proc. R. Soc. Med.*, 29:89–95.

22. Freedman, D. A., and Schental, J. E. (1953): A par-
enchymatous cerebellar syndrome following protracted high body temperature. *Neurology (Minneap.)*,
3:513–516.

23. Haack, D. W., Abel, J. H., and Jaenke, R. S. (1975):
Effects of hypoxia on the distribution of calcium in
arterial' smooth muscle cells of rats and swine. *Cell
Tissue Res.*, 157:125–140.

24. Hackenbrock, C. R., and Caplan, A. I. (1969): Ion-
induced ultrastructural transformations in isolated mitochondria. The energised uptake of calcium. *J. Cell
Biol.*, 42:221–234.

25. Heinemann, U., Lux, H. D., and Gutnick, M. J. (1977):
Extracellular free calcium and potassium during par-
oxysmal activity in the cerebral cortex of the cat. *Exp.
Brain Res.*, 27:237–243.

26. Herndon, R. M., and Coyle, J. T. (1977): Selective
destruction of neurons by a transmitter agonist. *Science*, 198:71–72.

27. Horton, R. W., Chapman, A. G., and Meldrum, B. S.
(1978): Regional changes in cerebral GABA concentration and convulsions produced by D- and L-allyl-
glycine. *J. Neurochem.*, 30:1501–1504.

28. Horton, R. W., Meldrum, B. S., Pedley, T. A., and
McWilliam, J. R. (1980): Regional cerebral blood flow
in the rat during prolonged seizure activity. *Brain
Res.*, 192:399–402.

29. Jenkins, L. W., Povlishoch, J. T., Becker, D. P., Miller,
J. P., and Sullivan, H. G. (1979): Complete cerebral
ischaemia. An ultrastructural study. *Acta Neuropathol. (Berl.)*, 48:113–125.

30. Johansson, B., and Nilsson, B. (1977): The pathophysiology of the blood-brain barrier dysfunction induced by severe hypercapnia and by epileptic brain
activity. *Acta Neuropathol. (Berl.)*, 38:153–158.

31. Kameyama, T., and Etlinger, J. D. (1979): Calcium
dependent regulation of protein synthesis and degradation in muscle. *Nature*, 279:344–346.

32. Kandel, E. R., and Spencer, W. A. (1961): Excitation
and inhibition of single pyramidal cells during hippocampal seizure. *Exp. Neurol.*, 4:162–179.

33. Kusano, K., Miledi, R., and Stinnakre, J. (1975):
Postsynaptic entry of calcium induced by transmitter
action. *Proc. R. Soc. Lond. (Biol.)*, 189:49–56.

34. Levy, D. E., and Brierley, J. B. (1979): Delayed pentobarbital administration limits ischaemic brain damage in gerbils. *Ann. Neurol.*, 5:59–66.

35. Lindenberg, R. (1955): Compression of brain arteries
as pathogenic factor for tissue necroses and their areas
of predilection. *J. Neuropathol. Exp. Neurol.*, 14:223–
243.

36. Ljunggren, B., Schutz, H., and Siesjö, B. K. (1974):
Changes in energy state and acid-base parameters of
the rat brain during complete compression ischaemia.
Brain Res., 73:277–289.

37. Llinas, R., and Hess, R. (1976): Tetrodotoxin-resistant dendritic spikes in avian Purkinje cells. *Proc.
Natl. Acad. Sci. U.S.A.*, 73:2520–2523.

38. Lowry, O. H., Passonneau, J. V., Hasselberger, F. X.,
and Schulz, D. W. (1964): Effect of ischemia on known
substrates and cofactors of the glycolytic pathway in
brain. *J. Biol. Chem.*, 239:18–30.

39. Margerison, J. H., and Corsellis, J. A. N. (1966):
Epilepsy and the temporal lobes. *Brain*, 89:499–530.

40. McGeer, E. G., McGeer, P. L., and Sigh, K. A. (1978):
Kainate induced degeneration of neostriatal neurons:
Dependency on the cortico-spinal tract innervation.
Brain Res., 139:381–383.

41. Meldrum, B. S. (1975): Present views on hippocampal
sclerosis. In: *Modern Trends in Neurology*, edited by
D. Williams, pp. 223–239. Butterworth, London.

42. Meldrum, B. S. (1975): Epilepsy and GABA-mediated inhibition. *Int. Rev. Neurobiol.*, 17:1–36.

43. Meldrum, B. S. (1976): The secondary pathology of
febrile and experimental convulsions. In: *IBRO Mono-
graphs, Vol. 2, Brain Dysfunction in Infantile Febrile
Convulsions*, edited by M. A. Brazier, pp. 213–222.
Raven Press, New York.

44. Meldrum, B. (1978): Physiological changes during
prolonged seizures and epileptic brain damage. *Neuropaediatrie*, 9:203–212.

45. Meldrum, B. (1981): Metabolic effects of prolonged
epileptic seizures and the causation of epileptic brain
damage. In: *Metabolic Disorders of the Nervous System*, edited by F. C. Rose, pp. 175–187. Pitman Medical, London.

46. Meldrum, B. (1981): unpublished data.

47. Meldrum, B. S., Balzano, E., Gadea, M., and Naquet, R. (1970): Photic and drug induced epilepsy in
the baboon *(Papio papio)*: The effects of isoniazid,
thiosemicarbizide, pyridoxine, and amino-oxyacetic
acid. *Electroencephalogr. Clin. Neurophysiol.*, 29:333–
347.

48. Meldrum, B. S., and Brierley, J. B. (1973): Prolonged
epileptic seizures in primates: Ischaemic cell change
and its relation to ictal physiological events. *Arch.
Neurol.*, 28:10–17.

49. Meldrum, B. S., and Horton, R. W. (1971): Convulsive effects of 4-deoxypyridoxine and of bicuculline
in photosensitve baboons *(Papio papio)* and in rhesus
monkeys *(Macaca mulatta)*. *Brain Res.*, 35:419–436.

50. Meldrum, B. S., and Horton, R. W. (1973): Physiology of status epilepticus in primates. *Arch. Neurol.*,
28:1–9.

51. Meldrum, B. S., Horton, R. W., and Brierley, J. B.
(1974): Epileptic brain damage in adolescent baboons
following seizures induced by allylglycine. *Brain*,
97:417–428.

52. Meldrum, B. S., Horton, R. W., Pedley, T., and
McWilliam, J. (1980): Regional cerebral blood flow
during generalised and focal seizures in the rat. In:
Circulation Cérébrale, edited by A. Bees and G. Gér-
aud, pp. 211–213. Imp. Fournié, Toulouse.

53. Meldrum, B. S., and Nilsson, B. (1976): Cerebral
blood flow and metabolic rate early and late in prolonged epileptic seizures induced in rats by bicuculline. *Brain*, 99:523–542.

54. Meldrum, B. S., Papy, J. J., Touré, M. F., and Brierley, J. B. (1975): Four models for studying cerebral
lesions secondary to epileptic seizures. In: *Advances
in Neurology, Vol. 10*, edited by B. S. Meldrum and
C. D. Marsden, pp. 147–161. Raven Press, New York.

55. Meldrum, B. S., Pedley, T., and Corsellis, J. A. N.
(1981): Unpublished data.

56. Meldrum, B. S., Vigouroux, R. A., and Brierley, J. B.
(1973): Systemic factors and epileptic brain damage.
Prolonged seizures in paralysed artificially ventilated
baboons. *Arch. Neurol.*, 29:82–87.

57. Menini, C., Meldrum, B. S., Riche, D. S., Silva-Comte, C., and Stutzmann, J. M. (1980): Sustained limbic seizures induced by intra-amygdaloid kainic acid in the baboon; symptomatology and neuropathological consequences. *Ann. Neurol.*, 8:501–509.

58. Nadler, J. V., and Cuthbertson, G. J. (1980): Kainic acid neurotoxicity toward hippocampal formation: Dependence on specific excitatory pathways. *Brain Res.*, 195:47–56.

59. Nadler, J. V., Perry, B. W., and Cotman, C. W. (1978): Intraventricular kainic acid preferentially destroys hippocampal pyramidal cells. *Nature*, 271:676–677.

60. Nayler, W. G., Fassold, E., and Yepez, C. (1978): Pharmacological protection of mitochondrial function in hypoxic heart muscle: Effect of verapamil, propranolol and methylprednisolone. *Cardiovasc. Res.*, 12:152–161.

61. Nicholson, C., Ten Bruggencate, G., Steinberg, R., and Stöckle, H. (1977): Calcium modulation in brain extracellular microenvironment demonstrated with ion-selective micropipette. *Proc. Natl. Acad. Sci. U. S. A.*, 74:1287–1290.

62. Olney, J. W., Fuller, T., and De Gubareff, T. (1979): Acute dendrotoxic changes in the hippocampus of kainate treated rats. *Brain Res.*, 176:91–100.

63. Olney, J. W., Rhee, V., and Ho, O. L. (1974): Kainic acid: A powerful neurotoxic analogue of glutamate. *Brain Res.*, 77:507–512.

64. Peiffer, J. (1963): Morphologische Aspekte der Epilepsien. *Monogr. Gesamtgeb. Neurol. Psychiatr. (Berlin)*, 100:1–185.

65. Penfield, W., Von Santha, K., and Cipriani, A. (1939): Cerebral blood flow during induced epileptiform seizures in animals and man. *J. Neurophysiol.*, 2:257–267.

66. Pfleger, L. (1880): Boebachtungen über Schrumpfung und Sklerose des Ammonshorns bei Epilepsie. *Allgemeine Zeitschrift Psychiatrie*, 36:359–365.

67. Publicover, S. J., Duncan, C. J., and Smith, J. L. (1978): The use of A23187 to demonstrate the role of intracellular calcium in causing ultrastructural damage in mammalian muscle. *J. Neuropathol. Exp. Neurol.*, 37:554–557.

68. Ribak, C. E. (1978): Aspinous and sparsely-spinous stellate neurons in the visual cortex of rats contain glutamic acid decarboxylase. *J. Neurocytol.*, 7:461–478.

69. Rubinson, K. A., and Baker, P. F. (1979): The flow properties of axoplasm in a defined chemical environment: Influence of anions and calcium. *Proc. R. Soc. Lond. [Biol.]*, 205:323–345.

70. Rushmer, D. S., Roberts, W. J., and Augter, G. K. (1976): Climbing fiber responses of cerebellar Purkinje cells to passive movement of the cat forepaw. *Brain Res.*, 106:1–20.

71. Schanne, F. A. X., Kane, A. B., Young, E. E., and Farber, J. L. (1979): Calcium dependence of toxic cell death: A final common pathway. *Science*, 206:700–702.

72. Scholz, W. (1951): *Die Krampfschädigungen des Gehirns.* Springer-Verlag, Berlin.

73. Scholz, W. (1959): The contribution of pathoanatomical research to the problem of epilepsy. *Epilepsia*, 1:36–55.

74. Schwartzkroin, P. A., and Prince, D. A. (1978): Cellular and field potential properties of epileptogenic hippocampal slices. *Brain Res.*, 147:117–130.

75. Schwartzkroin, P. A., and Prince, D. A. (1980): Changes in excitatory and inhibitory synaptic potentials leading to epileptogenic activity. *Brain Res.*, 183:61–76.

76. Schwartzkroin, P. A., and Wyler, A. R. (1979): Mechanisms underlying epileptiform burst discharges. *Ann. Neurol.*, 7:95–107.

77. Schwob, J. E., Fuller, T., Price, J. L., and Olney, J. W. (1980): Widespread patterns of neuronal damage following systemic or intracerebral injections of kainic acid: A histological study. *Neuroscience*, 5:991–1014.

78. Seil, F. J., Blank, N. K., and Leiman, A. L. (1979): Toxic effects of kainic acid on mouse cerebellum in tissue culture. *Brain Res.*, 161:253–265.

79. Shinozaki, H. (1978): Discovery of novel actions of kainic acid and related compounds. In: *Kainic Acid as a Tool in Neurobiology*, edited by E. G. McGeer, J. W. Olney, and P. L. McGeer, pp. 17–35. Raven Press, New York.

80. Siemkowicz, E. (1980): Improvement of restitution from cerebral ischaemia in hyperglycemic rats by pentobarbital or diazepam. *Acta Neurol. Scand.*, 61:368–376.

81. Sloper, J. J., Johnson, P., and Powell, T. P. S. (1980): Selective degeneration of interneurons in the motor cortex of infant monkeys following controlled hypoxia: A possible cause of epilepsy. *Brain Res.*, 198:204–209.

82. Sommer, W. (1880): Erkrankungen des Ammonshorns als aetiologisches Moment der Epilepsie. *Arch. Psychiatr. Nervenkr.*, 10:631–675.

83. Spielmeyer, W. (1922): *Histopathologie des Nervensystems.* Springer-Verlag, Berlin.

84. Spielmeyer, W. (1927): Die Pathogenese des epileptischen Krampfes. *Z. Neurol. Psychiatr.*, 109:501–520.

85. Stauder, K. H. (1935): Epilepsie und Schläfenlappen. *Arch. Psychiatr. Nervenkr.*, 104:181–211.

86. Streit, P., Stella, M., and Cuenod, M. (1980): Kainate-induced lesion in the optic tectum: Dependency upon optic nerve afferents or glutamate. *Brain Res.*, 187:47–57.

87. Sulakhe, P. V., and St. Louis, P. J. (1980): Passive and active calcium fluxes across plasma membranes. *Prog. Biophys. Mol. Biol.*, 35:135–195.

88. Traub, R. D. (1979): Neocortical pyramidal cells: A model with dendritic calcium conductance reproduces repetitive firing and epileptic behaviour. *Brain Res.*, 173:243–257.

89. Vogt, C., and Vogt, O. (1922): Erkrankungen der Groszhirnrinde im Lichte der Topistik, Pathoklise, und Pathoarchitektonik. *J. Psychol. Neurol. (Leipzig)*, 28:1–171.

90. Wong, R. K. S., and Prince, D. A. (1978): Participation of calcium spikes during intrinsic burst firing in hippocampal neurons. *Brain Res.*, 159:385–390.

91. Wong, R. K. S., Prince, D. A., and Basbaum, A. I. (1979): Intradendritic recordings from hippocampal neurons. *Proc. Natl. Acad. Sci. U. S. A.*, 76:986–990.

92. Wrogemann, K., and Pena, S. D. J. (1976): Mitochondrial calcium overload: A general mechanism for cell-necrosis in muscle diseases. *Lancet*, 1:672–674.

93. Wuerthele, S. M., Lovell, K. L., Jones, M. Z., and Moore, K. E. (1978): A histological study of kainic acid-induced lesions in the rat brain. *Brain Res.*, 149:489–497.

Advances in Neurology, Vol. 34: Status
Epilepticus, edited by A.V. Delgado-Escueta,
C.G. Wasterlain, D.M. Treiman, and R.J. Porter.
Raven Press, New York © 1983.

25

Status Epilepticus in the Limbic System: Biochemical and Pathological Changes

Robert C. Collins, Eric W. Lothman, and John W. Olney

Temporal lobe seizures (psychomotor seizures, complex partial seizures) are the most common form of epilepsy in adults. This probably reflects in part the extreme epileptogenicity of the limbic system in general and the hippocampus in particular. Despite this, status epilepticus in the limbic system has received little attention. Only in recent years has there been clear documentation of the clinical and EEG features of complex partial status epilepticus (9,20,21,48). Because the prolonged confusional state and automatism of this condition are not as dramatic as in generalized status epilepticus, it has not been as easily recognized or as well studied. It is known, however, that in patients with temporal lobe epilepsy, many of the epileptic discharges in deep limbic structures occur with little or no clinical manifestations and no abnormalities on conventional surface EEG recordings. In addition, over half of patients with temporal lobe seizures studied pathologically have shown characteristic neuropathological changes (19). The pathophysiological relationship among isolated epileptic discharges in the hippocampus, the development of limbic system status, and the neuropathological changes of hippocampal sclerosis remain unknown.

In the last several years we have been studying two chemical agents that on systemic administration preferentially activate limbic circuits, giving rise to both limbic status seizures and limbic brain damage. Kainic acid (KA), a potent excitatory and neurotoxic structural analogue of glutamate (Fig. 1), has received the most attention (1,7,8,16,17, 29,30,37). Although the mechanism of KA neurotoxicity is not fully understood, it is believed to involve a sustained depolarizing action at glutamate synaptic receptors (14,22,30). Glutamate is a leading transmitter candidate in several limbic pathways, including the perforant, commissural, and mossy fiber inputs to the hippocampus (26,43,44,49). We have found that KA given intravenously initiates epileptic discharges in the hippocampus that are first recordable in the ventral CA3 hippocampal region. These discharges build up progressively, spread, capture the entire limbic system in sustained seizure activity, and result in a distinctive limbic pattern of neuropathological changes (29,37). Quite to our surprise, an entirely different chemical, dipiperidinoethane (DPE), a tertiary amine (Fig. 1), was also found to cause

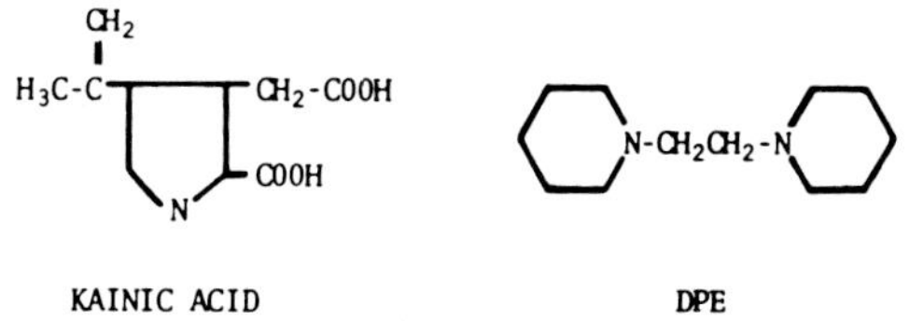

KAINIC ACID   DPE

FIG. 1. KA is a rigid analogue of glutamic acid. DPE is the most potent of a series of dipiperidine compounds in which lengthening of the hydrocarbon chain or substitutions within the piperidine rings reduce potency (15).

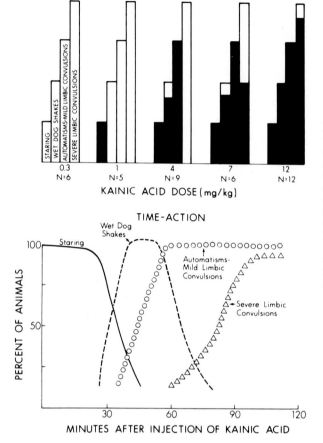

FIG. 2. Dose-response and time-action relationships of intravenous KA. **Top:** Dose-response relationship. Each bar corresponds to one of the behavioral changes seen after KA injections. Total length represents 100% of animals observed, and blackened portion indicates percent of animals that displayed the behavior. Bars are scaled to reflect clinical severity of phenomena. Numbers of animals receiving each dose are indicated below. **Bottom:** Time-action relationship. The percentages (ordinate) of animals ($N = 12$) showing the particular behaviors (different symbols) are plotted for times (abscissa) after injection of a dose of KA (12 mg/kg i.v.).

the same type of convulsions (6,28). We investigated the epileptic properties of this compound when we noticed that the gross neuropathological effects reported for DPE (15) were similar in distribution to those for KA (37).

EXPERIMENTAL PROCEDURES

Sprague-Dawley albino rats weighing 280 to 350 g were used for most experiments. Rats were anesthetized with halothane, and depending on the particular experimental design, catheters were placed in the femoral artery and/or vein. Others had surface and depth electrodes placed for recording EEGs. Limbic recording sites included the dorsal and ventral hippocampus, entorhinal cortex, dorsal subiculum, and amygdala. Animals were then fasted overnight and studied the next day. In all cases animals were unanesthetized and freely mobile. We used the quantitative ^{14}C-2-deoxyglucose (DG)

autoradiographic technique (40) to measure local changes in cerebral glucose metabolism. Because glucose uptake increases dramatically with seizures (5), this method allowed indentification of the anatomical sites of discharges for correlation with depth electrode recordings. KA (Sigma) and DPE (Aldrich) were dissolved in saline and neutralized to pH 7.3 to 7.4 before intravenous injection. DG was given after different doses of each convulsant and at different times after high doses to study the dose-response and time-action relationships. These data were correlated with recordings of electrographic discharges and behavioral changes. A similar design was used to study local changes in brain protein metabolism. In this case we used a new autoradiographic method to measure rates of incorporation of ^{14}C-L-leucine into protein (39).

In parallel experiments, animals were given DPE or KA, and changes in arterial blood gases, glucose

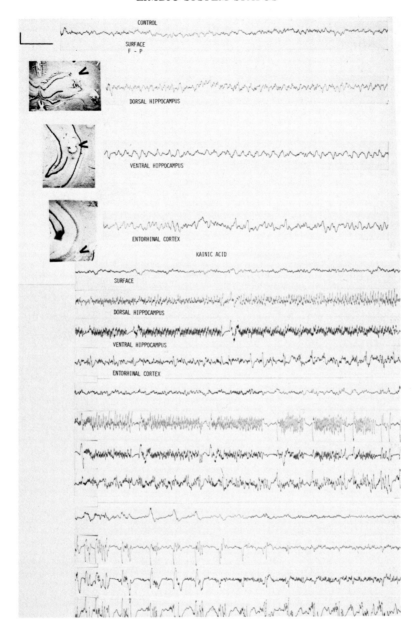

FIG. 3. Comparison of KA seizure activity in depth and surface leads. Records obtained in the control state *(top)* and 15 min after KA (12 mg/kg) *(below)*. Strips of EEG taken after KA show electrical activity at beginning (2nd), during (3rd), and at end *(bottom panels)* of an electrical seizure. Voltage calibration: 1,000 μV for surface, ventral hippocampus, and entorhinal cortex in the control; 1,250 μV for dorsal hippocampus in the control; 400 μV for entorhinal cortex and surface after KA; 625 μV for dorsal hippocampus after KA; 2,200 μV for ventral hippocampus after KA. Time calibration: 1 sec throughout.

and blood pressure were followed for up to six hours. These animals were then killed with pentobarbital, perfused and fixed with buffered 1.5% glutaraldehyde/1% paraformaldehyde for light and electron microscopy (27). These studies allowed observations on the possible role of systemic physiological changes in the development of neuropathological effects.

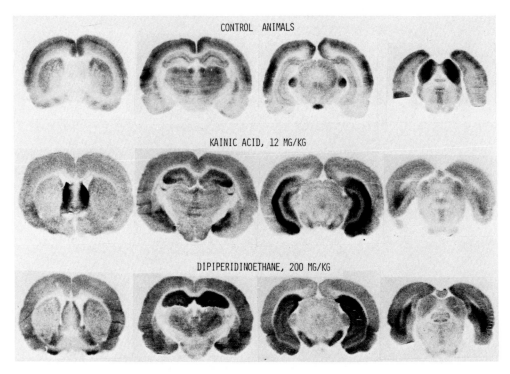

FIG. 4. Local changes in glucose metabolism during limbic seizures induced by KA (12 mg/kg) or DPE (200 mg/kg): rearing, forelimb clonus, salivation. Quantitative measurements of local DG metabolism (6,16) revealed twofold to sixfold increases in areas of increased optical density above control. This occurred in limbic areas: hippocampus, amygdala, pyriform and entorhinal cortex, and subcortical connections, especially lateral septum, N. accumbens, and substantia nigra. There were decreases in metabolic rate in many primary sensory and neocortical areas. Note especially the decreases in density in medial geniculate bodies and inferior colliculi and the dropout of cortical layer IV during seizures with both KA and DPE.

RESULTS

Limbic Seizures

Intravenous injections of KA yielded evidence of highly reproducible dose-response and time-action relationships (Fig. 2). Increasing doses resulted progressively in staring, wet-dog shakes, sniffing, head bobbing, and stereotyped "convulsions." The latter consisted of 15 to 60 sec of rearing, forelimb clonus, salivation, and occasionally falling over, identical with other forms of limbic seizures (33). At high doses (12 mg/kg) these latter episodes occurred progressively more often until animals were in a continuous state of behavioral convulsions.

Electrical recording showed that these behavioral changes were manifestations of epileptic activity in limbic structures. The EEG changes in the hippocampus occurred earlier and with lower doses than in other centers. The behavioral man-

ifestations of these isolated hippocampal discharges were subtle and were best appreciated when compared with those in a control animal, who would sleep quietly in a corner despite the same amount of manipulation. Animals with isolated hippocampal discharges looked alert, remained relatively motionless, exhibited mild hyperventilation (*vide infra*), and were hyporesponsive to tactile or auditory stimuli. As these seizures built up, other limbic structures, like the amygdala, began to show discharges at the time animals exhibited rearing, forelimb clonus, and salivation. In contrast, surface EEG tracings remained relatively normal until late in these events, when convulsions were severe (Fig. 3).

The dose-response and time-action relationships for DPE were more complex. Following a subcutaneous dose of 400 mg/kg, approximately 80% of animals had convulsions (rearing, forelimb clonus, salivation) by 4 to 6 hr. Intravenous doses above 50 mg/kg given in less than 15 sec caused

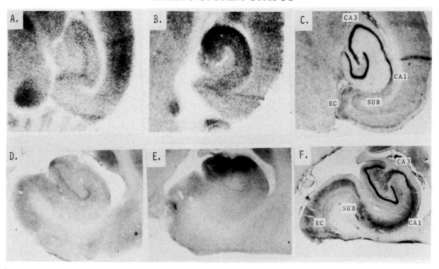

FIG. 5. Changes in glucose metabolism in hippocampus during limbic seizures. The top row are horizontal sections through the rat's hippocampus. **A:** Normal pattern of DG metabolism. The line of accentuated metabolism overlies the perforant pathway terminal field. **B:** Increase in DG metabolism during limbic seizures is greatest in the CA3 region. **C:** Thionin stain showing hippocampal fields of rat. The second row shows coronal sections through the hippocampus of monkey. **D:** Normal DG pattern with accentuation along perforant pathway input into dentate gyrus. **E:** Increased DG metabolism during KA-induced limbic seizures occurs in CA3 and CA4. **F:** Thionin stain of hippocampal fields of monkey. The CA1 region appears wider than normal due to staining artifact.

an immediate tonic-clonic convulsion that resembled a pentylenetetrazol-induced seizure. If many small doses were given slowly (25 mg/kg i.v. over 30 sec, every 15 min), the behavioral response in the first 2 hr was nearly identical with the behavior following a single dose of KA. Often, however, DPE-treated animals returned to normal for 2 to 4 hr only to have a second series of severe convulsions later. Tentatively, we suspect that there may be two actions of DPE. High doses given intravenously may involve a direct but diffuse epileptogenic action, whereas the cumulative effect of repetitive low intravenous doses and the delayed response to high subcutaneous doses suggest a slowly evolving epileptogenic action on limbic structures (kindling?). Depth electrode recordings following intravenous doses have revealed a slow buildup of discharges in limbic structures prior to behavioral convulsions. Conversely, or in addition, DPE may be slowly metabolized to a more active compound by the liver. Direct injections of DPE into the amygdala caused none of the excitotoxic effects that were seen with KA (28).

Metabolic Correlates of Limbic Seizures

Metabolic studies using DG showed essentially the same anatomical pattern of activity following either KA (12 mg/kg i.v.) or DPE (400 mg/kg s.c. or 200 mg/kg i.v. over 2 hr). Both groups of animals were having behavioral limbic convulsions during the 45 min of DG circulation. Compared with controls, the autoradiograms of seizure animals revealed threefold to sixfold increases in glucose utilization in limbic structures (Fig. 4). This was especially prominent in hippocampus, amygdala, pyriform cortex, entorhinal cortex, and subcortical connections in septum, reticular nuclei, and substantia nigra. Animals were also studied following low doses of KA (4 mg/kg) or immediately after injections of high doses (12 mg/kg). These animals exhibited only quiet staring, whereas depth electrode recordings revealed hippocampal discharges. Autoradiograms demonstrated increases in glucose utilization confined to the hippocampus, with the greatest activity in the CA3 subregion (Fig. 5).

In a separate series of experiments, we injected KA stereotactically through recording cannulae into the posterior hippocampus in primates *(Macaca fascicularis)*. At low doses, depth electrodes showed discharges at the site of injection and the ipsilateral amygdala, whereas surface leads remained normal. Even during profound electrical seizures, animals exhibited only slight and often equivocal decreases in responses to stimuli. DG studies dur-

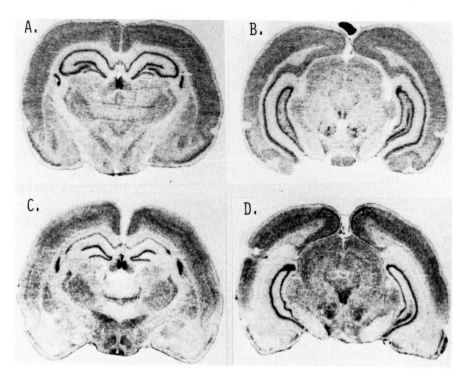

FIG. 6. Regional protein synthesis has been studied using ^{14}C-L-leucine autoradiography (39). The densities of the images in the control animals illustrated in **A** and **B** are proportional to the rate of protein synthesis. **C** and **D** are comparable sections from an animal studied during limbic status. There is essentially no incorporation of leucine into protein in the hippocampal pyramidal neurons (note exception in CA2 resistant zone in dorsal hippocampus of **C**). The severity of inhibition in particular limbic sites correlates with the intensity of glucose utilization studied in separate animals (Fig. 4).

ing this period revealed increased metabolism in hippocampus, predominantly in the CA3 region. This change was greatest in the neuropil above and below the pyramidal cell bodies (Fig. 5).

Limbic seizures were also found to disrupt protein synthesis. The rate of incorporation of ^{14}C-L-leucine into protein remained normal following low doses of KA (4 mg/kg), or during mild discharges. During severe limbic convulsions, however, there was marked inhibition of incorporation in the pyramidal cell layer of the hippocampus, pyriform cortex, amygdala, and some of their connections (Fig. 6). In general, areas that showed the greatest decreases in protein synthesis were those that had shown the most intense increases in glucose metabolism (Fig. 4).

Neuropathological Consequences of Limbic Seizures

Following systemic injections of KA or DPE, morphological changes could be recognized in the hippocampus once behavioral convulsions became manifest. One of the earliest and most subtle changes was a laminar vacuolation of the tissue seen along the zones of input of the commissural and perforant pathway onto CA1 pyramidal neurons and along the input of mossy fibers from dentate gyrus onto CA3 pyramids (Fig. 7). Electron microscopic studies identified these vacuoles as swollen dendrites (29). In addition, there was early swelling of the astrocytes, which were packed tightly among the CA3 and CA1 pyramids. At this early stage, presynaptic profiles remained normal, but a few neurons displayed mild swelling or disruption of cytoplasmic organelles, whereas others underwent dark cell changes. Animals studied further into the seizure process revealed more severe changes, with shrinkage and argyrophilia of neurons, tissue edema, and necrosis. Breakdown in the blood-brain (^{14}C-alpha-aminoisobutyrate or Evans blue dye) occurred in these areas of tissue necrosis (53). Neuronal loss and gliosis were the final results with greatest changes in hippocampal pyramidal cells (both CA3 and CA1), subiculum and olfactory cor-

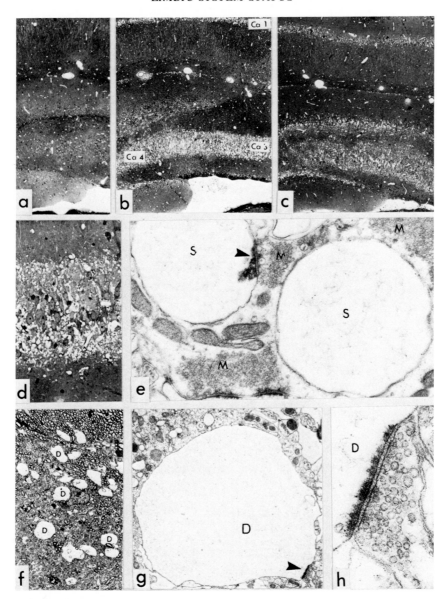

FIG. 7. Light micrographic scenes from the hippocampus of a normal rat (**a**) and rats treated 2 to 4 hr previously with KA (**b**) or DPE (**c**). Both **b** and **c** experienced status limbic seizures for about 1 hr before sacrifice. Note the laminar pattern of acute edematous changes affecting predominantly dendritic processes of CA1, CA3, and CA4 neurons or astroglia closely associated with these neurons. The acute reaction seen typically in the CA3 region following either KA or DPE treatment is magnified in **d** and the dendrotoxic component of that reaction is depicted electromicrographically in **e**. Note that the mossy fiber *(M)* is invaginated by two massively swollen dendritic spines *(S)*, one of which is in synaptic contact *(arrowhead)* with the mossy terminal. The acute dendrotoxic reaction seen typically in the CA1 basilar dendritic field after KA or DPE is shown in **f–h**. A cluster of massively swollen dendrites (D) is depicted in **f**, one of which is magnified in **g**, with a further magnification of a synaptic complex *(arrowhead)* shown in **h**; a–c = ×405; **d** = ×162; **e** = ×19,800; **f** = ×900; **g** = ×5,400; **h** = ×43,200.

TABLE 1. *Changes in systemic factors during limbic seizures*

Animal groups	PaO_2 (mm Hg)	$PaCO_2$ (mm Hg)	apH	Glucose (mg/ml)
Kainic acid (12 mg/kg i.v.)				
Control period ($N = 6$)	82.9 ± 2.2	32.8 ± 1.3	7.46 ± 0.01	1.27 ± 0.10
Staring—WDS ($N = 3$)	92.3 ± 4.7*	24.3 ± 1.0**	7.54 ± 0.02**	1.59 ± 0.04*
Mild convulsions ($N = 9$)	90.2 ± 2.8	23.6 ± 0.9**	7.54 ± 0.02**	1.97 ± 0.40
Severe convulsions ($N = 3$)	92.3 ± 2.1*	23.3 ± 1.0**	7.50 ± 0.03	2.06 ± 0.10
Dipiperidinoethane (200 mg/kg i.v.)				
Control period ($N = 5$)	82.6 ± 2.2	34.6 ± 0.1	7.46 ± 0.01	1.44 ± 0.15
Sniffing—WDS ($N = 9$)	91.1 ± 2.6*	31.1 ± 0.7**	7.46 ± 0.01	1.50 ± 0.20
Mild convulsions ($N = 5$)	99.4 ± 4.4**	25.6 ± 2.1**	7.49 ± 0.01	
Severe convulsions ($N = 20$)	90.2 ± 4.7*	26.5 ± 1.9*	7.46 ± 0.2	1.35 ± 0.10

*$p < 0.05$.
**$p < 0.01$.

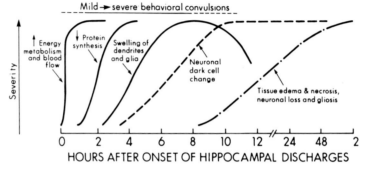

FIG. 8. Summary of the behavioral, metabolic, and neuropathological effects following a single injection of KA (12 mg/kg).

tex and usually less severe pathological changes in amygdala and subcortical limbic nuclei (37).

Physiological studies have suggested that changes in systemic factors during convulsions play little or no role in the pathogenesis of limbic lesions. KA and DPE caused hyperventilation and mild respiratory alkalosis (Table 1). Arterial oxygen tension actually was higher than in controls, even during severe limbic seizures. Blood pressure and body temperature remained normal. Blood glucose remained normal or increased. The brains of these animals studied physiologically were submitted for blind neuropathological analysis, and animals that had had repeated behavioral convulsions were found to have the characteristic cytopathological changes in limbic regions. The possibility that the hyperventilation and hypocarbia might reduce cerebral blood flow is being investigated using the ^{14}C-iodoantipyrine autoradiographic method. Preliminary results have shown an increase in blood flow throughout the limbic system during convulsions.

DISCUSSION

These studies indicate that systemic administration of KA or DPE can be used experimentally to initiate seizure discharges in the limbic system that build in intensity until continuous behavioral convulsions or "limbic system status" occurs. Despite the marked difference in chemical structures, these compounds are similar in selectively exciting the limbic system, as is evidenced in depth electrode recordings, pattern of behavioral convulsions, changes in glucose metabolism, and site and type of subcellular and cellular neuropathological changes. The sequence of events during these limbic seizures has been most thoroughly studied using KA (Fig. 8). Our current working hypothesis suggests the following sequence of events: Seizures begin in the hippocampus by excitation through glutamate synapses on pyramidal neurons, particularly in the CA3 region. DG and leucine autoradiography, depth electrode recordings, and neuropathological studies all indicate that the ear-

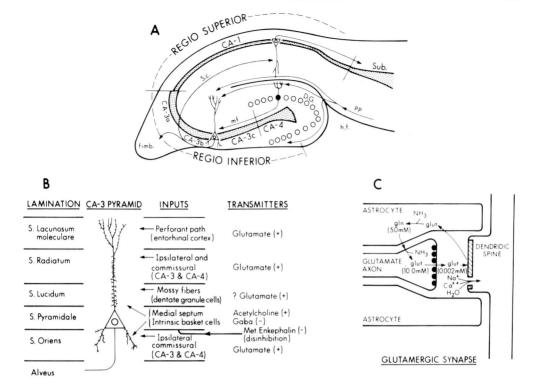

FIG. 9. Organization of hippocampus. **A:** Schematic view of the dorsal hippocampus of the rat is divided into regio superior (CA1, which includes most of the classic Sommer sector h1) and regio inferior (CA3 and CA4, which include the end folium h3–5). The location of CA2 and h2 is problematical and probably represents small transition zones between CA1 and CA3 and h1–h3, respectively. A "feed-forward" excitatory circuit in the hippocampus is indicated by arrows and includes the perforant pathway (pp) from the entorhinal cortex synapsing on the dentate granule cells, the mossy fiber (mf) synapse on the CA3 pyramid, and the Schaffer collateral (S.c.) input into CA1 (34). Other abbreviations: fimb. = fimbria; h.f. = hippocampal fissure. **B:** The classic lamination of Cajal and Lorente de No in the CA3 region has been successfully studied with respect to the source of synaptic connections (34,42,45,46) and the probable neurotransmitters involved (44). In many cases it has not been possible to differentiate glutamate from aspartate. The influence of both dicarboxylic amino acids on neuronal excitability is prominent (13). Inhibitory circuits using GABA and methionine enkephalin are also indicated. The latter actually disinhibits pyramidal neurons by inhibiting GABA neurons (52). The potentiating effect of morphine on KA seizures probably occurs here (10). **C:** Neuropharmacological studies of glutamate point out the very high level of intracellular glutamate (10.0 mM) compared with the very low synaptic levels (0.002 mM) (38). The release of small additional amounts, or an inhibition of reuptake by glia, would lead to excessive postsynaptic depolarization and burst firing at the soma. Calcium currents play an important role here (47). If synaptic action by glutamate is prolonged, there will likely be local shifts of cations and water resulting in dendritic swelling (4,13,25).

liest changes occur there. Behavioral convulsions occur in the 2- to 6-hr interval, and the severity of subsequent local metabolic and neuropathological changes roughly correlates with the frequency and intensity of these seizures. Systemic factors do not seem to play a role as they are believed to in generalized status epilepticus (3,23,24). If behavioral convulsions are blocked with barbiturates or anticonvulsants, then neuropathological changes are largely prevented (2,51). Diazepam is the most potent in this respect.

The convulsant mechanism of action of DPE is not yet known. Metabolic and neuropathological changes in the limbic system are essentially identical with those from KA once behavioral convulsions become manifest. Ongoing experimental studies at earlier times following intravenous DPE, or using smaller doses, have not yet indicated a selective activation at a particular locus in the limbic system. In this respect, it may have a different initial mechanism of action but a similar end result. The emphasis here should shift our attention away from the action of particular convulsants toward an understanding of common mechanisms of limbic seizures. Indeed, there are a great many experimental methods for initiating limbic seizures:

electrical kindling (11,33), systemic methoxy-pyridoxine (32), lidocaine kindling (31), intraventricular endorphins and enkephalins (12), intra-amygdaloid KA (1).

One common denominator for many causes of limbic seizures is the sensitivity of the CA3 and CA4 region, whether studied electrically, metabolically, or morphologically. Neuropathological studies of patients dying with temporal lobe epilepsy have revealed a high incidence of sclerosis of the end folium, or Somer's sector 3–5, which contains these subregions of hippocampus (Fig. 9). Electrophysiological studies of CA3 pyramidal cells have shown that the neurons there have a high propensity toward "epileptic" burst firing (41,50). This activity appears to be an inherent membrane property of these cells that can be triggered by movement of calcium ions into dendrites (47). It is especially intriguing that dendrites of these neurons have a high density of excitatory inputs (glutamate or aspartate) in specific laminated regions (36,43,44). It is likely that small or persistent changes in levels of excitatory transmitters at these synaptic sites might initiate burst firing of pyramidal neurons. KA might act, either by itself or in concert with glutamate, at these laminated sites. Using stereotactic injections of colchicine to make selective lesions of dentate gyrus cells, we found that the behavioral and DG responses to KA were greatly attenuated, indicating that the mossy fibers play a critical role in the initiation of epileptic activity in CA_3 pyramidal cells (18). Because of the "feed-forward" excitatory circuits through these hippocampal synapses, it is likely that seizure activity initiated elsewhere in the limbic system will be amplified here. Any prolonged effect of excitatory amino acid neurotransmitters could conceivably lead to dendritic swelling. Both glutamate and aspartate have excitotoxic potential (4,25,27). This hypothesis may be one explanation for the high incidence of dendritic pathological changes seen in surgical specimens from patients with temporal lobe epilepsy (35). These considerations should not overlook a possible role for changes in inhibitory circuits during hippocampal seizures, especially because recurrent axon collateral from pyramidal neurons (glutamatergic?) synapse on GABAergic basket cells. These concepts are summarized in Fig. 9.

ACKNOWLEDGMENTS

This work was supported in part by grants NS-14834, NS-095156, and RSA MH-38894 from the National Institutes of Health.

REFERENCES

1. Ben-Ari, Y., Tremblay, E., and Ottersen, O. P. (1980): Injections of kainic acid into the amygdaloid complex of the rat: An electrographic, clinical, and histological study in relation to the pathology of epilepsy. *Neuroscience*, 5:515–528.
2. Ben-Ari, Y., Tremblay, E., Ottersen, O. P., and Naquet, R. (1979): Evidence suggesting secondary epileptogenic lesions after kainic acid: Pretreatment with diazepam reduces distant but not local brain damage. *Brain Res.*, 165:362–365.
3. Blennow, G., Brierley, J. B., Meldrum, B. S., and Siesjö, B. K. (1978): Epileptic brain damage—The role of systemic factors that modify cerebral energy metabolism. *Brain*, 101:687–700.
4. Chan, P.-H., Fishman, R. A., Lee, J. L., and Chandelise, L. (1979): Effects of excitatory neurotransmitter amino acids in swelling of rat brain cortical slices. *J. Neurochem.*, 33:1309–1315.
5. Collins, R. C. (1978): Use of cortical circuits during focal penicillin seizures: An autoradiographic study with [^{14}C]-deoxyglucose. *Brain Res.*, 150:487–501.
6. Collins, R. C., Lothman, E. W., and Olney, J. W. (1981): Dipiperidinoethane causes limbic seizures. *Epilepsia, Abstr.*, 22:225.
7. Collins, R. C., McLean, M., Lothman, E. W., Klunk, W., and Olney, J. (1980): Kainic acid causes limbic seizures. *Epilepsia*, 21:186.
8. Collins, R. C., McLean, M., and Olney, J. (1980): Cerebral metabolic response to systemic kainic acid: 14-C-deoxyglucose studies. *Life Sci.*, 27:855–862.
9. Engel, J., Ludwig, B. I., and Fetell, M. (1978): Prolonged partial complex status epilepticus: EEG and behavioral observations. *Neurology (Minneap.)*, 28:863–869.
10. Fuller, T. A., and Olney, J. W. (1979): Effects of morphine or naloxone on kainic acid neurotoxicity. *Life Sci.*, 24:1793–1798.
11. Goddard, G. U., McIntyre, D. C., and Leech, C. K. (1969): A permanent change in brain functioning resulting from daily electrical stimulation. *Exp. Neurol.*, 25:295–330.
12. Hendrickson, S. J., Bloom, F. E., Ling, N., and Guilleman, R. (1978): Induction of limbic seizures by endorphins and opiate alkaloids: Electrophysiological correlates. *Neurosci. Abstr.*, 4:293.
13. Hosli, L., Andres, P. F., and Hosli, E. (1976): Ionic mechanisms associated with the depolarization by glutamate and aspartate on human and rat spinal neurones in tissue culture. *Pfluegers Arch.*, 363:43–48.
14. Johnson, G. A. R., Kennedy, S. M. E., and Twitchen, B. (1979): Action of the neurotoxin kainic acid on

high affinity uptake of L-glutamic acid in rat brain slices. *J. Neurochem.*, 32:121–127.

15. Levine, S., and Sowinski, R. (1980): Lesions of amygdala, pyriform cortex, and other brain structures due to dipiperidinoethane intoxication. *J. Neuropathol. Exp. Neurol.*, 39:56–64.

16. Lothman, E. W., and Collins, R. C. (1981): Kainic acid induced limbic seizures: Metabolic, behavioral, electroencephalographic and neuropathologic correlates. *Brain Res.*, 218:299–318.

17. Lothman, E. W., Collins, R. C., and Ferrendelli, J. A. (1981): Kainic acid induced limbic seizures: Electrophysiological studies. *Neurology (Minneap.)*, 31:806–812.

18. Lothman, E. W., Collins, R. C., Zucker, D. K., and Wooten, G. F. (1981): Mossy fiber lesions attenuate kainic acid-induced limbic seizures. *Epilepsia*, 22:229–230.

19. Margerison, J. H., and Corsellis, J. A. N. (1966): Epilepsy and the temporal lobes. *Brain*, 89:499–530.

20. Markland, O. N., Wheeler, G. L., and Pollack, L. P. (1978): Complex partial status epilepticus (psychomotor status). *Neurology (Minneap.)*, 28:189–196.

21. Mayeux, R., and Lueders, H. (1978): Complex partial status epilepticus: Case report and proposal for diagnostic criteria. *Neurology (Minneap.)*, 28:957–961.

22. McGeer, E. G., McGeer, P. L., and Singh, K. (1978): Kainate-induced degeneration of neostriatal neurons: Dependence upon corticostriatal tract. *Brain Res.*, 139:381–383.

23. Meldrum, B. S., and Brierley, J. B. (1973): Prolonged epileptic seizures in primates—Ischemic cell change and its relation to ictal physiological events. *Arch. Neurol.*, 28:10–17.

24. Meldrum, B. S., and Horton, R. W. (1973): Physiology of status epilepticus in primates. *Arch. Neurol.*, 28:1–9.

25. Mollgard, K., Moller, M., Lund-Andersen, H., and Hertz, L. (1974): Concordance between morphological and biochemical estimates of fluid spaces in rat brain cortex slices. *Exp. Brain Res.*, 22:299–314.

26. Nadler, J. V., Vaca, K. W., White, W. F., Lynch, G. S., and Cotman, C. W. (1976): Aspartate and glutamate as possible neurotransmitters of excitatory hippocampal afferents. *Nature*, 260:538–540.

27. Olney, J. W. (1971): Glutamate-induced neuronal necrosis in the infant mouse hypothalamus. An electron microscopic study. *J. Neuropathol. Exp. Neurol.*, 30:75–90.

28. Olney, J. W., Fuller, T., Collins, R. C., and deGubareff, T. (1980): Systemic dipiperidinoethane mimics the convulsant and neurotoxic actions of kainic acid. *Brain Res.*, 200:231–235.

29. Olney, J. W., Fuller, T., and deGubareff, T. (1979): Acute dendrotoxic changes in the hippocampus of kainate treated rats. *Brain Res.*, 176:91–100.

30. Olney, J. W., Rhee, V., and Ho, O. L. (1974): Kainic acid: A powerful neurotoxic analogue of glutamate. *Brain Res.*, 77:507–512.

31. Post, R. M., Kennedy, C., Shinohara, M., Squillace, K., Miyaoka, M., Suda, S., Ingvar, D. H., and Sokoloff, L. (1979): Local cerebral glucose utilization in lidocaine-kindled seizures. *Neurosci. Abstr.*, 5:196.

32. Purpura, D. P., and Gonzalez-Monteagudo, O. (1960): Acute effects of methoxypyridoxine on hippocampal end-blade neurons: An experimental study of "special pathoclisis" in the cerebral cortex. *J. Neuropathol. Exp. Neurol.*, 19:421–432.

33. Racine, R. (1980): Kindling: The first decade. *Neurosurgery*, 3:234–252.

34. Raisman, G., Cowan, W. M., and Powell, T. P. S. (1965): The intrinsic afferent, commissural and association fibers of the hippocampus. *Brain*, 88:963–995.

35. Scheibel, A. B. (1980): Morphological correlates of epilepsy: Cells in the hippocampus. In: *Antiepileptic Drugs, Mechanisms of Action*, edited by G. H. Glaser, J. K. Penry, and D. M. Woodbury, pp. 49–63. Raven Press, New York.

36. Schwartzkroin, P. A., and Andersen, P. (1975): Glutamic acid sensitivity of dendrites in hippocampal slices *in vitro. Adv. Neurol.*, 12:45–51.

37. Schwob, J. E., Fuller, T., Price, J. L., and Olney, J. W. (1980): Widespread patterns of neuronal damage following systemic or intracerebral injections of kainic acid: A histological study. *Neuroscience*, 5:991–1014.

38. Shank, R. P., and Aprison, M. H. (1979): Biochemical aspects of the neurotransmitter function of glutamate. In: *Glutamic Acid: Advances in Biochemistry and Physiology*, edited by L. J. Fuller, S. Garattine, M. R. Kare, W. A. Reynolds, and R. J. Wurtman, pp. 139–150. Raven Press, New York.

39. Smith, C. B., Patlak, C., Pettigrew, K., and Sokoloff, L. (1980): An autoradiographic method for the measurement of local rates of protein synthesis in the central nervous system. *(in preparation)*.

40. Sokoloff, L., Reivich, M., Kennedy, C., Des Rosiers, M. H., Patlak, C. S., Pettigrew, K. D., Sakurada, O., and Shinohara, M. (1977): The [14-C]deoxyglucose method for the measurement of local cerebral glucose utilization: Theory, procedures, and normal values in the conscious and anesthetized albino rat. *J. Neurochem.*, 28:897–916.

41. Spencer, W. A., and Kandel, E. R. (1961): Electrophysiology of hippocampal neurons. IV. Fast pre-potentials. *J. Neurophysiol.*, 24:272–285.

42. Steward, O. (1976): Topographic organization of the projections from the entorhinal area to the hippocampal formation of the rat. *J. Comp. Neurol.*, 167:285–314.

43. Storm-Mathisen, J. (1977): Glutamic acid and excitatory nerve endings: Reduction of glutamic acid uptake after axotomy. *Brain Res.*, 120:379–386.

44. Storm-Mathisen, J. (1977): Localization of neurotransmitter substances in the brain: The hippocampal formation as a model. *Prog. Neurobiol.*, 8:119–181.

45. Swanson, L. W., and Cowan, W. M. (1977): An autoradiographic study of the organization of the efferent

connections of the hippocampal formation in the rat. *J. Comp. Neurol.*, 172:49–84.

46. Swanson, L. W., Wyss, J. M., and Cowan, W. M. (1978): An autoradiographic study of the organization of intrahippocampal association pathways in the rat. *J. Comp. Neurol.*, 181:681–716.

47. Traub, R. D., and Llinas, R. (1979): Hippocampal pyramidal cells: Significance of dendritic ion conductances for neuronal function and epileptogenesis. *J. Neurophysiol.*, 42:476–496.

48. Weiser, H. G. (1980): Temporal lobe or psychomotor status epilepticus. A case report. *Electroencephalogr. Clin. Neurophysiol.*, 48:558–572.

49. White, W. F., Nadler, J. V., Hamberger, A., and Cotman, C. W. (1977): Glutamate as transmitter of hippocampal perforant path. *Nature*, 270:1228–1231.

50. Wong, R. K. S., and Prince, D. A. (1979): Dendritic mechanisms underlying penicillin-induced epileptiform activity. *Science*, 204:1228–1231.

51. Zaczek, R., Nelson, M. F., and Coyle, J. T. (1978): Effects of anesthetics and anticonvulsants on the action of kainic acid in the rat hippocampus. *Eur. J. Pharmacol.*, 52:323–327.

52. Zieglgansberger, W., French, E. D., Siggins, G. R., and Bloom, F. F. (1979): Opioid peptides may excite hippocampal pyramidal neurons by inhibiting adjacent inhibitory interneurons. *Science*, 205:415–417.

53. Zucker, D., Lothman, E. W., and Wooten, G. F. (1980): Neuropathologic and blood brain barrier changes in kainic acid induced limbic seizures. *Neurosci. Abstr.*, 10:400.

Advances in Neurology, Vol. 34: Status Epilepticus, edited by A.V. Delgado-Escueta, C.G. Wasterlain, D.M. Treiman, and R.J. Porter. Raven Press, New York © 1983.

26

Brain Protein and DNA Synthesis During Seizures

Antonio Giuditta, Salvatore Metafora, Maurizio Popoli, and Carla Perrone-Capano

PROTEIN SYNTHESIS

Polysomal Disaggregation

The first indication that cerebral seizures are associated with disaggregation of brain polysomes was provided by an experiment on rabbits in 1968 (25). After a series of six electroconvulsive shocks (ECSs) given at intervals of approximately 10 min, the polysomal profile of the cerebral cortex appeared considerably modified. The size of the monomer peak increased, whereas the area occupied by polysomes was correspondingly reduced. From 10 experiments the mean monomer increase was approximately 70%.

The appearance of the ribosomal pattern and, more compellingly, the lack of nascent peptide chains in the monomer region (Fig. 1) argued against attributing the observed effect to an activation of cerebral RNAase. These findings supported the view that the rate of mRNA binding to free ribosomes was impaired (25). The possibility of enzymatic breakdown of polysomes was further excluded in later experiments that showed that monomers isolated from the cortex in ECS-treated rabbits were readily dissociable into subunits (17). The presence of mRNA fragments would have stabilized free ribosomes in the dissociating conditions. Similar behavior was reported for monomers

and dimers separated from rat cerebral cortex after administration of 100 consecutive ECSs (26). Determination of RNAase activity in the postmitochondrial supernatant of rabbit cerebral cortex failed to reveal any activation after ECS treatment (17).

Disaggregation of cerebral polysomes induced by ECS has been observed in other mammalian species. In mice, after a single ECS, the effect was less evident than in rabbits (9,14). In the rat, a condition resembling status epilepticus induced by repetitive administration of ECS was accompanied by an increase in free ribosomes and dimers and by a corresponding reduction in the content of larger polysomes (26).

Inhibition of Protein Synthesis

The disaggregation of brain polysomes observed after ECS (25) strongly suggested the occurrence of a corresponding inhibition in the process of cerebral protein synthesis. This was shown by direct analysis using short periods of incorporation of radioactive amino acids (4,5,8,9). In mice, after a single ECS, the inhibition of cerebral protein synthesis reached values in excess of 50% (5,8), a finding at variance with the smaller effect noted on polysomes (9,14). The degree of inhibition attained levels comparable to those prevailing in po-

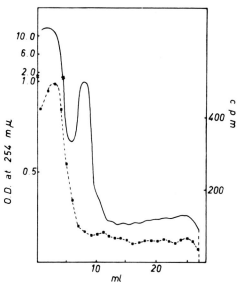

FIG. 1. Polysomal profile obtained from the cerebral cortex of a rabbit subjected to a series of six ECSs given at intervals of 12 to 15 min and killed immediately after the last seizure. Twenty microcuries of a mixture of ^{14}C-labeled amino acids were injected subarachnoidally 5 min before decapitation to label the nascent peptide chains. Solid line: optical density at 254 nm. Dash line: TCA-insoluble radioactivity. Direction of sedimentation to the right. Note the low concentration of polysomes and the abnormally high amount of monomers. Nascent peptide chains did not accumulate in the monomer region, a finding at variance with what would be expected if the disaggregation of polysomes were produced by RNAase hydrolysis of mRNA. (From Vesco and Giuditta, ref. 25, with permission.)

lysomes when the data were corrected for the specific radioactivity of the precursor (4).

Kinetics of the Effect

A kinetic study of the process of cerebral polysomal disaggregation was initially reported in the mouse subjected to a single ECS (14). The disaggregation increased with time. After reaching a minimum (17% below the control level) about 12 min after ECS, the polysome/single-ribosome ratio then rose to control values at 20 min and peaked at 17% above the control level at 30 min. The ratio then gradually returned to the control level at about 45 min.

A similar time course was observed for the inhibition of cerebral protein synthesis (4,8,9). Maximal inhibition occurred soon after administration of ECS, and by 10 to 15 min there was no difference between ECS animals and control animals. A suggestion of minor enhancement of the incor-

poration rate was observed between 15 and 30 min (9), in accordance with the temporary rebound observed in the ratio of polysomes to free ribosomes (14).

In the rabbit, soon after a single ECS, the disaggregation of cerebral polysomes appeared to be quite limited: the maximal effect was reached after about 10 min (17) (Fig. 2). A nonsignificant tendency to recovery occurred at 20 min, which was followed by a further decrease in the content of polysomes at 30 min. Normal polysomal profiles were attained after approximately 2 hr (21). On the whole, the process of recovery appeared to require considerably more time than the process of disaggregation.

In rats subjected to 50 ECSs given at intervals of 30 sec, the polysomal profile was still abnormal 30 min after the last ECS, despite the disappearance of EEG seizures. The polysomal patterns returned to normal 3 hr later (26). When the number of ECSs was raised to 100, the polysomal profile remained extensively disaggregated, and self-sustained seizures persisted for 3 hr after the last ECS. Only 5 hr later the pattern of cerebral polysomes showed signs of recovery.

A still more prolonged inhibition of cerebral protein synthesis was observed in mice injected with ^{14}C-glucose after a single ECS (7). The decrease in the ratio of ^{14}C in the protein fraction to that in the isolated amino acids (mostly glutamic and aspartic acids) averaged 13% and lasted from 45 min to 24 hr.

Mechanism of the Inhibition

The temporary hypoxia that follows ECS is not strictly related to the disaggregation of cerebral polysomes. Paralyzed rats subjected to a series of 50 or 100 consecutive ECSs under conditions of artificial ventilation with O_2 developed signs of polysomal disaggregation (26). The effect disappeared when the ECS was given under halothane anesthesia, which blocked cerebral seizures (26).

In mice, ether anesthesia failed to suppress the inhibition of cerebral protein synthesis produced by ECS, and in unanesthetized mice the inhibition persisted after administration of a current of subconvulsive intensity (4). In the same species, however, there was a high correlation between the intensity of the current and the degree of inhibition of cerebral protein synthesis (5,9). All these observations support the notion that polysomal dis-

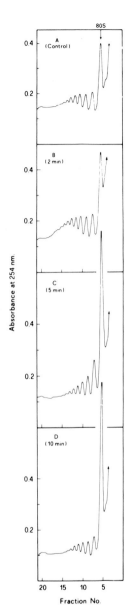

FIG. 2. Polysomal profiles obtained from the cerebral cortex of a control rabbit **(A)** and rabbits subjected to one ECS and killed at different times thereafter **(B, C, D)**. Direction of sedimentation to the left. Note the essentially normal pattern present 2 min after ECS and the marked rises in monomers observed after 5 min and after 10 min. The minor but clear increase in dimers occurring after 5 min was no longer apparent after 10 min. This sequence of events is consistent with a gradual runoff of monomers from polysomes and with their progressive accumulation as free ribosomes resulting from an impairment in the process of peptide chain initiation. (From Metafora et al., ref. 17, with permission.)

aggregation and the associated inhibition of protein synthesis reflect the presence of cerebral seizures.

The rapid utilization of cerebral energy reserves accompanying overt convulsions has suggested that polysomal disaggregation may be causally linked to the decrease in concentration of tissue ATP. Some support for this view has come from the inverse correlation existing between cerebral ATP level and current intensity (6). A similar inverse correlation has been noted between current intensity and cerebral protein synthesis (5,9). However,

the ATP level does not decrease in convulsing well-oxygenated animals (3), and the inhibition of protein synthesis persists in subconvulsive conditions (4,5,9). In addition, the decrease in cerebral ATP is fully reversed long before the peak of polysomal disaggregation is reached. Recovery from the inhibited state may take up to 2 hr in the rabbit (21).

A more likely mechanism for cerebral protein inhibition might involve the enhanced release of neurotransmitters such as dopamine and serotonin, which are known to produce disaggregation of cerebral polysomes (27). Other neurotransmitters (e.g., GABA) are known to influence brain protein synthesis (23) and may be contributing to the disaggregating effect of ECS.

Still another possibility is offered by consideration of the ion imbalance that follows cerebral seizures, in particular the increase in extracellular concentration of K[+] ions. It is known that cerebral protein synthesis is inhibited by cortical application of potassium chloride (2). In the squid, the synthesis of axoplasmic proteins in the isolated giant axon is particularly sensitive to high concentrations of K[+] ions added to the outer medium (19). This finding appears to support the view that the inhibitory effect of ECS may prevail in the neuronal periphery (9).

At the level of the protein synthetic machinery, the inhibitory effect of ECS has been pinpointed to the step of peptide chain initiation. This conclusion, suggested by our initial observations (25), has been borne out by an exhaustive series of *in vitro* experiments (17). In brief, ribosomes of ECS-treated rabbits were found to be markedly impaired in their ability to synthesize proteins (Fig. 3) but to retain their full capacity to release free monomers in the course of a synthetic run (Fig. 4). This suggested that the steps of elongation, termination, and release of peptide chains remain essentially normal. In separate assays it has been established that the concentration of the soluble factors required for protein synthesis and specifically for elongation is not affected by ECS. By excluding these sites of attack, our findings have restricted the locus of ECS inhibition to the process of peptide chain initiation. The same control site appears to be responsible for polysomal disaggregation in eukaryotic cells subjected to a number of different metabolic downshifts.

Subcellular Site of the Inhibition

In an *in vitro* assay it was found that the protein synthetic capacity of membrane-bound ribosomes isolated from the cortex in ECS-treated rabbits was consistently more inhibited than that of free ribosomes (17). The degree of inhibition reached 55% in the former fraction but only 29% in free ribosomes. A comparable differential effect was observed in the degree of polysomal disaggregation. After ECS, the ratio of monomers to polysomes increased 56% in free ribosomes and 82% in membrane-bound ribosomes. On the other hand, no significant difference was noted in the types of proteins synthesized by a cell-free system and released in soluble form (17). This result implied a lack of substantial differences in the populations of mRNA, at least at the peak of polysomal disaggregation (10 min). Direct estimation of the content of poly(A)-containing mRNA in different ribosomal fractions confirmed this conclusion. The

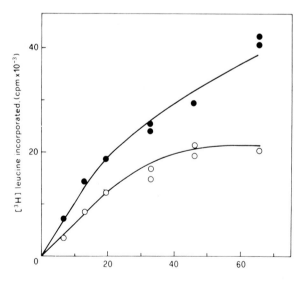

FIG. 3. *In vitro* synthesis of protein by total ribosomes isolated from the cerebral cortex in a control rabbit (filled circles) and a rabbit treated 10 min earlier with one ECS (open circles). The incubation mixture was supplemented with an excess of soluble factors obtained from rat brain cortex. The impaired rate of synthesis observed after ECS indicates that the inhibitory site is on ribosomes. (From Metafora et al., ref. 17, with permission.)

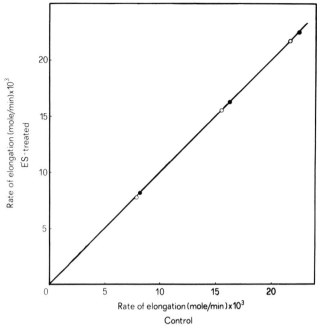

Control

FIG. 4. Relationship between the rate of peptide chain elongation, termination, and release displayed *in vitro* by cortical polysomes of a control rabbit and the corresponding rate determined in cortical polysomes of analogous size distribution isolated from a rabbit treated with one ECS 10 min earlier. The rate of elongation (mol of rRNA in monomers released per minute per 1,000 mol of polysomal rRNA present at time 0) was measured by the amount of monomers released from polysomes incubated at 37°C in a medium sustaining cell-free protein synthesis. Filled and open circles denote different experiments. The observed straight line with a slope of 1 indicates that control and ECS-treated rabbits have the same rate of peptide chain elongation and release. (From Metafora et al., ref. 17, with permission.)

size of the poly(A) moiety analyzed by gel electrophoresis and by zonal sedimentation was likewise not affected by ECS (17).

An attempt to determine the subcellular distribution of the ECS-inhibited, newly synthesized proteins was carried out in mice injected intraperitoneally with ³H- or ¹⁴C-leucine (8). Although nuclear and synaptosomal proteins appeared to be preferentially inhibited, interpretation of the results was made difficult by the possibility that the observed changes were due to the different transit times required by the labeled proteins to reach their respective subcellular compartments.

Involvement of Other Organs

The process of ECS-induced polysomal disaggregation is not limited to the cerebral cortex but involves other organs (24). This preliminary observation has recently been confirmed and studied in some detail (21). In rabbit liver, after a single ECS, the extent of the disaggregation is comparable to that in the cerebral cortex, but it follows

a different time course. The maximal effect occurs at 10 min; it is followed by a brief period of remission. A second episode of disaggregation takes place after 40 min and is not completed after 2 hr. A similar biphasic sequence is present in the kidney, except that control values appear to be regained after 2 hr.

DNA SYNTHESIS

The occurrence of a process of DNA synthesis superimposed on the processes of replication and repair has been suggested in eukaryotic cells by the work of Pelc (18). In the nervous system, a high rate of thymidine incorporation into DNA has been reported in the adult mammalian brain on the basis of biochemical studies (15,16) and autoradiographic evidence (13). The former authors have reported that a sizable fraction of the radioactive DNA is rapidly lost from the brain, and they have attributed this finding to repair processes enhanced by the radiation damage elicited by the incorporated radioactivity. More recent experiments by

Kimberlin et al. (12) have confirmed these findings but have shown that the metabolically active DNA fraction is larger in adult rats than in newborn rats, despite the substantially lower rate of incorporation of radioactive precursor in the former group. This finding does not support the view that the turnover of brain DNA is due to repair processes.

We reached similar conclusions in a recent study of rats weighing approximately 100 g (20). After a single intracerebral injection of ^{3}H-thymidine, the brain concentration of radioactive DNA reached a maximum after 5 hr and rapidly decreased to substantially lower values at later times. During the same time period, the liver concentration of radioactive DNA remained essentially unchanged. Again, these results fail to support the view that the turnover in brain DNA is due to repair processes. DNA turnover also occurs in nerve cells, as indicated by a kinetic experiment carried out with a fraction of purified neuronal perikarya (20) (Fig. 5).

Using rats of 100 to 150 g injected intracerebrally with ^{3}H-thymidine for brief periods, we observed (11) that ECS inhibited the process of cerebral DNA synthesis. After a single ECS, the inhibition reached a maximum after 10 to 15 min and disappeared after 50 to 60 min. A comparable degree of inhibition was observed in unanesthetized rats receiving ^{3}H-thymidine by intraperitoneal injection. This finding excludes the possible interferences attributable to the ether anesthesia or to the intracerebral route of injection.

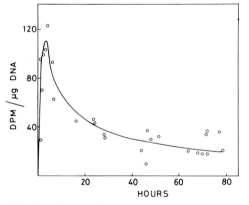

FIG. 5. Kinetics of labeling of neuronal DNA in the cerebral cortex in rats weighing approximately 100 g after intracranial injection of 50 μCi of [^{3}H-methyl]thymidine. A fraction of purified neuronal perikarya was isolated at each time interval according to the method of Satake and Abe [*J. Biochem. (Tokyo)*, 59:72–75, 1966]. (From Perrone-Capano et al., ref. 20, with permission.)

CONCLUSIONS

The intellectual deterioration that may follow status epilepticus and the state of confusion and memory disturbance associated with postictal periods may find their origin in the disturbance of macromolecular metabolism detected after ECS treatment. In particular, the retrograde amnesia produced by ECS may be attributable to an inhibitory action on cerebral protein synthesis analogous to the effects of specific inhibitory compounds that also induce retrograde amnesia (1,10). This view finds some support in the similar correlations between cerebral seizures and inhibition of protein synthesis and between cerebral seizures and retrograde amnesia (4,5,9). The less conspicuous inhibition of protein synthesis induced by ECS in comparison with the effect of specific inhibitors may be attributed to a hypothetical preferential effect of ECS on nerve terminals (9).

The prolonged impairment in cerebral protein synthesis that has been observed in rats after repetitive administration of consecutive ECSs (26) and in ECS-treated mice after injection of ^{14}C-glucose (7) may be considered a possible factor in the long-term intellectual deterioration that accompanies status epilepticus, particularly in infancy and early childhood (i.e., at times when cerebral protein synthesis is particularly high). An additional deranging factor may be identified in the disaggregation of polysomes in the liver and kidney after ECS (21). The relevance of the latter effect to brain function remains to be established. It should be pointed out that a supporting role for liver in maintaining satisfactory brain function has long been suspected.

Of some potential interest is the reversible inhibition of cerebral DNA synthesis induced by ECS. This result may be related to the report that learning induces an enhancement of brain DNA labeling (22). However, until the latter claim is substantiated and until the nature of brain metabolic DNA is clarified, the relevance of this observation to the biological effects of ECS will remain uncertain.

REFERENCES

1. Barondes, S. (1970): Is the amnesic effect of cycloheximide due to specific interference with a process of memory storage? In: *Protein Metabolism of the Nervous System*, edited by A. Lajtha, pp. 545–553. Plenum Press, New York.
2. Bennett, G. S., and Edelman, G. M. (1969): Amino acid incorporation into rat brain proteins during spreading cortical depression. *Science*, 163:393–395.

3. Collins, R. C., Posner, J. B., and Plum, F. (1970): Cerebral energy metabolism during electroshock seizures in mice. *Am. J. Physiol.*, 218:943–950.

4. Cotman, C. W., Banker, G., Zornetzer, S. F., and McGaugh, J. L. (1971): Electroshock effects on brain protein synthesis: Relation to brain seizures and retrograde amnesia. *Science*, 173:454–456.

5. Dunn, A. (1971): Brain protein synthesis after electroshock. *Brain Res.*, 35:254–259.

6. Dunn, A. (1973): The dependence of brain ATP content on cerebral electroshock current. *Brain Res.*, 61:442–445.

7. Dunn, A., and Giuditta, A. (1971): A long-term effect of electroconvulsive shock on the metabolism of glucose in mouse brain. *Brain Res.*, 27:418–421.

8. Dunn, A., Giuditta, A., and Pagliuca, N. (1971): The effect of electroconvulsive shock on protein synthesis in mouse brain. *J. Neurochem.*, 18:2093–2099.

9. Dunn, A., Giuditta, A., Wilson, J. E., and Glassman, E. (1974): The effect of electroshock on brain RNA and protein synthesis and its possible relationship to behavioral effects. In: *Psychobiology of Convulsive Therapy*, edited by M. Fink, J. L. McGaugh, S. Kety, and T. A. Williams, pp. 185–197. V. H. Winston and Sons, Washington, D.C.

10. Flexner, L. B., Flexner, J. B., and Stellar, E. (1965): Memory and cerebral protein synthesis in mice as affected by graded amounts of puromycin. *Exp. Neurol.*, 13:264–272.

11. Giuditta, A., Abrescia, P., and Rutigliano, B. (1978): Effect of electroshock on thymidine incorporation into rat brain DNA. *J. Neurochem.*, 31:983–987.

12. Kimberlin, R. H., Shirt, D. B., and Collis, S. C. (1974): The turnover of isotopically labeled DNA *in vivo* in developing, adult and scrapie-affected mouse brain. *J. Neurochem.*, 23:241–248.

13. Linden, I., and Smith, B. H. (1968): Neuronal uptake of ³H-thymidine. *Curr. Mod. Biol.*, 2:274–282.

14. MacInnes, J. W., McConkey, E. H., and Schlesinger, K. (1970): Changes in brain polyribosomes following an electro-convulsive seizure. *J. Neurochem.*, 17:457–460.

15. Merits, I., and Cain, J. (1969): Rapid loss of labeled DNA from rat brain due to radiation damage. *Biochim. Biophys. Acta*, 174:315–321.

16. Merits, I., and Cain, J. C. (1970): Loss of labeled DNA from rat brain following injections of precursors with high specific radioactivity. *Biochim. Biophys. Acta*, 209:327–338.

17. Metafora, S., Persico, M., Felsani, A., Ferraiuolo, R., and Giuditta, A. (1977): On the mechanism of electroshock-induced inhibition of protein synthesis in rabbit cerebral cortex. *J. Neurochem.*, 28:1335–1346.

18. Pelc, S. R. (1972): Metabolic DNA in ciliated protozoa, salivary gland chromosomes, and mammalian cells. *Int. Rev. Cytol.*, 32:327–355.

19. Pepe, I. M., Cimarra, P., and Giuditta, A. (1975): Inhibition of neuronal protein synthesis in the giant fibre system of the squid by a high potassium concentration. *J. Neurochem.*, 24:1271–1273.

20. Perrone-Capano, C., D'Onofrio, G., and Giuditta, A. (1982): DNA turnover in rat cerebral cortex. *J. Neurochem.*, 38:52–56.

21. Popoli, M., and Giuditta, A. (1980): Effect of electroconvulsive shock on polysomes of rabbit brain, liver, and kidney. *J. Neurochem.*, 35:1319–1322.

22. Reinis, S. (1972): Autoradiographic study of ³H-thymidine incorporation into brain DNA during learning. *Physiol. Chem. Phys.*, 4:391–397.

23. Sandoval, M.-E., Palacios, R., and Tapia, R. (1976): Studies on the relationship between GABA synthesis and protein synthesis in brain. *J. Neurochem.*, 27:667–672.

24. Scalenghe, F., Romano, M., and Giuditta, A. (1970): Effect of electroconvulsive shock on polysomes of rabbit brain and liver. Unpublished manuscript.

25. Vesco, C., and Giuditta, A. (1968): Disaggregation of brain polysomes induced by electroconvulsive treatment. *J. Neurochem.*, 15:81–85.

26. Wasterlain, C. G. (1972): Breakdown of brain polysomes in status epilepticus. *Brain Res.*, 39:278–284.

27. Weiss, B. F., Liebschutz, J. L., Wurtman, R. J., and Munro, H. N. (1975): Participation of dopamine- and serotonin-receptors in the disaggregation of brain polysomes by L-DOPA and L-5-HTP. *J. Neurochem.*, 24:1191–1195.

Advances in Neurology, Vol. 34: Status Epilepticus, edited by A.V. Delgado-Escueta, C.G. Wasterlain, D.M. Treiman, and R.J. Porter. Raven Press, New York © 1983.

27

Regulation of Brain Protein Synthesis During Status Epilepticus

Barney E. Dwyer and Claude G. Wasterlain

Sustained seizure activity causes profound physiological changes in humans (39,46,49,69), cats (66), rodents (7,10,42), and primates (41). Seizures result in markedly increased metabolic rate in cerebral tissue (7,10,42) and, when prolonged, lead to brain damage in the adult (40,43) and retarded brain growth in the neonate (56,67). Subsequent cerebral lesions are often ascribed to hypoxia resulting from reduced ventilation during seizure activity combined with increased demand for energy substrates both in brain and in peripheral tissues. However, there is evidence in primates that seizure activity in the absence of hypoxia and convulsions is also detrimental (43). In this chapter we shall concentrate on the mechanism by which seizures can affect the translation of new protein in brain and on the role of altered protein synthesis in cellular abnormalities following status epilepticus.

SEIZURES INHIBIT BRAIN PROTEIN SYNTHESIS

Brain protein synthesis is severely inhibited by seizures. Early studies showed that brain polyribosomes were dissociated after a series of electroconvulsive seizures in the rabbit (60) or a single electroconvulsive seizure in the mouse (38). Leucine incorporation into mouse brain protein following electroconvulsive shock was inhibited (14, 21). All of these studies employed freely convulsing animals, and so it is difficult to assess the effect of seizure activity on brain protein synthesis as distinct from the effects of peripheral involvement and transient hypoxia.

TABLE 1. *Brain protein synthesis in status epilepticus[a]*

	0 to 5 min of seizures		25 to 30 min of seizures		55 to 60 min of seizures	
	Leucine (cpm/μM)	Protein (cpm/mg)	Leucine (cpm/μM)	Protein (cpm/mg)	Leucine (cpm/μM)	Protein (cpm/mg)
Control group ± SEM	3,786 ± 137	654 ± 41	3,792 ± 147	699 ± 18	3,838 ± 172	666 ± 36
Electroconvulsive shock group ± SEM	6,278 ± 218	471 ± 11	6,264 ± 199	424 ± 14	6,093 ± 204	338 ± 25
p	<0.001	<0.001	<0.001	<0.001	<0.001	<0.001

[a] ^{3}H-leucine incorporation into cerebral proteins after 5-min pulses (500 μCi/kg) injected during repetitive electroconvulsive seizures in paralyzed oxygen-ventilated rats.

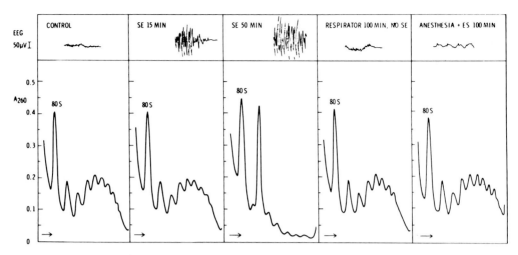

FIG. 1. Effects of status epilepticus (SE) on rat brain polysomal profiles. Rats were paralyzed with succinylcholine, then tracheotomized and ventilated with 100% O_2. Electroshock (ES) seizures were induced every 30 sec. The "anesthesia + ES" group received the same electrical stimulation as status epilepticus rats plus 2% halothane anesthesia. EEGs were recorded immediately before sacrifice. Specific details are given by Wasterlain (68).

This problem was addressed in later studies (64,68). Prolonged status epilepticus, induced electrically, in paralyzed rats ventilated with 100% oxygen resulted in the dissociation of brain polyribosomes (Fig. 1). In the same model (65), incorporation of leucine into brain protein of seizing rats was reduced up to 50% over control values (Table 1). This was not the result of an effect on amino acid transport, because leucine specific activity was greater in seizing animals. These studies demonstrated that paroxysmal central activity, when prolonged, even in the absence of hypoxia and muscle convulsions, could directly inhibit brain protein synthesis.

SEIZURES DISSOCIATE BRAIN POLYSOMES

Seizures dissociated brain polyribosomes into monomers and dimers (Fig. 1). The structural integrity of these ribosomes was not altered by prolonged seizures, as evidenced by their ability to synthesize polyphenylalanine using a polyuridylic acid (poly-U) template (Table 2). Polyribosome dissociation was not due to activation of ribonuclease activity, as measured by the hydrolysis of [^{3}H]poly-U. Furthermore, ribosomal monomers and dimers were dissociable into subunits in buffers containing 0.5-M potassium salts, indicating they were formed by runoff of polyribosomes. Ribosomes formed by RNase action are not dissociable in high-salt buffers. The polyribosome dissociation

TABLE 2. *Radioactivity incorporated into acid-precipitable material by cell-free systems from control and status epilepticus brains[a]*

	5 min	10 min	15 min
Control	1,290	2,075	2,622
Status (50 min)	681	1,046	1,112
Control + poly-U	1,625	2,591	3,014
Status + poly-U	1,816	2,760	3,311

[a] Radioactivity incorporated into TCA-precipitable material by brain postmitochondrial supernatant. Final concentrations of the assay system: 50-mM Tris HCl, pH 7.4 at 0°C; 25-mM KCl; 12-mM MgCl$_2$; 0.25-M sucrose; 2-mM creatine phosphate; 1-mM ATP; 1-mM GTP; creatine kinase (0.1 mg/ml); 1 mg of ribosomes; 2 mg of pH-5 enzymes; 1 μCi of [^{3}H]phenylalanine (sp. act. 2 Ci/mmole); and 0.5 A$_{260}$ unit of poly-U where indicated. Values represent the means of five experiments (each done in triplicate). See Wasterlain (68) for further details.

was reversible. Polyribosomes reformed 3 hr after status epilepticus lasting 50 min and more quickly when the duration of status was shorter (Fig. 2). This might not require the synthesis of new messenger RNA (mRNA), because reassociation occurred in animals treated with actinomycin D, an inhibitor of RNA synthesis. These observations are suggestive of a block in the initiation of new proteins while elongating chains continue to be processed, terminating in "runoff" dimers. Inhibition of initiation was also suggested by Metafora et al. (45). There is substantial evidence that initiation

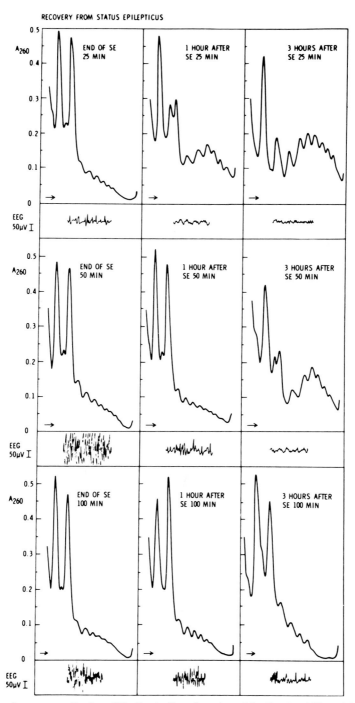

FIG. 2. Recovery from status epilepticus (SE). For details, refer to legend for Fig. 1 and Wasterlain (68).

is a major site of regulation of protein synthesis in other eukaryotic cells (2). Protein synthesis initiation is a complex, highly regulated process.

For our purposes, protein synthesis may be divided into two components: transcription and translation. Transcription refers to events in the nucleus that result in the synthesis and processing of new mRNA molecules. Translation refers to the reactions through which cytoplasmic mRNA is bound to ribosomes and amino acids are brought together and polymerized to form new polypeptides. Both of these processes are dependent on high-energy phosphates. Translational events may be further subdivided into three phases: (a) initiation (31), (b) elongation (12), and (c) termination of the polypeptide chain (9). A sequence for the assembly of an active 80S ribosome initiation complex, based on information obtained from the reticulocyte system (5), is illustrated in Fig. 3.

The first step in the translation of mRNA into protein is the formation of a ternary complex among initiation factor eIF-2, GTP, and the initiator species of methionyl tRNA (met-tRNA$_i$). We have recently shown that initiation factor eIF-2 activity is present in the brain (22). The ternary complex then binds to a 40S ribosomal subunit associated with initiation factor eIF-3, which presumably acts as a dissociation factor to prevent 40S and 60S ribosomal subunits from aggregating and may also

promote binding of ternary complex and mRNA to the 40S subunit (3,5,58). Binding of mRNA requires, in addition, the aid of several other factors and hydrolysis of ATP (5). The resulting complex is designated the 48S preinitiation complex (28,53). The 48S preinitiation complex joins to a 60S ribosomal subunit with the aid of initiation factor eIF-5, resulting in the formation of a competent 80S ribosomal initiation complex capable of elongating the peptide chain. The joining of the 40S and 60S subunits is accompanied by hydrolysis of GTP and the release of bound initiation factors (5).

THE ENERGY STATE OF THE CELL REGULATES INITIATION OF BRAIN PROTEIN SYNTHESIS THROUGH THE GDP/GTP RATIO

Convulsive seizures profoundly deplete the brain's energy reserves. Even in brain tissue of paralyzed oxygen-ventilated animals following prolonged seizure activity there is a small but significant decrease in ATP level, with a concomitant increase in ADP level (11,19,30). This alteration, which occurs soon after the onset of seizure activity, is maintained for the duration of the seizure and correlates precisely with polyribosome dissociation. How might such a change affect protein synthesis?

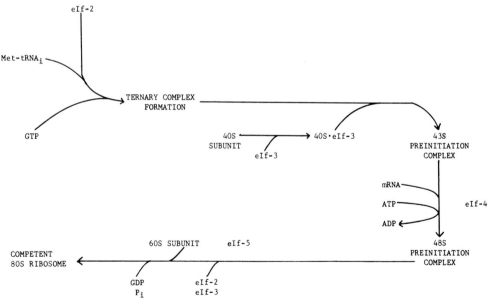

FIG. 3. The sequence of reactions of protein synthesis initiation in the reticulocyte.

In brain, as in other tissues, ternary-complex formation is specific for GTP (Table 3). Of all the nucleotides we tested, only the nonhydrolyzable artificial GTP analogue guanosine 5'-(β,γ-imino) triphosphate [GMP-P(NH)P] proved able to substitute for GTP.

We found that GDP is a potent inhibitor of ternary-complex formation. GDP can bind to the α subunit of eIF-2 in a manner that prevents binding of met-tRNA$_i$. When the ratio of GDP to GTP is 1:10 (close to the physiological range), ternary-complex formation is inhibited between 40% and 50% (Fig. 4). This occurs over a 30-fold concentration range of GTP (22). This inhibition is specific for GDP. When GDP is replaced by ADP, UDP, or CDP *in vitro*, ternary-complex formation is inhibited, but this is because of the formation of GDP in the assay mixture via the enzyme nucleoside diphosphate kinase (EC 2.7.4.6) present in the brain extract (22). This enzyme catalyzes the reaction $XTP + YDP \rightleftarrows XDP + YTP$, where X and Y can be adenosine, guanosine, cytidine, or uridine. Adenylate kinase, which catalyzes the formation of ADP from AMP and ATP, may contribute to the formation of GDP from AMP and GTP. We have evidence for this reaction in brain (22), but ADP is much more effective in promoting inhibition of ternary-complex formation than AMP.

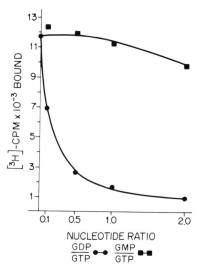

FIG. 4. Effects of GDP and GMP on GTP-dependent ternary-complex formation. Ternary-complex formation was assayed by retention of radioactivity on nitrocellulose filters (22). GTP was present in the assay mixture at 1.5 mM, and various amounts of GDP or GMP were added to give the desired concentration ratio. GTP-independent binding was subtracted from all determinations.

SIGNIFICANCE OF REGULATION OF PROTEIN SYNTHESIS INITIATION BY GDP

We can now describe a mechanism that relates inhibition of protein synthesis in brain to the increased energy demand by the cell during prolonged seizures. Seizure activity results in an elevated ratio of ADP to ATP, which increases the ratio of GDP to GTP by the enzyme nucleoside diphosphate kinase. Presumably this acts as an amplification system whereby small decreases in ATP result in large increases in GDP relative to GTP. The result is reduced ternary-complex formation and inhibition of protein synthesis. Small reductions in the adenylate energy charge result in the inhibition of energy-intensive macromolecule synthesis and allow energy resources to be used for such things as maintaining ion gradients, which are essential to cell survival.

More than 10 years ago Atkinson (1) proposed that the adenylate energy charge of the cell could regulate the enzymes involved in energy-requiring biosynthetic processes. Thompson and Atkinson (57) showed that the adenylate energy charge could regulate the nucleoside diphosphate kinase reaction. Walton and Gill (61–63) have proposed that the adenylate energy charge can regulate ternary-complex formation and hence protein synthesis via

TABLE 3. *Nucleotide substitution of GTP in ternary-complex formation*[a]

Nucleotide	Ternary-complex formation (% of complete system)
GTP (complete system)	100
GMP-P(NH)P	173
GMP-P(CH$_2$)P	15
ATP	12
CTP	12
UTP	8
ADP	3
GDP	2
UDP	1
CDP	1
AMP	0
GMP	1
UMP	0
CMP	0

[a] The ternary complex was assayed by retention of radioactivity on nitrocellulose filters. When replacing GTP, nucleotides were present at a concentration of 1.5 mM in the incubation mixture. GTP-independent binding was subtracted from all determinations.

this enzyme in reticulocytes, and this mechanism has also been proposed to operate in rat thymic lymphocytes during glucose deficiency (44). Our findings suggest that the same mechanism exists in brain to curtail protein synthesis when excess energy demand threatens cell survival. This may explain in part the inhibition of protein synthesis by prolonged seizures and would be applicable to any situation where the energy state of cells may be perturbed, as, for example, hypoxia (6,8,54,55), ischemia (20,37), and ethanol consumption (51). Restoration of the normal adenylate energy charge should reverse this block. How status epilepticus may affect the adenylate energy charge in various cell populations is not known. The situation may be more complex if there is compartmentation of GTP in brain, as has been suggested in other tissues (33).

PHOSPHORYLATION OF INITIATION FACTORS

Several protein synthesis initiation factors, including eIF-2 from reticulocytes, have been shown to be phosphorylated both *in vivo* (3) and *in vitro* (3,32,59). There is abundant evidence that inhibition of protein synthesis in reticulocyte lysates deficient in heme is in some way mediated by the phosphorylation of the α subunit of eIF-2 by a kinase (designated the heme-controlled repressor, HCR). The mechanism by which phosphorylation mediates inhibition is not certain, but the result is a reduction in 40S met-tRNA initiation complexes (13,28,34,47,48,50), although the activated HCR may also interfere with subunit joining (27). Phosphorylation of eIF-2α can also be stimulated by oxidized glutathione (23), heat and pressure (29), double-stranded RNA (23,36), and possibly by cyclic AMP via a cyclic-AMP-dependent protein kinase (16–18). This latter pathway has been disputed (25,35). Specific phosphoprotein phosphatases that dephosphorylate the α subunit of eIF-2 have also been described (15,26,52). Thus, protein synthesis initiation in the reticulocyte may be regulated by a phosphorylation-dephosphorylation cycle. Whether or not such a pathway exists in brain is not known.

SIGNIFICANCE OF PROTEIN SYNTHESIS INHIBITION IN BRAIN

Inhibition of protein synthesis could affect the brain in several ways. Reduced rates of protein synthesis may affect cell viability by altering the synthesis of key enzymes, structural proteins, or proteins with very short half-lives that may be required to prevent irreversible cell damage resulting from status epilepticus. In the developing brain, reduced rates of protein synthesis may prolong the cell cycle time in actively dividing cell populations and affect normal cell growth and differentiation, resulting in reduced cell populations, aberrant dendritic patterns, and abnormal synaptic organization in key brain regions. This is extremely critical in the developing brain, because once the strictly defined periods of cell division and differentiation have been bypassed, recovery is often not possible, and permanent morphological and behavioral deficits can result.

We have suggested one mechanism by which protein synthesis initiation is inhibited during status epilepticus, i.e., regulation of protein synthesis initiation by GDP, and ultimately by the adenylate energy charge of the cell. This is an important protective mechanism in brain, where there is very little margin for survival when energy reserves are depleted. However, should inhibition of protein synthesis be prolonged, as during status epilepticus, dire consequences for the brain and organism may result.

ACKNOWLEDGMENTS

This work was supported by research grant NS-13515 from the National Institute of Neurological and Communicative Disorders and Stroke and by the Research Service of the Veterans Administration.

REFERENCES

1. Atkinson, D. E. (1968): The energy charge of the adenylate pool as a regulatory parameter. Interaction with feedback modifiers. *Biochemistry,* 7:4030–4034.
2. Austin, S. A., and Clemens, M. J. (1980): Control of the initiation of protein synthesis in mammalian cells. *F.E.B.S. Lett.,* 110:1–7.
3. Benne, R., Edman, J., Traut, R. R., and Hershey, J. W. B. (1978): Phosphorylation of eukaryotic protein synthesis initiation factors. *Proc. Natl. Acad. Sci. U.S.A.,* 75:108–112.
4. Benne, R., and Hershey, J. W. B. (1976): Purification and characterization of initiation factor IF-E3 from rabbit reticulocytes. *Proc. Natl. Acad. Sci. U.S.A.,* 73:3005–3009.
5. Benne, R., and Hershey, J. W. B. (1978): The mechanism of action of protein synthesis initiation factors from rabbit reticulocytes. *J. Biol. Chem.,* 253:3078–3087.

6. Berlet, H. (1976): Hypoxic survival of normogly-caemic young adult and adult mice in relation to cerebral metabolic rates. *J. Neurochem.*, 26:1267–1274.

7. Borgstrom, L., Chapman, A. G., Siesjö, B. K. (1976): Glucose consumption in the cerebral cortex of rat during bicuculline-induced status epilepticus. *J. Neurochem.*, 27:971–973.

8. Broniszewska-Ardelt, B., and Jongkind, J. F. (1971): Effect of hypoxia on substrate levels in the brain of the adult mouse. *J. Neurochem.*, 18:2237–2240.

9. Caskey, C. T. (1980): Peptide chain termination. *Trends in the Biochemical Sciences*, 5:234–237.

10. Chapman, A. G., Meldrum, B. S., and Siesjö, B. K. (1976): Cerebral blood flow and cerebral metabolic rate during prolonged epileptic seizures in rats. *J. Physiol.*, 254:61–62.

11. Chapman, A. G., Meldrum, B. S., and Siesjö, B. K. (1977): Cerebral metabolic changes during prolonged epileptic seizures in rats. *J. Neurochem.*, 28:1025–1035.

12. Clark, B. (1980): The elongation step of protein biosynthesis. *Trends in the Biochemical Sciences*, 5:207–210.

13. Clemens, M. J., Henshaw, E. C., Rahamimoff, H., and London, I. M. (1974): Met-tRNA$_f$ binding to 40S ribosomal subunits: A site for the regulation of initiation of protein synthesis by hemin. *Proc. Natl. Acad. Sci. U.S.A.*, 71:2946–2950.

14. Cotman, C. W., Banker, G., Fornetzer, S. F., and McGaugh, J. L. (1971): Electroshock effects on brain protein synthesis: Relation to brain seizures and retrograde amnesia. *Science*, 173:454–456.

15. Crouch, D., and Safer, B. (1980): Purification and properties of eIF-2 phosphatase. *J. Biol. Chem.*, 255:7918–7924.

16. Datta, A., DeHaro, C., and Ochoa, S. (1978): Translational control by hemin is due to binding to cAMP-dependent protein kinase. *Proc. Natl. Acad. Sci. U.S.A.*, 75:1148–1152.

17. Datta, A., DeHaro, C., Sierra, J. M., and Ochoa, S. (1977): Role of 3′:5′-cyclic-AMP-dependent protein kinase in regulation of protein synthesis in reticulocyte lysates. *Proc. Natl. Acad. Sci. U.S.A.*, 74:1463–1467.

18. Datta, A., DeHaro, C., Sierra, J. M., and Ochoa, S. (1977): Mechanism of translational control by hemin in reticulocyte lysates. *Proc. Natl. Acad. Sci. U.S.A.*, 74:3326–3329.

19. Duffy, T. E., Howse, D. C., and Plum, F. (1975): Cerebral energy metabolism during experimental status epilepticus. *J. Neurochem.*, 24:925–934.

20. Duffy, T. E., Nelson, S. R., and Lowry, O. H. (1972): Cerebral carbohydrate metabolism during acute hypoxia and recovery. *J. Neurochem.*, 19:959–977.

21. Dunn, A., Giuditta, A., and Pagliuca, N. (1971): The effect of electroconvulsive shock on protein synthesis in mouse brain. *J. Neurochem.*, 18:2093–2099.

22. Dwyer, B. E., and Wasterlain, C. G. (1980): Regulation of the first step of the initiation of brain protein synthesis by guanosine diphosphate. *J. Neurochem.*, 34:1639–1647.

23. Ernst, V., Levin, D. H., and London, I. M. (1979): In situ phosphorylation of the alpha subunit of eukaryotic initiation factor 2 in reticulocyte lysates inhibited by heme deficiency, double-stranded RNA,

24. Fando, J. L., Conn, M., and Wasterlain, C. G. (1979): Brain protein synthesis during neonatal seizures: An experimental study. *Exp. Neurol.*, 63:220–228.

25. Grankowski, N., Kramer, G., and Hardesty, B. (1979): No effect of cAMP on protein synthesis in reticulocyte lysates. *J. Biol. Chem.*, 254:3145–3147.

26. Grankowski, N., Lehmusvirta, D., Kramer, G., and Hardesty, B. (1980): Partial purification and characterization of reticulocyte phosphatase with activity for phosphorylated peptide initiation factor 2. *J. Biol. Chem.*, 255:310–317.

27. Gross, M. (1979): Control of protein synthesis by hemin. Evidence that the hemin-controlled translational repressor inhibits formation of 80S initiation complexes from 48S intermediate initiation complexes. *J. Biol. Chem.*, 254:2370–2377.

28. Gross, M. (1979): Regulation of protein synthesis by hemin: Evidence that the hemin-controlled translational repressor inhibits the rate of formation of 40S-Met-tRNA$_f$ complexes directly. *J. Biol. Chem.*, 254:2378–2383.

29. Henderson, A. B., Miller, A. H., and Hardesty, B. (1979): Multistep regulatory system for activation of a cyclic AMP-independent eukaryotic initiation factor 2 kinase. *Proc. Natl. Acad. Sci. U.S.A.*, 76:2605–2609.

30. Howse, D. C. N. (1979): Metabolic responses to status epilepticus in the rat, cat and mouse. *Can. J. Physiol. Pharmacol.*, 57:205–212.

31. Hunt, T. (1980): The initiation of protein synthesis. *Trends in the Biochemical Sciences*, 5:178–181.

32. Issinger, O.-G., Benne, R., Hershey, J. W. B., and Traut, R. R. (1976): Phosphorylation *in vitro* of eukaryotic initiation factors IF-E2 and IF-E3 by protein kinases. *J. Biol. Chem.*, 251:6471–6474.

33. Johnson, G. S., and Mukku, V. R. (1979): Evidence in intact cells for an involvement of GTP in the activation of adenylate cyclase. *J. Biol. Chem.*, 254:95–100.

34. Legon, S., Jackson, R. J., and Hunt, T. (1973): Control of protein synthesis in reticulocyte lysates by haemin. *Nature [New Biol.]*, 241:150–152.

35. Levin, D., Ernst, V., and London, I. M. (1979): Effects of the catalytic subunit of cAMP-dependent protein kinase (type II) from reticulocytes and bovine heart muscle on protein phosphorylation and protein synthesis in reticulocyte lysates. *J. Biol. Chem.*, 254:7935–7941.

36. Levin, D., and London, I. M. (1978): Regulation of protein synthesis: Activation by double-stranded RNA of a protein kinase that phosphorylates eukaryotic initiation factor 2. *Proc. Natl. Acad. Sci. U.S.A.*, 75:1121–1125.

37. Lowry, O. H., Passonneau, J. V., Hasselberger, F. X., and Schulz, D. W. (1964): Effect of ischemia on known substrate and cofactors of the glycolytic pathway in brain. *J. Biol. Chem.*, 239:18–30.

38. MacInnes, J. W., McConkey, E. H., and Schlesinger, K. (1970): Changes in brain polyribosomes following an electroconvulsive seizure. *J. Neurochem.*, 17:457–460.

gers the lipid effect cannot be determined at this time. The rise in the free fatty acid pool in the central nervous system in bicuculline-treated rats may be due to the activation of a membrane phospholipid degradative enzyme.

It has been suggested by our colleagues that there are two pathways to explain the lipid effect of convulsions (3,8). The reactions are as follows:

PI → 1-stearoyl-2-arachidonoyldiglycerol + phosphorylinositol (I)

1-stearoyl-2-arachidonoylglycerol → free arachidonic acid + 1-stearoylglycerol (II)

1-stearoylglycerol → free stearic acid + glycerol (III)

PI → free arachidonic acid + monoacyl PI (IV)

These reactions seem also to be affected in the brain by early ischemia (2,4,7). The simultaneous production of arachidonoyldiglycerols and free arachidonic acid may be due to the activation of a phospholipase C (I), followed by the activation of a diglyceride lipase (II). To account for the release of free stearic acid, either a second lipase may be activated (III) or the enzyme catalyzing reaction II may hydrolyze both acyl chains. Alternatively, deacylation of phosphatidylinositol may be by phospholipases A_2 (IV). The transiently increased free arachidonic acid (as well as other fatty acids) represents the overshooting of enzymatic reactions that may play a key role in modulating membrane permeability. Ischemia and trauma also stimulate the production of brain free fatty acids (1,5, 14,19,28). Because lesser increases in these lipids are found when there is stronger resistance to anoxia (e.g., newborn mammals, poikilothermic animals), it has been suggested that this pathway may

be linked to the establishment of irreversible brain damage (7,14). If such enzymes are also altered during status epilepticus, deranged membrane function may arise, yielding a persistently high content of free fatty acids. This change may have a bearing on the establishment of epileptic brain damage (Fig. 1). The loss of the diacylphospholipid and the accumulation of free fatty acids and metabolites may play active roles in the pathogenesis of such lesions. Prostaglandins (20,24,25, 31,35) and lipid peroxides (18,23,30,33) are formed under these conditions.

The trigger, at least partially, may be a neurotransmitter of the catecholamine type, because α-methyl-*p*-tyrosine inhibits by 25% the effect of bicuculline (Table 2). Cyclic nucleotides (29,32) and adenosine (30) show early changes during convulsions and seem to involve membrane receptors. However, the roles played by these regulatory metabolites in membrane phospholipid dynamics are not known. Because ischemia or anoxia also produces a similar release of free fatty acids in the nervous system (1,5,7,19,26,28), there remains to be studied in detail the role that hypoxia or circulatory disturbances at the onset of seizures play in the lipid changes described. These data will be needed to clarify the intimate mechanism involved and to lead to new lines of research with drugs in an effort to diminish the selective breakdown of membrane lipids that occurs during convulsions.

CONCLUSIONS

Membrane alterations in status epilepticus may involve phospholipid breakdown, giving rise to free arachidonic acid, other free fatty acids, and arachidonoyldiglycerols. Bicuculline greatly enhances this lipid pool in rat cerebrum. α-Methyl-

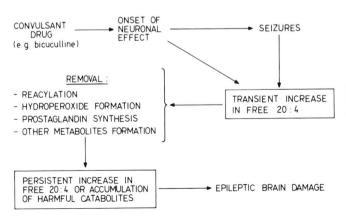

FIG. 1. Outline of brain changes involving membrane lipids that may lead to brain damage in status epilepticus.

p-tyrosine prevents the electroshock-induced effect on brain free fatty acids, but it inhibits by only about 25% the bicuculline-stimulated production of cerebral free fatty acids. In status epilepticus induced by bicuculline, the largest changes in cerebral free fatty acids are observed in free arachidonic acid. Relatively larger changes in free docosahexaenoic acid and smaller increments in all other free fatty acids take place in cerebellum.

The release of free arachidonic acid and of arachidonoyldiglycerols in cerebrum from rats with bicuculline-induced status epilepticus is a selective process. Phosphatidylinositol from neuronal membranes may be the source of the lipids augmented. The accumulation of arachidonic acid, the formation of metabolites, and the breakdown of a membrane phospholipid pool may be involved in the pathogenesis of epileptic brain damage.

REFERENCES

1. Aveldaño, M. I., and Bazán, N. G. (1975): Differential lipid deacylation during brain ischemia in a homeotherm and poikilotherm. Content and composition of FFA and triacylglycerols. *Brain Res.*, 100:99–110.
2. Aveldaño, M. I., and Bazán, N. G. (1975): Rapid production of diacylglycerols enriched in arachidonate and stearate during early brain ischemia. *J. Neurochem.*, 25:919–920.
3. Aveldaño de Caldironi, M. I., and Bazán, N. G. (1979): α-Methyl-*p*-tyrosine inhibits the production of free arachidonic acid and diacylglycerols in brain after a single electroconvulsive shock. *Neurochem. Res.*, 4:213–221.
4. Banschbach, M. W., and Geison, R. L. (1974): Postmortem increase in rat cerebral hemisphere diglyceride pool size. *J. Neurochem.*, 23:875–877.
5. Bazán, N. G., Jr. (1970): Effects of ischemia and electroconvulsive shock on free fatty acid pool in the brain. *Biochim. Biophys. Acta*, 218:1–10.
6. Bazán, N. G., Jr. (1971): Changes in free fatty acids of brain by drug-induced convulsions, electroshock and anaesthesia. *J. Neurochem.*, 18:1379–1385.
7. Bazán, N. G. (1976): Free arachidonic acid and other lipids in the nervous system during early ischemia and after electroshock. In: *Function and Metabolism of Phospholipids in the Central and Peripheral Nervous Systems*, edited by G. Porcellati, L. Amaducci, and C. Galli, pp. 317–335. Plenum Press, New York.
8. Bazán, N. G., Aveldaño de Caldironi, M. I., Cascone de Suárez, G. D., and Rodríguez de Turco, E. B. (1980): Transient modifications in brain free arachidonic acid in experimental animals during convulsions. In: *Neurochemistry and Clinical Neurology*, edited by L. Battistin, G. Hashim, and A. Lajtha, pp. 167–179. Alan R. Liss, New York.
9. Bazán, N. G., and Bazán, H. E. P. (1975): Analysis of free and esterified fatty acids in neural tissues using gradient-thickness thin-layer chromatography (GT-
TLC). In: *Research Methods in Neurochemistry, Vol. 3*, edited by N. Marks and R. Rodnight, pp. 309–324. Plenum Press, New York.
10. Bazán, N. G., Jr., de Bazán, H. E. P., Kennedy, W. G., and Joel, C. D. (1971): Regional distribution and rate of production of free fatty acids in rat brain. *J. Neurochem.*, 18:1387–1393.
11. Bazán, N. G., and Giusto, N. M. (1980): Docosahexaenoyl chains are introduced in phosphatidic acid during de novo synthesis in retinal microsomes. In: *Membrane Fluidity: Biophysical Techniques and Cellular Regulation*, edited by M. Kates and A. Kuksis, pp. 223–236. Humana Press, Clifton, New Jersey.
12. Bazán, N. G., Morelli de Liberti, S., and Rodríguez de Turco, E. B. (1982): Arachidonic acid and arachidonoylidiglycerols increase in rat cerebrum during bicuculline-induced status epilepticus. *Neurochem. Res.*, 7:839–843.
13. Bazán, N. G., Jr., and Rakowski, H. (1970): Increased levels of brain free fatty acids after electroconvulsive shock. *Life Sci.*, 9:501–507.
14. Bazán, N. G., and Rodríguez de Turco, E. B. (1980): Membrane lipids in the pathogenesis of brain edema: Phospholipids and arachidonic acid, the earliest membrane components changed at the onset of ischemia. *Adv. Neurol.*, 28:197–205.
15. Breckenridge, W. C., Gombos, G., and Morgan, I. G. (1971): The docosahexaenoic acid of the phospholipids of synaptic membranes, vesicles and mitochondria. *Brain Res.*, 33:581–583.
16. Chapman, A. G., Meldrum, B. S., and Siesjö, B. K. (1977): Cerebral metabolic changes during prolonged epileptic seizures in rats. *J. Neurochem.*, 28:1025–1035.
17. Delgado-Escueta, A. V., and Horan, M. P. (1980): Brain synaptosomes in epilepsy: Organization of ionic channels and the Na^+-K^+ pump. *Adv. Neurol.*, 27:85–126.
18. Flamm, E. S., Demopoulos, H. B., Seligman, M. L., Poser, R. G., and Ransohoff, J. (1978): Free radicals in cerebral ischemia. *Stroke*, 9:445–447.
19. Galli, C., and Spagnuolo, C. (1976): The release of brain free fatty acids during ischaemia in essential fatty acid-deficient rats. *J. Neurochem.*, 26:401–404.
20. Gaudet, R. J., and Levine, L. (1979): Transient cerebral ischemia and brain prostaglandins. *Biochem. Biophys. Res. Commun.*, 86:893–901.
21. Glass, J. D., Fromm, G. H., and Chattha, A. S. (1980): Bicuculline and neuronal activity in motor cortex. *Electroencephalogr. Clin. Neurophysiol.*, 48:16–24.
22. Hirata, F., and Axelrod, J. (1980): Phospholipid methylation and biological signal transmission. *Science*, 209:1082–1090.
23. Majewska, J., Strosznajder, J., and Lazarewicz, J. (1978): Effect of ischemic anoxia and barbiturate anesthesia on free radical oxidation of mitochondrial phospholipids. *Brain Res.*, 158:423–434.
24. Marion, J., Pappius, H. M., and Wolfe, L. S. (1979): Evidence for the use of a pool of the free arachidonic acid in rat cerebral cortex tissue for prostaglandin $F_{2\alpha}$ synthesis in vitro. *Biochim. Biophys. Acta*, 573:229–237.
25. Marion, J., and Wolfe, L. S. (1978): Increase in vivo of unesterified fatty acids, prostaglandin $F_{2\alpha}$ but not

thromboxane B_2 in rat brain during drug induced convulsions. *Prostaglandins*, 16:99–110.

26. Marion, J., and Wolfe, L. S. (1979): Origin of the arachidonic acid released post-mortem in rat forebrain. *Biochim. Biophys. Acta*, 574:25–32.

27. Pascual de Bazán, H. E., and Bazán, N. G. (1976): Phospholipid composition and [^{14}C]glycerol incorporation into glycerolipids of toad retina and brain. *J. Neurochem.*, 27:1051–1057.

28. Porcellati, G., De Medio, G. E., Fini, C., Floridi, A., Goracci, G., Horrocks, L. A., Lazarewicz, J. W., Palmerini, C. A., Strosznajder, J., and Trovarelli, G. (1978): Phospholipid and its metabolism in ischemia. In: *Proceedings of the European Society for Neurochemistry*, edited by V. Neuhoff, pp. 285–302. Verlag Chemie, Weinheim.

29. Rehncrona, S., Siesjö, B. K., and Westerberg, E. (1978): Adenosine and cyclic AMP in cerebral cortex of rats in hypoxia, status epilepticus and hypercapnia. *Acta Physiol. Scand.*, 104:453–463.

30. Sattin, A., Rall, T. W., and Zanella, J. (1975): Regulation of cyclic adenosine 3′,5′-monophosphate lev-
els in guinea-pig cerebral cortex by interaction of alpha adrenergic and adenosine receptor activity. *J. Pharmacol. Exp. Ther.*, 192:22–32.

31. Spagnuolo, C., Galli, C., Omini, C., and Folco, G. C. (1978): Antipyretic action of mepacrine without blockade of prostaglandin (PG) synthesis in the C.N.S. *Pharmacol. Res. Commun.*, 10:779–786.

32. Wasterlain, C. G., and Csiszar, E. (1980): Cyclic nucleotide metabolism in mouse brain during seizures induced by bicuculline or dibutyryl cyclic guanosine monophosphate. *Exp. Neurol.*, 70:260–268.

33. Westerberg, E., Åkesson, B., Rehncrona, S., Smith, D. S., and Siesjö, B. K. (1979): Lipid peroxidation in brain tissue *in vitro*: Effects on phospholipids and fatty acids. *Acta Physiol. Scand.*, 105:524–526.

34. Woodbury, D. M. (1980): Convulsant drugs: Mechanisms of action. *Adv. Neurol.*, 27:249–303.

35. Zatz, M., and Roth, R. H. (1975): Electroconvulsive shock raises prostaglandins F in rat cerebral cortex. *Biochem. Pharmacol.*, 24:2101–2103.

Advances in Neurology, Vol. 34: Status Epilepticus, edited by A.V. Delgado-Escueta, C.G. Wasterlain, D.M. Treiman, and R.J. Porter. Raven Press, New York © 1983.

29

Effects of Seizures on Ion Transport and Membrane Protein Phosphorylation

Antonio V. Delgado-Escueta and Michael Horan

Since 1938, electroshock (ES) convulsion has been used as an experimental model to study the effects of depolarization and seizures. After a single maximal convulsion, transient changes result. ADP and phosphocreatine decrease (27), and the whole-brain sodium concentrations rise, whereas potassium concentrations remain unchanged (59). Brain polysomes break down, but free monomers increase acutely (55), probably as a result of selective inhibition of peptide chain initiation (15, 38,55,56). ES convulsions also transiently increase inosine, hypoxanthine (31), and the number of ^{3}H-diazepam (benzodiazepine) receptors, focusing attention on the benzodiazepine-GABA receptor complex and its associated chloride ionophore (51). Longer-lasting effects can also result after repeated ES convulsions. Brain weight, norepinephrine turnover (26), and monoamine oxidase and acetylcholinesterase activities (42) increase after daily seizures for 4 to 20 weeks. Free fatty acids, mainly arachidonic acid and diacylglycerols enriched in arachidonate, also increase within the brain, especially in the hypothalamus and brainstem (1).

Pentylenetetrazol (pentamethylenetetrazol, Metrazol®, PTZ) convulsions, in contrast to ES convulsions, have been used as an experimental model to study generalized absence seizures. Although its mechanism of action is still unknown, PTZ selectively antagonizes GABA-mediated postsynaptic inhibition in dissociated mouse spinal cord neurons grown in tissue culture (34). It decreases by 50% the fast inhibitory responses that result from the increase in chloride conductance induced by iontophoretic application of GABA or other transmitters to neurons of *Aplysia californicus* (41). PTZ also attenuates cholinergic inhibitory postsynaptic potentials without marked effects on excitatory postsynaptic potentials in the same neuron. In addition to its synaptic effects, PTZ has direct effects on membrane properties, produces a negative-resistance region in the *I-V* relation of the neuron (58), and modifies its resistance and ionic conductances (6), notably increasing K^+ permeability and neuronal firing (28). PTZ inhibits cerebral cortex $Na^+K^+ATPase$ and decreases $HCO_3^-ATPase$ activity (a mitochondrial enzyme that is mainly localized in glial cells of the CNS and is involved in active chloride transport into glial cells) (60). PTZ also inhibits brain acetylcholinesterase (37), phosphorylase (3), and glutamic acid decarboxylase (32).

Because of the foregoing differences in ES convulsions and PTZ seizures, we used both models in studying the relationship of ion transport to membrane protein phosphorylation. Single tonic-clonic seizures were produced daily in 18- to 30-day-old Sprague-Dawley rats by a clinical electroshock apparatus capable of delivering up to 300 V of 60-Hz alternating current, with stimulus durations of 0.1 to 1 sec. Shocks were delivered through ear electrodes with currents of 70 to 120 V for 0.4 to 0.6 sec, necessary to produce a long extensor tonic phase and a short flexor component (maximal ES convulsions). For controls, electroshock electrodes were placed on the ears of rats, but the current was not turned on.

PTZ was injected intraperitoneally at 70 mg/kg to induce repeated myoclonic jerks that evolved into one clonic-tonic-clonic seizure.

Although Lust et al. (33) suggested sacrificing animals by cryogenic techniques to minimize postmortem changes in brain metabolism, animals were sacrificed by decapitation instead of immersion in liquid nitrogen. Previous experiments from our laboratories had shown that freezing alters the state of membrane fractions and prevents us from analyzing pump and leak systems for ions. Because we were interested in relating ion transport to membrane protein phosphorylation, we decapitated the animals at the end of clonic jerks and 24 hr after the end of convulsions. For both ionic experiments and protein phosphorylation studies it was critical to decapitate the animals quickly, dissect the brains rapidly in ice at 4°C, and homogenize the brain as soon as possible.

SEIZURES AND Ca^{2+} TRANSPORT

Immediately after isolation of synaptosomes, internal calcium (Ca_i), potassium (K_i), and sodium (Na_i) were measured using a rapid filtration technique and atomic absorption spectrophotometry as previously described (9,10). Transient changes in Na^+, K^+, and Ca^{2+} were observed after a single tonic-clonic seizure. Na^+ and Ca^{2+} rose 45% and 50%, respectively, whereas K^+ dropped by 37%. Twenty-four hours later, ions were measured to be normal, and no significant alterations in endogenous synaptosome ion content were observed. When animals were subjected to daily convulsions, K^+ content decreased gradually until it dropped by 40% on the sixth day of daily convulsions, whereas Ca^{2+} and Na^+ rose by 37% (Fig. 1).

Previous analyses of the [Na^+K] pump, the Na^+K^+ATPase, and the Na^+ and K^+ leak systems had shown that the downhill movements of Na^+ and K^+ were responsible for the observed changes (9,10). No abnormalities in active Na^+ or K^+ transport were detected. Analysis of Ca^{2+} influx and outflux revealed that the elevated Na_i after convulsions was responsible for the enhanced Ca^{2+}

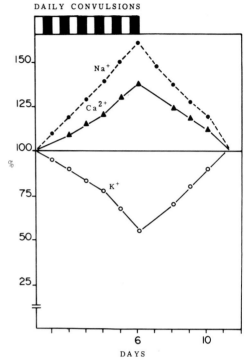

FIG. 1. Immediately after a single tonic-clonic seizure, Na^+ and Ca^{2+} rose 45% and 55%, respectively, and K^+ dropped by 37%; 24 hr later, ions were measured to be normal. After daily seizures for 6 days, K^+ content dropped by 40%, and Ca^{2+} and Na^+ rose by 37%. Four days after the last convulsion, ion content had returned to base-line levels.

influx and decreased Ca^{2+} outflux, combining to produce a net increase in Ca^{2+} content.

Table 1 shows that a high internal sodium content accelerated calcium influx and increased Ca_i. In these experiments the internal sodium content of synaptosomes was altered by suspension in 0.1-mM p-chloromercuriphenyl sulfonic acid (PCMBS) (Sigma), varying concentrations of Na^+, 1-mM $MgCl_2$, 0.1-M sucrose, and 0.066-M Tris chloride, pH 7.4 (11). Table 1 shows that this loading method can also alter the internal concentrations of Na^+ in convulsed animals, where Na_i will have had a high base-line value (first column in Table 1). PCMBS at 5°C obviously encouraged the efflux of Na^+ when the loading medium was free of Na^+. When 162-mM Na^+ was present in the loading medium, more Na^+ appeared to enter synaptosomes harvested from convulsed animal. Although calcium appeared to move at a considerably higher rate in convulsed animals (average 1.94 ± 0.04) than in controls (average 1.54 ± 0.030), the dif-

TABLE 1. *Calcium influx: stimulation by Na$_i$ after PCMBS loading*[a]

Loading medium	Na$_i$ (μmole/mg protein)	$^{45}Ca^{2+}$ influx (μmole/g protein/min)	
		Total influx	Na$_i$-dependent
Control			
0 Na$^+$	(a) 0.12 ± 0.01	0.44 ± 0.03	
	(b) 0.08 ± 0.01	0.38 ± 0.01	
	(c) 0.10 ± 0.01	0.40 ± 0.02	
	(d) 0.11 ± 0.01	0.40 ± 0.10	
80-mM Na$^+$	(a) 0.60 ± 0.01	1.2 ± 0.04	0.8
	(b) 0.54 ± 0.01	1.0 ± 0.03	0.62
	(c) 0.59 ± 0.01	1.2 ± 0.05	0.8
162-mM Na$^+$	(a) 0.90 ± 0.008	2.0 ± 0.06	1.56
	(b) 0.80 ± 0.006	1.9 ± 0.06	1.52
	(c) 0.88 ± 0.008	2.0 ± 0.06	1.50
ES-convulsed			
0 Na$^+$	(a) 0.10 ± 0.01	0.40 ± 0.02	
	(b) 0.12 ± 0.01	0.40 ± 0.05	
	(c) 0.16 ± 0.01	0.40 ± 0.10	
	(d) 0.14 ± 0.01	0.40 ± 0.06	
162-mM Na$^+$	(a) 0.96 ± 0.008	2.27 ± 0.10	1.87
	(b) 1.04 ± 0.006	2.32 ± 0.13	1.92
	(c) 1.10 ± 0.01	2.4 ± 0.08	1.98
	(d) 1.08 ± 0.01	2.38 ± 0.16	1.98

[a]After synaptosomes from control and ES-convulsed animals were loaded with varying concentrations of Na$^+$, intrasynaptosomal sodium was measured; then $^{45}Ca^{2+}$ influx was measured. Na$_i$ values represent arithmetic means ± SD obtained from four determinations. $^{45}Ca^{2+}$ influx represents the mean of three determinations ± SD. The letters designate synaptosomes from control and ES-convulsed animals prepared simultaneously.

ference in rates was accounted for by the difference in Na$_i$ values. These differences in calcium influx were observed only in a K$^+$-free Na-free external choline medium.

Increasing the Na$^+$ content of synaptosomes by convulsions slowed the rate of calcium outflow by 34%. The inhibitory effect of Na$_i$ on calcium outflow was also observed when Na$_i$ within synaptosomes was altered by the PCMBS method (Table 2). In both control and ES-convulsed animals, low Na$_i$ accelerated Ca^{2+} outflow, and high Na$_i$ retarded Ca^{2+} outflow. Our series of experiments on calcium transport (Tables 1 and 2) therefore favor the concept that Ca$_i$ increases within synaptosomes after convulsions because elevated Na$_i$ doubles the rate of calcium influx while it decreases calcium efflux by 34% (9).

MEMBRANE PROTEIN PHOSPHORYLATION

For analysis of membrane protein phosphorylation, submitochondrial fractions or P$_2$ fractions were prepared according to previously described methods (9–11). P$_2$ fractions were resuspended in 6-mM Tris solution (pH 8.1) and allowed to stand for a minimum of 90 min. A pellet was obtained from this suspension and homogenized in a solution containing 5-mM magnesium acetate in 100-mM Tris, pH 7.45. This homogenate was then used in 60-μl incubations at 37°C with 3-μM (4–32P) ATP, magnesium acetate, calcium chloride, and sufficient water to equalize the volume. Phosphorylation was stopped by a solution of 6% sodium dodecyl sulfate (SDS), 10% BME, and 12% sucrose in 0.06-M Tris (pH 6.8).

Aliquots of proteins were separated electrophoretically using Laemmli's method and a vertical gel electrophoresis apparatus by BioRad (10). A separating gel of 10% acrylamide:BIS (33:0.08), 0.2% SDS, 0.1% ammonium persulfate, and 0.038% TEMED in 0.375-M Tris was used.

Figure 2 shows the densitogram of endogenously phosphorylated proteins in P$_2$ membrane fractions from rats subjected to a single PTZ sei-

TABLE 2. *Calcium outflow: inhibition by Na_i after PCMBS loading* [a]

Loading medium	Na_i (μmole/mg protein)	Total $^{45}Ca^{2+}$ outflow (μmole/g protein/min)
Control		
0 Na⁺	(a) 0.01 ± 0.01	0.30 ± 0.01
	(b) 0.12 ± 0.01	0.32 ± 0.01
	(c) 0.10 ± 0.01	0.30 ± 0.02
	(d) 0.14 ± 0.01	0.31 ± 0.01
80-mM Na⁺	(a) 0.60 ± 0.01	0.23 ± 0.01
	(b) 0.58 ± 0.01	0.24 ± 0.01
	(c) 0.60 ± 0.01	0.24 ± 0.01
	(d) 0.59 ± 0.01	0.24 ± 0.01
162-mM Na⁺	(a) 0.88 ± 0.01	0.15 ± 0.02
	(b) 0.90 ± 0.008	0.15 ± 0.01
	(c) 0.88 ± 0.01	0.13 ± 0.01
	(d) 0.80 ± 0.01	0.15 ± 0.01
ES-convulsed		
0 Na⁺	(a) 0.10 ± 0.01	0.30 ± 0.01
	(b) 0.11 ± 0.01	0.30 ± 0.02
	(c) 0.14 ± 0.01	0.33 ± 0.02
	(d) 0.15 ± 0.01	0.31 ± 0.01
162-mM Na⁺	(a) 0.92 ± 0.01	0.14 ± 0.01
	(b) 1.04 ± 0.008	0.14 ± 0.01
	(c) 1.08 ± 0.01	0.13 ± 0.01
	(d) 1.08 ± 0.01	0.12 ± 0.01

[a] Synaptosomes were simultaneously isolated from control and ES-convulsed animals and processed separately. The letters designate synaptosomes prepared simultaneously. Values of $^{45}Ca^{2+}$ outflow represent the means of three determinations ± SD. Four separate experiments are represented in which external Tris medium with 50-mM Na⁺ and 10-mM K⁺ was used.

zure (nine experiments). In all experiments performed, significant elevations in phosphorylation were observed in proteins with apparent molecular weights (MW) of 18,000 to 21,000. Small and insignificant changes were noted in phosphorylation of proteins with apparent MW of 50,000 and 60,000.

Quantitative analyses of the effects of ES convulsions and PTZ seizures are shown in Figs. 3 and 4 and Table 3. Percentage differences in phosphorylation were calculated after autoradiographs of P_2 fractions from control and convulsed animals were scanned. Specific areas on the densitogram representing the endogenous phosphorylation of proteins of 18,000 MW (18K proteins) were obtained for each experimental condition. The averages of six separate experiments were then used to obtain *p* values that indicated similarity or differences from the state of phosphorylation of re-

spective control animals. Figure 3 represents animals that were decapitated immediately after ES convulsions. The state of phosphorylation was optimally enhanced after 90 sec of incubation with 10-mM Mg^{2+} (64.8%) and/or 10-mM Ca^{2+} (64.4%). Enhanced phosphorylation could be detected even with 20 sec of incubation with 5-mM Mg^{2+} and no calcium (35%), 1-mM Ca^{2+} (44.9%), or 10-mM Ca^{2+} (31.1%). Interestingly, the percentage enhancement in phosphorylation of 18K proteins was not as marked when animals had daily seizures for 6 consecutive days.

Figure 4 shows that PTZ convulsions enhanced phosphorylation of membrane proteins considerably more than did ES convulsions. After 90 sec of incubation with 10-mM Mg^{2+}, phosphorylation of 18K proteins increased by 80% in the absence of external Ca^{2+}, by 136% with 1-mM Ca^{2+}, and by 148% with 10-mM Ca^{2+}. In contrast with the findings in ES convulsions, phosphorylation continued to be enhanced when animals had daily seizures for 6 consecutive days. For example, Fig. 4 shows that after 90 sec of incubation, phosphorylation was still elevated by 80% in the absence of external Ca^{2+}.

The persisting state of enhanced phosphorylation after PTZ seizures was more evident when animals were sacrificed 24 hr after a single convulsion or after the last of six daily convulsions (Fig. 5). Phosphorylation continued to be increased after 90 sec of incubation with 10-mM Mg^{2+} and no Ca^{2+} (by 57.6%), with 1-mM Ca^{2+} (by 83.6%), or with 10-mM Ca^{2+} (by 109.9%).

Additional differences were noted between ES convulsions and PTZ clonic-tonic-clonic seizures when periods of incubation were varied: 5-mM Mg^{2+} and 1-mM Ca^{2+} increased phosphorylation of 18K proteins by 55% in P_2 fractions from both controls and ES-convulsed animals after 20 sec of incubation. The enhanced state of phosphorylation induced by 5-mM Mg^{2+} and 1-mM Ca^{2+} had decreased after 90 sec of incubation. In contrast to these observations, 5-mM Mg^{2+} and 1-mM Ca^{2+} stimulated protein phosphorylation in PTZ seizures after 20 sec and 90 sec of incubation. These findings, in explaining the marked differences in phosphorylation between the control state and PTZ convulsions noted after 90 sec, also provide a reason for the quantitative differences noted between ES convulsions and PTZ seizures.

Of further importance is the enhancement in protein phosphorylation when PTZ (10^{-6}-M) was in-

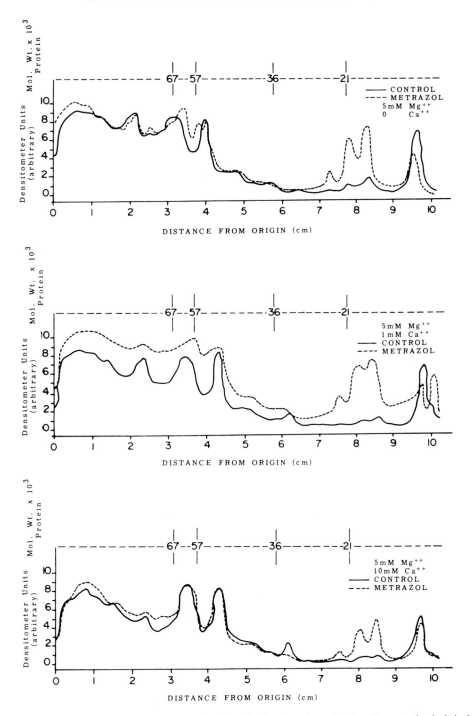

FIG. 2. Densitogram of endogenously phosphorylated proteins in P_2 membrane fractions from rats that had single PTZ clonic-tonic-clonic seizure (nine experiments). Similar experiments were performed in rats subjected to ES convulsions (five experiments). In all experiments, significant elevations in phosphorylation were observed in proteins with apparent molecular weights of 18,000 to 20,000.

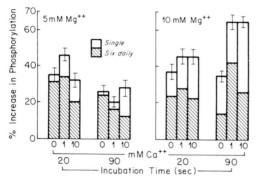

FIG. 3. Quantitative analysis of the effects of ES convulsions. Animals were decapitated immediately after convulsions. The state of phosphorylation was optimally enhanced after 90 sec of incubation with 10-mM Mg^{2+} (by 64.8%) and/or 10-mM Ca^{2+}. Enhanced phosphorylation could be detected even in the absence of calcium in the external medium. Note that stimulation of phosphorylation was not as marked when single convulsions were administered daily for 6 days.

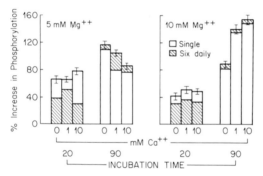

FIG. 4. Quantitative analysis of the effects of PTZ seizures. PTZ seizures enhanced protein phosphorylation considerably more than did ES convulsions. After 90 sec of incubation with 10-mM Mg^{2+}, phosphorylation of 18K proteins increased by 80% in the absence of external Ca^{2+}, by 136% with 1-mM Ca^{2+}, and by 148% with 10-mM Ca^{2+}. In contrast with the findings in ES convulsions, phosphorylation continued to be enhanced at a similar level after 6 days of seizures.

cubated *in vitro* with the membrane fractions. Stimulation of protein phosphorylation was maximal with 5-mM Mg^{2+} and 10-mM Ca^{2+} after 20 sec of incubation (Table 3).

DISCUSSION AND OUTLOOK

Our results show that repeated ES convulsions increased the calcium content in presynaptic terminals (9). We do not know the exact mechanism for this phenomenon. There are two possible explanations: First, the synaptosomal membrane may

be porous specifically to calcium ions. Second, the changes in calcium transport could be secondary to another primary ion event. Or both circumstances could be operative. After daily single convulsions for 6 days, the calcium transport system within synaptosomes appeared healthy and functional. No changes were observed in the ability of ATP or glutamate to stimulate calcium uptake. Modifying K_0, Na_0, or K_i produced identical results in controls and in convulsed animals. The only significant factor that appeared to explain the changes in the influx and efflux processes of calcium was the elevated concentration of sodium in synapses. When Na_i was increased by preincubating synaptosomes in a high-Na^+ medium, calcium influx proportionately increased in controls and ES-convulsed animals. Although more calcium moved inward in membranes from ES-convulsed rats, the accelerated influx could be explained by the higher baseline concentrations of Na_i. Increased base-line Na_i also accounted for the decreased calcium efflux from synaptosomes of ES-convulsed animals. Our results, therefore, favor the suggestion that Ca_i increased within synapses after *in vivo* ES convulsions secondary to a primary ionic event, namely an elevated Na_i. The rise in internal sodium *in vivo* then accelerated calcium influx while it decreased calcium outflow. Our results, however, do not rule out the possibility that calcium influx into synapses increased independently of Na_i during *in vivo* convulsions.

Raising Na_i promoted *in vitro* calcium influx while it antagonized calcium outflow. Raising Na_0 also antagonized calcium influx. Sigmoidal curves depicted the relationship between calcium outflow and external sodium concentrations in both convulsed and control states. This suggests that in both controls and convulsed animals the efflux of one Ca^{2+} ion was activated by more than a single Na^+—perhaps two or three, as suggested for barnacle and squid axons and synaptosomes (4,5,9). The preservation of this exchange system could have been responsible for the subsequent increase in calcium content within synapses when internal sodium rose after convulsions.

The increased calcium content of synaptic terminals produced by *in vivo* convulsions could have increased the *in vitro* net phosphorylation of 18K to 21K proteins of P_2 fractions. Ehrlich and associates were the first to show that protein band H-4 (MW 18,000) markedly and transiently increased [32P]-phosphate incorporation during ES

TABLE 3. *Effects of ES convulsions and PTZ in vivo and in vitro on phosphorylation of membrane proteins*[a]

	N/S[b]	20 sec						90 sec					
		5-mm Mg²⁺			10-mm Mg²⁺			5-mm Mg²⁺			10-mm Mg²⁺		
		0 Ca²⁺	1-mm Ca²⁺	10-mm Ca²⁺	0 Ca²⁺	1-mm Ca²⁺	10-mm Ca²⁺	0 Ca²⁺	1-mm Ca²⁺	10-mm Ca²⁺	0 Ca²⁺	1-mm Ca²⁺	10-mm Ca²⁺
ES[c]	1/0	+35	+44.9	+31.1	+36.5	+45.4	+45.3	+26.0 (<.05)[f]	+20 (<.02)	+30	+34.7	+64.8	+64.4
	1/24	−5.7 (ns)[e]	−10.1 (ns)	−27.8	−17.0	−13.1 (<0.02)	−20.5	−1.5 (ns)	−8.8 (ns)	−13.1 (ns)	−17.0	−4.4 (ns)	−10.9 (ns)
	6/0	+30.3	+34.2	+19.5 (<0.05)	+23.4	+27.7	+22.4	+22.9 (<0.02)	+16.0 (ns)	+12.1 (ns)	+14.2	+42.2	+26.0
	6/24	+20.6	+12.0 (<0.05)	+7.2 (ns)	+15.0	+19.2	+13.1	+22.6	+12.0 (ns)	+14.7 (ns)	+14.7	+24.0	+33.1
PTZ[d]	1/0	+64.1	+64.2	+76.1 (0.05)	+41.4	+49.7	+49.1	+111.0	+78.2 (ns)	+75.7 (ns)	+83.2	+135.9	+147.8
	1/24	−0.8 (ns)	+3.3 (ns)	−17.2 (0.05)	+7.0 (ns)	+0.2 (ns)	+1.9 (ns)	+0.7 (ns)	+0.8 (ns)	+2.6 (ns)	+7.6 (ns)	+4.4 (ns)	+29.8
	6/0	+38.2	+50.8	+29.4	+29.8	+34.5	+33.4	+113.4 (ns)	+104.4 (ns)	+85.2 (ns)	+88.0 (ns)	+137.7 (ns)	+150.7
	6/24	+21.3	+31.7	+16.5 (<0.05)	+21.5	+20.3	+20.5	+23.0	+28.4	+34.7	+57.6	+83.6	+109.9
PTZ *in vitro*		+30.3	+55.8	+79.1	+22.6	+29.2	+35.0	+0.7 (ns)	+5.3 (ns)	−1.1 (ns)	+6.1 (ns)	+3.7 (ns)	+2.8 (ns)

[a]Results pertain to percentage change in control.
[b]N = number of seizures; S = sacrificed immediately (0) or 24 hr after last convulsion.
[c]ES = electroshock convulsions.
[d]PTZ = pentylenetetrazol convulsions.
[e]ns = not statistically significant.
[f]p values are <0.001 unless noted.

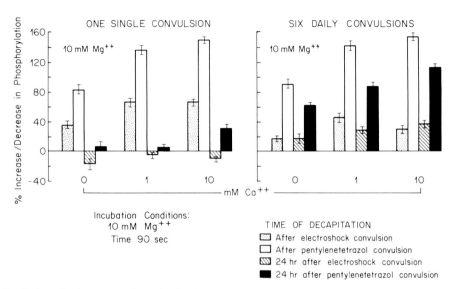

FIG. 5. Prolonged enhancement of protein phosphorylation after PTZ seizures. Twenty-four hours after a seizure or after the last of six daily convulsions, phosphorylation continued to be increased after 90 sec of incubation with 10-mM Mg^{2+} and no Ca^{2+} (by 57.6%), with 1-mM Ca^{2+} (by 83.6%), or with 10-mM Ca^{2+} (by 110%).

convulsions (16,18). Ehrlich's reports in 1978 also constituted the first demonstration of reversible changes in the phosphorylation of specific proteins in response to seizures (18). Our studies, in confirming his results on ES seizures, extend these findings to PTZ seizures and demonstrate, in addition, a prolonged state of enhanced phosphorylation after ES and PTZ seizures (11). The magnitude and longevity of this seizure-induced effect was remarkable, not only by itself but also because of its time relation to the demonstrated transmembrane shifts of Ca^{2+}. The increase in intrasynaptic Ca^{2+} content and the stimulated state of phosphorylation of 18K to 21K proteins were both reversible. Both conditions disappeared or were less evident when the time interval between the last convulsion and the actual sacrifice of the animal was lengthened. When rats were sacrificed 2 to 3 days after their last convulsions, calcium content and protein phosphorylation were still higher than control values. However, when animals were sacrificed 4 days after their last maximal seizures, the previously observed increased calcium content and protein phosphorylation were no longer evident. The close association and parallel behavior of both synaptic events lead us to suspect that the elevated calcium within synapses enhanced phsophorylation of the 18K to 21K proteins (10). One of the most fundamental properties of endogenous phosphorylation systems in brain fractions is their de-

pendence on Mg^{2+} and Ca^{2+}. Independent experiments from various laboratories (12,18,48), including ours, have shown inactivation of phosphorylatiòn of 18K membrane proteins in the presence of EGTA and restoration of phosphorylation with the addition of Mg^{2+} and Ca^{2+}.

Another reason we think the seizure-induced elevations in internal calcium stimulated the *in vitro* phosphorylation of proteins is the enhanced state of protein phosphorylation noted in the absence of Ca^{2+} in the external medium. This observation can be attributed to the presence of elevated and sufficient amounts of endogenous calcium to support protein phosphorylation. Synaptosomes and synaptic plasma membranes, in fact, contain significant concentrations of intrinsic calcium even in the absence of convulsions (11).

Of interest, in this regard, is the slight reduction in enhanced net phosphorylation of proteins after PTZ seizures noted when increasing calcium concentrations (1 to 10 mM) are added to the external medium. It is possible that higher calcium concentrations are by themselves inhibitory. Alternatively, calcium ATPase could have been activated, which would reduce the amount of [^{32}P]ATP available for stimulated phosphorylation.

Although these results suggest that the search in other experimental models of epilepsy now be directed toward a calcium-sensitive phosphorylation system in neural membranes, the possibility that the enhanced protein phosphorylation resulted from neuropeptide regulation should also be considered. Methionine-enkephalins and human β-endorphins inhibit phosphorylation of synaptic proteins *in vitro*, and it has been suggested that the accelerated release of peptides during convulsions inhibits phosphorylation of 18K proteins *in vivo* (17,18). This inhibition during seizure activity *in vivo* would be manifested by an apparent increase in ^{32}P-phosphate incorporation *in vitro*. The latter is in keeping with the studies of Weller and Rodnight (57), which have shown that the amount of phosphate transferred *in vitro* from ATP to membrane-bound proteins depends on the *in vivo* state of phosphorylation of these proteins. According to this explanation, increased phosphorylation of proteins *in vitro* reflects increased numbers of available phosphorylation sites due to decreased phosphorylation *in vivo*. We do not subscribe to this interpretation because of the correlative changes we observed in Ca^{2+} levels and membrane protein phosphorylation. The observations of *in vitro* PTZ stimulating protein phosphorylation also argue against this interpretation.

Is the phosphorylation of 18K membrane proteins a concomitant of calcium entry *in vivo*? Or is the enhanced ^{32}P-phosphate incorporation a reflection of regulation of calcium flux, rather than a consequence of calcium entry? Are calcium-mediated phosphorylations of membrane proteins parts of subsequent intrasynaptic events that lead to neurotransmitter release and possible repeated depolarizations? Are 18K proteins breakdown products of higher-molecular-weight proteins? What are their relationships, if any, to the various proteins described by Greengard and associates (30,54), DeLorenzo et al. (12–14), and Gordon et al. (19,20,21)? What are the relationships of 18K proteins to cyclic nucleotides (Table 3)?

Since Rall (44) first suggested adenosine 3':5'-monophosphate (cyclic AMP, cAMP) as the second messenger translating extracellular messages of circulating hormones into entracellular responses (44), an increasing body of evidence has shown that both cyclic AMP and cyclic GMP (guanosine 3':5'-monophosphate) translate neurotransmitter signals into appropriate cellular responses. Mediation of the inhibitory action of dopamine by cyclic AMP and the excitatory muscarinic action of acetylcholine by cyclic GMP is probably best documented in the superior cervical ganglion (24,25). The mediation of inhibitory action of norepinephrine by cyclic AMP in the cerebellar Purkinje cells is also well known (50).

In 1969, Kuo and Greengard hypothesized that the physiological effects of cyclic AMP in various tissues were mediated through regulation (by the cyclic nucleotide) of the phosphorylation of specific membrane proteins (30,54). These authors further proposed that cyclic-nucleotide-mediated protein phosphorylation, in turn, regulated membrane permeability to ions. To prove this point, correlative experiments between protein phosphorylation and physiological responses were performed in the toad bladder and avian erythrocytes. The toad bladder responds to antidiuretic hormone (ADH) with increased transepithelial sodium transport. This response results from an increase in passive membrane permeability to sodium and is mediated by cyclic AMP (40). DeLorenzo et al. (14) found that ADH caused a marked change in the level of phosphorylation of a specific protein in the toad bladder, and the time course of this ADH-induced biochemical effect was similar to the time course of the ADH-induced increase in sodium transport (Table 4). In avian erythrocytes, Rudolph and Greengard found that the β-adrenergic agonist isoproterenol increased ^{32}P incorporation into a single protein band of membrane origin (apparent MW 240,000) and that this effect of isoproterenol was mimicked by cyclic AMP. The dose-response curve for the phosphorylation of this protein was similar to the dose-response curve for cation fluxes. In addition, the time required (6 min) for a half-maximal increase in phosphorylation of this protein was similar to that for the half-maximal increase in cation flux (47). Since then, phosphorylation of various membrane proteins of differing molecular weights (Table 4) has been associated with increased Na^+ influx, as in red blood cell ghosts from myotonic dystrophy patients (46), and with increased calcium influx, as in synaptosomes (29) and synaptic vesicles (13). Interestingly, in the latter preparations, the association of membrane protein phosphorylation and ion fluxes has not been dependent on cyclic AMP.

In an effort to better understand the functions of these polypeptide substrates of different molecular weights, Uno, Ueda, and Greengard solubilized and purified the endogenous cAMP-dependent protein kinase of synaptic membrane fractions. They found them to require a divalent cation for significant activity; Mg^{2+}, Mn^{2+}, and Co^{2+} were considerably effective in supporting the phosphorylation

TABLE 4. *Correlations between protein phosphorylation and membrane ion flux*

Membrane	^{32}P incorporation	Protein MW	Effects of cAMP	Associated ion flux	References
Epithelium of toad bladder	↓ [a] with ADH[c]	50,000	↑	↑ Na$^+$ influx is stimulated by ADH	14
RBC (turkey)	↑ [b] with isoproterenol	240,000	↑	↑ Na$^+$ influx is stimulated by isoproterenol	47
RBC ghosts	→	100,000	ɸ[a]	↑ Na$^+$ influx	46
Muscle from myotonic dystrophy patients	→	50,000 (component 2)	ɸ	↑ Na$^+$ influx	46
	→	30,000 (component 2)	ɸ	↑ Na$^+$ influx	46
Synaptosomes	↑	80,000	ɸ	↑ Ca^{2+} influx	29
		86,000	ɸ	↑ Ca^{2+} influx	
Synaptic vesicles	↑ (inhibited by phenytoin)	60–63,000 (DPH-L)	ɸ	↑ Ca^{2+} influx is inhibited by phenytoin	13
	↑ (inhibited by phenytoin)	50–54,000 (DPH-M)	ɸ	↑ Ca^{2+} influx is inhibited by phenytoin	13
Mitochondria	↑ with EDTA	41,000	ɸ	Independent of Ca^{2+} influx	36
Crude mitochondrial fractions	↑ (inhibited by β-endorphin)	18,000	ɸ	↑ Ca^{2+} influx	11,17,18

[a] ↓ = inhibited.
[b] ↑ = stimulated.
[c] ADH = antidiuretic hormone.
[d] ɸ = not dependent on cAMP.

reaction (54). These investigators then found that of all the natural substrate proteins, only one, namely "protein 1" (MW 80,000 and 86,000), was specific to synaptic membranes, whereas "protein 2" had a widespread tissue distribution and was in fact the regulatory subunit of the cAMP-dependent protein kinase (MW 52,000) (54).

DeLorenzo also described several proteins weighing 60,000 to 63,000 and 50,000 to 54,000 that appear to be endogenous to the synaptic terminal more specifically to the synaptic vesicles. These proteins were designated DPh-L and DPh-M, respectively, because diphenylhydantoin or phenytoin inhibited phosphorylation. These protein phosphorylations have been suggested to be Ca^{2+}-stimulated and calmodulin-dependent (12,13).

Protein kinase activity and protein kinase substrates have also been demonstrated in membrane fractions enriched in the acetylcholine receptor (from the electric organ of *Torpedo californica*). In these fractions, phosphorylation of the 65,000-dalton component was maximally stimulated at 1-mM Na^+ and 100-mM K^+. Higher concentrations of Na^+ were less effective or inhibitory, whereas K^+ at low concentrations had no effect (19,20,21).

Thus, polypeptide substrates of differing molecular weights as the substrates of the brain protein kinase have been found in both innervated and noninnervated tissues, and the exact relationship between synaptic membrane phosphorylation and specific ionic permeability is still unclear. The wide distribution of the phosphorylation/dephosphorylation system for proteins and their purported roles in the synthesis, storage, and release of neurotransmitters (12), ion transport (13), and responses to depolarizing and hyperpolarizing stimuli (7,8, 45,48,49) have led to suggestions that there may be a common cellular mechanism in the various seizure processes. Potassium depolarization, electrical stimulation, and A23187 ionophore addition all facilitate calcium-dependent protein phosphorylation and neurotransmitter release (29). The relationship of protein phosphorylation to neurotransmitter release also raises the question whether or not the phosphorylation of low-molecular-weight proteins we observe is exclusively presynaptic. Pharmacological and immunocytochemical studies of phosphorylated higher-molecular-weight proteins IA and IB (86,000 and 80,000 MW, respectively) by Greengard and associates have localized these proteins to the synaptic vesicle (22). PTZ and picrotoxin also increase the state of phospho-

rylation of these proteins (53). In contrast, phenytoin has been shown to inhibit the phosphorylation of a 65K MW polypeptide of acetylcholine-receptor-enriched membranes purified from the electric organ of *T. californica* (21). The 18K protein has been observed in both P_2 and synaptosome fractions by Ehrlich et al. and in our laboratories. However, studies on these fractions have repeatedly indicated the possibility of postsynaptic membrane contamination. Postsynaptic dendritic processes, in addition to nerve terminals, may break off during homogenization and form resealed structures similar to light synaptosomes in their behavior on density-gradient centrifugation (2,35). Thus, more studies are needed to accurately determine if these 18K proteins are exclusively presynaptic or if they are also present in postsynaptic membranes (35,39) and glial cells (43,52).

REFERENCES

1. Bazan, N. G. (1971): Changes in free fatty acids of brain by drug-induced convulsions, ECT and anaesthesia. *J. Neurochem.*, 18:1379–1385.
2. Behrman, R. F., Huelihan, J. P., Kinnier, W. J., and Wilson, E. R. (1980): Phosphorylation of synaptic membranes. *J. Neurochem.*, 34:431–437.
3. Biswas, C., and Talwar, G. P. (1968): Effect of pentamethylene tetrazol (Metrazol) on rat brain phosphorylaze in vitro. *J. Neurochem.*, 15:107–113.
4. Blaustein, M. P., Johnson, E. M., Jr., and Needleman, P. (1972): Calcium-dependent norepinephrine release from presynaptic nerve endings in vitro. *Proc. Natl. Acad. Sci. U.S.A.*, 69:2237–2240.
5. Blaustein, M. P., and Osborn, C. J. (1975): The influence of sodium on calcium fluxes in pinched-off nerve terminals in vitro. *J. Physiol. (Lond.)*, 247:657–686.
6. David, R. J., Wilson, R. A., and Delgado-Escueta, A. V. (1974): Voltage clamp analysis of pentylenetetrazol effects on *Aplysia* neurones. *Brain Res.*, 67:549–554.
7. de Belleroche, J. S., and Bradford, H. F. (1972): The stimulus-induced release of acetylcholine from synaptosome beds and its calcium dependence. *J. Neurochem.*, 19:1817–1819.
8. de Belleroche, J. S., and Bradford, H. F. (1972): Metabolism of beds of mammalian cortical synaptosomes: Response to depolarizing influences. *J. Neurochem.*, 19:585–602.
9. Delgado-Escueta, A. V., Davidson, D., and Victor, S. (1980): The effects of seizures on calcium transport within synaptosomes. *J. Neurochem.*, 34:1140–1148.
10. Delgado-Escueta, A. V., and Horan, M. P. (1980): Brain synapses in epilepsy. In: *Mechanism of Action of Antiepileptic Drugs*, edited by G. Glazer, J. K. Penry, and D. Woodbury, Raven Press, New York.
11. Delgado-Escueta, A. V., and Horan, M. P. (1982): The effects of pentylenetetrazol and electroshock con-

vulsions on phosphorylation of cerebral cortical membrane proteins. *J. Neurochem.*, *(in press)*.

12. DeLorenzo, R. J. (1976): Calcium-dependent phosphorylation of specific synaptosomal fraction proteins: Possible role of phosphoproteins in mediating neurotransmitter release. *Biochem. Biophys. Res. Commun.*, 71:590–597.

13. DeLorenzo, R. J., and Freedman, S. D. (1978): Calcium dependent neurotransmitter release and protein phosphorylation in synaptic vesicles. *Biochem. Biophys. Res. Commun.*, 80:183–192.

14. DeLorenzo, R. J., Walton, K. G., Curran, P. F., and Greengard, P. (1973): Regulation of phosphorylation of a specific protein in toad-bladder membrane by antidiuretic hormone and cyclic AMP and its possible relationship to membrane permeability changes. *Proc. Natl. Acad. Sci. U.S.A.*, 79:880.

15. Dunn, A. N., Giuditta, A., and Pagliuca, N. (1971): The effect of electroconvulsive shock on protein synthesis in mouse brain. *J. Neurochem.*, 18:2093–2099.

16. Ehrlich, Y. H. (1979): Phosphoproteins as specifiers for mediators and modulators in neuronal function. *Adv. Exp. Med. Biol.* 116:75–101.

17. Ehrlich, Y. H., Davis, L. G., Keen, P., and Brunngraber, E. G. (1980): Endorphin-regulated protein phosphorylation in brain membranes. *Life Sci.*, 26:1795–1772.

18. Ehrlich, Y. H., Reddy, M. V., Keen, P., Davis, L. G., Daugherty, J., and Brunngraber, E. G. (1980): Transient changes in the phosphorylation of cortical membrane proteins after electoconvulsive shock. *J. Neurochem.*, 34:1327–1330.

19. Gordon, A. S., Davis, C. G., Milfay, D., Kaur, J., and Diamond, I. (1980): Membrane-bound protein kinase activity in acetylcholine receptor-enriched membranes. *Biochim. Biophys. Acta*, 600:421–431.

20. Gordon, A. S., Milfay, D., Davis, C. G., and Diamond, I. (1979): Protein phosphatase activity in acetylcholine receptor-enriched membranes. *Biochem. Biophys. Res. Commun.*, 87:876–883.

21. Gordon, A. S., Milfay, D., and Diamond, I. (1979): Phosphorylation of the membrane-bound acetylcholine receptor: Inhibition by diphenylhydantoin. *Ann. Neurol.*, 5:201–203.

22. Greengard, P. (1978): *Cyclic Nucleotides, Phosphorylated Proteins and Neuronal Function.* Raven Press, New York.

23. Hefti, F., and Lichtensteiger,W. (1978): Subcellular distribution of dopamine in substantia nigra of the rat brain: Effect of γ-butyrolactone and destruction of noradrenergic afferents suggest formation of particles from dendrites. *J. Neurochem.*, 30:1217–1230.

24. Kebabian, J. W., and Greengard, P. (1971): Dopamine sensitive adenyl cyclase: Possible role in synaptic transmission. *Science*, 174:1346.

25. Kebabian, J. W., Steiner, A. L., and Greengard, P. (1975): Muscarinic cholinergic regulation of cyclic guanosine 3'5'-monophosphate in autonomic ganglia: Possible role in synaptic transmission. *J. Pharmacol. Exp. Ther.*, 193:474.

26. Kety, S. S., Javoy, F., Thierry, A. R., Julou, L., and Glowinski, J. A. (1967): A sustained effect of electroconvulsive shock on the turnover of norepinephrine in the central nervous system of the rat. *Proc. Natl. Acad. Sci. U.S.A.*, 58:1240.

27. King, L. J., Lowry, O. H., and Passoneau, J. V. (1976): Effects of convulsants on energy reserves in cerebral cortex. *J. Neurochem.*, 14:599–611.

28. Klee, M., Faber, D., and Heiss, W. (1973): Strychnine and pentylenetetrazol-induced changes of excitability in *Aplysia* neurons. *Science*, 179:1133–1136.

29. Krueger, B. K., Form, J., and Greengard, P. (1977): Depolarization-induced phosphorylation of specific proteins, mediated by calcium ion flux in rat brain synaptosomes. *J. Biol. Chem.*, 252:2764–2773.

30. Kuo, F. J., and Greengard, P. (1969): Cyclic nucleotide-dependent protein kinases. IV. Widespread occurrence of adenosine 3'5'-monophosphate-dependent protein kinase in various tissue and phyla of the animal kingdom. *Proc. Natl. Acad. Sci. U.S.A.*, 64:1349.

31. Lewin, E. (1976): Endogenously released adenine derivatives: A possible role in epileptogenesis. *Trans. Am. Neurol. Assoc.*, 101:192–195.

32. Loscher, W., and Frey, H. H. (1977): Effect of convulsant and anticonvulsant agents on level and metabolism of γ-aminobutyric acid in mouse brain. *Naunyn Schmiedebergs Arch. Pharmacol.*, 296:263–269.

33. Lust, W. D., Goldberg, N. D., and Passoneau, J. V. (1976): Cyclic nucleotides in murine brain: The temporal relationship of changes induced in adenosine 3'5' monophosphate and guanosine 3'5' monophosphate following maximal electroshock or decapitation. *J. Neurochem.*, 26:5–10.

34. MacDonald, R. L., and Barker, J. L. (1977): Penicillin and pentylenetetrazol selectively antagonize GABA-mediated postsynaptic inhibition of cultured mammalian neurons. *Neurology (Minneap.)*, 27:337.

35. Madeira, V. M. C., and Artunes-Madeira, M. C. (1973): Interaction of Ca^{2+} and Mg^{2+} with synaptic plasma membranes. *Biochim. Biophys. Acta*, 232:369–407.

36. Magilen, G., Gordon, A., Au, A., and Diamond, I. (1981): Identification of a mitochondrial phosphoprotein in brain synaptic membrane preparation. *J. Neurochem.*, 36:1861–1865.

37. Mahon, P. J., and Bruik, J. J. (1970): Inhibition of acetylcholinesterase in vitro by pentylenetetrazol. *J. Neurochem.*, 17:949–953.

38. Metafora, S., Persico, M., Felsani, A. Ferraiulo, R., and Giuditta, A. (1977): On the mechanism of electroshock-induced inhibition of protein synthesis in rabbit cerebral cortex. *J. Neurochem.*, 28:1335–1346.

39. Ng, M., and Matus, A. (1979): Protein phosphorylation in isolated plasma membranes and postsynaptic junctional structures from brain synapses. *Neuroscience*, 4:169–180.

40. Orloff, J., and Handler, J. (1967): The role of adenosine 3'5'-phosphate in the action of antidiuretic hormone. *Am. J. Med.*, 42:751.

41. Pellmar, T. C., and Wilson, W. A. (1977): Synaptic mechanism of pentylenetetrazol: Selectivity for chloride conductance. *Science*, 197:912–914.

42. Pryor, G. T., and Otis, L. S. (1969): Brain biochemical and behavioral effects of 1, 2, 4, or 8 weeks electroshock treatment. *Life Sci.*, 118:387.

43. Raine, C. S., Wisniewski, H. M., Iobal, K., Grundkelobal, J., and Nerton, W. T. (1977): Studies on the encephalitogenic effects of purified preparations of

human and bovine oligodendrocytes. *Brain Res.*, 120:269–286.

44. Rall, T. W. (1972): Roll of adenosine 3'5'-monophosphate (cyclic AMP) in actions of catecholamines. *Pharmacol. Rev.*, 24:399.

45. Redburn, D. A., Shelton, D., and Cotman, C. W. (1976): Calcium dependent release of exogenously loaded γ-amino ¹⁴-C-butyrate from synaptosomes: Time course of stimulation by potassium, veratridine and the calcium ionophore A23187. *J. Neurochem.*, 26:297–303.

46. Roses, A. D., and Appel, S. H. (1974): Muscle membrane protein kinase in myotonic muscular dystrophy. *Nature*, 250:245–247.

47. Rudolph, S. A., and Greengard, P. (1974): Regulation of protein phosphorylation and membrane permeability by β-adrenergic agents and cyclic adenosine 3'5'-monophosphate in the avian erythrocyte. *J. Biol. Chem.*, 249:5684.

48. Schulman, H., and Greengard, P. (1978): Stimulation of brain membrane protein phosphorylation by calcium and an endogenous heat-stable protein. *Nature*, 271:478–479.

49. Sieghart, W., Forn, L., Schwarcz, R., Coyle, J. T., and Greengard, P. (1978): *Brain Res.*, 156:345–350.

50. Siggins, G. R., Oliver, A. P., Hoffer, B. J., and Bloom, F. E. (1971): Cyclic adenosine monophosphate and norepinephrine: Effects on transmembrane properties of cerebellar Purkinje cells. *Science*, 171:192.

51. Skolnick, P., Syapin, P., Paugh, B., Moncada, V., Marangos, P., and Paul, S. (1979): Inosine, an endogenous ligand of the brain benzodiazepine receptor antagonizes PTZ-induced seizures. *Proc. Natl. Acad. Sci. U.S.A.*, 76:1515–1518.

52. Steck, A., and Appel, S. H. (1977): Phosphorylation of myelin basic protein. *J. Biol. Chem.*, 249:5415–5420.

53. Strombom, U., Forn, J., Dolphin, A. C., and Greengard, P. (1979): Regulation of the state of phosphorylation of specific neuronal proteins in mouse brain by in vivo administration of anaesthetic and convulsant agents. *Proc. Natl. Acad. Sci. U.S.A.*, 76:4687–4690.

54. Uno, I., Ueda, T., and Greengard, P. (1977): Adenosine 3'5'-monophosphate-regulated phosphoprotein system of neuronal membranes. II. Solubilization, purification and some properties of an endogenous adenosine 3'5'-monophosphate-dependent protein kinase. *J. Biol. Chem.*, 252:5164–5174.

55. Vesco, C., and Giuditta, A. (1968): Disaggregation of brain polysomes induced by electroconvulsive treatment. *J. Neurochem.*, 15:81–85.

56. Wasterlain, C. G. (1977): Effects of epileptic seizures on brain ribosomes: Mechanism and relationship to cerebral energy metabolism. *J. Neurochem.*, 29:707–716.

57. Weller, M., and Rodnight, R. (1973): The state of phosphorylation in vivo of membrane-bound phosphoproteins in rat brain. *Biochem. J.*, 133:387–389.

58. Wilson, W. A., and Delgado-Escueta, A. V. (1974): Common synaptic effects of pentylenetetrazol and penicillin. *Brain Res.*, 72:168–171.

59. Woodbury, D. M. (1958): Effects of diphenylhydantoin on electrolytes and radiosodium turnover in brain and other tissues of normal, hyponatremic and postictal rats. *J. Pharmacol. Exp. Ther.*, 115:74–95.

60. Woodbury, D. M. (1980): Convulsant drugs: Mechanism of action. In: *Antiepileptic Drugs: Mechanism of Action*, edited by G. H. Glaser, J. K. Penry, and D. M. Woodbury, Raven Press, New York.

Advances in Neurology, Vol. 34: Status
Epilepticus, edited by A.V. Delgado-Escueta,
C.G. Wasterlain, D.M. Treiman, and R.J. Porter.
Raven Press, New York © 1983.

30

Calcium-Calmodulin Protein Phosphorylation in Neuronal Transmission: A Molecular Approach to Neuronal Excitability and Anticonvulsant Drug Action

Robert John DeLorenzo

The name epilepsy refers to the many varieties of recurrent seizures produced by paroxysmal excessive neuronal discharges in different parts of the brain (28,29,31). Status epilepticus represents an extreme situation in which seizures occur so frequently that there is little if any time between seizures (27,50).

Study of the epilepsies has revealed that this condition really refers to numerous situations that produce seizures (29). There are many types of epilepsy, and the possible causes of seizures are numerous. Thus, no one simple approach will allow us to fully understand the nature of this complex clinical phenomenon.

In an attempt to develop a biochemical approach to epilepsy (11), it is important to focus on a particular aspect of neuronal function that might be related to seizure activity and study it in detail. Because the synapse is a major site for neuronal communication, excitatory and inhibitory synaptic transmissions are believed to regulate ongoing neuronal discharges in the brain (23). Thus the synapse is a major site where control of neuronal activity can be exerted. Alterations in "normal" synaptic activity can produce an overly excitable neuronal population, representing the substrate for seizure discharge (23–25). The importance of synaptic activity in relation to epilepsy and the actions of anticonvulsant drugs have been well reviewed (23).

A MOLECULAR APPROACH TO NEURONAL EXCITABILITY

Experiments in our laboratory have been directed at understanding specific biochemical processes that relate to synaptic function (7–19). Calcium ions play a major role in regulating synaptic activity (21,31,34,35,41,43), and several of the excitatory effects of calcium on synaptic function have been shown to be antagonized by the anticonvulsant phenytoin (22,26,30,39,44–47,54). Thus, synaptic biochemical processes that are stimulated by calcium and inhibited by phenytoin are of considerable interest, because they may represent a molecular process that modulates neuronal excitability.

Numerous enzyme systems were studied in our laboratory in the early 1970s in an attempt to find a calcium-stimulated phenytoin-inhibited process. We identified a unique calcium-stimulated protein phosphorylation system in brain that was also inhibited by phenytoin (7,8,11,12). It is important to emphasize that this calcium kinase system is a protein phosphorylation system distinct from the well-described brain cyclic AMP protein kinases (3). Thus, efforts in our laboratory have been directed at determining the role of calcium-dependent protein phosphorylation in modulating synaptic function and neuronal excitability. The following sections present the evidence for involvement of the calcium-calmodulin protein kinase system in modulating synaptic excitability and anticonvulsant drug action.

EFFECTS OF PHENYTOIN AND CALCIUM ON PROTEIN PHOSPHORYLATION IN THE PRESYNAPTIC NERVE TERMINAL

The effect of phenytoin on calcium-dependent phosphorylation in whole-brain preparations was shown to be present in preparations enriched in presynaptic nerve terminals, synaptosomes (8,14). Calcium caused a dramatic increase in the level of endogenous phosphorylation of proteins DPH-L and DPH-M, with molecular weights of 60,000 to 63,000 and 50,000 to 54,000, respectively (8,14). These phosphoproteins in the synaptosomal preparation migrated and behaved indentically as proteins DPH-L and DPH-M from homogenate preparations. Phenytoin inhibited the calcium-dependent phosphorylation of proteins DPH-L and DPH-M by more than 40% to 50%. These results demonstrate that the calcium-dependent phosphorylation of proteins DPH-L and DPH-M is observed in synaptosomal preparations and that phenytoin can inhibit this phosphorylation in therapeutic concentrations.

Because synaptosome preparations have been shown to be heterogeneous in composition, it is important to demonstrate that the calcium-dependent phosphorylation of proteins DPH-L and DPH-M occurs within the presynaptic nerve endings, not in the membrane, glial cell fragments, or mitochondrial contaminations of this synaptosomal fraction. Attempts were made to determine if synaptosomal phosphoproteins DPH-L and DPH-M 0could be clearly localized within the presynaptic nerve terminal. Following osmotic shock, presynaptic nerve terminal preparations were subfractionated into synaptic membrane and synaptosome mitochondria by previously established techniques (Table 1). Synaptosome soluble protein and a highly purified synaptic vesicle fraction were obtained by our previously described procedure (1). The composition of each synaptosome subfraction was con-

firmed by electron microscopy and enzyme markers. The composition of the synaptic vesicle fraction demonstrated that this fraction was highly purified, containing both plain and coated synaptic vesicles and less than 4% to 5% contamination by small membrane fragments. The synaptic membrane fraction was free of mitochondria, but contained a small percentage of synaptic vesicles. The synaptosomal mitochondria fraction was enriched in mitochondria, but also contained some unbroken synaptosomes and large membrane fragments.

The effects of calcium and phenytoin on the net levels of phosphorylation of proteins DPH-L and DPH-M in each synaptosomal subfraction were determined. The specific activity of the calcium-stimulated phosphorylation of proteins DPH-L and DPH-M was highly enriched in the synaptic vesicle fraction. The calcium-dependent phosphorylation of these synaptic-vesicle-associated proteins was significantly inhibited by phenytoin. The effects of DPH and calcium on the phosphorylation of synaptic-vesicle-associated proteins DPH-L and DPH-M were independent of ATP concentration over the range 0.5 to 50 μM. The soluble synaptosomal fraction showed significant calcium-stimulated phosphorylation.

Proteins DPH-L and DPH-M are clearly present in highly purified synaptic vesicle preparations. Calcium and phenytoin have the same antagonistic effects on the levels of these synaptic vesicle proteins as on proteins DPH-L and DPH-M in the synaptosome preparation. Because synaptic vesicles are localized within the presynaptic nerve terminal and are not found in glial or other synaptosome fraction contaminations, these results demonstrate that the antagonistic actions of DPH and calcium on brain protein phosphorylation occur within the presynaptic nerve terminal in close association with the synaptic vesicles. The localization of phosphoproteins DPH-L and DPH-M within the presynaptic nerve terminal indicates that the antagonistic effects of phenytoin and calcium on the levels of phosphorylation on these presynaptic nerve terminal proteins could account for the opposing effects of phenytoin and calcium on the release of neurotransmitter from the presynaptic nerve ending.

DEVELOPMENT OF A MORE PHYSIOLOGICALLY ACTIVE SYNAPTIC VESICLE PREPARATION

To study neurotransmitter release from synaptic vesicles, it was important to develop a vesicle

TABLE 1. *Effects of calcium and phenytoin on the net level of phosphorylation of proteins DPH-L and DPH-M in synaptosomal subfractions*[a]

Synaptosomal subfraction	Protein DPH-L			Protein DPH-M		
	Calcium	Calcium + phenytoin		Calcium	Calcium + phenytoin	
Synaptic vesicle fraction	356[b]	903	479	423	1,466	739
Synaptic membrane fraction	178	271	205	391	516	451
Synaptosome mitochondria fraction	206	349	266	363	526	427
Synaptosome soluble fraction	332	632	427	416	703	598

[a]Reactions were conducted under standard conditions except for the presence or absence of calcium ions (10 μM) or DPH (80 μM). Each value represents the mean from six experiments. The largest range about the mean was ±33 counts per minute, and thus the ranges were omitted for clarity.
[b]Counts per minute above background per 300 μg of subfraction protein.

preparation that was stable and as physiologically active as possible. Experiments were initiated to prepare synaptic vesicles under numerous preparation conditions to determine if methods of preparation could affect the physiological viability of vesicles (15,17). The first set of experiments demonstrated that the norepinephrine content of synaptic vesicles isolated from whole brain was significantly influenced by the methods of preparation (15,17). Vesicles were isolated under isotonic and hypotonic conditions, at different pH values, and under different techniques of preparation.

Preparations of presynaptic nerve terminals (synaptosomes) were isolated by standard techniques (18). Synaptic vesicles are traditionally isolated from synaptosomes, by inducing osmotic shock of the synaptosome preparation and isolating the vesicles by differential centrifugation (20). The hypotonic and nonphysiological conditions that result during these procedures produce synaptic vesicle preparations that have low neurotransmitter content.

Several support solutions (Table 2) were used to attempt to restore a more physiological intracellular environment following osmotic shock and release of synaptic vesicles. One of these physiological support media developed in this investigation, designated Iso-KCl medium, produced the highest norepinephrine content. Isotonic sucrose was not as good. Hypotonic buffered media were also not as good support solutions. Standard hypotonic methods for isolating synaptic vesicles from brain caused a significant reduction in norepinephrine content of vesicles, and the vesicles were very unstable in such solutions in the absence of added soluble protein. In addition to support media, it as shown that more vigorous homogenization during osmotic shock of the P$_2$ pellet, prolongation of the preparation time, and increasing or decreasing pH significantly affected the neurotransmitter content of the vesicles.

These experiments developed an isolation procedure for synaptic vesicles that produced significantly higher vesicle neurotransmitter content. This vesicle preparation was then employed to study the possible role of calcium-dependent protein phosphorylation in neurotransmitter release.

CALCIUM-DEPENDENT NEUROTRANSMITTER RELEASE AND PROTEIN PHOSPHORYLATION IN SYNAPTIC VESICLES

The effect of calcium on the release of neurotransmitter substances from synaptic vesicles was investigated. Calcium ions caused a marked decrease in the norepinephrine content of vesicles prepared in Iso-KCl medium, but had much less effect on the release on neurotransmitter from vesicles prepared in sucrose or hypotonic medium (Table 2).

In the standard vesicle preparation (Iso-KCl), calcium caused a significant decrease in norepinephrine content of synaptic vesicles and a corresponding increase in the amount of norepinephrine released from the vesicles. The action of calcium on neurotransmitter release was dependent on the presence of magnesium. The calcium ion concentration required to produce a half-maximal increase in norepinephrine release under standard conditions was approximately 10 μM.

TABLE 2. *Effects of calcium and calmodulin on norepinephrine content and protein phosphorylation in synaptic vesicles prepared under different conditions[a]*

Preparation conditions	Norepinephrine content (%)		Protein DPH-M phosphorylation (%)	
	Control	Calcium	Control	Calcium
Physiologic medium (Iso-KCl)	100	55.6	9.3	100
Prolonged preparation time	89.6	81.7	4.2	8.3
Tris-maleate, 10 mM, pH 6.5	42.1	39.7	3.9	8.3
Distilled water	38.2	35.6	3.1	9.1

[a]Synaptic vesicles were isolated for protein phosphorylation and neurotransmitter release as described previously (18). Vesicles were isolated by centrifugation from osmotically shocked synaptosomes. Following osmotic shock of synaptosomes with distilled water, samples were centrifuged directly or after suspension in physiological medium or Tris-maleate buffer. Brains were homogenized within 15 sec of decapitation. For prolonged preparation times, brains were homogenized 5 min after decapitation (3). Each value represents the mean of eight determinations and is expressed as percentage of the maximal value or maximal stimulation (100%). Maximal values (100%) for morepinephrine content and protein DPH-M phosphorylation were 5.78 ng/ mg (protein) and 2,333 cpm/500 μg (protein), respectively. Largest ± SEM was ±5.1%.

The effects of calcium ions on the level of endogenous phosphorylation of synaptic vesicle proteins were simultaneously studied in the same preparation employed to investigate calcium-dependent norepinephrine release (Fig. 1). Calcium caused a dramatic increase in the phosphorylation of synaptic-vesicle-associated proteins with half-maximal Ca^{2+} levels of 0.8 and 0.9 μM, respectively. Calcium ion concentrations were determined employing a Ca^{2-}-EGTA buffer solution as described previously (10). Calcium ions stimulated both the initial rate and the net level of phosphorylation of synaptic-vesicle-associated proteins DPH-L and DPH-M and caused a greater percentage stimulation in the level of phosphorylation of proteins DPH-L and DPH-M in this preparation than in the hypotonic Tris-maleate preparation of synaptic vesicles. The effects of calcium ions on the phosphorylation of proteins DPH-L and DPH-M were dependent on magnesium ions. Proteins DPH-L and DPH-M demonstrated only minimal magnesium-dependent phosphorylation.

PHENYTOIN INHIBITION OF CALCIUM-DEPENDENT PROTEIN PHOSPHORYLATION AND NEUROTRANSMITTER RELEASE

Phenytoin has been shown to inhibit calcium-dependent neurotransmitter release in several preparations (22,30,39,44–47,54). If synaptic vesicle protein phosphorylation mediates calcium-dependent release of neurotransmitter from the nerve terminal, phenytoin might be expected to inhibit this calcium-dependent protein phosphorylation and norepinephrine release in synaptic vesicle preparations.

To further elucidate the role of synaptic-vesicle-associated phosphoproteins in neurotransmitter release, it would be important to demonstrate that calcium ions stimulated both neurotransmitter release and protein phosphorylation in the same preparation. The following results from this investigation suggested a more direct relationship between synaptic-vesicle-associated protein phosphorylation and neurotransmitter release by simultaneously determining the effects of phenytoin and calcium ions on neurotransmitter release and protein phosphorylation in the same preparation of highly purified synaptic vesicles isolated from rat brain.

Phenytoin was shown to inhibit both the calcium-dependent release of neurotransmitter and stimulation of protein phosphorylation in synaptic vesicles (11). The concentrations of phenytoin required to produce half-maximal inhibition of calcium-stimulated norepinephrine release and protein phosphorylation were 8×10^{-5} and 9.5×10^{-5} M, respectively. Phenytoin inhibited both the net level and the rate of calcium-dependent release and phosphorylation. These effects of phenytoin on neurotransmitter release and protein phosphorylation in synaptic vesicles were shown to be independent of ATP concentration.

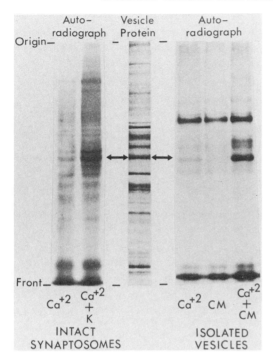

FIG. 1. Phosphorylation of vesicle protein. Effects of calmodulin (CM) and Ca^{2+} on protein phosphorylation in isolated calmodulin-depleted synaptic vesicles *(right)* and of depolarization-dependent Ca^{2+} uptake on protein phosphorylation of synaptic vesicles isolated from ^{32}P-labeled intact synaptosomes *(left)*. For experiments with isolated vesicles, γ-^{32}P-ATP was added to the reaction mixture and incubated for 1 min in the presence and/or absence of Ca^{2+} (free $[Ca^{2+}]$, 10 μM) and CM (5 μg). For experiments with intact synaptosomes, synaptosomes were preincubated with ^{32}P and then incubated with Ca^{2+} (1 mM) or Ca^{2+} (1 mM) plus K^+ (65 mM). Following incubation, synaptic vesicles were rapidly isolated from each incubated synaptosome reaction and analyzed for vesicle protein phosphorylations (10). Protein DPH-M is designated by arrows. (From DeLorenzo, ref. 10, with permission.)

BIOCHEMICAL MECHANISM MEDIATING CALCIUM'S ACTIONS ON SYNAPTIC VESICLE PREPARATIONS: CALMODULIN

Calcium's role in neurotransmitter release from the presynaptic nerve terminal has been a subject of great interest in the neurosciences, but little is known about the molecular mechanisms of Ca^{2+} in stimulating neurotransmitter release or its other physiological functions in the nerve terminal. Recent studies have suggested that some of calcium's effects on nerve function may be modulated by a heat-stable Ca^{2+} receptor protein with specific and strong binding affinity for Ca^{2+}. These results plus the presence of calmodulinlike proteins in a wide variety of mammalian and invertebrate tissues have suggested that many of calcium's physiological functions may be mediated by Ca^{2+}-receptor proteins such as calmodulin (6,38).

It would be of great importance to demonstrate that calmodulin or calmodulinlike proteins play a role in mediating calcium's effect on depolarization-dependent neurotransmitter release. Our approach to this question has been to study the physiologically active preparation of synaptic vesicles that has been developed in our laboratory, demonstrating both Ca^{2+}-dependent neurotransmitter release and protein phosphorylation. The vesicle preparation offers distinct advantages for studying the effects of calmodulin on these Ca^{2+}-dependent vesicle functions and may offer new insights into the molecular mechanism of neurotransmitter release from the intact nerve terminal.

It has been shown that the removal of an endogenous heat-stable protein fraction from synaptic vesicle preparations abolishes calcium's effects on neurotransmitter release and protein phosphorylation in this preparation (18). Calcium's ability to stimulate release and phosphorylation was restored to the treated vesicle preparation when synaptic vesicle extract (SVE) or boiled SVE was added back to the vesicle preparation (Table 3). SVE did not significantly stimulate calcium's effects on release and phosphorylation in plain or washed synaptic vesicle preparation, indicating that these preparations were saturated with endogenously bound activator. Heat-stable SVE did not exhibit endogenous Ca^{2+}- or Mg^{2+}-dependent protein phosphorylation, nor did it show protein kinase activity with the artificial substrates histone, casein, or protamine. Characterization of SVE by treatment with heat, dialysis, DNase, RNase, and trypsin demonstrated that the active factor in SVE responsible for restoring calcium-dependent norepinephrine release and protein phosphorylation to treated vesicles was heat-stable and protein in nature.

CALMODULIN AND CALCIUM ACTIVATE SYNAPTIC VESICLE NOREPINEPHRINE RELEASE AND PROTEIN PHOSPHORYLATION

The heat stability and the properties of the stimulating factor in SVE suggested a possible relationship to calmodulin that modulates adenylate

TABLE 3. *Effects of phenytoin, SVE, and calmodulin on calcium-stimulated synaptic vesicle neurotransmitter release and protein phosphorylations*[a]

Condition	Calcium-stimulated norepinephrine release		Calcium-stimulated protein DPH-M phosphorylation	
	ng	%	cpm	%
Plain vesicles	28	53.1	1,131	303
+ phenytoin	16	20.2	521	126
Washed vesicles	22	43.2	1,078	297
+ phenytoin	14	18.6	492	110
Treated vesicles	5	9.3	143	36
+ SVE	21	46.3	1,129	313
+ SVE + phenytoin	11	21.4	512	154
+ Calmodulin	23	47.8	1,158	325
+ Calmodulin + phenytoin	15	24.6	631	173

[a]Plain, washed, or treated synaptic vesicles were incubated for 1 min under standard conditions (18) to study neurotransmitter release (10 mg of vesicle protein containing 4.3–5.6 ng of norepinephrine per milligram of protein) and protein phosphorylation (1 mg of vesicle protein) with or without the addition of SVE (20 μg), calmodulin (20 μg), or phenytoin (9 $\times$ 10^{-5} M) in the presence or absence of calcium. The reactions were terminated by centrifugation at 4°C, and vesicle norepinephrine content and protein DPH-M phosphorylation were measured. Endogenous Ca^{2+}-stimulated norepinephrine release and protein DPH-M phosphorylation are expressed as the difference between control and Ca^{2+}-stimulated reactions in vesicle norepinephrine content (nanograms released) and protein DPH-M phosphorylation (cpm of ^{32}P-phosphate incorporated per 100 μg of reaction protein); percentage Ca^{2+}-stimulated release and phosphorylation are expressed compared to control conditions. Total recovery of released and bound norepinephrine was 95% to 100%. Results qualitatively similar to those for DPH-M were obtained for protein DPH-L and other protein bands shown in Fig. 1. Data are the means of five determinations, representative of four separate experiments. The largest SEM values for release, phosphorylation, percentage release, and percentage phosphorylation were 4 ng, 122 cpm, 8%, and 23% respectively, and were omitted for clarity. Data from DeLorenzo (11).

cyclase and cyclic-nucleotide-dependent phosphodiesterase activities (10,18). Thus, calmodulin was purified to homogeneity from bovine and rat brain preparations to test its effect on the vesicle preparation (10). Bovine and rat preparations of calmodulin migrated as single bands of essentially identical molecular weights on SDS-polyacrylamide-gel electrophoresis (Fig. 2). Both preparations of calmodulin were as effective as SVE in restoring calcium's ability to stimulate norepinephrine release and protein phosphorylation (Fig. 1) when added to treated vesicle preparations. Calmodulin-depleted cyclic-nucleotide-dependent phosphodiesterase was prepared from rat brain by DEAE-cellulose-column chromatography to determine if SVE was as effective as calmodulin in activating this enzyme system. Calmodulin and boiled SVE were equally effective in stimulating activator-deficient phosphodiesterase. These results indicate that SVE and calmodulin are functionally equivalent in their abilities to stimulate calcium-dependent phosphodiesterase activity, synaptic vesicle protein kinase activity, and synaptic vesicle norepinephrine release (Table 3).

The major protein component seen on the electrophoretic pattern of boiled SVE, representing approximately 65% to 80% of the total protein in SVE, co-migrated identically with calmodulin, molecular weight 17,000 to 19,000 (10). The major protein staining component of SVE, like calmodulin, was also extremely heat-stable, sensitive to trypsin, and resistant to dialysis, RNase, and DNase, suggesting that the active fraction in SVE is a vesicle-bound calmodulinlike protein. Therefore, we recently purified to homogeneity and characterized this major protein component in SVE and demonstrated that this heat-stable vesicle-bound protein was the stimulating factor in SVE and was

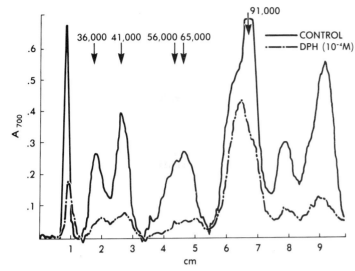

FIG. 4. Effect of phenytoin (10^{-4} M) on endogenous phosphorylation in AChR-enriched membranes. Polypeptides having molecular weights of 41,000, 56,000, and 65,000 have been identified as components of the postsynaptic AChR (9).

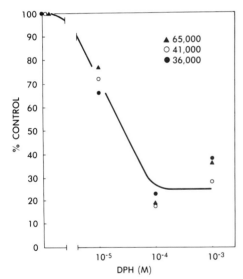

FIG. 5. Effects of phenytoin on the phosphorylation of several polypeptides in AChR-enriched membranes as a function of phenytoin concentration (9).

5×10^{-5} M. This is about 10 times less than the concentration of phenytoin that produces half-maximal inhibition of the phosphorylation of brain proteins (2).

Inhibition of membrane protein phosphorylation by phenytoin could be due to an effect of the drug on membrane protein kinase activity or on the availability of membrane substrates for the phosphorylation reaction. To help differentiate between these two possibilities, the effect of phenytoin on

membrane protein kinase activity was studied using casein as a soluble exogenous substrate. Phenytoin did not inhibit the phosphorylation of casein over a concentration range from 10^{-6} through 10^{-3} M (9).

CONCLUSIONS

These studies open a new avenue for investigating the role of anticonvulsants at the synapse. In most studies of synaptic membrane phosphorylation, the identity of the phosphorylated protein is unknown. In our studies, however, the AChR substrate for the phosphorylation-dephosphorylation reaction is an identified protein, the AChR, and the function of this receptor has been well studied in many systems (10). A major advantage to using receptor-enriched membranes to study phosphorylation of AChR *in situ* is that the level of phosphorylation can be correlated with receptor function. The AChR in these membranes has been well characterized with respect to its affinity for cholinergic agonists and antagonists (10). Changes in binding affinity (desensitization) of this response have also been observed *in vitro* (11). Therefore, it will be possible to determine the effects of phosphorylation and dephosphorylation of the AChR on receptor affinity for agonists as well as receptor-mediated ion fluxes. Such an approach offers a unique advantage in studying the functional significance of receptor phosphorylation and dephosphorylation at the synapse.

Low concentrations of phenytoin inhibit phosphorylation of membrane-bound AChR by an endogenous membrane protein kinase. Phenytoin might either inhibit membrane protein kinase activity in these membranes or interfere with the availability of membrane protein substrate for the phosphorylation reaction. These alternatives cannot be investigated readily because the substrate and enzyme are located in the same membrane preparation. However, it seems likely that phenytoin does not affect membrane kinase activity directly, because phosphorylation of casein by the membrane kinase was not inhibited by phenytoin. Therefore, phenytoin appears to have a direct effect on the availability of postsynaptic membrane protein substrates for the phosphorylation reaction. This occurs at concentrations of phenytoin about 10 times lower than therapeutic levels in the brain.

Epilepsy is characterized by excessive synaptic activity. This could be due to failure of normal desensitization mechanisms in the postsynaptic membrane. We have proposed that desensitization could be regulated by reversible phosphorylation and dephosphorylation of neuroreceptors. Because phenytoin inhibits AChR phosphorylation, phenytoin may effect receptor desensitization. This could be important for the therapeutic effect of the drug in patients.

ACKNOWLEDGMENTS

This work was supported by grants from the National Institutes of Health, the National Science Foundation, the Muscular Dystrophy Associations of America, and the Los Angeles and California chapters of the Myasthenia Gravis Foundation.

REFERENCES

1. Converse, C. A., and Papermaster, D. (1975): Membrane protein analysis by two-dimensional immunoelectrophoresis. *Science*, 189:469–472.

2. DeLorenzo, R. J. (1977): Antagonistic action of diphenylhydantoin and calcium in the level of phosphorylation of particular rat and human brain proteins. *Brain Res.*, 134:125–138.

3. DeLorenzo, R. J. (1978): Calcium dependent neurotransmitter release and protein phosphorylation in synaptic vesicles. *Biochem. Biophys. Res. Commun.*, 80:183–192.

4. Gordon, A. S., Davis, C. G., and Diamond, I. (1977): Phosphorylation of membrane proteins at a cholinergic synapse. *Proc. Natl. Acad. Sci. U.S.A.*, 74:263–267.

5. Gordon, A. S., Davis, C. G., Milfay, D., and Diamond, I. (1977): Phosphorylation of the acetylcholine receptor by an endogenous membrane protein kinase in receptor-enriched membranes of *Torpedo californica*. *Nature*, 267:539–540.

6. Gordon, A. S., Davis, C. G., Milfay, D., Kaur, J., and Diamond, I. (1980): Membrane-bound protein kinase activity in acetylcholine receptor-enriched membranes. *Biochim. Biophys. Acta*, 600:421–431.

7. Gordon, A. S., Guillory, R., Diamond, I., and Hucho, F. (1979): ATP-binding proteins in acetylcholine receptor-enriched membranes. *F.E.B.S. Lett.*, 108:37–39.

8. Gordon, A. S., Milfay, D., Davis, C. G., and Diamond, I. (1979): Protein phosphatase activity in acetylcholine receptor-enriched membranes. *Biochem. Biophys. Res. Commun.*, 87:876–883.

9. Gordon, A. S., Milfay, D., and Diamond, I. (1979): Phosphorylation of the membrane-bound acetylcholine receptor: Inhibition by diphenylhydantoin. *Ann. Neurol.*, 5:201–203.

10. Heidmann, T., and Changeux, J. P. (1978): Structural and functional properties of the acetylcholine receptor protein in its purified and membrane-bound states. *Ann. Rev. Biochem.*, 47:317–357.

11. Weber, M., David-Pfeuty, T., and Changeux, J. P. (1975): Regulation of binding properties of the nicotinic receptor protein by cholinergic ligands in membrane fragments from *Torpedo marmorata*. *Proc. Natl. Acad. Sci. U.S.A.*, 72:3443–3447.

Advances in Neurology, Vol. 34: Status Epilepticus, edited by A.V. Delgado-Escueta, C.G. Wasterlain, D.M. Treiman, and R.J. Porter. Raven Press, New York © 1983.

32

Protein Phosphorylation, Neuronal Receptors, and Seizures in the Central Nervous System

Yigal H. Ehrlich

ROLES OF SPECIFIC PHOSPHOPROTEINS IN NEURAL FUNCTION

A large body of evidence has been accumulated demonstrating that the phosphorylation-dephosphorylation cycles of proteins play important and ubiquitous roles in the regulation of numerous physiological processes; for reviews, see all the chapters in the work edited by Rosen and Krebs (20). Thus, it has been shown that the phosphorylation of nuclear proteins is involved in DNA and RNA synthesis; the phosphorylation of ribosomal proteins and of initiation factors regulates protein synthesis; the phosphorylation of cytoplasmic and microsomal enzymes controls the metabolism of carbohydrates, lipids, catecholamines, etc.; the phosphorylation of membrane-bound proteins has been correlated with changes in membrane permeability to cations (K^+, Na^+, Ca^{2+}), changes in uptake and transport, and changes in the regulation of various membrane-bound enzymes such as ATPase and adenylate cyclase. In addition to these processes that operate in all eukaryotic cells, protein phosphorylation has been implicated in the regulation of several functions characteristic of neural tissues. These include the synthesis, storage, and release of neurotransmitters, axonal transport, determination of receptor sensitivity, and the responses of membranes to de-

polarizing and hyperpolarizing stimuli. Recent reviews are available (4,17,29).

In spite of the great diversity of metabolic and physiological events regulated by protein phosphorylation, only a few different types of protein kinase have been isolated from brain tissue (17). The first clue to the question of the source of specificity in this mode of regulation was provided by studies in the laboratory of Greengard and associates (18,25), who reported that preparations of synaptic membranes from rat cerebrum contained two specific proteins whose phosphorylation was regulated by cyclic AMP. Our initial studies (14,21) confirmed those reports and identified six additional proteins in synaptic membranes whose phosphorylation and dephosphorylation are carried out by kinase(s) and phosphatase(s) that constitute part of the structure of these membranes (Fig. 1). Subsequent studies (4,9) revealed the presence of over 20 different membrane-bound phosphoproteins and over 40 different soluble phosphoproteins in brain tissue, distributed differentially among various subcellular fractions. The great heterogeneity of cells in the brain raised the possibility that different phosphoproteins are located in different cells. However, studies using a homogeneous population of neuroblastoma cells differentiated in culture provided evidence that an individual nerve cell can contain a multiplicity of endogenously phosphorylated proteins (7,11). Differences in phosphor-

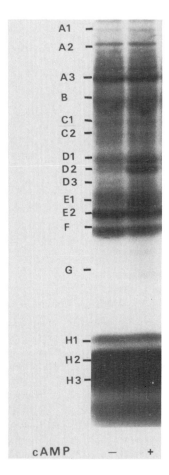

FIG. 1. Endogenously phosphorylated proteins of cortical synaptic membranes. Synaptosomal preparations from rat cerebral cortex were lysed in a hypo-osmotic buffer containing 50-μM CaCl$_2$, and membrane fractions were obtained as decribed previously (9,14). Aliquots containing 40 μg protein were incubated for 10 sec at 30°C with 3-μM γ-^{32}P-ATP in the presence (+) and absence (−) of 5-μM cyclic AMP. Assays were stopped by solubilizing the membranes in sodium dodecyl sulfate (SDS), followed by slab-SDS-gel electrophoresis and autoradiography (7,9,11,12,14). In the autoradiograph shown, band intensity is proportional to the amount of ^{32}P-phosphate incorporated into specific proteins. Note that whereas the phosphorylation of two proteins (designated D1 and D2) (9) is stimulated by cyclic AMP, the others are unaffected by the addition of this cyclic nucleotide to the reaction medium.

ylative properties, subcellular locations, and responses to various regulatory factors between these phosphoprotein substrates could account for the specificity in the diverse physiological functions regulated by even a few protein kinases (4). It is possible, therefore, that only certain specific

phosphoproteins are involved in the responses of neurons to seizure-producing stimuli. Subsequent studies attempted to identify these phosphoproteins.

PROTEIN PHOSPHORYLATION AND SEIZURE ACTIVITY IN THE CNS

Early studies of brain tissue *in situ* detected an increase in phosphate incorporation into neuronal membrane proteins in response to electrical and neurohumoral stimulation (28). However, which of the numerous endogenously phosphorylated proteins that are present in synaptic membranes (Fig. 1) is involved in this process has not been determined. We have found that analysis of phosphorylative activity in membranes prepared from rats killed by cryogenic methods (8) can reveal the identity of specific proteins whose phosphorylation is altered by environmental or pharmacological stimulations of the intact animal (6,12). This investigative approach had been used to determine the effects of electroconvulsive shock (ECS) on protein phosphorylation in cortical membranes (13,19). The methods used were described in detail previously (13). Briefly, male albino rats (120–140 g) were administered ECS transaurically and manifested generalized tonic-clonic seizures. They were killed by rapid head freezing in liquid nitrogen during the tonic (9–11 sec after shock) or clonic (28–32 sec after shock) phase of the convulsions. Two additional groups were killed during behavioral recovery: One group was killed when the convulsions had ceased (2 min after shock), and the other group was killed when the rats began running about the cage (4 min after shock). Sham-shocked rats served as controls. Preparations containing synaptic membranes from the cerebral cortex were incubated with γ-^{32}P-ATP and subjected to SDS-gel electrophoresis for analysis of phosphorylation of specific proteins (Fig. 1).

Marked changes in the phosphorylation of proteins in the molecular-weight range of 10,000 to 20,000 were seen in cortical membranes from convulsing rats. These proteins constitute a group of seven phosphorylated bands designated H-1 through H-7 (9,13,14). The results of quantitative analyses of the effects of ECS on the phosphorylation of protein band H-4 (MW 18,000) are shown in Fig. 2. It can be seen that ECS induced transient changes in ^{32}P-phosphate incorporation into this cortical membrane protein. The increase is characterized

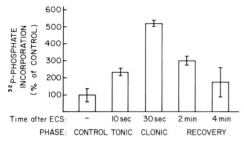

FIG. 2. Effects of ECS on the phosphorylation of a specific protein in cortical membranes. Rats were delivered ECS as described in the text and killed by head immersion in liquid N_2 at various phases, as indicated in the figure. Cortical membranes were prepared and assayed for endogenous phosphorylation of specific proteins as described for Fig. 1. Phosphate incorporation into protein bands of the group designated H (see Fig. 1) showed temporal changes that paralleled the behavioral effects of the ECS (13). Depicted are the results obtained for band H-4 (MW 18,000). Data from Ehrlich et al. (13,19).

by a rapid onset; it reaches a maximum during tonic seizures and gradually returns to control levels on behavioral recovery from the effects of the ECS. To our knowledge, these reports (13,19) constitute the first demonstration of reversible changes in the phosphorylation of specific proteins in response to a stimulus with transient effects on neuronal activity. It is important to note here that Delgado-Escueta and Horan (see Chapter 29) recently found a net increase in the *in vitro* phosphorylation of an 18,000-dalton protein after administration of convulsive doses of pentylenetetrazol. The magnitude of this drug-induced effect (fivefold increase) was identical with the maxima found in our studies ($514\% \pm 21\%$) (Fig. 2). Additional support for the involvement of this specific phosphoprotein in seizure activity comes from investigation of *in vitro* endogenous phosphorylation of brain proteins in a hereditary model of epilepsy. High seizure susceptibility in epileptic fowl is due to an autosomal recessive mutation. Homozygotes (epileptics) develop spontaneous seizures, whereas heterozygotes (carriers) do not. Tuchek et al. (24) reported recently that of all the membrane-bound phosphoproteins in this avian brain, only one, estimated at 16,000 daltons, showed significant differences in phosphorylation between samples from the epileptic and carrier fowls. The good agreement in findings between studies from three separate laboratories serves to focus attention on phosphoproteins in the group we have designated H in relation to seizures in the CNS.

NEUROPEPTIDE REGULATION OF Ca²⁺-STIMULATED PHOSPHORYLATION IN NEURAL MEMBRANES

The studies we have described enabled us to identify specific proteins whose phosphorylation is involved in seizure activity, but they did not provide a clue as to the mechanism underlying their role in this phenomenon. As pointed out in a review of early studies on protein phosphorylation by Rubin and Rosen (22), characterization of the phosphorylative properties that different phosphoproteins exhibit *in vitro* can serve as an indicator of their functional roles *in vivo*. The most fundamental property of endogenous phosphorylation systems in brain membranes is their dependence on divalent cations, notably Mg^{2+} and Ca^{2+}. All our studies of endogenous protein phosphorylation in synaptic membranes were carried out using membranes prepared from synaptosomes subjected to hypo-osmotic lysis in the presence of 50-μM $CaCl_2$ (14). The saturation of Ca^{2+}-binding sites in the membranes during this procedure is the most likely reason for our ability to detect phosphorylation of specific proteins that were not seen by Ueda et al. (25). Indeed, DeLorenzo (3) and later Schulman and Greengard (23), using EGTA buffers, demonstrated Ca^{2+} stimulation of Mg^{2+}-dependent phosphorylation of specific proteins in synaptic membranes and its regulation by calmodulin. We recently reported (13) that inactivation of phosphorylative activity in Ca^{2+}-saturated membranes required prolonged dialysis against EGTA. However, as demonstrated in Fig. 3, addition of Mg^{2+} ions or Ca^{2+} ions or both to the phosphorylation assay medium restored the activity to predialysis levels. Optimal endogenous phosphorylative activity in synaptic membranes *in vitro* requires 5- to 10-mM Mg^{2+} (14,18,21,25) but only micromolar levels of free Ca^{2+} ions (3,13,23). Addition of boiled synaptoplasm to the reaction medium enhanced the phosphorylation of several proteins larger than 50,000 daltons (Fig. 3, lanes marked + sup.), presumably because of the effects of calmodulin (23) (see Chapter 30). However, the same addition also inhibited Ca^{2+}-stimulated phosphorylation of proteins in the range of 10,000 to 20,000 daltons, namely, the H bands. Thus, brain extracts contain factor(s) that exert inhibitory effects on the phosphorylation of those synaptic phosphoproteins found to be the most susceptible to seizure-producing stimulation.

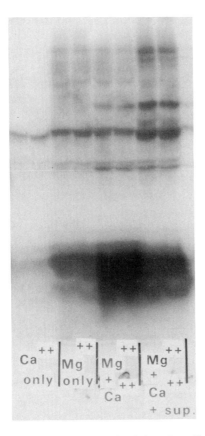

FIG. 3. Ca²⁺-regulated phosphorylation of specific proteins in cortical membranes. Preparations containing synaptic membranes from rat cerebral cortex (see Fig. 1) were dialysed against 0.6-mM EGTA to chelate all Ca²⁺ ions out of the membranes. Aliquots were assayed for endogenous protein phosphorylation (see Fig. 1) in a buffer containing 20-mM Tris-HCl (pH 7.4) + 0.6-mM EGTA and 0.8-mM CaCl₂ (Ca²⁺ only) or 10-mM MgCl₂ (Mg²⁺ only) or Mg²⁺ + Ca²⁺ (at concentrations as above) or Mg²⁺ + Ca²⁺ + a trace of boiled synaptoplasmic supernatant (sup.), which contains calmodulin (23) and other peptides (2,10). Note that the phosphorylation of only one protein band is supported by Ca²⁺ in the absence of Mg²⁺. The phosphorylation of many proteins is dependent on Mg²⁺ and stimulated by Ca²⁺. The cytosol contains heat-stable components that enhance the phosphorylation of high-MW proteins and inhibit the Ca²⁺-dependent phosphate incorporation into bands of low MW (the H group at the bottom of the gel).

daltons. In another line of investigation, we found that the exposure of rats to chronic morphine treatment resulted in decreased phosphorylation of H proteins in neostriatal membranes (6). These findings have raised the possibility that enkephalins and/or endorphins, the endogenous ligands of opiate receptors, are the peptides exerting the inhibitory effects depicted in Fig. 3. Indeed, studies reported in detail elsewhere (10) have confirmed this contention. Addition of methionine-enkephalin in the micromolar concentration range, or human β-endorphin in the nanomolar range, to assay mixtures used to measure endogenous phosphorylation in synaptic membranes produced a 70% to 80% decrease in phosphate incorporation into bands of group H and 40% to 60% inhibition of phosphorylation of another protein band, designated F (MW 47,000) (Fig. 4).

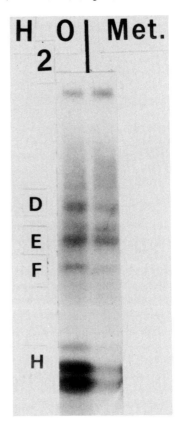

FIG. 4. Methionine-enkephalin inhibition of protein phosphorylation. Autoradiograph depicting the pattern of endogenously phosphorylated proteins in neostriatal membranes incubated in vitro in the presence (Met.) and absence (H₂O added instead) of 100-μM methionine-enkephalin. Experimental details have been published (10).

Fractionations and partial characterization of the endogenous factors in brain that inhibit the phosphorylation of H-band proteins in synaptic membranes were carried out using aqueous extracts of synaptosomes and of synaptic membranes (2). Preliminary results have indicated that these factors are small peptides in the range of 500 to 2,000

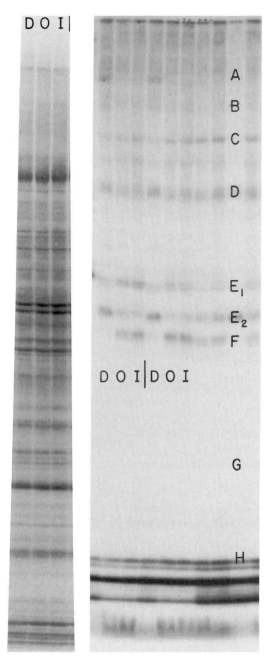

FIG. 5. Catecholamine-regulated protein phosphorylation in synaptic membranes. Synaptosomal preparations (P_2) from rat neostriatum were osmotically shocked in the presence of 50-μM $CaCl_2$ and then washed in a buffer containing 50-mM KCl. Aliquots containing 60 μg protein were incubated (30 sec at 30°C) with 1-μM γ-^{32}P-ATP and 10-mM $MgCl_2$ without additions (O) or with 10-μM dopamine (D). Stock solutions of dopamine (Sigma) in 1-mN HCl were stored at -20°C, thawed, and diluted before the assays. SDS-solubilized reaction products were separated in a 30-cm-long slab-polyacrylamide-gel gradient (10%–16%, exponential), stained with Coomassie blue (left), and autoradiographed (right). In the autoradiograph, note the multiple effects of dopamine on different phosphoproteins; e.g., dopamine stimulated the phosphorylation of bands A, D, and E_2, but inhibited bands C, E_1, and F. Addition of 10-μM ($-$)isoproterenol (I), a noradrenergic ligand, had minimal effects on the neostriatal membranes used here, but it was inhibitory in phosphorylation assays carried out with cortical membranes (5,27).

It has been reported that intraventricular administration of opioid peptides induces epileptogenic seizures (15). It is therefore of particular interest that the same peptides exert direct effects on the Ca^{2+}-stimulated phosphorylation of phosphoproteins implicated in seizure activity. The discrepancy between the finding that endorphins inhibit *in vitro* the phosphorylation of the same proteins that show an apparent increase in phosphorylation after ECS administered *in vivo* has been explained (13) by the finding that increased ^{32}P-phosphate incorporation *in vitro* reflects increased numbers of available phosphorylation sites due to decreased phosphorylation *in vivo*. Thus, the mechanism that operates to bring about the observed effects of ECS on protein phosphorylation (Fig. 2) may involve accelerated release of peptides that inhibit the phosphorylation of proteins in group H. This inhibition during seizure activity *in vivo* would be manifested by an apparent increase in ^{32}P-phosphate incorporation *in vitro*.

PROTEIN PHOSPHORYLATION AND RECEPTOR FUNCTION

Endorphins are not the only endogenous ligands in brain that may exert some of their effects on neural function by regulating Ca^{2+}-stimulated phosphorylation in synaptic membranes. In fact, we have found (5) that the most recently discovered ligands of neuronal receptors, the benzodiazepines, also exert inhibitory effects on protein phosphorylation (see Chapter 30). In this context, it may be mentioned that Davis and Cohen (1) identified an endogenous peptide ligand for the benzodiazepine receptor. This peptide was isolated from an aqueous supernatant of synaptosomes that also contained peptides that inhibited the phosphorylation of H proteins (Fig. 3) (2). Moreover, "classic" putative neurotransmitters of the CNS, and not only neuropeptides, were shown to affect protein phosphorylation in synaptic membranes. Thus, carbachol inhibits the endogenous phosphorylation of specific proteins in acetylcholine-receptor-enriched membranes from the electric organ of *Torpedo californica* (16) (see Chapter 31). Regulation of protein phosphorylation by catecholamines in the mammalian CNS is exemplified here in Fig. 5, depicting the multiple effects of dopamine on endogenous phosphorylation of different proteins in rat neostriatal membranes. The effects of adrenergic ligands, such as norepinephrine and isoproterenol, were best seen in preparations of

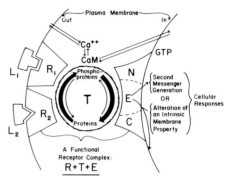

FIG. 6. Hypothetical role for protein phosphorylation in receptor function. The interaction of receptor ligands (L) with recognition sites (R) localized on the outer surface of plasma membranes results in activation or inhibition of an effector site (E) that initiates the chain of events leading to cellular responses. R confers specificity to the binding of ligands. E may be, e.g., adenylate cyclase (containing a catalytic subunit C and GTP-binding sites N) or an intrinsic membrane activity such as ion channels. A transducing mechanism (T) is needed for the coupling of R with E. A Ca^{2+}-calmodulin-(CaM)-dependent phosphorylation-dephosphorylation system that is regulated by neurohormones (L) can confer reversible conformational changes that carry a signal from R to E. There is no requirement of specificity from T. A phosphorylation system that plays a role in the transducing mechanism may, therefore, also play a modulatory role in balancing the responses to two (L_1, L_2) or more hormones interacting with several receptors (R_1, R_2) present on the same cell.

cortical membranes (5,27). All these findings support the suggestion (4) that neurotransmitter-regulated protein phosphorylation may play an important role in receptor-mediated functions at the synapse, as depicted in Fig. 6.

The main function of receptors is the transduction of signals through plasma membranes. The regulation of intracellular adenylate and guanylate cyclase activities represents extensively studied neuronal responses to extracellular ligands. Recent studies in our laboratory (27) have demonstrated that preincubation of synaptic membranes under phosphorylating conditions alters the activity of adenylate cyclase in these membranes, measured in a reincubation phase of the assay. The presence or absence of free Ca^{2+} ions in the preincubation determines whether cyclic AMP formation in the reincubation is increased or decreased. Moreover, inclusion of a neurotransmitter, such as $(-)$iso-proterenol, in the preincubation inhibits the phosphorylation of specific proteins and results in altered cyclase activity in the reincubation (26). It is well established that seizures are associated with altered regulation of cyclic AMP and cyclic GMP levels in the CNS (see Chapter 33). Our observations suggest that the activity of adenylate cyclase in the CNS is regulated, at least in part, by neurotransmitter-sensitive Ca^{2+}-dependent phosphorylation of specific proteins in synaptic membranes. Future studies should investigate whether or not a primary defect in such an endogenous phosphorylation system may be a cause of certain types of epilepsy and status epilepticus.

SUMMARY

Several lines of investigation indicate that the phosphorylation of proteins localized in synaptic membranes plays a role in the electrogenic response of neurons to stimulation by neurotransmitterrs. Our previous studies demonstrated that massive stimulation of the CNS by electroconvulsive shock produces rapid and reversible changes in the phosphorylation of specific proteins localized in synaptic membranes of rat cerebral cortex. The most affected phosphoproteins were of MW 15,000–20,000, and maximal changes (500%) coincided with the phase of clonic convulsions. The phosphorylation of these proteins returned to preseizure levels on behavioral recovery of the animals from the effects of the electroshock. The studies reported here investigated the role of phosphoproteins in mechanisms underlying seizure activity, by examining the possibility that neurotransmitters exert direct regulatory effects on the phosphorylation of specific proteins in synaptic membranes, It was found that addition of neurotransmitters (e.g., endorphins, catecholamines) to assays used to measure endogenous phosphorylation in synaptic membranes *in vitro* causes selective alterations in the Ca^{2+}-dependent phosphorylation of different proteins. One of the functional consequences of these interactions was tested by analyzing adenylate cyclase activity as a function of the phosphorylation state of membrane-bound proteins. These assays revealed that neurotransmitter-induced alterations in the phosphorylation of specific protein may cause changes in the activity of adenylate cyclase. These findings support the hypothesis that conformational changes induced by altered protein phosphorylation may constitute a transducing mechanism triggered by the interaction of neurotransmitters with membrane-localized receptors. This process may, therefore, play a crucial role in the initiation, maintenance, and/or propagation of epileptogenic seizures in the CNS.

ACKNOWLEDGMENTS

Some of the studies described here were supported by USPHS grant DA-02747 from the National Institute on Drug Abuse and by a research award from the Epilepsy Foundation of America.

REFERENCES

1. Davis, L. G., and Cohen, R. K. (1980): Identification of an endogenous peptide-ligand for the benzodiazepine receptor. *Biochem. Biophys. Res. Commun.*, 92:141–148.
2. Davis, L. G., and Ehrlich, Y. H. (1979): Opioid peptides and protein phosphorylation. *Adv. Exp. Med. Biol.*, 116:233–244.
3. DeLorenzo, R. J. (1976): Calcium-dependent phosphorylation of specific synaptosomal fraction proteins: Possible role of phosphoproteins in mediating neurotransmitter release. *Biochem. Biophys. Res. Commun.*, 71:590–597.
4. Ehrlich, Y. H. (1979): Phosphoproteins as specifiers for mediators and modulators in neuronal function. *Adv. Exp. Med. Biol.*, 116:75–101.
5. Ehrlich, Y. H. (1980): Protein phosphorylation: A potential "action site" of membrane-localized receptors. *Soc. Neurosci. Abstr.*, 6:498.
6. Ehrlich, Y. H., Bonnet, K. A., Davis, L. G., and Brunngraber, E. G. (1978): Decreased phosphorylation of specific proteins in neostriatal membranes from rats after long-term narcotic exposure. *Life Sci.*, 23:137–146.
7. Ehrlich, Y. H., Brunngraber, E. G., Sinah, P. K., and Prasad, K. N. (1977): Specific alterations in phosphorylation of cytosol proteins from differentiating neuroblastoma cells grown in culture. *Nature*, 265:238–240.
8. Ehrlich, Y. H., Davis, L. G., and Brunngraber, E. G. (1978): Effects of decapitation stress on protein phosphorylation in cortical membranes. *Brain Res. Bull.*, 3:251–256.
9. Ehrlich, Y. H., Davis, L. G., Gilfoil, T., and Brunngraber, E. G. (1977): Distribution of endogenously phosphorylated proteins in subcellular fractions of rat cerebral cortex. *Neurochemical Res.*, 2:533–548.
10. Ehrlich, Y. H., Davis, L. G., Keen, P., and Brunngraber, E. G. (1980): Endorphin-regulated protein phosphorylation in brain membranes. *Life Sci.*, 26:1795.
11. Ehrlich, Y. H., Prasad, K. N., Davis, L. G., Sinah, P. K., and Brunngraber, E. G. (1978): Endogenous phosphorylation of specific proteins in subcellular fractions from malignant and cAMP-induced differentiated neuroblastoma cells in culture. *Neurochemical Res.*, 3:803–813.
12. Ehrlich, Y. H., Rabjohns, R., and Routtenberg, A. (1977): Experiential-input alters the phosphorylation of specific proteins in brain membranes. *Pharmacol. Biochem. Behav.*, 5:169–174.
13. Ehrlich, Y. H., Reedy, M. V., Keen, P., Davis, L. G., Daugherty, J., and Brunngraber, E. G. (1980): Tran-

sient changes in the phosphorylation of cortical membrane proteins after electroconvulsive shock. *J. Neurochem.*, 34:1327–1330.

14. Ehrlich, Y. H., and Routtenberg, A. (1974): Cyclic AMP regulates phosphorylation of three proteins of rat cerebral cortex membranes for thirty minutes. *F.E.B.S. Lett.*, 45:237–243.

15. Frenk, H., McCarty, B. C., and Liebeskind, J. C. (1978): Different brain areas mediate the analgesic and epileptic properties of enkephalin. *Science*, 200:335–337.

16. Gordon, A. S., and Diamond, I. (1979): Phosphorylation of the acetylcholine receptor. In: *Modulators, Mediators and Specifiers in Brain Function*, edited by Y. H. Ehrlich, J. Volavka, L. G. Davis, and E. G. Brunngraber, pp. 175–198. Plenum Press, New York.

17. Greengard, P. (1978): *Cyclic Nucleotides, Phosphorylated Proteins and Neuronal Function.* Raven Press, New York.

18. Johnson, E. M., Ueda, T., Maeno, H., and Greengard, P. (1972): Cyclic AMP-dependent phosphorylation of a specific protein in synaptic membranes. *J. Biol. Chem.*, 247:5650–5652.

19. Reddy, M. V., Ehrlich, Y. H., Davis, L. G., Daugherty, J., and Brunngraber, E. G. (1978): Altered phosphorylation of cortical membrane proteins after ECS. *Soc. Neurosci. Abstr.*, 4:146.

20. Rosen, O. M., and Krebs, E. G. (editors) (1981): *Protein-phosphorylation: Proceedings of the 8th Cold Spring Harbor Conference on Cell Proliferation.* CHS Publication, New York.

21. Routtenberg, A., and Ehrlich, Y. H. (1975): Endogenous phosphorylation of four proteins in cerebral cortex membranes. Role of cyclic nucleotides, ATP and divalent cations. *Brain Res.*, 92:415–430.

22. Rubin, C. S., and Rosen, O. M. (1975): Protein phosphorylation. *Annu. Rev. Biochem.*, 44:831–887.

23. Schulman, H., and Greengard, P. (1978): Stimulation of brain membrane protein phosphorylation by calcium and an endogenous heat-stable protein. *Nature*, 271:478–479.

24. Tuchek, J. M., Johnson, D. D., and Crawford, R. D. (1980): Abnormalities in endogenous phosphorylation in a hereditary model of epilepsy. *Soc. Neurosci. Abstr.*, 6:444.

25. Ueda, T., Maeno, H., and Greengard, P. (1973): Regulation of endogenous phosphorylation of specific proteins in synaptic membrane fractions from rat brain by adenosine 3′,5′-monophosphate. *J. Biol. Chem.*, 248:8295–8305.

26. Whittemore, S. R., Lenox, R. H., and Ehrlich, Y. H. (1981): Protein phosphorylation mediates effects of isoproterenol on adenylate cyclase activity in rat cortical membranes. *Neurochem. Res.*, 7:777–787.

27. Whittemore, S. R., Lenox, R. H., Hendley, E. D., and Ehrlich, Y. H. (1981): Membrane protein phosphorylation regulated adenylate cyclase activity. *Trans. Am. Soc. Neurochem.*, 12:125.

28. Williams, M., Pavlik, A., and Rodnight, R. (1974): Turnover of protein phosphorus in respiring slices of guinea pig cerebral cortex: Cellular localization of phosphoprotein sensitive to electrical stimulation. *J. Neurochem.*, 22:373–376.

29. Williams, M., and Rodnight, R. (1977): Protein phosphorylation in nervous tissue. *Prog. Neurobiol.*, 8:183–250.

Advances in Neurology, Vol. 34: Status Epilepticus, edited by A.V. Delgado-Escueta, C.G. Wasterlain, D.M. Treiman, and R.J. Porter. Raven Press, New York © 1983.

33

Relationship Between Seizures and Cyclic Nucleotides in the Central Nervous System

James A. Ferrendelli

At the present time it is difficult, if not impossible, to ascertain the biochemical basis of epilepsy, because our knowledge of the molecular and cellular mechanisms of nervous tissue function is extremely limited. Nevertheless, it is possible to establish relationships between certain normal and abnormal neural functions and some biochemical processes, and defining these relationships may provide important information concerning pathophysiological mechanisms of seizure disorders. For this reason we have attempted to determine the influence of seizure activity on specific biochemical systems in the CNS and vice versa. Our recent studies have explored the relationships between seizures and cyclic nucleotides (adenosine 3',5'-monophosphate, cyclic AMP, and guanosine 3',5'-monophosphate, cyclic GMP) in the brain. This chapter summarizes the available data on this subject and describes a hypothesis suggesting roles for these nucleotides in seizure mechanisms.

CYCLIC NUCLEOTIDES IN CNS

Prior to considering relationships between seizures and cyclic nucleotides, it would be useful to summarize briefly the current concepts of cyclic AMP and cyclic GMP biochemistry in nervous tissue. For original references and a more detailed account of this subject, the reader is referred to several review articles (2,3,19,22).

Cyclic AMP

This nucleotide exists throughout mammalian CNS at a concentration of approximately 1 μM (10 μmole/kg protein), and there is little regional variation in its level. Cyclic AMP is formed from ATP by the enzyme adenylate cyclase and is metabolized to 5'-AMP by cyclic AMP phosphodiesterase(s). This appears to be its only pathway of synthesis and degradation in biological tissues. Adenylate cyclase is a membrane-bound enzyme under complex regulation. Both ATP and Mg^{2+} are required for its activity. Calcium at high concentrations inhibits its activity and at low concentrations produces activations via calmodulin. Fluoride ions and guanine nucleotides also are activators of adenylate cyclase. There is substantial evidence indicating that adenylate cyclase is linked to receptors of certain neurotransmitters or neuroregulators, including dopamine, norepinephrine, prostaglandins, adenosine, and others. Thus, the actions of these substances include activation of adenylate cyclase and accumulation of cellular levels of cyclic AMP. It has been suggested that the neuroregulatory effects of several of these substances are mediated by cyclic AMP. This action of cyclic AMP, as well as its reported effects on several cellular functions and biochemical processes, is believed to occur as a result of activation of cyclic-AMP-dependent protein kinases. Thus, cyclic AMP is an intracellular regulatory substance or "second messenger." Intracellular levels of cyclic AMP may also be regulated by phosphodiesterase. There appear to be several enzymes with cyclic AMP-phosphodiesterase activity in CNS, with different activities and affinities for cyclic AMP, and their activities are influenced by several endogenous and exogenous substances.

Cyclic GMP

In most regions of mammalian CNS, cyclic GMP exists at a concentration of 0.1 μM, an order of magnitude lower than that of cyclic AMP. However, in cerebellum the level of cyclic GMP is near 1 μM, and in retinal photoreceptor cells it is an order of magnitude higher. Thus, there are marked regional variations in cyclic GMP concentrations in CNS. Cyclic GMP is formed from GTP by guanylate cyclase(s) and is metabolized to $5'$-GMP by the action of phosphodiesterase. There appear to be at least two guanylate cyclases, a soluble enzyme and a particulate enzyme, in CNS; a third, and probably unique, guanylate cyclase is present in retinal photoreceptors. Several phosphodiesterases capable of acting on cyclic GMP have been identified in nervous tissue, and all of these have different kinetic properties. At present, it is unclear whether or not guanylate cyclases or cyclic GMP phosphodiesterases or both are primarily responsible for regulating cellular cyclic GMP levels. In contrast to adenylate cyclase, guanylate cyclase activity is not influenced by neuroregulatory substances (neurotransmitters or neurohormones). Some of the more potent activators of guanylate cyclases are Ca^{2+}, detergents, azide, and nitro compounds, and these have different effects on the soluble and particulate enzymes. Cyclic GMP phosphodiesterases in CNS, similar to the phosphodiesterases that act on cyclic AMP, may be influenced by exogenous and endogenous substances. Calmodulin is a potent activator of cyclic GMP phosphodiesterase as well as an activator of adenylate cyclase. The function or functions of cyclic GMP in tissues are poorly understood. Cyclic GMP-dependent protein kinases have been identified, and it is believed that cyclic GMP produces actions, yet unidentified, through these enzymes. At the present time, most authorities consider cyclic GMP to be an intracellular regulatory substance or second messenger similar to cyclic AMP. However, there are striking and substantial differences between the two nucleotides, as noted earlier, and more infor-

mation is needed to establish a probable role for cyclic GMP.

REGULATION OF CYCLIC NUCLEOTIDES IN EPILEPTIC BRAIN

Several different convulsant drugs and stimuli have been reported to elevate CNS levels of cyclic AMP or cyclic GMP or both (1,5,6,8–10, 15,17,18,20,24,25). Thus, it appears that changes in cyclic nucleotide levels are associated with seizure activity or some closely related process and are independent of the processes that initiate the seizure activity. Moreover, seizures produce elevations in cyclic nucleotides in paralyzed ventilated animals, indicating that the biochemical changes are related to CNS processes and are not the results of systemic alterations such as increased motor activity or hypoxia. Also, partial or focal seizures appear to alter cyclic nucleotide levels only in those regions of brain where seizure discharges occur, further indicating a direct relationship between the two phenomena (23,28).

Some studies have attempted to determine the temporal relationships between seizure discharges and changes in levels of cyclic nucleotides in brain *in vivo* (1,5,15,16,18,25). The results of these investigations have demonstrated that cyclic AMP increases only after the onset of clinically evident seizure activity or after the appearance of epileptiform EEG activity. In contrast, cyclic GMP levels have been reported to increase prior to the onset of clinical seizure, and subconvulsant doses (insufficient to produce clinically evident seizures or epileptiform EEG activity) as well as convulsant doses of drugs elevate cyclic GMP levels in brain. This indicates that cyclic AMP elevations are a consequence of seizure activity and that elevations of cyclic GMP are related to, but can occur independently of, seizure discharges.

Several drugs modify the effects of seizures on cyclic nucleotide levels in brain. Anticonvulsants such as phenytoin, phenobarbital, ethosuximide, valproic acid, and others attenuate or block seizure-induced accumulation of both cyclic AMP and cyclic GMP (6,8,16). However, these effects of anticonvulsant drugs are directly proportional to their ability to prevent seizures, indicating that the inhibitory effects of anticonvulsant drugs on seizure-induced accumulation of cyclic nucleotides are secondary to their antiepileptic actions and are not a result of some direct effect on cyclic nucleotide formation or degradation.

Drugs other than anticonvulsants can modify cyclic nucleotide accumulation induced by seizures. Sattin (25) first demonstrated that theophylline or caffeine inhibited accumulation of cyclic AMP in mouse forebrain after maximal electroshock or after induction of seizures with hexafluorodiethyl ether. Lust et al. (15) reported that amphetamine, diphenhydramine, and trifluoroperazine all partially inhibited electroshock-induced elevation of cyclic AMP in mouse cerebral cortex. The increase in cyclic AMP levels in mouse cerebral cortex produced by seizures induced with 3-mercaptopropionic acid were reported to be attenuated by pretreatment of animals with propranolol (9). We examined the effects of several drugs, purported to alter noradrenergic influence in CNS, on pentylenetetrazol-induced seizure activity and regulation of cyclic nucleotide levels in cerebral cortex and hippocampus in mice (11,12). Depletion of brain stores of norepinephrine with reserpine or treatment of neonatal mice with 6-OH-dopamine decreases seizure latency and/or threshold and diminishes seizure-induced accumulation of cyclic AMP in brain. Propranolol, a β-adrenergic receptor antagonist, and yohimbine, an α_2-adrenergic receptor antagonist, have effects qualitatively similar to those of reserpine and 6-OH-dopamine, but phentolamine, an α_1-adrenergic antagonist, increased seizure threshold and latency and did not reduce accumulation of cyclic AMP. Imipramine and *d*-amphetamine, drugs that increase noradrenergic influence in brain, had dissimilar actions. The former prevented tonic seizures, but lowered the threshold and latency for clonic seizures; the latter worsened all seizure activity. Neither of these two drugs altered the elevations in cyclic AMP levels. Aminophylline, a methylxanthine with multiple actions, but most likely producing blockade of adenosine receptors in the CNS at the doses used in our experiments, also inhibited the accumulation of cyclic AMP in several regions of the brain and caused tonic seizures to develop sooner. None of the foregoing drugs inhibited accumulation of cyclic GMP in pentylenetetrazol-treated animals, and some augmented its increase slightly when seizure activity was more severe.

Thus, the available data indicate that seizures increase cyclic AMP and cyclic GMP levels by two different mechanisms. With regard to cyclic AMP, it appears that biogenic amines, particularly norepinephrine, and perhaps adenosine, which are released from intracellular stores by the seizure discharge, activate adenylate cyclases and produce much, or perhaps all, of the increase of cyclic AMP levels. Furthermore, it appears that when the influence of norepinephrine or adenosine in the CNS is diminished, seizure discharges spread and become sustained more rapidly, and tonic seizures occur more quickly. An attractive possibility is that the reduction in cyclic AMP accumulation and the change in seizure activity are somehow related. The mechanism or mechanisms responsible for the elevation of cyclic GMP levels have not been defined. However, we suggest that an increase in the free intracellular concentration of calcium, which is known to occur during cellular depolarization and would certainly take place in brain tissue undergoing a seizure discharge, probably activates guanylate cyclase and produces at least some of the accumulation of cyclic GMP seen in epileptic brain. In support of this contention are the observations that cellular depolarization of brain tissue, *in vitro*, causes marked elevations in cyclic GMP levels, and this effect appears to be secondary to an augmented influx of calcium into cells (4,7). In addition, soluble guanylate cyclase in brain has been reported to be activated by calcium (27). Regardless of the mechanisms regulating cyclic GMP levels in epileptic brain, it is apparent that cyclic AMP and cyclic GMP are regulated differently, which suggests that the two cyclic nucleotides are involved in different pathophysiological events during seizures.

EFFECTS OF CYCLIC NUCLEOTIDES ON SEIZURES

There has been little attempt to directly assess the effects of cyclic nucleotides on seizure discharges, but the few studies reported have generated interesting data. Hoffer and colleagues have demonstrated that iontophoresis of cyclic GMP, or stable derivatives of this substance, powerfully excites and even produces epileptic activity in pyramidal neurons in hippocampus transplanted and maintained in the anterior chamber of the eye (13,14). These investigators also observed that phosphodiesterase inhibitors potentiated this response.

We have examined the effects of derivatives of cyclic AMP and cyclic GMP on evoked and spontaneous electrical activity in slices of guinea pig hippocampus maintained *in vitro*. 8-Br-cyclic GMP (0.03–0.1 μM) increased the duration of evoked potentials twofold to threefold and markedly increased the amount of spontaneous activity in the slices; in some, it produced spontaneous epileptiform activity. In contrast, 8-Br-cyclic AMP (0.1–10 μM) always depressed evoked potentials and spontaneous activity. Isobutylmethylxanthine (100 μM) or concentrations of K^+ between 6 and 9 mM, which simultaneously elevated endogenous tissue levels of cyclic GMP and depressed cyclic AMP, also increased the duration of evoked potentials and markedly increased spontaneous activity.

POSSIBLE ROLES OF CYCLIC NUCLEOTIDES IN PATHOPHYSIOLOGICAL MECHANISMS OF EPILEPSY

Although there is insufficient information to make any definitive statement concerning the roles of cyclic AMP and cyclic GMP in pathophysiological mechanisms of epilepsy, the available data do allow the formation of a hypothesis, which will be outlined next.

There is much evidence implicating cyclic AMP as the mediator of neurotransmitter-evoked changes in neuronal activity. Adenosine and the biogenic amines have been shown to be inhibitory when iontophoresed in the vicinity of most central neurons and also have been shown to markedly elevate cyclic AMP levels in incubated brain slices. Iontophoretically applied cyclic AMP also causes hyperpolarization of many central neurons. In addition, cyclic AMP depresses electrical activity in incubated hippocampal slices. All these data are consistent with the hypothesis that cyclic AMP may be the second messenger for biogenic amines and/or adenosine and may, in fact, be responsible for the inhibitory actions of these compounds. Our studies have demonstrated that both a reduction in the norepinephrine influence in the CNS, probably at beta receptors, and blockade of adenosine receptors in the CNS inhibit seizure-induced cyclic AMP elevations and concomitantly hasten the appearance of tonic seizures after pentylenetetrazol injection (vide supra). Together, these data suggest a close relationship among neurotransmitter actions, accumulation of cyclic AMP, and seizure activity. We suggest that seizure discharges cause a release, from intracellular stores, of biogenic amines and adenosine and that these substances then act at synaptic sites to increase intracellular cyclic AMP levels. Cyclic AMP, in turn, may act at membranes to alter ion permeability, as well as

having other actions. Thus, elevated cyclic AMP levels in brain may have an antiepileptic effect and may perhaps have some role in mechanisms inhibiting the spread and/or duration of seizure discharges.

Cyclic GMP, unlike cyclic AMP, has not been definitely linked to any individual neurotransmitter system, but it has been shown to be related to neuronal activity. Many stimuli that produce cellular depolarization elevate levels of cyclic GMP in brain. Moreover, cyclic GMP has been shown to alter neuronal activity in nervous tissue. Phillis (21) reported that iontophoretic application of cyclic GMP onto unidentified cat cerebral cortex cells increased their firing rate 51%. Similar percentages of rat pyramidal tract neurons were activated by iontophoretically applied cyclic GMP (26). More recently, it has been demonstrated that cyclic GMP can produce seizure discharges in hippocampal explants and increase electrical activity in hippocampal slices. These results are particularly intriguing, and in association with the data on the effects of seizures on cyclic GMP levels, they suggest that cyclic GMP may be involved in mechanisms responsible for initiating and/or maintaining seizure discharges.

This hypothesis obviously is overly simplistic, but it is considered to be only a first approximation, and it may be useful for directing future research to eventually determine the significance of cyclic nucleotides in pathophysiological mechanisms of seizures.

ACKNOWLEDGMENT

This work was supported in part by grant NS-14834 from the National Institutes of Health.

REFERENCES

1. Berti, F., Bernareggi, V., Folco, G. C., Fumagalli, R., and Paoletti, R. (1976): Prostaglandin E_2 and cyclic nucleotides in rat convulsions and tremors. In: Advances in Biochemical Psychopharmacology, Vol. 15, First and Second Messengers—New Vistas, edited by E. Costa, E. Giacobini, and R. Paoletti, pp. 367–377. Raven Press, New York.
2. Bloom, F. E. (1975): The role of cyclic nucleotides in central synaptic function. Rev. Physiol. Biochem. Pharmacol., 74:1–103.
3. Daly, J. (1977): Cyclic Nucleotides in the Nervous System. Plenum Press, New York.
4. Ferrendelli, J. A. (1976): Cellular depolarization and cyclic nucleotide content in central nervous system. In: Advances in Biochemical Psychopharmacology, Vol. 15, First and Second Messengers—New Vistas,

edited by E. Costa, E. Giacobini and R. Paoletti, pp. 303–313. Raven Press, New York.

5. Ferrendelli, J. A., Blank, A. C., and Gross, R. A. (1980): Relationships between seizure activity and cyclic nucleotide levels in brain. *Brain Res.*, 200:93–103.

6. Ferrendelli, J. A., and Kinscherf, D. A. (1977): Cyclic nucleotides in epileptic brain: Effects of pentylenetetrazol on regional cyclic AMP and cyclic GMP levels *in vivo. Epilepsia*, 18:525–531.

7. Ferrendelli, J. A., Rubin, E. H., and Kinscherf, D. A. (1976): Influence of divalent cations on regulation of cyclic GMP and cyclic AMP levels in brain tissue. *J. Neurochem.*, 264:741–748.

8. Folbergrová, J. (1975): Cyclic 3′,5′-adenosine monophosphate in mouse cerebral cortex during homocysteine convulsions and their prevention by sodium phenobarbital. *Brain Res.*, 92:165–169.

9. Folbergrová, J. (1977): Changes of cyclic AMP and phosphorylase a in mouse cerebral cortex during seizures induced by 3-mercaptopropionic acid. *Brain Res.*, 135:337–346.

10. Folco, G. C., Longiave, D., and Bosisio, E. (1977): Relations between prostaglandin E_2, $F_{2\alpha}$, and cyclic nucleotide levels in rat brain and induction of convulsions. *Prostaglandins*, 13:893–900.

11. Gross, R. A., and Ferrendelli, J. A. (1979): Effects of reserpine, propranolol and aminophylline on seizure activity and CNS cyclic nucleotides. *Ann. Neurol.*, 6:296–301.

12. Gross, R. A., and Ferrendelli, J. A. (1982): Relationships between norepinephrine and cyclic nucleotides in brain and seizure activity. *Neuropharmacology*, 21:655–661.

13. Hoffer, B., Seiger, A., Freedman, R., Olson, L., and Taylor, D. (1977): Electrophysiology and cytology of hippocampal formation transplants in the anterior chamber of the eye. II. Cholinergic mechanisms. *Brain Res.*, 119:108–132.

14. Hoffer, B. J., Seiger, A., Taylor, D., Olson, L., and Freedman, R. (1977): Seizures and related epileptiform activity in hippocampus transplanted to the anterior chamber of the eye. I. Characterization of seizures, interictal spikes, and synchronous activity. *Exp. Neurol.*, 54:233–250.

15. Lust, W. D., Goldberg, N. D., and Passonneau, J. V. (1976): Cyclic nucleotides in murine brain: The temporal relationship of changes induced in adenosine 3′,5′-monophosphate and guanosine 3′,5′-monophosphate following maximal electroshock or decapitation. *J. Neurochem.*, 26:5–10.

16. Lust, W. D., Kupferberg, H. J., Yonekawa, W. D., Penry, J. K., Passonneau, J. V., and Wheaton, A. B. (1978): Changes in brain metabolites induced by convulsants or electroshock: Effects of anticonvulsant agents. *Mol. Pharmacol.*, 14:347–356.

17. Mao, C. C., Guidotti, A., and Costa, E. (1974): The regulation of cyclic guanosine monophosphate in rat cerebellum: Possible involvement of putative amino acid neurotransmitters. *Brain Res.*, 79:510–514.

18. Mao, C. C., Guidotti, A., and Costa, E. (1975): Evidence for an involvement of GABA in the mediation of the cerebellar cGMP decrease and the anticonvulsant action of diazepam. *Naunyn Schmiedebergs Arch. Pharmacol.*, 289:367–378.

19. Nathanson, J. A. (1977): Cyclic nucleotides and nervous system function. *Physiol. Rev.*, 57:157–256.

20. Palmer, G. C., Jones, D. J., Medina, M. A., and Stavinoha, W. B. (1979): Anticonvulsant drug actions on *in vitro* and *in vivo* levels of cyclic AMP in the mouse brain. *Epilepsia*, 29:95–104.

21. Phillis, J. W. (1974): Evidence for cholinergic transmission in the cerebral cortex. *Adv. Behav. Biol.*, 10:57–77.

22. Phillis, J. W. (1977): The role of cyclic nucleotides in the CNS. *Can. J. Neurol. Sci.*, 4:151–195.

23. Raabe, W., Nicol, S., Gumnit, R. J., and Goldberg, N. D. (1978): Focal penicillin epilepsy increases cyclic GMP in cerebral cortex. *Brain Res.*, 144:185–188.

24. Rehncrona, S., Siesjö, B. K., and Westerberg, E. (1978): Adenosine and cyclic AMP in cerebral cortex of rats in hypoxia, status epilepticus and hypercapnia. *Acta Physiol. Scand.*, 104:453–463.

25. Sattin, A. (1971): Increase in the content of adenosine 3′,5′-monophosphate in mouse forebrain during seizures and prevention of the increase by methylxanthines. *J. Neurochem.*, 18:1087–1096.

26. Stone, T. W., Taylor, D. A., and Bloom, F. E. (1975): Cyclic AMP and cyclic GMP may mediate opposite neuronal responses in the rat cerebral cortex. *Science*, 187:845–847.

27. Troyer, E. W., Hall, I. A., and Ferrendelli, J. A. (1978): Guanylate cyclases in CNS: Enzymatic characteristics of soluble and particulate enzymes from mouse cerebellum and retina. *J. Neurochem.*, 31:825–833.

28. Walker, J. E., Lewin, E., Sheppard, J. R., and Cromwell, R. (1973): Enzymatic regulation of adenosine 3′,5′-monophosphate (cyclic AMP) in the freezing epileptogenic lesion of rat brain and in homologous contralateral cortex. *J. Neurochem.*, 21:79–85.

Advances in Neurology, Vol. 34: Status Epilepticus, edited by A.V. Delgado-Escueta, C.G. Wasterlain, D.M. Treiman, and R.J. Porter. Raven Press, New York © 1983.

34

Role of Benzodiazepine Receptors in Seizures

Phil Skolnick, Paul J. Marangos, and Steven M. Paul

The benzodiazepines are the most widely prescribed class of drugs in current therapeutic use (37). Diazepam (Valium®) and clonazepam (Clonopin®) are considered the drugs of choice for treatment of status epilepticus and are also efficacious for treatment of other types of seizure disorders, including absence and clonic seizures (3,6,19), myoclonic spasms of infancy, and minor myoclonic and akinetic seizures in children.

The discovery of high-affinity, saturable, stereospecific binding sites for benzodiazepines in the mammalian central nervous system (CNS) (20, 35,38) has radically altered our concepts of the molecular mechanisms of benzodiazepine action. These recognition sites for benzodiazepines are now believed to be pharmacological receptors. The binding of a benzodiazepine (or endogenous ligand) to this site may be the first step in a cascade of events that results in a therapeutic effect. Furthermore, the recent demonstration that these receptors are altered following electrically or chemically (18,24) induced seizures suggests these receptors may be of fundamental importance in physiological control of seizure activity. The presence in brain tissue of endogenous substances capable of either binding to the benzodiazepine recognition site (e.g., purines such as inosine and hypoxanthine) or modulating receptor affinity (e.g., GABA) has also prompted studies of their possible relationships to seizure mechanisms. In this chapter, we shall attempt to relate recent information obtained in our laboratory and other laboratories implicating benzodiazepine recognition sites in the anticonvulsant actions of the benzodiazepines and in physiological control of seizure activity.

EVIDENCE IMPLICATING BENZODIAZEPINE RECEPTORS IN THE ANTICONVULSANT ACTIONS OF BENZODIAZEPINES

One of the most striking observations made during the initial characterization of the benzodiazepine receptor (13,35) was that "classic" neurotransmitters (e.g., dopamine, acetylcholine, serotonin, glycine, GABA), synthetic agonist and antagonist derivatives of these compounds, many peptidergic hormones, as well as a large number of psychoactive compounds could not displace radiolabeled diazepam from these CNS binding sites. Only other benzodiazepines were able to competitively displace radioactive diazepam from these sites. When the relative receptor affinities of a series of benzodiazepines for these binding sites *in vitro* were compared with the abilities of the same series of compounds to antagonize pentylenetetrazol-(PTZ)-induced seizures in mice (21), an excellent correlation ($r = 0.90$, $p < 0.001$) was obtained between these two parameters (Table 1). This correlation is even more remarkable because pharmacokinetic factors such as differential metabolism of compounds as well as differences in lipid solubility would tend to confound such *in vivo/in vitro* comparisons. Highly significant correlations were also obtained for the muscle relaxant, anxiolytic, and antiaggressive properties of benzo-

TABLE 1. *Relationship between the anti-PTZ effects of benzodiazepines and in vitro affinities for benzodiazepine receptor*

Benzodiazepine	K_i (nM)[a]	ED_{50} (μmole/kg)
Clonazepam	0.87	0.95
Flunitrazepam	2.2	0.32
Lorazepam	2.3	0.62
Diazepam	7.4	7.0
Nitrazepam	9.2	2.5
Flurazepam	11	4.7
Oxazepam	19	2.4
Bromazepam	21	2.2
Chlorazepate	44	5.7
DPXD	360	23.8
Medazepam	880	22.8
Ro 5-2181	5,300	33.1

[a]Data obtained from human cerebral cortex. Data abstracted from Mohler and Okada (20).

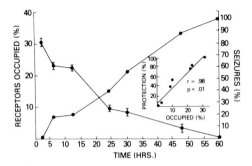

FIG. 1. Correlation between receptor occupation and the anticonvulsant properties of diazepam. Mice were injected with diazepam (4 mg/kg i.p.) at time 0, and the numbers of drug-occupied benzodiazepine receptors were correlated with its anticonvulsant activity over the next 60 hr. To determine the numbers of drug-occupied receptors, mice were killed by decapitation, and synaptosomal membranes were prepared from forebrain. The final synaptosomal pellet was resuspended in 40 volumes of ice-cold Tris HCl (pH 7.4, 50 mM) to a final protein concentration of about 1 mg/ml. Benzodiazepine receptors were measured in the lysed synaptosomal membrane fragments using a previously described technique (23). The percentage of receptors occupied by diazepam (plus metabolites) in synaptosomal membranes was determined by the following formula: % occupied = $R_c - R_d/B_{max} \times 100$, where R_c = [³H]diazepam bound in vehicle-treated mice; R_d = [³H]diazepam bound in diazepam-treated mice, and B_{max} = maximum number of binding sites in vehicle-treated mice (determined to be 1,213 fmole [³H]diazepam bound per milligram protein by Scatchard analysis). R_c and R_d were determined in the presence of 4.4-nM [³H]diazepam. At this concentration of diazepam, R_c = 653 ± 10 fmole [³H]diazepam bound per milligram protein (N = 18). To determine the number of mice seizing, half of the experimental group were injected with PTZ (80 mg/kg i.p.). Mice were counted as having had a seizure if generalized tonic-clonic movements were observed within 15 min of injection. This dose of PTZ produced seizures in more than 95% of vehicle-treated mice. (Adapted from Paul et al., ref. 25.)

diazepines (21). These correlations supported the hypothesis that binding sites were receptors mediating many if not all of the pharmacological effects of the benzodiazepines, and they provided indirect correlative evidence of a relationship between benzodiazepine receptors and the pharmacological properties of the benzodiazepines.

In a study designed to establish a relationship between benzodiazepine receptor occupancy by a drug and therapeutic action, we observed a highly significant direct correlation ($r = 0.96$, $p < 0.01$) (Fig. 1) between occupation of benzodiazepine receptors by diazepam and the protective effects of this drug against an ED_{99} of PTZ (25).

These studies suggest a direct participation of the benzodiazepine receptor in the anticonvulsant effects of diazepam and also imply that the convulsant actions of PTZ are mediated through this receptor. This hypothesis is supported by the recent finding (27) of a highly significant correlation ($r = 0.87$, $p < 0.01$) between the potencies of a series of tetrazol congeners (C_3–C_{11}) to displace [³H]diazepam from CNS receptor sites *in vitro* and their potencies as convulsants *in vivo*.

These data also revealed that only a relatively small number (less than 30%) of benzodiazepine receptors need be occupied to fully manifest an anticonvulsant effect of diazepam against PTZ-induced seizures (25). If these receptors are involved in the physiological regulation of seizure activity, it is tempting to speculate that a far smaller percentage would be needed for the tonic modulation of the neuronal activity. This hypothesis would not require an endogenous modulator of this receptor

to have a high affinity for the receptor, because occupation of only a small number of sites would be required for tonic regulation. A discussion of these hypotheses in the context of recent findings concerning putative endogenous ligand(s) or modulator(s) of this receptor will be presented.

PURINES AS ENDOGENOUS LIGANDS OF THE BENZODIAZEPINE RECEPTOR

Initial observations that only pharmacologically active benzodiazepines were capable of displacing radiolabeled benzodiazepines from CNS binding sites (13,35), coupled with the unique chemical structures of benzodiazepines that appeared to be unrelated to heretofore described compounds in the CNS, implied the existence of endogenous compounds that would physiologically subserve this receptor and prompted an intensive search for such factors.

Extraction of bovine brain with acidified acetone and subsequent chromatographic purification resulted in the isolation of two compounds that competitively inhibited [³H]diazepam binding to synaptosomal membrane fragments (15). These compounds were subsequently identified as the purines inosine and hypoxanthine (30). The affinities of these compounds for the benzodiazepine receptor are relatively low (K_i 836 and 982 μM for inosine and hypoxanthine, respectively) when compared with other classic endogenous ligands (e.g., norepinephrine, GABA). However, the small percentage of benzodiazepine receptor occupancy required to elicit a pharmacologic response, coupled with the relatively high brain concentrations of these compounds in brain (8,29) and the observation that inosine and hypoxanthine concentrations increase severalfold following electrically or chemically induced depolarization of neurons (26,36), suggests that these compounds may play a role as endogenous modulators or ligands of this receptor. The identification of these compounds as endogenous inhibitors of the benzodiazepine receptor has now been confirmed by several laboratories (1,22). In addition, Asano and Spector (1) have also demonstrated a cross-reactivity between these purines and a benzodiazepine-specific antibody, suggesting common areas of molecular recognition. Nonetheless, pharmacological examination of the effects of purines using several different paradigms is required to support *in vitro* binding studies that would not discriminate receptor agonists from antagonists.

Initial studies in our laboratories (31) examined the effects of inosine on PTZ-evoked seizures. Inosine was administered intraventricularly because this compound is readily transformed *in vivo* and does not readily cross the blood-brain barrier. Pretreatment of mice with up to 150 μg (0.56 μmole) of inosine did not afford frank protection from an ED$_{99}$ dose of PTZ administered intraperitoneally. However, mice administered this dose of inosine had a longer *latency* between the injection of PTZ and the development of tonic-clonic convulsions. This increased seizure latency was proportional to both the injection interval between inosine and PTZ and the dose of inosine administered (Fig. 2). In contrast, 7-methylinosine, which does not displace [³H]diazepam from receptor sites *in vitro* (16), did

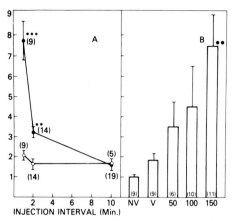

FIG. 2. Effects of intraventricularly administered inosine on PTZ-induced seizures. **A:** Effects of injection interval between inosine and PTZ on seizure latency; ***$p < 0.001$, **$p < 0.01$ compared with saline controls. **B:** Effects of varying doses of inosine (micrograms/mouse) on seizure latency; ●●$p < 0.01$ compared with vehicle alone. Ordinate: Seizure latency (min) defined as the interval between the PTZ challenge and the first appearance of tonic-clonic convulsions.

not alter seizure latency when administered in an equimolar dose. 2'-Deoxyinosine, which is three to four times as potent as inosine in displacing [³H]diazepam from receptor sites *in vitro* (16), was almost twice as potent in increasing the seizure latency as inosine. The transient protective effects of inosine may be partially due to pharmacokinetic factors, because after an equimolar dose of [¹⁴C]inosine was administered to mice, it was found that more than 80% of the radioactivity had left the CNS after 1 min. These data are suggestive of an action of inosine, at least when administered under these conditions, to be analogous to those of an "ultra-short-acting" benzodiazepine (31).

Other structurally related purines were examined for their potencies in displacing [³H]diazepam from these receptor sites. It was found that caffeine (16) was more potent than inosine, with a K_i value of approximately 284 μM. Caffeine has been described as a CNS stimulant that in high doses produces seizures. The concentrations of caffeine necessary to produce seizures in the human range from 8 to 12 g (28). Assuming distribution in total body water, brain concentrations of caffeine could theoretically occupy approximately 20% of the benzodiazepine receptors, a number that we have previously shown sufficient to elicit a pharmacological effect (25). This finding prompted us to examine the effects of purines and benzodiazepines on caffeine-evoked seizures. In these experiments, purines were administered parenterally, because Mohler et al. (22) had demonstrated that large (1,000 mg/kg) doses of parenterally administered inosine protected mice against convulsions induced by 3-mercaptopropionic acid (a GABA synthesis inhibitor). The dose of caffeine used (290 mg/kg) was sufficient to elicit seizures in approximately 90% of the mice. Inosine (500–1,000 mg/kg) protected animals against caffeine-induced seizures in a dose-dependent fashion (Fig. 3) and also increased seizure latency (14). 7-Methylinosine (1,000 mg/kg) did not protect animals from the convulsive effects of caffeine, nor did it alter seizure latency.

The electrophysiological effects of inosine have been examined in primary cultures of fetal mouse spinal neurons. These cultures possess "brain-type" benzodiazepine receptors (7) and are chemosensitive to benzodiazepines, amino acids, and convulsants (2,11). Application of inosine to these cells by either pressure ejection or iontophoresis elicited two types of transmitterlike membrane effects, a rapidly desensitizing excitatory response and a nondesensitizing inhibitory response. The benzodiazepine flurazepam (Dalmane®) elicited a similar excitatory response that displayed cross-desensitization with the excitatory response produced by inosine. The inhibitory response to inosine was blocked by flurazepam. These data suggest that inosine can activate two different conductances on spinal neurons and that flurazepam activates one of these conductances and antagonizes the other (12). In another series of experiments, MacDonald and Barker demonstrated that inosine can reverse the paroxysmal depolarizing

events produced by the convulsant picrotoxin (23). Benzodiazepines and barbiturates can also reverse the effects of picrotoxin. Lewin (9) reported that intracortical injections of adenosine, inosine, and hypoxanthine at concentrations from 10^{-4} to 10^{-8} M uniformly resulted in electroencephalographic seizures, and these effects were blocked by phenobarbital. These results would appear at variance with the apparent benzodiazepinelike effects of inosine observed in primary cultures. However, at least two different conductances were activated in spinal neurons in culture by inosine, and one appeared to be antagonized by flurazepam. In a recent study, Lewin and Bleck (10) measured purine levels postictally following electroshock in rat brain. These workers proposed that early increases in inosine and hypoxanthine following electroshock may be involved in seizure generation or propagation, whereas the higher levels observed during and after clinical recovery may be involved in the termination of epileptic activity. The proposed bimodal actions of inosine and hypoxanthine are consonant with recent biochemical findings from our laboratory that these purines are approximately 10-fold more potent in inhibiting GABA-enhanced [³H]diazepam binding than in inhibiting basal (non-GABA-enhanced) binding (17) and would suggest that relatively low concentrations of purines may be involved in the genesis or propagation of seizures by inhibiting GABA-benzodiazepine-receptor coupling, whereas higher concentrations of purines would terminate this effect by occupation of the benzodiazepine "recognition site" analogous to clinically active benzodiazepines (27). Recent behavioral studies from our laboratory and other laboratories

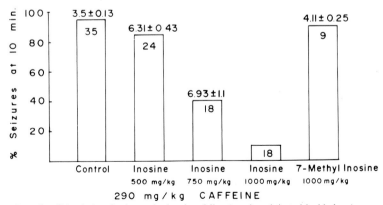

FIG. 3. Antagonism of caffeine-induced seizures by inosine. Mice (numbers injected inside bars) were pretreated with inosine or 7-methylinosine and 20 min later were treated with caffeine (290 mg/kg i.p.). The numbers of animals with tonic-clonic seizures within 10 min of injection were then noted. The numbers over the bars are seizure latency times (min). (Adapted from Marangos et al., ref. 14.)

(4,34) have suggested that in relatively low doses inosine antagonizes some of the behavioral actions of diazepam.

In toto, these data suggest that both inosine and hypoxanthine are involved in the physiological regulation of the benzodiazepine receptor. Certainly, further investigations are necessary to better define the precise roles of these purines.

REGULATION OF BENZODIAZEPINE RECEPTORS IN SEIZURE STATES

Direct evidence linking the benzodiazepine receptor to seizure states has been provided by the observations that benzodiazepine receptor numbers are altered as a result of either electrically (18,24) or chemically (24) induced seizures.

Electroshock (150 V ac, 1 sec) or PTZ (45 mg/kg i.p.) elicited rapid (maximum effect developed by 15 min postictally) and reversible (return to control levels by 60 min postictally) increases in [^{3}H]diazepam binding in rat cerebral cortex. Scatchard analysis of [^{3}H]diazepam binding revealed this increase in binding to be due to an increase in receptor number rather than an alteration in apparent receptor affinity (K_D). Administration of subconvulsive shock (70 V ac, 0.4 sec), argon-induced hypoxia, or a subconvulsive dose of PTZ did not elicit an alteration in [^{3}H]diazepam binding. McNamara et al. (18) reported persistent increases in benzodiazepine receptor numbers of 30% to 40% following kindling (14–19 stimulations) and 20% following electroshock (15–18 stimulations) in rat hippocampus. The effect was present at 24 hr after the last electrical stimulation, which was in marked contrast to the rapidly reversible increase in receptor number following a single electroshock seizure or PTZ.

Gallager et al. (5) recently reported a 35% increase in benzodiazepine receptor number 60 min after a single i.p. dose of diphenylhydantoin (DPH). This observation was confirmed using an *in vivo* labeling technique with [^{3}H]diazepam, as well as the more traditional *in vivo/in vitro* paradigm. Direct *in vitro* addition of DPH did not enhance diazepam binding, a finding consistent with electrophysiological data demonstrating a lack of effect following direct iontophoretic application of DPH. We have recently reported that a purine derivative with anticonvulsant properties, EMD 28422 (32,33), enhances receptor number both *in vivo* and *in vitro*. We have proposed that the observation of an increase in receptor number *in vitro* (at

4°C) suggests that this compound, as well as electroshock- and PTZ-induced seizures and DPH, may "unmask" receptors, perhaps by removing a factor that binds in a reversible but noncompetitive fashion. This hypothesis would explain the phenomenon of the rapid up-and-down regulation of this receptor that has been reported.

CONCLUSIONS

There is now sufficient experimental evidence to support a role for the benzodiazepine receptor in mediating the anticonvulsant actions of the benzodiazepines. Evidence also indicates that benzodiazepine receptors are altered as a result of seizure activity, but further investigation is necessary to precisely define the significance of postictal alterations in this receptor. The putative endogenous ligand(s) of the benzodiazepine receptor, inosine and hypoxanthine, have been demonstrated to both electrophysiologically and pharmacologically modify seizure activity. However, these studies suggest a bimodal action, and more rigorous experimentation is necessary before a precise role for these compounds in seizures can be determined. The modulation of benzodiazepine receptor affinity by GABA is now well established (37). The role of GABA as an inhibitory neurotransmitter and the induction of seizures by agents that interfere with GABA synthesis, receptors, and release have long been areas of intensive investigation. Future investigations will focus on the relationship of the benzodiazepine-GABA receptor complex (along with an associated chloride ionophore) and its role in seizures.

REFERENCES

1. Asano, T., and Spector, S. (1979): Identification of inosine and hypoxanthine as endogenous ligands for the brain benzodiazepine receptor binding sites. *Proc. Natl. Acad. Sci. U.S.A.*, 76:977–981.
2. Barker, J., and Ransom, B. (1978): Amino acid pharmacology of mammalian central neurons grown in tissue cultures. *J. Physiol. (Lond.)*, 280:331–354.
3. Browne, T. R., and Penry, J. K. (1973): Benzodiazepines in the treatment of epilepsy: A review. *Epilepsia*, 14:277–310.
4. Crawley, J., Marangos, P., Paul, S., Skolnick, P., and Goodwin, F. (1981): Purine-benzodiazepine interaction: Inosine reverses diazepam-induced stimulation of mouse exploratory behavior. *Science*, 211:725–727.
5. Gallager, D., Mallorga, P., and Tallman, J. (1980): Interaction of diphenylhydantoin and benzodiazepines in the CNS. *Brain Res.*, 185:209–220.
6. Greenblatt, D. J., and Shader, R. (1974): *Benzodiazepines in Clinical Practice.* Raven Press, New York.

7. Huang, A., Barker, J., Paul, S., and Skolnick, P. (1980): Characterization of benzodiazepine receptors in primary cultures of fetal mouse brain and spinal cord. *Brain Res.*, 190:485–492.

8. Kleihues, P., Kobayashi, K., and Hossmann, K. A. (1974): Purine metabolism in the cat brain after one hour of complete ischemia. *J. Neurochem.*, 23:417–425.

9. Lewin, E. (1976): Endogenously released adenine derivatives: A possible role in epileptogenesis. *Trans. Am. Neurol. Assoc.*, 101:1–3.

10. Lewin, E., and Bleck, V. (1980): Electroshock seizures: Effect on brain adenosine and its metabolites. *Trans. Am. Neurol. Assoc.*, 105:59–61.

11. MacDonald, J. R., and Barker, J. (1979): Enhancement of GABA-mediated postsynaptic inhibition in cultured mammalian spinal cord neurons: A common mode of anticonvulsant action. *Brain Res.*, 167:323–336.

12. MacDonald, J., Barker, J., Paul, S., Marangos, P., and Skolnick, P. (1979): Inosine may be an endogenous ligand for benzodiazepine receptors on cultured spinal neurons. *Science*, 205:715–717.

13. Mackerer, C., Kochman, R., Bierschenk, F., and Bremer, S. S. (1978): The binding of [³H]diazepam to rat brain homogenates. *J. Pharmacol. Exp. Ther.*, 206:405–413.

14. Marangos, P., Martino, A., Paul, S., and Skolnick, P. (1981): Benzodiazepines and inosine antagonize caffeine induced seizures. *Psychopharmacology*, 72:269–274.

15. Marangos, P., Paul, S., Greenlaw, P., Goodwin, F. K., and Skolnick, P. (1978): Demonstration of an endogenous competitive inhibitor of [³H]diazepam binding in bovine brain. *Life Sci.*, 22:1893–1900.

16. Marangos, P., Paul, S., Parma, A., Goodwin, F., Syapin, P., and Skolnick, P. (1979): Purinergic inhibition of diazepam binding to rat brain *(in vitro)*. *Life Sci.*, 24:851–858.

17. Marangos, P., Paul, S., Parma, A., and Skolnick, P. (1981): Inhibition of GABA stimulated [³H]diazepam binding by benzodiazepine receptor ligands. *Biochem. Pharmacol.*, 30:2171–2173.

18. McNamara, J., Peper, A., and Patrone, V. (1980): Repeated seizures induce long-term increase in hippocampal benzodiazepine receptors. *Proc. Natl. Acad. Sci. U.S.A.*, 77:3029–3033.

19. Millichap, J. G. (1972): General principles: Clinical efficacy and use. In: *Antiepileptic Drugs*, edited by D. M. Woodbury, J. K. Penry, and R. P. Schmidt, pp. 497–518. Raven Press, New York.

20. Mohler, H., and Okada, T. (1977): Benzodiazepine receptor: Demonstration in the central nervous system. *Science*, 198:849–851.

21. Mohler, H., and Okada, T. (1978): Biochemical identification of the site of action of benzodiazepines in human brain by [³H]diazepam binding. *Life Sci.*, 22:985–996.

22. Mohler, H., Polc, P., Cumin, R., Pieri, L., and Kettler, R. (1979): Nicotinamide is a brain constituent with benzodiazepine-like actions. *Nature*, 287:563–565.

23. Paul, S., Marangos, P., and Skolnick, P. (1980): CNS benzodiazepine receptors: Is there an endogenous ligand? In: *Psychopharmacology and Biochemistry of Neurotransmitter*, edited by R. W. Olsen and H. I. Yamamura, pp. 661–676. Elsevier/North-Holland, New York.

24. Paul, S. M., and Skolnick, P. (1978): Rapid changes in benzodiazepine receptors after experimental seizures. *Sciences*, 202:892–894.

25. Paul, S., Syapin, P., Paugh, B. A., Moncada, V., and Skolnick, P. (1979): Correlation between benzodiazepine receptor occupation and anticonvulsant effects of diazepam. *Nature*, 281:688–689.

26. Pull, I., and McIlwain, H. (1972): Adenine derivatives as neurohumoral agents in the brain. *Biochem. J.*, 130:975–981.

27. Rehavi, M., Skolnick, P., and Paul, S. (1982): Effects of tetrazole derivatives on [³H]diazepam binding *in vitro*: Correlation with convulsant potency. *Eur. J. Pharmacol.*, 78:353–356.

28. Ritchie, J. M. (1970): Central nervous system stimulants. II. The xanthine. In: *The Pharmacological Basis of Therapeutics*, edited by L. S. Goodman, and A. Gilman, pp. 358–370. Macmillan, New York.

29. Saugstad, O. D., and Schrader, H. (1978): The determination of inosine and hypoxanthine in rat brain during normothermic and hypothermic hypoxia. *Acta Neurol. Scand.*, 57:281–288.

30. Skolnick, P., Marangos, P., Goodwin, F. K., Edwards, M., and Paul, S. (1978): Identification of inosine and hypoxanthine as endogenous inhibitors of [³H]diazepam binding in the central nervous system. *Life Sci.*, 23:1473–1480.

31. Skolnick, P., Syapin, P., Paugh, B., Moncada, V., Marangos, P., and Paul, S. (1979): Inosine, an endogenous ligand of the brain benzodiazepine receptor antagonizes PTZ-induced seizures. *Proc. Natl. Acad. Sci. U.S.A.*, 76:1515–1518.

32. Skolnick, P., Lock, K. L., Paugh, B., Marangos, P., Windsor, R., and Paul, S. (1980): Pharmacologic effects of EMD 28422, a novel purine which enhances [³H]diazepam binding. *Pharmacol. Biochem. Behav.*, 12:685–689.

33. Skolnick, P., Lock, K., Paul, S., Marangos, P., Jonas, R., and Irmscher, K. (1980): Increased benzodiazepine receptor number elicited *in vitro* by a novel purine, EMD 28422. *Eur. J. Pharmacol.*, 67:179–186.

34. Slater, P., and Longman, D. (1979): Effects of diazepam and muscimol on GABA mediated neurotransmission: Interactions with inosine and nicotinamide. *Life Sci.*, 25:1963–1967.

35. Squires, R. F., and Braestrup, C. (1977): Benzodiazepine receptors in rat brain. *Nature*, 266:732–734.

36. Sun, M. C., McIlwain, H., and Pull, I. (1976): The metabolism of adenine derivatives in different parts of the brain of the rat, and their release from hypothalamic preparations on excitation. *J. Neurobiol.*, 7:109–122.

37. Tallman, J. F., Paul, S. M., Skolnick, P., and Gallager, D. W. (1980): Receptors for the age of anxiety: Pharmacology of the benzodiazepines. *Science*, 207:274–281.

38. Williamson, M., Paul, S., and Skolnick, P. (1978): Labeling of benzodiazepine receptors *in vivo*. *Nature*, 275:533–535.

Advances in Neurology, Vol. 34: Status Epilepticus, edited by A.V. Delgado-Escueta, C.G. Wasterlain, D.M. Treiman, and R.J. Porter. Raven Press, New York © 1983.

35

Inosine, Hypoxanthine, and Seizures

Edward Lewin

Inosine and hypoxanthine, the immediate metabolites of adenosine, may play some role in the epileptic process. Electroconvulsive shock produces marked increases in these purines in rat brain (6). Similarly, in the mouse, electroshock seizures result in a dramatic and progressive rise in inosine, peaking at 5 min, and a somewhat slower increase in hypoxanthine, reaching its maximum at 10 min (3). These increases are reduced in magnitude by prior administration of either phenytoin or phenobarbital, possibly secondary to seizure modification by these drugs. Recently, we found that a subconvulsive series of single electroshocks also produced an immediate elevation in brain inosine. This increase was completely blocked by both phenytoin and phenobarbital, a result suggesting a direct effect on inosine formation or release (2).

Inosine and hypoxanthine may have both epileptogenic and antiepileptic actions. The injection of inosine or hypoxanthine into rat cortex at concentrations down to 10^{-8} M produces epileptiform discharges and seizures (1). However, inosine injected intraventricularly in mice antagonizes pentylenetetrazol-induced seizures (8). In mouse spinal neurons grown in culture, inosine and hypoxanthine cause an early brief excitation followed by a more prolonged inhibitory response (4).

In the studies reported here, diazepam, a drug commonly used to treat status epilepticus, was administered prior to electroshock, and these purines were measured at intervals following the stimulus. Both a convulsive stimulus and a subconvulsive stimulus were used. In addition, the effect of a subconvulsive series of electroshocks on pentylenetetrazol-induced seizures was investigated, because this stimulus rapidly elevates brain inosine.

METHODS

Seizures were induced through electrodes applied to the shaved scalp just anterior to the ears. A 60-Hz square-wave current at 100 V with a pulse duration of 5 msec was applied for 5 sec. The subconvulsive stimulus consisted of 15 shocks given at 3 Hz with the same voltage and pulse duration. Mice were sacrificed for chemical studies by immersion in liquid nitrogen. Brains were removed and extracted as described previously (3), and inosine, hypoxanthine, and adenosine were determined enzymatically (5).

RESULTS

Control mice almost immediately developed tonic extension of the hindlimbs when the 60-Hz current was applied. Tonic extension persisted for 5 to 15 sec after the stimulus was removed and was followed by clonic movements, which continued for 5 to 10 sec. Animals became ambulatory at 40 to 80 sec. In mice receiving diazepam (10 mg/kg i.p. 10 min before electroshock), tonic extension appeared promptly but generally persisted for less than 5 sec after the stimulus was stopped. Clonic movements were also brief. However, these mice remained quietly on their sides and did not ambulate.

The brains of control mice contained low levels of inosine (Fig. 1) and somewhat higher concentrations of hypoxanthine (Fig. 2). Following the convulsive stimulus, inosine rose rapidly and continued to increase up to 5 min, the longest interval studied. Hypoxanthine increased more slowly. In the brains of mice receiving diazepam, the elevations in inosine were significantly reduced at 30 sec and thereafter, and increases in hypoxanthine were significantly less at 3 and 5 min.

Mice given the low-frequency stimulus manifested a myoclonic jerk with each shock, whether or not diazepam had been administered. The animals were immediately active after this series of stimuli.

In the brains of untreated mice, inosine was elevated immediately and at 60 sec (Table 1). Diazepam markedly inhibited this increase in inosine. Hypoxanthine was increased slightly in both untreated and treated mice (Table 2).

A series of 4 mice were given pentylenetetrazol (100 mg/kg i.p.), and the latency to onset of clonic jerks was measured. The mean latency was found to be 33 ± 2.6 sec (SEM). In a second group of 5 mice given the same injection of pentylenetetrazol followed immediately by the subconvulsive series of electroshocks, the latency was significantly increased to 92 ± 3.0 sec ($p < 0.001$).

DISCUSSION

Electroshock, both at 3 Hz and 60 Hz, produced a rapid rise in brain inosine, and the 60-Hz stimulus and resultant seizure were followed by a somewhat slower increase in brain hypoxanthine as well. Because inosine at low concentrations is epileptogenic (1), the early increase in inosine may be

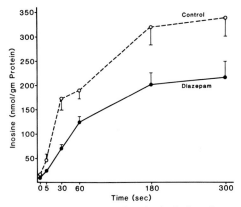

FIG. 1. Inosine concentrations in the brains of control mice and mice given diazepam following 60-Hz electroshock for 5 sec at 100 V and 5 msec pulse duration. Results are the means of four brains ± SEM.

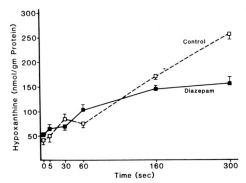

FIG. 2. Hypoxanthine concentrations in the brains of control mice and mice given diazepam following 60-Hz electroshock for 5 sec at 100 V and 5 msec pulse duration. Results are the means of four brains ± SEM.

TABLE 1. *Inosine concentration in mouse brain following subconvulsive electroshock*[a]

Drug	Control	Post shock	
		Sacrificed immediately	Sacrificed at 60 sec
None	14.9	63.7	188
	(3.75)	(5.18)	(31.6)
Diazepam	10.7	12.6	34.0
	(1.75)	(1.68)	(2.99)

[a]Fifteen stimuli given at 3 Hz, 5 msec pulse duration, and 100 V. Results expressed as nanomoles per gram of protein. Figures in parentheses are SEM. Values are the means of four experiments.

TABLE 2. *Hypoxanthine concentration in mouse brain following subconvulsive electroshock*[a]

Drug	Control	Post shock	
		Sacrificed immediately	Sacrificed at 60 sec
None	72.8	58.4	107
	(10.3)	(7.59)	(14.5)
Diazepam	52.7	62.9	74.2
	(3.93)	(6.85)	(4.75)

[a]Fifteen stimuli given at 3 Hz, 5 msec pulse duration, and 100 V. Results expressed as nanomoles per gram of protein. Figures in parentheses are SEM. Values are the means of four experiments.

involved in seizure generation. However, in the mice given the convulsive stimulus, both inosine and hypoxanthine reached their highest levels after the mice had apparently recovered from their seizures.

We have suggested that these two purines may participate in the termination of epileptic activity (3), perhaps by interacting with the benzodiazepine receptor for which they are ligands (7). The effectiveness of at least two benzodiazepines, diazepam and lorazepam (9), in the treatment of status epilepticus (i.e., in arresting ongoing and repeated seizures) supports the idea that the benzodiazepine receptor may play a role in stopping seizure activity.

Diazepam, unlike phenytoin and phenobarbital, did not prevent or delay the onset of tonic hindlimb extension produced by 60-Hz electroshock, but the duration of tonic extension following cessation of the stimulus was decreased. However, as found with phenytoin and phenobarbital, diazepam significantly reduced the increases in inosine and hypoxanthine produced by electroshock seizures and also markedly decreased the elevation in inosine evoked by the subconvulsive stimulus. The persistently high levels of inosine and hypoxanthine observed after tonic-clonic seizures induced by electroshock may result largely from the propagated seizure rather than from the electric stimulus alone, and the inhibition of these changes by diazepam may be secondary to its modification of the seizure pattern. However, diazepam also markedly reduced the rise in inosine evoked by the subconvulsive shock without apparently altering the accompanying myoclonic jerks. This result suggests that diazepam may have had a direct effect on inosine formation or release.

The time from injection to onset of pentylenetetrazol-induced seizures was significantly prolonged by the 3-Hz stimulus given for 5 sec immediately after injection. This increase in latency may have been mediated by the marked and rapid elevation in brain inosine evoked by the elec-

troshock. Skolnick et al. (8) have found that inosine injected intraventricularly lengthens the latency of onset of pentylenetetrazol seizures.

Status epilepticus may result in part from the failure of mechanisms that operate in the brain to stop epileptic activity once it has been initiated. The endogenous benzodiazepine receptor ligands, inosine and hypoxanthine, may be involved in one such mechanism.

REFERENCES

1. Lewin, E. (1976): Endogenously released adenine derivatives: A possible role in epileptogenesis. *Trans. Am. Neurol. Assoc.*, 101:192–195.
2. Lewin, E. (1981): Brain adenosine and its metabolites: Effects of electroshock and anticonvulsant drugs. In: *Chemisms of the Brain*, edited by R. Rodnight, H. Bachelard, and W. Stahl, pp. 276–280. Churchill Livingstone, Edinburgh.
3. Lewin, E., and Bleck, V. (1980): Electroshock seizures: Effect on brain adenosine and its metabolites. *Trans. Am. Neurol. Assoc.*, 59–61.
4. MacDonald, J. F., Barker, J. L., Paul, S. M., Marangos, P. J., and Skolnick, P. (1979): Inosine may be an endogenous ligand for benzodiazepine receptors on cultured spinal neurons. *Science*, 205:715–717.
5. Olsson, R. A. (1970): Changes in content of purine nucleoside in canine myocardium during coronary occlusion. *Circ. Res.*, 26:301–306.
6. Schultz, V., and Lowenstein, J. M. (1978): The purine nucleotide cycle: Studies of ammonia production and interconversions of adenine and hypoxanthine nucleotides and nucleosides by rat brain in situ. *J. Biol. Chem.*, 253:1938–1943.
7. Skolnick, P., Marangos, P. J., Goodwin, F. K., Edwards, M., and Paul, S. (1978): Identification of inosine and hypoxanthine as endogenous inhibitors of [³H]diazepam binding in the central nervous system. *Life Sci.*, 23:1473–1480.
8. Skolnick, P., Syapin, P. J., Paugh, B. A., Moncada, V., Marangos, P. J., and Paul, S. M. (1979): Inosine, an endogenous ligand of the brain benzodiazepine receptor, antagonizes pentylenetetrazole-evoked seizures. *Proc. Natl. Acad. Sci. U.S.A.*, 76:1515–1518.
9. Walker, J. E., Homan, R. W., Vasko, M. R., Crawford, I. L., Bell, R. D., and Tasker, W. G. (1979): Lorazepam in status epilepticus. *Ann. Neurol.*, 6:207–213.

Advances in Neurology, Vol. 34: Status Epilepticus, edited by A.V. Delgado-Escueta, C.G. Wasterlain, D.M. Treiman, and R.J. Porter. Raven Press, New York © 1983.

36

Role of Receptors for Neurotransmitters in Status Epilepticus

Anne M. Morin and Claude G. Wasterlain

The role that neurotransmitter receptors may play in status epilepticus has not been well explored. However, our knowledge of the adaptive properties of both peripheral and central receptor systems suggests that their responses to prolonged seizures are worthy of further study. Neurotransmitter receptors in the central nervous system have been shown to adjust their concentrations or physiological activities in response to changes in stimuli. These changes may be relatively long term, as in the case of denervation supersensitivity, or they may occur in a short-term period, with reestablishment of basal levels an intricate part of receptor regulation. Initial studies on the involvement of receptors in seizure models such as electroconvulsive shock or kindling have centered on measuring two aspects of receptors: changes in receptor density in a particular brain area or in whole brain and changes in receptor affinity for a radiolabeled ligand. Both aspects can be determined by Scatchard analysis of data on saturation binding of various ligands to membrane preparations. Given the limited data obtained by this approach, it would be beneficial to examine other aspects of receptor activity to understand receptor control mechanisms.

β-ADRENERGIC RECEPTOR REGULATION

β-adrenergic receptors have been studied in peripheral systems such as lymphocytes (19), in cul-tured cell lines (9), and in brain slices and homogenates (4,10,21). Certain basic features such as desensitization or hypersensitivity may serve as examples of receptor adaptation to changes in stimuli. The β-adrenergic receptors studied in lymphocytes respond to prolonged exposure to agonists by decreasing the apparent number of binding sites available for binding of radiolabeled agonist (e.g., [^{3}H]hydroxybenzylisoproterenol). Exposure to antagonist does not cause this decrease and in fact blocks the "desensitization" of the receptor by agonist. The decrease in agonist binding sites is accompanied by a decrease in the responsiveness of adenylate cyclase to catecholamines, thus indicating a decrease in receptor activity. Interestingly, this loss of agonist receptor binding is not reflected equally in the loss of binding of antagonists (39), a fact that may be of some importance when studies are carried out in membranes from convulsing animals; see the review of Hoffman and Lefkowitz (14).

The mechanism of desensitization is not known, but different examples of desensitization appear to share some common features. Receptors must usually be agonist-occupied, with impairment of the capacity for formation of a "high-affinity" form of the receptor. There is a loss of receptor binding sites, possibly by internalization within the cell or by conformational changes. The loss of physiological responsiveness often precedes actual loss of binding sites, as has been shown in cultured astrocytoma cells (13).

REGULATION OF β-ADRENERGIC RECEPTORS: SUPERSENSITIVITY

Increased sensitivity (supersensitivity) to agonists has been shown to follow decreased exposure to agonist. Rats treated with reserpine have depleted endogenous norepinephrine. Cortical membranes from such animals show enhanced cyclic AMP production in response to norepinephrine (10). Supersensitivity is also produced after lesions of noradrenergic pathways or treatment with 6-hydroxydopamine, which depletes catecholamines. Desensitization and supersensitivity share common features. Changes in receptor response appear to be related to sustained changes in exposure to neurotransmitter. Decreased exposure appears to lead to postsynaptic hypersensitivity, whereas an increase leads to hyposensitivity or desensitization. The responses are rapid, recovery is relatively slow, and the intensity of each response appears to be related to the duration of stimuli (30).

β-ADRENERGIC RECEPTORS IN MODELS OF EPILEPSY

The binding capacity of the β-adrenergic receptor has been measured in several experimental models of seizures. Depletion of endogenous catecholamines (2,8) facilitated the development of seizures in the "kindling" model of Goddard (11). Examination of [³H]dihydroalprenolol binding immediately after a kindled seizure (15 hr) showed no change in specific binding (22); however, 3 days later there was a decrease in receptor concentration.

β-adrenergic receptor concentration, but not that of α-adrenergic or serotonin receptors, was decreased after seven daily single electroconvulsive shocks (ECS) in rats (5). There was no change in receptor affinity ($K_d = 2.7$ nM), but the number of binding sites (B_{max}) rose from 10.9 to 7.8 pmole/g.

β-ADRENERGIC RECEPTORS IN STATUS EPILEPTICUS

[³H]dihydroalprenolol binding to β receptors (1) in forebrain membranes of mice subjected to 30 consecutive seizures (simulating status epilepticus) has been measured in our laboratory. Adult C57 black mice were subjected to ECS every 30 sec

using a Woodbury-Davenport apparatus. The first stimulation delivered electrical current (25 mA, 60 Hz ac) through alligator clips attached to the ears. Whenever a clinical seizure failed to occur, the intensity of the next and subsequent electroshocks was increased by 1 mA. In most mice, the threshold of generalized clonic seizures was 26 mA. The average animal required an intensity of 28 mA after 10 min and 29 mA after 20 min. Higher initial intensities resulted in high mortality. The animals were allowed to rest for 15 min after their last seizure and were then killed by cervical dislocation. Preliminary data (6 animals per group) indicate a significant loss ($p < 0.05$) of binding sites from 78 ± 7 fmole/mg protein in controls to 58 ± 5 fmole/mg protein ($\downarrow 26\%$) in the ECS group. There was no change in affinity (K_d), which was 2.3 ± 0.5 nM in controls and 2.4 ± 0.5 nM in the ECS group.

Cyclic AMP concentrations were measured by radioimmunoassay (34) in the forebrains of mice killed by microwave fixation during status epilepticus. Interestingly, the concentrations were markedly elevated with the first seizure (26.7 ± 3.5 pmole/mg protein as compared with 8.1 ± 0.9 pmole/g protein in controls). By the 50th seizure, however, the concentrations had decreased to 12.4 ± 2.7 pmole/mg protein. It is not known whether or not desensitization of β-adrenergic receptors plays a role in the fall of cyclic AMP response to seizures during status epilepticus. Investigations of norepinephrine stimulation of adenylate cyclase are in progress.

MUSCARINIC RECEPTOR REGULATION

Much of the information concerning the regulation of muscarinic receptors has been accumulated in studies of cell cultures and appears to hold true for brain as well (6,16–18). Receptor exposure to agonist results in downward regulation. The concentration of receptor as measured by [³H]quinuclidinylbenzilate (QNB) binding is decreased inversely to agonist concentration. Antagonists such as atropine block this response (31,32). Affinity for antagonist does not change, whereas agonist affinity does. Recovery of receptor concentration requires protein synthesis (16). Alternatively, Richelson (29) characterized "short-term" desensitization in mouse neuroblastoma cells (NIE-115), as measured by agonist-stimulated cyclic GMP production. Desensitization to agonist occurred rapidly (within 3–4 min), with recovery following quickly (1 hr). There were no detectable changes in [³H]QNB binding, indicating that antagonist binding was not altered.

MUSCARINIC RECEPTORS IN EPILEPSY

Measurements of radiolabeled-ligand binding to muscarinic receptors in some experimental situations related to epilepsy have shown fluctuations in receptor concentration. Depolarizing electrical stimulations of synaptosomes resulted in a 50% decrease in [³H]methylatropine binding. The overall loss of binding appeared to be correlated with persistent openings of the Na⁺ channels and was proportional to the intensity of the stimulus (18).

We have measured [³H]QNB binding (40) in the brains of electrically (11) and chemically (37) kindled rats. Long-term alterations in the concentration or affinity of muscarinic receptors have not been found (38), but there is evidence of a decrease shortly after a kindled seizure (22).

MUSCARINIC RECEPTORS IN STATUS EPILEPTICUS

In the model of repetitive seizures in mice described earlier, we found no significant change in specific binding of antagonist ([³H]QNB) to mouse forebrain membranes, using the procedure of Yamamura and Snyder (40) (Table 1).

Desensitization or actual receptor loss (downward regulation) may be reflected in a decrease in agonist binding as opposed to binding of antagonist (16). When mice receiving repetitive ECS were compared with controls, there was no observable difference in the capacity of carbachol to displace [³H]QNB bound to forebrain membrane preparations, suggesting no change in receptor affinity for agonist.

Desensitization of muscarinic receptors has been shown to decrease carbamylcholine-stimulated cyclic GMP formation. We have measured the concentrations of cyclic GMP in whole forebrain of mice receiving repetitive seizures, according to the procedure of Steiner et al. (34). The concentration increased from a control value of 0.4 ± 0.04 pmole/mg protein to 1.32 ± 0.24 pmole/mg protein during the first seizure. The level remained high (1.45 ± 0.4 pmole/mg protein) even after 50 consecutive seizures. These data support a lack of desensitization of muscarinic-receptor-mediated cyclic GMP production during prolonged seizures.

GABA AND BENZODIAZEPINE RECEPTORS IN EPILEPSY

The involvement of both the GABA system (24,25) and the benzodiazepines in seizures (12) has been well documented. The finding that activation of the GABA postsynaptic receptor may cause an increase in the affinity of the benzodiazepine binding site for either [³H]diazepam or [³H]flunitrazepam (7,15,20,35) further suggests that this system may very well be involved in seizure suppression.

Paul and Skolnick (27) demonstrated an increase (21.2%) in binding of [³H]diazepam to cortical membranes prepared from rats subjected to a single convulsant electroshock or pentylenetetrazol-induced seizures. They observed an increase in the number rather than in the affinity of the benzodiazepine binding sites. The increase was transient, appearing within 15 min of the seizure and disappearing after 60 min. Likewise, examination of [³H]diazepam binding to membranes prepared from the brains of spontaneously seizing gerbils indicated that there was increased specific binding in cerebral cortex, hippocampus, brainstem, and striatum. However, the increase in binding in striatum appears to be a result of increased affinity of the receptor, not in total concentration of binding sites (3). Paul et al. (28) showed excellent correlation between receptor occupancy and degree of protection against pentylenetetrazol-induced seizures in rats. McNamara et al. (23) demonstrated that daily ECS in rats produced a 19% increase in [³H]diazepam binding sites in hippocampus when measured 24 hr after the last seizure. The increase was observed in rats receiving a large number of shocks (17 seizures) but was not apparent in animals receiving fewer daily shocks (7 seizures).

We have measured [³H]diazepam binding to cerebral membranes (26,33) prepared from mice given repetitive ECS at 29 mA/sec in 30-sec intervals for 15 min and allowed to rest for 15 min before sacrifice. Crude membrane fractions were washed three times to decrease the amount of residual endogenous GABA. There were no differences in specific [³H]diazepam binding in whole forebrain, cortex, or hippocampus. We also measured [³H]diazepam binding in the presence of 10-μM GABA, a concentration that will increase the affinity of the benzodiazepine binding site (7,20).

TABLE 1. *Receptor binding in mouse brain after repetitive ECS[a]*

Ligand	Area	Control ($N = 6$)	ECS ($N = 6$)
		(10^{-15} mole/mg protein $\pm$ SE)	
[³H]QNB (1.5 nM)	Forebrain	1,621.1 $\pm$ 48.6	1,557.8 $\pm$ 111.9
	Cortex	1,813.9 $\pm$ 80.2	1,770.6 $\pm$ 38.7
	Hippocampus	1,391.0 $\pm$ 157.5	1,365.7 $\pm$ 43.7
	Striatum	2,254.4 $\pm$ 228.5	2,195.1 $\pm$ 203.0
[³H]diazepam (1.6 nM)	Forebrain	367.7 $\pm$ 18.6	399.6 $\pm$ 24.0
	+ GABA (10 μM)	531.9 $\pm$ 21.7	546.7 $\pm$ 21.7
	Cortex	456.5 $\pm$ 21.5	475.5 $\pm$ 21.0
	+ GABA (10 μM)	636.7 $\pm$ 23.5	656.3 $\pm$ 23.4
	Hippocampus	268.0 $\pm$ 24.5	264.8 $\pm$ 5.5
	+ GABA (10 μM)	380.3 $\pm$ 24.5	388.8 $\pm$ 9.9
[³H]muscimol (14 nM)	Forebrain	792.9 $\pm$ 78.1	674.0 $\pm$ 66.8
[³H]dihydrolalprenolol (0.05–5.0 nM)	Forebrain	78 $\pm$ 7	58 $\pm$ 5[b]

[a]Mice (C57 black males) were given a series of repetitive ECS (26 mA/sec, 30-sec intervals of 15 min and rested 15 min prior to death by cervical dislocation). Crude membrane fractions were prepared by centrifugation (1,000 $\times$ g, 10 min) of homogenates (20%, w/v) of whole right forebrains or specific areas dissected from the intact left hemispheres. Supernatants were centrifuged (50,000 $\times$ g, 10 min). The pellets were washed twice, resuspended in buffer, and stored frozen ($-25°C$) prior to use.
[b]$p = 0.05$ when compared with controls.

There was no difference in percentage stimulation of the benzodiazepine binding site by exogenous GABA when the whole forebrain (137.7 $\pm$ 4.7%), cortex (138.4 $\pm$ 3.1%), and hippocampus (147.1 $\pm$ 5.3%) obtained from the seizing animals ($N = 6$) were compared to corresponding structures from controls ($N = 6$) (forebrain, 144.9 $\pm$ 2.4%; hippocampus, 145.1 $\pm$ 12.5%; cortex, 140.0 $\pm$ 4.8%). Measurement of binding of [³H]muscimol to the GABA receptor in the areas mentioned did not indicate any alteration of the binding properties of this receptor. The results of *in vitro* receptor binding assays do not necessarily reflect receptor function *in vivo*. It would seem probable that increased GABA release during prolonged seizure activity may be instrumental in increasing the affinity of the benzodiazepine binding site for an endogenous ligand. Whether or not the binding of the endogenous ligand(s) promotes an anticonvulsant effect is not known as yet.

In summary, these studies failed to show any change in GABA or benzodiazepine receptors during status epilepticus. The increases observed by others after a single seizure (27) or after multiple daily seizures (23) were not found after multiple seizures. We speculate that this may result from the severe inhibition of protein synthesis observed in status epilepticus (36) and that the failure of benzodiazepine binding sites to increase in sta-

tus epilepticus may in fact explain why anticonvulsants control single seizures more readily than the multiple seizures of status epilepticus.

In conclusion, recent studies suggest that receptors for neurotransmitters may play an important role in the changes in cerebral excitability that are so obvious in status epilepticus and may offer a fertile area for future investigations.

ACKNOWLEDGMENTS

The authors wish to thank Inga L. Anderson and Patricia Shamblin for assistance in the preparation of this manuscript, as well as Eva Csiszer and Iris Tanaka for their skilled technical help. This work was supported by the Research Service of the Veterans Administration and by research grant NS-13227 from the National Institute of Neurological and Communicative Disorders and Stroke.

REFERENCES

1. Alexander, R. W., Williams, L. T., and Lefkowitz, R. J. (1975): Identification of cardiac beta adrenergic receptors by [³H]-dihydroalprenolol. *Proc. Natl. Acad. Sci. U.S.A.*, 72:1564–1568.
2. Arnold, P., Racine, R., and Wise, R. (1973): Effect of atropine, reserpine, 6-hydroxy-dopamine and handling on seizure development in rat. *Exp. Neurol.*, 40:457–460.
3. Asano, T., and Mizutani, A. (1980): Brain benzodiazepine receptors and their rapid changes after sei-

zures in the mongolian gerbil. *Jpn. J. Pharmacol.*, 30:783–788.

4. Baudry, M., Martres, M. P., and Schwartz, J. C. (1976): Modulation in the sensitivity of noradrenergic receptors in the CNS studied by the responsiveness of the cyclic AMP system. *Brain Res.*, 116:111–124.

5. Bergstrom, D., and Kellar, K. (1979): Effect of electroconvulsant shock on monoaminergic receptor binding sites in rat brain. *Nature*, 278:464–465.

6. Birdsall, N. J. M., and Hulme, E. C. (1976): Biochemical studies on muscarinic acetylcholine receptors. *J. Neurochem.*, 27:7–16.

7. Briley, M. S., and Langer, S. Z. (1978): Influence of GABA receptor agonists and antagonists on the binding of [³H]-diazepam to the benzodiazepine receptor. *Eur. J. Pharmacol.*, 52:129.

8. Corcoran, M. E., Fibiger, H. C., McCaughran, J. A., and Wada, J. A. (1974): Potentiation of amygdaloid kindling and metrazol-induced seizures by 6-hydroxydopamine in rats. *Exp. Neurol.*, 45:118–133.

9. deVellis, J., and Brooker, G. (1974): Reversal of catecholamine refractoriness by inhibitors of RNA and protein synthesis. *Science*, 186:1221–1223.

10. Dismukes, K., and Daly, J. W. (1974): Norepinephrine-sensitive systems generating adenosine 3'5'-monophosphate. Increased responses in cerebral cortical slices from reserpine-treated rats. *Mol. Pharmacol.*, 10:933–940.

11. Goddard, G. V. (1967): Development of epileptic seizures through brain stimulation at low intensity. *Nature*, 214:1020–1021.

12. Haefely, W. E. (1980): GABA and the anticonvulsant action of benzodiazepines and barbiturates. In: *GABA Neurotransmission: Current Developments in Physiology and Neurochemistry*, edited by H. Lal, S. Fielding, J. Malick, E. Roberts, N. Shah, and E. Usdin, pp. 873–878. Ankho, Fayetteville, N.Y.

13. Harden, T. K., Su, Y. F., and Perkins, J. P. (1979): Catecholamine-induced desensitization involves an uncoupling of beta adrenergic receptors and adenylate cyclase. *J. Cycl. Nucl. Res.*, 5:99–106.

14. Hoffman, B., and Lefkowitz, R. J. (1980): Radioligand binding studies of adrenergic receptors: New insights into molecular and physiological regulations. *Annu. Rev. Pharmacol. Toxicol.*, 20:581–608.

15. Karobath, M., and Sperk, G. (1979): Stimulation of benzodiazepine receptor binding by γ-aminobutyric acid. *Proc. Natl. Acad. Sci. U.S.A.*, 76:1004.

16. Klein, W. (1980): Regulation of muscarinic acetylcholine receptors. *Proc. West. Pharmacol. Soc.*, 23:449–458.

17. Klein, W. L., Nathanson, N., and Niremberg, M. (1979): Muscarinic acetylcholine receptor regulation by accelerated rate of receptor loss. *Biochem. Biophys. Res. Commun.*, 90:506–516.

18. Luqmani, Y. A., Bradford, H. F., Birdsall, N. J. M., and Hulme, E. C. (1979): Depolarization induced changes in muscarinic cholinergic receptors in synaptosomes. *Nature*, 277:481–483.

19. Makman, M. H. (1971): Properties of adenylate cyclase of lymphoid cells. *Proc. Natl. Acad. Sci. U.S.A.*, 68:885–889.

20. Martin, I. L., and Candy, J. M. (1978): Facilitation of benzodiazepine binding by sodium chloride and GABA. *Neuropharmacology*, 17:993.

21. Martres, M. P., Baudry, M., and Schwartz, J. C. (1975): Subsensitivity of noradrenaline-stimulated cyclic AMP accumulation in brain slices of *d*-amphetamine-treated mice. *Nature*, 255:731–733.

22. McNamara, J. O. (1978): Muscarinic cholinergic receptors participate in the kindling model of epilepsy. *Brain Res.*, 154:415–420.

23. McNamara, J. O., Peper, A. M., and Patrone, V. (1980): Repeated seizures induce long-term increase in hippocampal benzodiazepine receptors. *Proc. Natl. Acad. Sci. U.S.A.*, 77:3029–3032.

24. Meldrum, B. (1975): Epilepsy and GABA-mediated inhibition. *Int. Rev. Neurobiol.*, 17:1–13.

25. Meldrum, B. (1979): Convulsant drugs, anticonvulsants and GABA-mediated neuronal inhibition. In: *GABA-Neurotransmitters*, edited by P. Krogsgaard-Larsen, J. Scheel-Krüger, and H. Kofod, pp. 390–405. Munksgaard, Copenhagen.

26. Möhler, H., and Okada, T. (1977): Benzodiazepine receptor: Demonstration in the central nervous system. *Science*, 198:849–851.

27. Paul, S. M., and Skolnick, P. (1978): Rapid changes in brain benzodiazepine receptors after experimental seizures. *Science*, 202:892–893.

28. Paul, S. M., Syapin, P. J., Paugh, B. A., Moncada, V., and Skolnick, P. (1979): Correlation between benzodiazepine receptor occupation and anticonvulsant effects of diazepam. *Nature*, 281:688–689.

29. Richelson, E. (1978): Desensitization of muscarinic receptor-mediated cyclic GMP formation by cultured nerve cells. *Nature*, 272:366–368.

30. Schwartz, J. C., Costentin, J., Martres, M. P., Protais, P., and Baudry, M. (1978): Modulation of receptor mechanisms in the CNS: Hyper- and hyposensitivity to catecholamines. *Neuropharmacology*, 17:665–685.

31. Shifrum, G. S., and Klein, W. L. (1980): Regulation of muscarinic acetylcholine receptor concentration in cloned neuroblastoma cells. *J. Neurochem.*, 34:993–999.

32. Simon, R. G., and Klein, L. (1979): Cholinergic activity regulates muscarinic receptors in central nervous system cultures. *Proc. Natl. Acad. Sci. U.S.A.*, 76:4141–4145.

33. Squires, R. F., and Braestrup, C. (1977): Benzodiazepine receptors in rat brain. *Nature*, 26:732–734.

34. Steiner, A. L., Parker, C. W., and Kipnis, D. M. (1972): Radioimmunoassay for cyclic nucleotides. *J. Biol. Chem.*, 247:1106–1113.

35. Wastek, G. J., Speth, R. C., Reisine, T. D., and Yamamura, H. I. (1978): The effect of γ-aminobutyric acid [³H]-flunitrazepam in rat brain. *Eur. J. Pharmacol.*, 50:445.

36. Wasterlain, C. G. (1974): Inhibition of cerebral protein synthesis by epileptic seizures without manifestations. *Neurology (Minneap.)*, 24:175–180.

37. Wasterlain, C. G., and Jonec, V. (1980): Transsynaptic generation of a chronic seizure focus. *Life Sci.*, 26:387–391.

38. Wasterlain, C. G., and Morin, A. M. (1980): Electrical kindling in the amygdala: Evidence against a muscarinic mechanism. *Ann. Neurol.*, 8:93.
39. Wessels, M. R., Mullikin, D., and Lefkowitz, R. J. (1978): Differences between agonist and antagonist binding following beta-adrenergic receptor desensitization. *J. Biol. Chem.*, 253:3371–3373.
40. Yamamura, H., and Snyder, S. H. (1974): Muscarinic cholinergic binding in rat brain. *Proc. Natl. Acad. Sci. U.S.A.*, 71:1725–1729.

Treatment

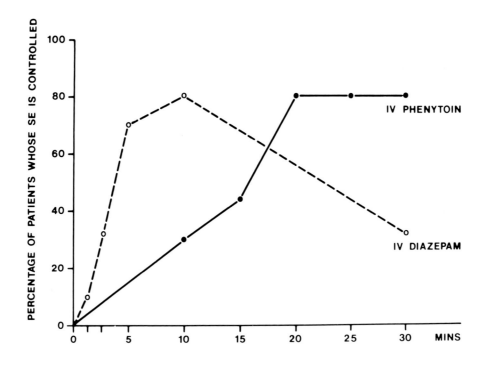

The single ideal pharmacological agent for convulsive status epilepticus does not exist. Hence, both intravenous diazepam and intravenous phenytoin should be used. Intravenous diazepam stops convulsions in 70% of patients within 3 min. As the acute effects of diazepam decline 10 min after intravenous bolus injection, the antiepileptic effects of intravenously infused phenytoin become evident. Eighty percent of patients are protected against recurrence of seizures 20 min after phenytoin infusion.

Advances in Neurology, Vol. 34: Status
Epilepticus, edited by A.V. Delgado-Escueta,
C.G. Wasterlain, D.M. Treiman, and R.J. Porter.
Raven Press, New York © 1983.

37

General Principles of Treatment: Responsive and Intractable Status Epilepticus in Adults

David M. Treiman

Status epilepticus is a neurological emergency that requires immediate effective treatment to avoid severe permanent brain damage or death. The longer that generalized convulsive status epilepticus continues before effective treatment, the higher the morbidity and mortality. Recent experimental and clinical evidence suggests that focal convulsive status and nonconvulsive status also require immediate effective treatment in order to prevent permanent neuronal damage and subsequent neurological dysfunction, such as hemiparesis or chronic impairment of recent memory.

Understanding the mechanisms of such brain damage following status epilepticus is essential in consideration of the general principles of treatment.

EFFECTS OF STATUS EPILEPTICUS: PHYSIOLOGY

A number of physiological changes take place during status epilepticus. Those secondary to the violent motor activity of generalized tonic-clonic seizures are summarized in Table 1. However, during status epilepticus, there are other physiological responses that appear to be related to the abnormal neuronal discharges, as evidenced by their persistence during curarization of subjects. There are initial increases in blood pressure (18,41) and heart rate due to increased sympathetic activity that can be stopped by ganglionic blockade (16). Late in

status epilepticus the systemic blood pressure drops to hypotensive levels (18).

Within 1 to 2 sec after the onset of generalized seizures, cerebral blood flow increases markedly because of decreased cerebral vascular resistance. A comparable increase in cerebral blood flow in the seizure focus may also be observed shortly after the onset of focal seizures (19,41). If generalized or focal cerebral vasodilation persists into the late stages of status epilepticus, inadequate arterial perfusion may result because of the associated systemic hypotension. These events may help explain why prolonged status produces permanent neurological damage. There is also a dramatic rise in cerebral venous pressure to levels greater than 1,000 mm H_2O during tonic seizures in experimental animals (18). White et al. (41) recorded a twofold to threefold increase in cerebrospinal fluid (CSF) pressure in paralyzed ventilated subjects during pentylenetetrazol-induced seizures. Inadequate arterial perfusion, together with the increase in venous pressure, may account for the petechial hemorrhages observed in subpial cortex after status epilepticus (16).

Compromise of respiration may occur in status epilepticus as the result of three mechanisms (16). In generalized convulsive seizures there may be mechanical impairment of respiration. However, even in nonconvulsive seizures and in experimental seizures with subjects paralyzed and artificially ventilated, there are two other mechanisms of res-

TABLE 1. *Physiological changes in major motor status*

Transient or early (0–30 min)	Late (after 30 min)
Arterial hypertension	Arterial hypotension
Cerebral venous pressure (CVP) raised	CVP raised or normal
Arterial P_{O_2} low or normal	Arterial P_{O_2} low or normal
Arterial P_{O_2} high	Arterial P_{O_2} normal
CV P_{O_2} (low or high)	CV P_{O_2} normal or low
CV P_{CO_2} high	CV P_{CO_2} normal (or high)
Cerebral blood flow (CBF) increased	CBF increased, normal, or decreased
Hyperglycemia	Normoglycemia, hypoglycemia
Hyperkalemia	Hyperkalemia
Hemoconcentration	
Lactic acidosis	Hyperpyrexia (secondary)

Adapted from Meldrum (16).

piratory embarrassment. Brainstem respiratory centers may be inhibited by the abnormal electrical discharges. Massive autonomic discharges also occur, at least in generalized tonic seizures. These result in excessive bronchial secretions and bronchial constriction, and thus the arterial P_{O_2} drops as the P_{CO_2} rises (20).

Other autonomic effects are the composite result of simultaneous activation of the sympathetic and parasympathetic nervous systems. Meldrum (16) has cited evidence that the cerebrovascular vasodilatation seen in generalized seizures is mediated by parasympathetic discharges.

Another physiological consequence of status epilepticus is an increase in the cerebral metabolic rate. Meldrum and Nilsson (19) have demonstrated a twofold to threefold increase in cerebral oxygen consumption during 2 hr of bicuculline-induced status epilepticus in artificially ventilated rats. Borgstrom et al. (4) have shown similar increases in glucose consumption. The increase in cerebral metabolic rate observed in paralyzed but ventilated animals is due to excessive neuronal activity, not to secondary effects associated with increased muscle activity. Blennow et al. (2) deliberately produced hypoxia, arterial hypotension, or hyperthermia in rats subjected to 2 hr of bicuculline-induced status epilepticus. They found no decrease in the phosphorylation state of the adenine nucleotide pool, as compared with rats with uncomplicated status epilepticus.

These experiments support the view of Meldrum's group and Siesjö's group that neuronal damage following prolonged status epilepticus is due to excessive metabolic activity of vulnerable neurons in the presence of adequate energy supplies.

An opposite explanation for neuronal damages following prolonged status epilepticus has been provided by Kreisman et al. (see Chapter 22), who have shown that during experimental serial seizures in rats there is a transition from increased tissue P_{O_2} to decreased tissue P_{O_2} and a transition from oxidation of cytochrome a,a_3 to reduction of cytochrome a,a_3 in cerebral cortex. These authors have suggested that this transition from oxygen sufficiency to insufficiency is probably related to deteriorating or inappropriate vascular reactivity that results in decreased ability to deliver oxygen to focal areas of metabolically hyperactive cerebral tissue. Thus neuronal damage could occur directly as a result of the episodes of transient local hypoxia that occur during seizures following the transition.

EFFECTS OF STATUS EPILEPTICUS: PATHOLOGY

There is now considerable evidence, such as that cited earlier, that prolonged status epilepticus produces profound neuronal damage even in paralyzed, artificially ventilated animals. Pathological changes in the brains of children and adults dying shortly after status epilepticus have been well documented by Fowler (10), Scholtz (28), and Norman (21). Ischemic neuronal changes are seen in the Sommer sector (field h_1) of the hippocampus, in layers 3, 5, and 6 of the cerebral cortex, in the Purkinje cells of the cerebellum, in the thalamus and basal ganglia, and in the hypothalamus (13,35). The distribution of the pathological changes induced by status epilepticus is similar to that seen following cerebral hypoxia or severe hypoglycemia (16). However, Söderfeldt et al. (see Chapter 16) have recently demonstrated that the electron microscopic appearance of neurons following bicuculline-induced status epilepticus in paralyzed, artificially ventilated rats is different from the appearance of neurons subjected to ischemic cell damage. This suggests that neuronal damage following status epilepticus must be caused by factors other than cerebral hypoxia alone.

Although the precise molecular mechanisms of brain dysfunction during and following status epilepticus are not known, it is likely that both increases in neuronal metabolic activity and decreases in energy substrates contribute to the development of permanent neurological dysfunction in prolonged status epilepticus.

Most clinical and experimental studies of the consequences of status epilepticus have dealt with the results of generalized tonic-clonic status. However, it is important to recognize newly developed evidence that prolonged complex partial status epilepticus may also produce permanent neuronal damage manifested as chronic loss of memory (see Chapter 7). There is also evidence that prolonged focal status may result in permanent neuronal damage. Knopman and his colleagues (14) reported diffuse neuronal necrosis limited to the left hemisphere in a patient who died after 4 weeks of continuous clonic activity of the right arm and leg.

Although it is probably true that systemic changes in homeostasis do play some role in the development of brain damage in generalized tonic-clonic status epilepticus, the occurrence of profound memory deficits following prolonged psychomotor status and local neuronal necrosis after prolonged focal motor status provides evidence that abnormal neuronal electrical activity must play a role in the development of neurological deficits following both convulsive status and nonconvulsive status. Recognition of this important concept should lead us to change a frequently stated misconception that focal motor and nonconvulsive status epilepticus need not be treated with the same urgency as generalized tonic-clonic status.

In addition to neuronal damage, status epilepticus may give rise to a number of systemic complications. Rhabdomyolysis and acute myoglobinuria may lead to renal failure (31,40), hyperkalemia (39) and acute intravascular coagulation (8). In patients with preexisting systemic disease, status epilepticus may exacerbate the original condition. Cardiopulmonary compromise may be exacerbated as a result of status. Acute pulmonary edema has been reported as a complication of status epilepticus in a patient with rheumatic heart disease (32) and may also occur on a neurogenic basis. For detailed discussions of the medical complications of status epilepticus, see Chapters 39 and 40.

Both clinical evidence and experimental evidence dictate rapid termination of epileptogenic paroxysms in status epilepticus if permanent brain damage is to be prevented. In a study of major status epilepticus, Rowan and Scott (25) found the mean duration of episodes of status epilepticus to be 2 hr 45 min. The longer the duration of the status, the more frequently severe neurological sequelae occurred. In 30 patients who had no neurological sequelae, the median duration of status was 90 min. On the other hand, the mean duration for 11 patients with neurological sequelae was 10 hr. The duration for patients who died as a result of status was 13 hr. In the nonfatal cases, the median interval between onset of status and the initiation of treatment was 90 min; in the fatal cases, the median interval was 15 hr. Whitty and Taylor (42) also found an onset–treatment interval of 90 min in their nonfatal cases of status and an interval of 4 hr in their fatal cases. In experimental studies, Meldrum and Brierley (17) subjected adolescent baboons to generalized seizures induced by bicuculline. The duration of status in these experiments was important. Seizures that lasted less than 90 min produced no pathological changes, whereas status that lasted longer than 90 min resulted in ischemic cell changes in the hippocampus, neocortex, and cerebellum. These same experiments were repeated in paralyzed, artificially ventilated animals and resulted in similar, though less severe, pathological changes (20).

DIAGNOSIS

Although rapid and vigorous treatment of status epilepticus is essential once the diagnosis is made, it is equally important not to initiate emergency therapy until the diagnosis of status epilepticus is confirmed.

Status epilepticus is generally defined as a state in which a patient suffers from a series of seizures without fully recovering consciousness between these seizures. Recently, the term has also been applied to continuous clinical or electrical seizures, or both, lasting at least 30 min even if consciousness is not impaired. This definition thus includes (a) repeated generalized tonic-clonic seizures in which the patient does not recover to a normal alert state between attacks, (b) prolonged attacks of nonconvulsive seizures, such as absence status and complex partial status, where the clinical presentation is a prolonged "twilight" state, and (c) continuous focal motor seizure activity, even when there is no alteration of consciousness. In practice, the diagnosis of status epilepticus should not be made until the physician has witnessed at least one generalized tonic-clonic seizure occurring in a patient with a depressed state of consciousness who has a history of repeated seizures without awakening fully between the seizures. In the case of nonconvulsive or focal motor status, the diagnosis should not be made until 30 min of continuous seizure activity has been observed. Following such criteria should preclude inappropriate emergency parenteral administration of large doses of potentially toxic drugs.

TREATMENT

Once the diagnosis of status epilepticus is made, treatment with appropriate intravenous medication should be initiated as rapidly as possible and a search for precipitating causes undertaken. Status epilepticus may be precipitated by alcoholic debauch (5,26), infectious hepatitis (12), polio encephalitis (15), congenital syphilis (29), African trypanosomiasis (9), DDT and BHC poisoning (7), theophylline intoxication (1), and treatment with intrathecal penicillin (36), cortisone (33), isoniazid (37), and electroconvulsive therapy (24). Myoclonic status epilepticus has been reported after chloralose anesthesia (3), and generalized tonic-clonic status has been reported after neuroleptic anesthesia (27).

From the preceding considerations, it becomes apparent that the goals in managing status epilepticus should be the following:

1. Terminate electrical and clinical seizure activity as soon as possible, preferably within 30 min.
2. Prevent recurrences of seizures.
3. Ensure adequate cardiorespiratory function and brain oxygenation.
4. Correct any precipitating factors such as hypoglycemia, electrolyte imbalance, or fever.
5. Stabilize metabolic balance by prevention or correction of lactic acidosis, electrolyte imbalance, and dehydration.
6. Prevent or correct any other systemic complications.

7. Evaluate and treat possible causes of status epilepticus.

Rapid termination of the seizure activity of status epilepticus requires detailed knowledge of the pharmacokinetics of the antiepileptic drugs that might be used. Ideally, the most potent drug should be used. It should be administered intravenously to ensure effective serum and brain tissue concentrations so as to stop the seizures. The drug used must be able to cross the blood-brain barrier rapidly. Treatment should not be started with intramuscular or oral administration, because absorption by these routes is too slow and too variable. Furthermore, because of the rapid redistribution from the circulation that occurs with some drugs, serum concentrations adequate to stop ongoing seizures may never be achieved. Caution should be used in selecting the rate of intravenous infusion in order to avoid hypotension, cardiac arrhythmias, and respiratory depression. When therapy is started, sufficiently high doses should be used and adequate time allowed for the drug to enter the brain before changing to a second drug.

As soon as the seizures are stopped, an adequate loading dose of a long-acting maintenance antiepileptic drug should be given intravenously in order to prevent recurrence of seizures, and this should be followed by maintenance therapy.

CHOICE OF DRUGS

A variety of drugs have been used successfully in the management of status epilepticus. Tables 2 and 3 summarize the pharmacological properties of anticonvulsants important in the management of status epilepticus. No consensus yet exists as to the drug of choice with which to initiate treatment of status. One reason that a drug of choice cannot be defined is that, as yet, none of the antiepileptic drugs available for the management of status epilepticus fulfills the requirement for an ideal drug for the management of status. Table 4 outlines some of these properties.

A review of the pharmacokinetics of drug entry into the brain illustrates the reason for listing these characteristics of an ideal drug for the treatment of status epilepticus.

Obviously, for a drug to be considered ideal for the treatment of status, it must rapidly terminate the recurrent seizures. Thus, intravenous administration is essential to ensure that the drug is rapidly available to enter the brain. When a drug is

GENERAL PRINCIPLES OF TREATMENT   381

TABLE 2. *Properties of drugs of importance in treating status epilepticus*

Property	Diazepam	Phenytoin	Phenobarbital	Paraldehyde	Valproate
Route of administration	i.v.	i.v.	i.v.	i.v.	i.v., rectal
Time to enter brain	10 sec	1 min	20 min	<2 min	1 min
Time to enter peak brain concentration		15–30 min	30 min	20 min	
Effective serum concentration in status epilepticus (μg/ml)	0.2–0.8	25	45	150–120	50
Time to stop status	1 min	5–30 min	20 min	?	?
Effective half-life (hr)	0.25	22+	50–120	6	12
Brain/plasma ratio		0.6–1.4	0.6–0.9	0.61	
pKa	3.4	8.3	7.41		4.5
Partition coefficient[a]		295.1	26.3	32.6	1.36
Protein binding	96%	87–93%	45–50%		80–94%
Volume of distribution	1–2 liter/kg	0.5–0.8 liter/kg	0.7 liter/kg	0.9 liter/kg	0.13–0.16 liter/kg

[a]Octanol/water, pH 7.5 (data from Cornford and W.H. Oldendorf, *personal communication*).
Adapted from Treiman and Delgado-Escueta (34).

TABLE 3. *Drugs of importance in treating status epilepticus: clinical parameters*

Parameter	Diazepam	Phenytoin	Phenobarbital	Paraldehyde
Indications	Most forms of status	Phenytoin withdrawal, intracranial bleed	Phenobarbital withdrawal	Ethanol withdrawal
Loading dose	0.25 mg/kg up to 20 mg	18 mg/kg	20 mg/kg	0.1 ml/kg
Rate of administration	2 mg/min	50 mg/min	100 mg/min	
Potential side effects				
Depression of consciousness	10–30 min	None	>0.5 g	
Respiration	0.5–1 min	None	>0.5 g	
Hypotension	Occasional	50% of patients		
Atrial fibrillation	None		None	None
Cardiac arrest	Rare		>2 g	

Adapted from Treiman and Delgado-Escueta (34).

TABLE 4. *Properties of an ideal drug for treatment of status epilepticus*

1. Rapidly effective against all types of status
2. Available for intravenous administration
3. Potent, so that small volumes can be given rapidly
4. Safe: no cardiorespiratory depression, no depression of consciousness, no systemic side effects
5. Rapidly enter the brain
6. Long distribution half-life
7. Short elimination half-life
8. Useful in oral form as a chronic antiepileptic drug

given intravenously, it requires about 10 sec for the first bolus to reach the brain and about 1 min for dispersal of the drug throughout the blood volume.

Once a compound enters brain capillaries, brain uptake can be shown to be either carrier-mediated or lipid-mediated. Carrier mediation, where a specific transport mechanism exists to facilitate penetration of the blood-brain barrier by lipophobic substances, is important in neurochemistry because most metabolic substrates are polar substances and thus lipid-insoluble. On the other hand, lipid mediation is important in pharmacology because lipid solubility determines the ability of drugs to penetrate the blood-brain barrier (22). Lipid solubility is determined by the physicochemical properties of the drug, including degree of ionization and extent of hydrogen binding, which in turn is a function of the polarity of the molecule.

In addition to blood-brain barrier permeability, brain concentrations of a drug after intravenous administration will be affected by plasma protein binding, accumulation of the drug by liver, kidney, or other tissues, the rate of systemic degradation of the drug, and the degree of brain tissue binding (22).

The ideal drug is one that is rapidly taken up by the brain but that will remain in the brain sufficiently long to provide protection from further seizures until a steady-state level can be achieved. The length of time a drug remains in the brain can be determined experimentally by measuring brain washout, assuming a small initial dose and thus no continuing uptake. However, two other factors determine brain residence time in the therapeutic situation where large doses are given: drug binding by brain compounds and the length of time the drug remains in the blood, or distribution half-life. The distribution half-life, in turn, is influenced by the physical properties of the drug. Highly lipid soluble drugs with a high partition coefficient will rapidly enter the body lipid pools; blood concentrations drop, and drug leaves the brain. An example of this phenomenon is the case of diazepam, which is rapidly effective in stopping status but that frequently is associated with recurrent seizures 15 to 30 min after administration. This is because as the drug redistributes in the body fat, the drug leaves the brain, and thus the protective effect is lost. On the other hand, the elimination half-life is quite long, and thus the drug remains in the body for a prolonged period of time. Ideally, a drug given for an acute CNS effect, such as stopping status epilepticus, should have a lipid/water partition coefficient high enough to allow rapid penetration of the blood-brain barrier but low enough to prevent significant depot fat accumulation. Oldendorf (23) has suggested that an optimum partition coefficient (olive oil:water) for a relatively short acting centrally active drug is between about 0.1 and 1.0.

Penetration of the blood-brain barrier and uptake by the brain are at least partially determined by the degree of ionization of the drug. If a drug is largely un-ionized at pH 7.4, its entry into the brain is favored (6,11). This can be predicted by the pKa or dissociation constant of the drug. When pH equals pKa, 50% of the drug will be ionized and 50% un-ionized. For acidic drugs (drugs that serve as proton donors when dissociated into ionized form), if the pH is less than the pKa, then the drug will be largely un-ionized and will thus more easily cross lipid membranes. On the other hand, a basic drug (a drug that serves as a proton acceptor when

dissociated) becomes more ionized if the pH falls below the pKa of the drug. Because blood pH is quite stable and can shift only about ± 0.5, changes in blood pH ordinarily do not play a significant role in altering the penetration of a drug through the blood-brain barrier (22). However, if a drug used for status epilepticus has a pKa near 7.4 (as does phenobarbital), then relatively small shifts in the blood pH due to the lactic acidosis usually encountered during status may produce a considerable change in the degree of ionization of the drug and thus the extent of penetration of the blood-brain barrier. Waddell and Butler (38) have shown in dogs that the brain concentration of phenobarbital changes in the opposite direction to the blood pH. Thus, in their experiments, the normal brain/plasma concentration ratio of 0.9 rose to 1.4 in acidotic animals and fell to 0.7 in alkalotic animals. These effects should be considered when designing new drugs for use in status epilepticus.

Cerebral blood flow may also influence the rate of entry of drugs into brain, especially for lipid-mediated drugs. Simon et al. (30) have recently reported a 10.5-fold increase in the amount of lidocaine entering the brain during experimental status in rats, as compared with controls. When potentially cerebrotoxic drugs such as lidocaine (which may cause seizures in high concentrations) are used in the management of status, these effects must be considered.

These considerations illustrate the need for a thorough understanding of pharmacokinetic principles that influence the behavior of cerebroactive drugs. Unfortunately, little is yet known about the pharmacokinetics of drug entry into the brain and how these parameters may be modified by changes from the normal physiological state such as occur during status epilepticus. Further knowledge of the pharmacokinetics of these drugs and their mechanisms of action should lead to the development of more effective drugs for the management of status epilepticus and provide more rational guidelines for their use.

REFERENCES

1. Begue, P., and Lasfargues, G. (1970): Neurological complications of theophylline and piperazine. *Rev. Prat. (Paris)*, 20:5319–5321 *(Epilepsy Abstr., 4/1066)*.
2. Blennow, G., Nilsson, B., and Siesjö, B. K. (1977): Sustained epileptic seizures complicated by hypoxia, arterial hypotension or hyperthermia: Effects on cerebral energy state. *Acta Physiol. Scand.*, 100:26–128.
3. Bodouresques, J., Roger, J., Naquet, R., Bille, J., Guin, P., Vigouroux, R., and Gosset, A. (1966): Acute

chloralose intoxication. Status myoclonicus. Electroencephalographic control of evolution. *Rev. Neurol. (Paris)*, 114:312–317 *(Epilepsy Abstr.*, R/5251).

4. Borgstrom, L., Chapman, A. G., and Siesjö, B. K. (1976): Glucose consumption in the cerebral cortex of rat during bicuculline-induced status epilepticus. *J. Neurochem.*, 27:971–973.

5. Boudin, G., Barbizet, J., Brion, S., Nivet, M., and Masson, S. (1959): Subintrant epilepsy and major insufficiency of the liver. A clinical, electroencephalographic and anatomic study of six cases of alcoholic cirrhosis with ascites and status epilepticus. *Bull. Soc. Med. Hop. Paris*, 75:301–313 *(Epilepsy Abstr.*, R/1028).

6. Brodie, B. B., Kurze, H., and Schauker, L. S. (1960): The importance of dissociation content and lipid solubility in influencing the passage of drugs into the cerebrospinal fluid. *J. Pharmacol. Exp. Ther.*, 130:20–25.

7. Eskanasy, J. J. (1972): Status epilepticus by dichlorodiphenyl trichlorethane and hexachlorcyclohexane poisoning. *Rev. Roum. Neurol.*, 9:435–442.

8. Fisher, S. P., Lee, J., Zatuchni, J., and Greenberg, J. (1977): Disseminated intravascular coagulation in status epilepticus. *Thromb. Hemostasis*, 38:909–913.

9. Forster, E. F. B. (1950): Status epilepticus: A syndrome complex of African trypanosomiasis. *Br. Med. J.*, 4686:987–988.

10. Fowler, M. (1957): Brain damage after febrile convulsions. *Arch. Dis. Child.*, 32:67–76.

11. Goldsworthy, P. D., Aird, R. B., and Becker, R. A. (1954): The blood-brain barrier—the effect of acidic dissociation constant on the permeation of certain sulfonamides into brain. *J. Cell. Comp. Physiol.*, 44:519–526.

12. Gortvai, P., and Hasan, N. (1973): Status epilepticus in infective hepatitis. *Br. J. Clin. Pract.*, 27:139–140.

13. Karlov, V. A., Gerber, E. L., and Voronkin, G. V. (1974): The pathomorphology of status epilepticus. *Zh. Nevropatol. Psikhiatr.*, 74:1659–1666 *(Epilepsy Abstr.*, 8/830).

14. Knopman, D., Margolis, G., and Reeves, A. G. (1977): Prolonged focal epilepsy and hypoxemia as a cause of focal brain damage: A case study. *Ann. Neurol.*, 1:195–198.

15. Lohmann, W. (1949): Contraction atelectasis and symptomatic epilepsy in poliomyelitis. *Arztl. Wochenschr.*, 4:570–572 *(Epilepsy Abstr.*, R/2326).

16. Meldrum, B. S. (1976): Neuropathology and pathophysiology. In: *A Textbook of Epilepsy*, edited by J. Laidlaw and A. Richens, pp. 314–354. Churchill Livingstone, Edinburgh.

17. Meldrum, B. S., and Brierley, J. B. (1973): Prolonged epileptic seizures in primates: Ischemic cell change and its relation to ictal physiological events. *Arch. Neurol.*, 28:10–17.

18. Meldrum, B. S., and Horton, R. W. (1973): Physiology of status epilepticus in primates. *Arch. Neurol.*, 28:1–9.

19. Meldrum, B. S., and Nilsson, B. (1976): Cerebral blood flow and metabolic rate early and late in prolonged epileptic seizures induced in rats by bicuculline. *Brain*, 99:523–542.

20. Meldrum, B. S., Vigouroux, R. A., and Brierley, J. B. (1973): Systemic factors and epileptic brain damage: Prolonged seizures in paralyzed artificially ventilated baboons. *Arch. Neurol.*, 29:82–87.

21. Norman, R. M. (1964): The neuropathology of status epilepticus. *Med. Sci. Law*, 4:46–51.

22. Oldendorf, W. H. (1974): Blood-brain barrier permeability to drugs. *Annu. Rev. Pharmacol.*, 14:239–248.

23. Oldendorf, W. H. (1975): Permeability of the blood-brain barrier. In: *The Nervous System, Vol. 1: The Basic Neurosciences*, edited by R. O. Brady, pp. 279–289. Raven Press, New York.

24. Roith, A. I. (1959): Status epilepticus as a complication of E.C.T. *Br. J. Clin. Pract.*, 13:711–712.

25. Rowan, A. J., and Scott, D. F. (1970): Major status epilepticus. *Acta. Neurol. Scand.*, 46:573–584.

26. Sarabia Alvarez Ude, J., Lopez Agreda, J. M., and Ortega Nunez, A. (1973): Functional status epilepticus in a severe liver disease. *Hosp. Gen. (Madrid)*, 13:471–482 *(Epilepsy Abstr.*, 7/1011).

27. Schiffter, R., and Straschill, M. (1977): A case report of a patient with sensory status epilepticus. *Nervenarzt*, 48:321–335 *(Epilepsy Abstr.*, 11/1428).

28. Scholtz, W. (1959): The contribution of patho-anatomical research to the problem of epilepsy. *Epilepsia*, 1:36–55.

29. Seger, J. E., and Kollrach, H. W. (1969): An unusual meningoencephalitic onset, with status epilepticus, of a juvenile paralysis. *Monatsschr. Kinderheilkd.*, 117:469–471 *(Epilepsy Abstr.*, 3/248).

30. Simon, R., Benowit, N., and Bronstein, J. (1981): Increased brain concentrations of lidocaine during status epilepticus. *Neurology (NY)*, 31:114 (abstract).

31. Singhal, P. C., Chugh, K. S., and Gulati, D. R. (1978): Myoglobinuria and renal failure after status epilepticus. *Neurology (NY)*, 28:200–201.

32. Sivriev, L., Trifinov, M., and Platikanov, N. (1968): Acute pulmonary edema induced by status epilepticus in a patient with valvulotomized mitral stenosis. *Vatr. Bol. Sofia*, 7:231–234 *(Epilepsy Abstr.*, 2/445).

33. Stephen, E. H. M., and Noad, K. B. (1951): Status epilepticus occurring during cortisone therapy. *Med. J. Aust.*, 2:334–335.

34. Treiman, D. M., and Delgado-Escueta, A. V. (1980): Status epilepticus. In: *Critical Care of Neurological and Neurosurgical Emergencies*, edited by R. A. Thompson and J. R. Green, pp. 55–99. Raven Press, New York.

35. Urechia, C. I., and Lichter, C. (1958): Histopathologic examination of the diencephalon in status epilepticus. *Neurologia Buc.*, 3:299–305 *(Epilepsy Abstr.*, R/2206).

36. Vallery-Radot, P., Millinez, P., Laroche, C., and Hazard, J. (1951): Fatal status epilepticus after an intrathecal injection of penicillin for meningococcal meningitis. *Bull. Soc. Med. Hop. Paris*, 67:769–771 *(Epilepsy Abstr.*, R/5329).

37. Vic-Dupont, Lissac, J., Pocidalo, J. J., and Sachs, C. (1965): A case of acute isoniazid poisoning. Status epilepticus associated with severe metabolic acidosis. *Bull. Soc. Med. Hop. Paris*, 116:613–618.

38. Waddell, W. J., and Butler, T. C. (1957): The distribution and excretion of phenobarbital. *J. Clin. Invest.*, 36:1217–1226.
39. Warden, J. C. (1966): Fatal hyperkalaemia in status epilepticus. *Med. J. Aust.*, 53:22–24.
40. Warren, D. J., Leitch, A. G., and Leggett, R. J. E. (1975): Hyperuricaemic acute renal failure after epileptic seizures. *Lancet*, 2:385–387.

41. White, P. T., Grant, P., Mosier, J., and Craig, A. (1961): Changes in cerebral dynamics associated with seizures. *Neurology (Minneap.)*, 11:354–361.
42. Whitty, C. W. M., and Taylor, M. (1949): Treatment of status epilepticus. *Lancet*, 2:591–594.

Advances in Neurology, Vol. 34: Status
Epilepticus, edited by A.V. Delgado-Escueta,
C.G. Wasterlain, D.M. Treiman, and R.J. Porter.
Raven Press, New York © 1983.

38

General Principles of Treatment: Status Epilepticus in Neonates

Michael J. Painter

Neonatal seizures constitute one of the most common and most distinctive neurological events seen in the nursery population. Seizures, per se, are not a specific diagnosis, but rather a symptom of central nervous system dysfunction. Seizures may be due to a primary central nervous system lesion or secondary to systemic disorders.

TYPES OF NEONATAL SEIZURES

Unlike seizure activity in the older child or adult, which is most often obvious and generalized, neonatal seizures frequently are subtle and covert. *Subtle seizure activity* is that most commonly seen in the newborn (30). It is characterized by tonic, horizontal, or vertical deviation of the eyes, with or without nystagmus, repetitive eye blinking, and repetitive oral buccolingual movements, such as sucking or swallowing. Subtle seizure activity may or may not be associated with tonic and/or clonic movements of the extremities. Apnea as a manifestation of seizure activity may occur as an isolated event or may be associated with subtle activity.

Generalized tonic seizures are characterized by tonic extension of the arms and legs, with the appearance of decerebrate or decorticate posturing. This seizure type usually indicates an underlying structural central nervous system cause and is characteristically seen in the premature infant with subependymal hemorrhage. This seizure type must be distinguished from uncal herniation and primary brain stem events.

Multifocal clonic seizure activity is characterized by clonic movements of the extremities, migrating from one body part to another in an unpredictable fashion. This seizure type is characteristic of the full-term infant and is the kind most commonly seen with an underlying metabolic abnormality, such as hypocalcemia.

Focal clonic seizure activity, which is characterized by localized clonic jerking of one of the extremities, is the most discrete seizure type seen in the newborn. Although this seizure type may be seen with underlying metabolic encephalopathies, it is most often seen in focal central nervous system lesions, such as cerebral contusions secondary to birth trauma.

Myoclonic seizures are relatively rare events in the neonatal period. These seizures are characterized by single or multiple jerks of flexion of the arms and legs. Myoclonic seizures may be seen following asphyxia and may be a precursor to the later development of infantile spasms associated with a hypsarrhythmic EEG pattern.

Status epilepticus is a particularly ominous event in the neonatal period and is arbitrarily defined as a repetition of clinical or electrical seizures of 30 min duration, with an impaired neurological state between seizures (19).

The covert nature of neonatal seizures is, no doubt, related to the immature cortical organization of the central nervous system. The newborn monkey is very much dependent on connections between cortical and deep gray matter for the propagation of focal paroxysmal activity, whereas the adult monkey is dependent on interconnections at the level of the superficial cortical gray matter for propagation of this activity (5). Indeed, in the human newborn, seizure activity with all the varieties of clinical manifestations described has been seen with hydranencephaly, indicating that the epileptic foci can originate at brainstem level (10).

Seizure activity in the newborn period must be distinguished from clonus or jitteriness that is not convulsive and does not respond to anticonvulsants. Clonus is rhythmic, and the alternating movements are of equal amplitudes; the alternating movements in seizure activity are of unequal amplitudes. Clonus may be precipitated by or ablated by changes in position; seizures are not particularly position-sensitive. Clonus is ablated by restraining the moving part; if this is attempted in seizure activity, underlying muscle contractions are felt. Most important, seizures frequently are associated with eye movements and sucking or swallowing activity, which is not seen with clonus.

DIAGNOSIS AND THERAPY

When confronted with the newborn who exhibits peculiar movements that may or may not represent seizure activity, the physician may find simultaneous EEG recording and clinical observation of value. However, parallelism between clinical and electrical seizure activity in the newborn is not absolute.

When seizure activity is documented, resuscitation equipment should be available, and the infant's airway should be protected. Because of the localized nature of neonatal seizures, respiratory arrest usually is not a problem, but it may occur during drug administration. The causes of neonatal seizures are many (Table 1), but every attempt should be made to determine the correct cause, bearing in mind that metabolic abnormalities often coexist with structural disease and must be treated. The metabolic abnormalities that should be evaluated first are hypoglycemia and hypocalcemia. Glucose concentration can be determined in minutes using a Dextrostix and then confirmed on whole blood or plasma by the standard glucose oxidase method. Hypoglycemia is defined as a whole-blood glucose concentration below 30 mg/dl in the term infant or below 20 mg/dl in the preterm infant, in the first 72 hr. The blood glucose concentration

TABLE 1. *Causes of neonatal seizures*

1. Trauma and anoxia
   a. Subdural hematoma
   b. Intracortical hemorrhage
   c. Cerebral necrosis
   d. Cortical vein thrombosis
   e. Intraventricular hemorrhage
   f. Asphyxia
2. Congenital anomalies (cerebral dysgenesis)
3. Metabolic disturbances
   a. Hypocalcemia (hypomagnesemia, high phosphate load, infant of a diabetic mother, hypoparathyroidism, maternal hyperparathyroidism, and idiopathic)
   b. Hypoglycemia (galactosemia, intrauterine growth retardation, infant of a diabetic mother, idiopathic, glycogen storage disease, and leucine-sensitive hypoglycemia)
   c. Electrolyte imbalance (hypernatremia and hyponatremia)
4. Infections
   a. Bacterial meningitis
   b. Cerebral abscess
   c. Herpes encephalitis
   d. Coxsackie meningoencephalitis
   e. Cytomegalovirus
   f. Toxoplasmosis
   g. Syphilis
5. Drug withdrawal
   a. Methadone
   b. Heroin
   c. Barbiturate
   d. Propoxyphene
6. Pyridoxine dependency
7. Amino acid disturbances
   a. Maple syrup urine disease
   b. Urea cycle abnormalities
   c. Nonketotic hyperglycinemia
   d. Ketotic hyperglycinemias
8. Kernicterus
9. Toxins
   a. Local anesthetics
   b. Isoniazid
   c. Indomethacin
10. Benign familial seizures

should be above 40 mg/dl in all infants more than 3 days old.

If there is any delay in determining the serum calcium concentration, an electrocardiogram can be obtained and a Q-oTc interval determined. This interval is determined by dividing the Q-oTc by the square root of the rate determined by the R interval, that is, the peak of the R wave to the peak of the next R wave. By the formula Q-oTc/(R-R), intervals greater than 0.21 sec in the preterm infant and 0.19 sec in the term infant support the diagnosis of hypocalcemia. The definitions of hypocalcemia vary. However, prolonged Q-oTc intervals usually are seen with serum calcium concentrations below 8 mg/dl in the term infant and below 7.5 mg/dl in the preterm infant. Hypocalcemia is treated with rapid intravenous infusion of calcium gluconate (200 mg/kg). When hypocalcemia is diagnosed, serum magnesium concentration should be determined, because a significant number of hypocalcemic infants are also hypomagnesemic, and hypomagnesemic hypocalcemia will not respond to calcium alone. A concentration less than 1 mEq/liter confirms the diagnosis of hypomagnesemia and is corrected by 1 to 2 cc of 50% magnesium sulfate given intramuscularly (28). Hypoglycemia is treated with 2 to 4 ml of 25% dextrose intravenously, followed by intravenous infusion of 8 to 10 mg/kg/min to maintain normal blood glucose concentration. If necessary, very hypertonic glucose infusions or steroids may be used. It is important to bear in mind that hypoglycemia may be an accompanying abnormality in infants who are asphyxiated or who have other underlying metabolic abnormalities, such as maple syrup urine disease, propionic acidemia, or methylmalonic acidemia. Infants of diabetic mothers and infants who are of low birth weight for gestational age are at particular risk for the development of hypoglycemia.

Asphyxiated low-birth-weight infants, infants of diabetic mothers, and infants with the DiGeorge syndrome are at risk for the development of early hypocalcemia. The DiGeorge syndrome is a congenital abnormality of the third and fourth pharyngeal pouches resulting in aplasia of the thymus and parathyroid glands and abnormalities of the great vessels. These infants often have hypertelorism, micrognathia, ear abnormalities, downslanting palpebral fissures, and a funnel-shaped mouth. Seizures due to hypocalcemia that occur beyond 7 days of age are most often due to high-phosphate formulas and are seen much more frequently in Great Britain than in the United States.

Following the evaluation of calcium and glucose metabolism, the cerebrospinal fluid should be examined, because seizures are not uncommonly the initial manifestation of central nervous system infections. The newborn may be infected *in utero*, during delivery, or in the immediate perinatal period. Primary maternal infection with rubella, cytomegalovirus, syphilis, toxoplasmosis, or herpes may result in neonatal infection. The neurological manifestations of congenital syphilis usually are delayed beyond the perinatal period, whereas the clinical manifestations of other infectious agents may present shortly after delivery. When central nervous system infections are found, it is important to monitor serum sodium concentration, because inappropriate ADH secretion may complicate meningitis. During the delivery process, an infant may become infected with group B streptococci, *E. coli*, or herpes simplex. Of course, early identification of infections with these agents is important, because specific therapy is available.

If an infant has a family history of neonatal seizures, a peculiar odor, milk intolerance, acidosis, alkalosis, or seizures unresponsive to conventional anticonvulsants, other primary metabolic causes should be sought. Maple syrup urine disease is due to inability to decarboxylate the branched-chain amino acids valine, leucine, and isoleucine. Newborns with this disorder appear well until the institution of protein feeding or until an insult that results in catabolism of protein. The clinical manifestations often are dramatic: vomiting, a shrill cry, hypotonia, and convulsions. To an astute observer, the odor of maple syrup may be detectable in the urine and other body secretions. When maple syrup urine disease is suspected, urine should be boiled briefly to remove nonspecific ketones and then mixed with equal parts of 2,4-dinitrophenylhydrazine; in the presence of the keto derivatives of the branched-chain amino acids, a fluffy yellow precipitate will occur. It is important to be aware that hypoglycemia may accompany maple syrup urine disease. Exchange transfusion and/or peritoneal dialysis have been used in the treatment of this disorder, but it appears that a high-calorie diet (150 calories/kg/day) must also be used to reduce the plasma concentration of leucine and correct the accompanying hypoglycemia (12). Plasma amino acid chromatography and analysis of the enzyme activity of fibroblasts are necessary to confirm the diagnosis.

The urea cycle disorders, including carbamyl phosphate synthetase (CPS), ornithine, transcarbamylase (OTC), citrullinemia, argininosuccinic aciduria, and argininemia, may present in the neonatal period with seizure activity. In addition, transient hyperammonemia may manifest with neonatal seizures (2). Manifestations of these disorders may appear very rapidly after delivery if enzyme deficiency is complete, or they may be delayed until later in infancy or childhood if enzyme deficiency is incomplete. The manifestations of the urea cycle disorders include vomiting, lethargy, hypotonia, coma, and intractable seizures. Respiratory alkalosis is often seen early in the course of these disorders. The diagnosis of urea cycle enzyme deficiencies is confirmed by the presence of an elevated blood ammonia concentration, which is extraordinarily high in male infants with CPS or OTC deficiency. Therapy for infants who present with urea cycle enzyme deficiencies is particularly difficult, consisting of exchange transfusion and/or peritoneal dialysis to lower blood ammonia concentrations. Recent data have demonstrated that peritoneal dialysis is superior to exchange transfusion, in that it removes body nitrogen in the form of glutamine, glutamate, and alanine (3). Because all patients with urea cycle enzyme deficiencies are hypoargininemic, arginine infusions are indicated. In the case of argininosuccinic aciduria, arginine supplementation may suffice to maintain normal ammonia metabolism. Sodium benzoate has also been of value in the treatment of hyperammonemia by increasing nitrogen removal through hippurate synthesis. During the acute phase of treatment of these disorders, protein is withheld, and high glucose concentrations are used as an energy source.

Infants with nonketotic hyperglycinemia may present very early in the neonatal period with hypotonia, lethargy, and myoclonic seizures. The seizures characteristically are quite stimulus-sensitive and are associated with an EEG pattern that consists initially of periodic paroxysmal bursts on an almost flat background (4). The EEG evolves later into a hypsarrhythmic pattern. Glycine concentrations in plasma and cerebrospinal fluid are markedly elevated. This disorder appears to be due to lack of a glycine cleavage enzyme, so that glycine is not metabolized to carbon dioxide, ammonia, and a one-carbon tetrahydrofolate fragment. This metabolic defect has been demonstrated in liver fibroblasts and brain tissue. Therapy directed at the nonketotic form of hyperglycinemia has included initial exchange transfusions to lower plasma concentrations of glycine and the use of strychnine sulfate (17), but these have not been particularly successful. This disorder is not always fatal in the immediate neonatal period, but the vast majority of survivors are significantly neurologically impaired.

The ketotic hyperglycinemias, including propionic acidemia and methylmalonic acidemia, may present very early in the neonatal period and are characterized by vomiting, dehydration, coma, and seizures. These disorders may respond to dietary therapy. In addition, vitamin-B_{12}-dependent forms of methylmalonic acidemia have been reported in the neonatal period. Ketone bodies in the urine of children with neonatal seizures, as well as acidosis and thrombocytopenia, are clues to the presence of these disorders. The finding of an elevated concentration of the appropriate short-chain organic acid in the urine confirms the diagnosis. Isovaleric acidemia is a very rare disorder that may present with seizure activity, vomiting, acidosis, and ketosis in the newborn period. Infants with this disorder have an offensive body odor.

Pyridoxine-dependency seizures characteristically appear in the newborn period. Although only about 50 patients with pyridoxine dependency have been described since this disorder was first recognized, the number is greater than 200 if relatives who have expired in the neonatal period are included. This disorder is due to the dependence of glutamic acid decarboxylase on high concentrations of pyridoxine. Glutamic acid decarboxylase is necessary for synthesis of the inhibitory neurotransmitter γ-aminobutyric acid (GABA). This disorder has been a suspected cause of intrauterine convulsions, and it is not uncommon for these infants to be delivered with meconium staining. The seizures are of the generalized tonic-clonic variety and may closely mimic those seizures due to asphyxia. The diagnosis can be confirmed and therapy provided when 100 mg of pyridoxine is given intravenously under EEG monitoring (6); the EEG will be dramatically abnormal, with generalized disorganization and spike and polyspike discharges. The clinical seizures will stop within minutes after pyridoxine administration, and the EEG will normalize within hours. These infants appear to require pyridoxine supplementation for life.

Newborns can become intoxicated with procaine derivatives used for maternal analgesia at the time of delivery, and in these circumstances seizures usually are of the generalized tonic-clonic variety and not infrequently are associated with cardiac arrhythmias and absence of brainstem reflexes. The brainstem abnormalities and cardiac arrhythmias help to distinguish these infants from infants who have seizures on a postasphyxic basis, in which brainstem abnormalities are less common and arrhythmias respond to oxygenation (14). A further clue to the cause is that mothers often note no pain relief at the time of administration of the procaine derivative. Most often, one notes a site of injection in the scalp of the infant immediately after delivery. Direct injections of local anesthetics into infants have been reported with the paracervical, pudendal, and saddle block routes of maternal administration. Treatment of infants with procaine-derivative intoxication consists in acidifying the urine, inducing diuresis, and administering conventional anticonvulsants. Diuresis of the procaine derivatives appears to be the most beneficial measure.

Neonatal seizures may be due to withdrawal from analgesics, narcotics, or hypnotic-sedatives used by the mother during pregnancy. Neonatal seizures are far more common following withdrawal of methadone than from heroin addiction. Herzlinger et al. (13) noted an incidence of 7.8% following methadone withdrawal, as compared with 1.2% when mothers were addicted to heroin. The usual time of onset of narcotic-withdrawal seizures in the neonate is 10 ± 8 days (range 3–34 days). Some investigators have noted a relationship to the amount and time of the mother's last dose of methadone or heroin and the onset of neonatal seizures. Herzlinger et al. (13) were unable to make this association. Neonatal seizures have also been described following maternal barbiturate addiction and subsequent withdrawal (7). Four agents have

been advocated for the treatment of withdrawal syndromes in the neonate: diazepam, phenobarbital, chlorpromazine, and paregoric. There appears to be no clear superiority of one agent over the other. However, chlorpromazine reduces seizure threshold, and it would not appear prudent to use this agent in the treatment of neonates with withdrawal symptoms.

ANTICONVULSANT THERAPY

When an underlying metabolic cause for neonatal seizure activity is not found, conventional anticonvulsants are used in the treatment of the seizure state. The aggressiveness with which therapy is approached in the neonatal period is currently a subject of controversy. Studies in the rat have demonstrated an increased susceptibility of the immature central nervous system to seizure activity, with subsequent impairment of brain growth and decreased DNA, RNA, protein, and cholesterol (33). In addition, there has been breakdown of brain polysomes and inhibition of cerebral protein synthesis noted in status epilepticus (31,32). The presence of neonatal seizures has been an ominous predictor in studies determining the outcome for categories of high-risk infants (11,20). Other investigators, however, have called attention to the possible impairment of brain growth following phenobarbital or valproic acid administration in rat

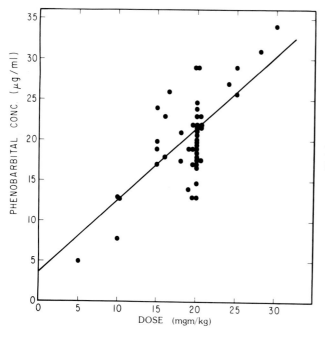

FIG. 1. Phenobarbital loading doses and plasma concentrations achieved.

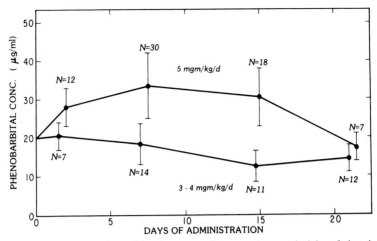

FIG. 2. Plasma concentrations achieved on two maintenance dosage schedules of phenobarbital.

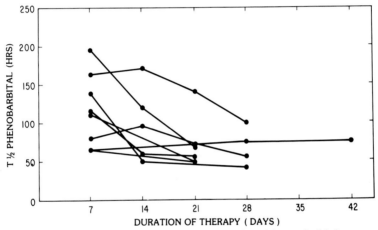

FIG. 3. Phenobarbital half-life relative to duration of therapy in 8 infants.

pups (8,9). Phenytoin appears to have an adverse effect on developing cortical neurons in fetal mouse cultures (27).

Anticonvulsants that have been used in the newborn include phenobarbital, phenytoin, diazepam, primidone, and paraldehyde.

Phenobarbital is probably the most commonly used anticonvulsant in the neonatal period. Studies by Jalling (15), Lockman et al. (16), and our group (22) have demonstrated that loading doses of phenobarbital should be used in treating neonatal seizure states in order to rapidly obtain therapeutically efficacious but nontoxic concentrations of the drug. The currently recommended dosage schedules in most standard textbooks result in less than therapeutic concentrations following initial administration, but toxic accumulation occurs if maintenance

dosage schedules are followed. The half-lives of phenytoin and phenobarbital are prolonged in the neonate as compared with the adult. We and Lockman's group assumed an arbitrary therapeutic concentration of phenobarbital of 20 μg/ml. Loading doses of 20 mg/kg are necessary to obtain concentrations within this range (Fig. 1). Maintenance dosages of more than 5 mg/kg/day would be expected to result in accumulation of phenobarbital and subsequent clinical intoxication (Fig. 2). The newborn, however, does improve in terms of ability to metabolize phenobarbital, and half-lives decline from more than 100 hr after 7 days of treatment to 60 to 70 hr after 28 days of therapy (Figs. 3 and 4). Neither the loading dose nor the maintenance dosage of phenobarbital appears to be influenced by gestational age or birth weight. The

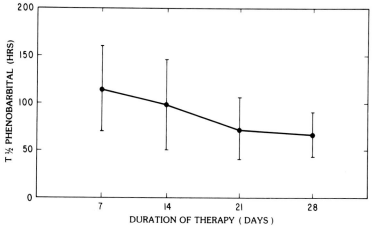

FIG. 4. Mean phenobarbital half-life and standard deviation relative to duration of therapy in 8 infants.

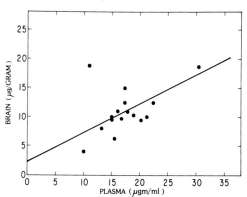

FIG. 5. Brain-to-plasma ratio of phenobarbital.

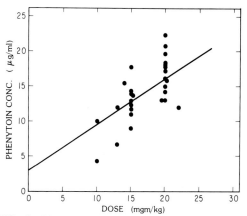

FIG. 6. Phenytoin loading doses and plasma concentrations achieved.

brain to plasma ratio of phenobarbital (Fig. 5) has been found to be 0.71 ± 0.21 (23), in general agreement with the brain to plasma ratios of phenobarbital reported in the adult, which vary from 0.59 to 0.91 (24.29). The brain-to-plasma ratio of phenobarbital increases with gestational age, but the drug does not accumulate in the brain with prolonged treatment (22). Clinical effectiveness of phenobarbital is uncommonly seen below a concentration of 16 μg/ml (16). Approximately 60% of high-risk newborns who are controlled with conventional anticonvulsants can be expected to be controlled with phenobarbital alone.

At the present time, the second most commonly used anticonvulsant in the neonatal period is *phenytoin*. If the therapeutic concentration of phenytoin is arbitrarily defined as 15 μg/ml, then loading doses of 20 mg/kg will be necessary to achieve this concentration (Fig. 6). If dosages of more than 5 mg/kg/day are used for maintenance, toxic accumulation of the drug can be expected to occur. Phenytoin does not appear to be reliably absorbed from the neonatal gastrointestinal tract, and the oral route is not acceptable for maintenance therapy. Intramuscular administration of phenytoin is irritating and results in unpredictable plasma concentrations. The intravenous route, therefore, is the only acceptable mode of administering the drug to the newborn. The brain-to-plasma ratio of phenytoin in the neonate (Fig. 7) is 1.28 ± 0.32 (23), which is in general agreement with the ratio of 0.75 to 1.5 recorded in the adult (29). In contrast with findings in adults, we did not note in newborns an influence of serum albumin concentration on the brain-to-plasma ratio of phenytoin. Data are not available concerning the clinical response seen with phenytoin alone in the treatment in neonatal seizures, but it is effective in neonates who are uncontrolled with phenobarbital. Care must be taken in administering phenytoin by the intravenous route,

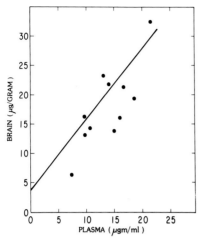

FIG. 7. Brain-to-plasma ratio of phenytoin.

because it has produced cardiac arrhythmias. As with phenobarbital, loading doses and maintenance dosages of phenytoin are not influenced by birth weight or gestational age.

Intravenous *diazepam* has been reported to be effective in the treatment of prolonged seizure activity in infants and neonates (26). Some investigators have become concerned with the use of diazepam in the treatment of neonatal seizures because of the possibility of its vehicle, sodium benzoate, uncoupling bilirubin from albumin and increasing the risk of kernicterus (30). This would not appear to be a significant problem in the infant without an increased bilirubin concentration, and diazepam has not been reported to cause kernicterus in the immediate perinatal period. Studies done in the Gunn rat would indicate that the amount of sodium benzoate delivered to an infant when using diazepam for treatment of neonatal seizures would have no effect on bilirubin metabolism (21). Indeed, because the degree of albumin binding of bilirubin is even greater in the human than in the Gunn rat, there appears to be minimal risk that diazepam doses used to treat seizures would cause kernicterus in the human newborn. In the rat, benzodiazepine receptors are present in the brain early in the gestational period, and they reach levels seen in the mature rat within 7 days following birth (1). We have no experience with using diazepam as an initial drug in the treatment of status epilepticus, but we have reported that it did not improve seizure control when used as a third agent (22). The presence of phenytoin, however, may have an adverse effect on benzodiazepine receptors (18). The ben-

zodiazepines should be evaluated as the initial agent in treating neonatal status epilepticus.

Paraldehyde has been advocated by some as an effective anticonvulsant in the newborn period, and it may be administered by the rectal route or as a 10% solution in an intravenous drip. However, it has produced pulmonary edema, pulmonary hemorrhage, and hypotension in older children (25), and therefore it should be used with caution in the neonate, particularly the neonate with respiratory disease.

We have used *primidone* as the third anticonvulsant in difficult seizure states and have found it effective. We have found, with preliminary observations, that the neonate does not appear to have the ability to convert primidone to phenobarbital; therefore, primidone at 20 mg/kg as a loading dose results in plasma concentrations of 8 to 15 μg/ml.

The causes of neonatal seizures are diverse. A successful therapeutic approach demands a correct

TABLE 2. *Diagnosis and therapy for neonatal seizures*

History
  Family history of neonatal seizures or deaths
  Maternal drug history
  Delivery history
  Maternal infections during pregnancy
Examination
  Chorioretinitis
  Needle marks on scalp
  Mental status
  Seizure type
  Skin lesions
  Fontanelle
Initial studies
  Na, BUN, glucose, Ca^{2+}, Mg^{2+}, bilirubin, NH_3, blood gases, screen urine with 2,4-DNPH, L-P
Symptomatic therapy
  Glucose
  Phenobarbital
  Phenytoin
  Paraldehyde
  Diazepam
  Primidone
  CT scan
  Torch titers
Specific therapy
  Pyridoxine
  Glucose
  Calcium
  Dialysis (maple syrup urine disease)
  Exchange transfusion (hyperammonemia)
  Vitamins (nonketotic hyperglycinemia)
  Hypertonic glucose (ketotic hyperglycinemia)
  Plasma amino acids
  Fibroblast assay

diagnosis and an understanding of the metabolic peculiarities of the newborn. Table 2 summarizes our approach to neonatal seizures.

REFERENCES

1. Baestrup, C., and Nielsen, M. (1978): Ontogenic development of benzodiazepine receptors in the rat. *Brain Res.*, 147:170–173.
2. Ballard, R. A., Vincur, B., Reynolds, J. W., Wennberg, R. P., Merritt, A., Sweetman, L., and Nyhan, W. L. (1978): Transient hyperammonemia of the preterm infant. *N. Engl. J. Med.*, 299:920–925.
3. Batshaw, M. L., and Brusilow, S. W. (1980): Treatment of hyperammonemia coma caused by inborn errors of urea synthesis. *J. Pediatr.*, 97:893–900.
4. Dalla Bernardina, B., Aicardi, J., Gautiers, F., and Plouin, P. (1979): Glycine encephalopathy. *Neuropaediatrie*, 10:200–225.
5. Caveness, W. F., Echlin, F., Kemper, T., and Motohiro, K. (1973): The propagation of focal paroxysmal activity in the *Macaca mulatta* at birth and at 24 months. *Brain*, 96:757–764.
6. Clarke, T. A., Saunder, B. S., and Fedlman, B. (1979): Pyridoxine dependent seizures requiring high doses of pyridoxine for control. *Am. J. Dis. Child.*, 133:963–965.
7. Desmond, M. M., Schwanecke, R. P., Wilson, G. S., Yasunaga, S., and Burgdoff, I. (1972): Maternal barbiturate utilization and neonatal withdrawal symptomatology. *J. Pediatr.*, 80:190–197.
8. Diaz, J., Schain, R. J., and Bailey, B. G. (1977): Phenobarbital-induced brain growth retardation in artificially reared rat pups. *Biol. Neonate*, 32:77–82.
9. Diaz, J., and Shields, W. D. (1978): Chronic administration of diapropylacetate early in life: Effects on brain development and behavior. *Ann. Neurol.*, 4:198.
10. Ferguson, J., Levinsohn, M., and Derakshan, I. (1974): Brainstem seizures in hydranencephaly. *Neurology (Minneap.)*, 24:1152–1157.
11. Fitzhardinge, P. M., Pape, K., Arstikaitis, M., Boyle, M., Ashby, S., Rowley, C., and Swyer, P. R. (1976): Mechanical ventilation of infants less than 1501 gm. birth: Health, growth, and neurologic sequelae. *J. Pediatr.*, 88:531–541.
12. Hammersen, G., Wille, L., Schmidt, H., Lutz, P., and Bickel, H. (1978): Maple syrup urine disease. Emergency treatment of the neonate. *Mongr. Hum. Genet.*, 9:84–89.
13. Herzlinger, R. A., Krandall, S. R., and Vaughan, H. G. (1977): Neonatal seizures associated with narcotic withdrawal. *J. Pediatr.*, 91:638–641.
14. Hillman, L. S., Hillman, R. E., and Dodson, W. E. (1979): Diagnosis, treatment, and follow-up of neonatal mepivacaine intoxication secondary to paracervical and pudendal blocks during labor. *J. Pediatr.*, 95:472–477.
15. Jalling, B. (1975): Plasma concentrations of phenobarbital in the treatment of seizures in the newborn. *Acta Paediatr. Scand.*, 64:514–524.
16. Lockman, L. A., Kriel, R., Zaske, D., Thompson, T., and Virnig, N. (1979): Phenobarbital dosage for control of neonatal seizures. *Neurology (Minneap.)*, 29:1445–1449.
17. MacDermot, K. D., Nelson, W., Reichert, C. M., and Schulman, J.D. (1980): Attempts at the use of strychnine sulfate in the treatment of non-ketotic hyperglycinemia. *Pediatrics*, 65:61–64.
18. Mimaki, T., Deshmukh, P. P., and Yamamura, H. I. (1980): Decreased benzodiazepine receptor density in rat brain following chronic phenytoin administration. *Ann. Neurol.*, 8:230.
19. Monod, N., Dreyfus-Brisac, C., and Sfaelo, Z. (1979): Appearance and prognosis of neonatal status epilepticus. A clinical and EEG study of 150 cases. *Arch. Fr. Pediatr.*, 26:1085–1102.
20. Mulligan, J. D., Painter, M. J., O'Donaghue, P., MacDonald, H., Allen, A., and Taylor, P. (1980): Neonatal asphyxia. II. Neonatal mortality and long term sequelae. *J. Pediatr.*, 96:903–907.
21. Nathenson, G., Cohen, M., and McNormora, H. (1975): The effect of Na benzoate on serum bilirubin in the Gunn rat. *J. Pediatr.*, 86:799–803.
22. Painter, M. J., Pippenger, C., MacDonald, H., and Pitlick, W. (1978): Phenobarbital and diphenylhydantoin levels in neonates with seizures. *J. Pediatr.*, 92:315–319.
23. Painter, M. J., Pippenger, C., Wasterlain, C., Barmada, M., Pitlick, W., Carter, G., and Abern, S. (1981): Phenobarbital and phenytoin in neonatal seizures, metabolism and tissue distribution. *Neurology (Minneap.)*, 31:1107–1112.
24. Sherwin, A. L., Eisen, A. A., and Sokolowski, C. D. (1973): Anticonvulsant drugs in human epileptogenic brain. Correlation of phenobarbital and diphenylhydantoin levels with plasma. *Arch. Neurol.*, 29:73–77.
25. Sinal, S., and Crowe, J. (1976): Cyanosis, cough, and hypotension following intravenous administration of paraldehyde. *Pediatrics*, 57:158–159.
26. Smith, B. T., and Masotti, R. E. (1971): Intravenous diazepam in the treatment of prolonged seizure activity in neonates and infants. *Dev. Med. Child Neurol.*, 13:630–634.
27. Swaiman, K. F., Schrier, B. K., Neale, E. A., and Nelson, P. G. (1980): Effects of chronic phenytoin and valproic acid exposure on fetal mouse cortical cultures. *Ann. Neurol.*, 8:230.
28. Tsang, R. C. (1972): Neonatal magnesium disturbances. *Am. J. Dis. Child.*, 124:282–293.
29. Vajda, F., Faith, F.M., Davidson, S., et al. (1974): Human brain, cerebrospinal fluid and plasma concentrations of DPH and phenobarbital. *Clin. Pharmacol. Ther.*, 15:597.
30. Volpe, J. (1977): Management of neonatal seizures. *Crit. Care Med.*, 5:43–49.
31. Wasterlain, C. G. (1972): Breakdown of brain polysomes in status epilepticus. *Brain Res.*, 39:278–284.
32. Wasterlain, C. G. (1974): Inhibition of cerebral protein synthesis by epileptic seizures without motor manifestations. *Neurology (Minneap.)*, 24:175–180.
33. Wasterlain, C. G., and Plum, F. (1973): Vulnerability of developing rat brain to electroconvulsive seizures. *Arch. Neurol.*, 29:38–45.

Advances in Neurology, Vol. 34: Status Epilepticus, edited by A.V. Delgado-Escueta, C.G. Wasterlain, D.M. Treiman, and R.J. Porter. Raven Press, New York © 1983.

39

Medical Complications of Status Epilepticus

Gilbert H. Glaser

Status epilepticus of generalized convulsions (grand mal) produces, in addition to the repetitive severe tonic-clonic seizures, a marked disturbance of generalized cerebral and bodily functions. The patient is usually comatose in the intervals between the generalized seizure activity, as well as during the repetitive seizures. The autonomic nervous system is usually overwhelmingly in a state of dysfunction. Cumulative anoxia occurs, both cerebral and systemic. The medical complications involve many systems, and uncontrolled they lead to high morbidity, further cerebral damage, and mortality.

This was recognized in 1667 by Thomas Willis (16), who wrote "whenas the fits are often repeated and every time grow more cruell, the animal function is quickly debilitated; and from thence by the taint, by degrees brought on the spirits and the nerves serving the Praecordia, the vital function is by little and little enervated, til at length the whole body languishing and the pulse being loosened and at length ceasing, at last the vital flame is extinguished."

However, it was not until the nineteenth century that further detailed attention was paid to the severe effects of generalized convulsions. In 1824, Calmeil (2), writing his thesis on epilepsy, stated: "le danger est pressant, beaucoup de malades succombent." Yet Gowers (3), in his landmark book on epilepsy, stated that, in his experience, a severe degree of status epilepticus was very rare and usually occurred in "asylums." There were no deaths under his own observation. However, he did report

that in some patients the pulse and respirations increased, the body temperature could rise to 107°F, and patients could die in a state of collapse. By 1907, Turner (14) indicated that in his own experience he observed at least 5% of patients in status epilepticus; under various conditions, and evaluating the experiences of others as well as his own, he reported mortality of 11% to 50%, especially in severe cases with prolonged coma. It is perhaps quite important to realize, as did Hunter (4) in 1959, that the incidence of status epilepticus has increased over the years and has become more severe since the beginning of the administration of antiepileptic drugs in the latter part of the nineteenth century. Mortality has remained between 10% and 45% (1,8,10,11,12). There is no doubt that many instances of status epilepticus have been precipitated by the manipulation and/or withdrawal of such medications (4). During the last 20 years there have been a number of important evaluations of status epilepticus, mainly with regard to its neurophysiology and its effect on the brain, with some indications of the medical complications contributing to the morbidity and mortality. These reports have been both clinical (1,5,8,11) and experimental (6,7,15).

In 1960, Lennox (5) described the serious medical condition of these patients, initially in stupor and then coma, with rising temperature, pulse, and respirations. He stated that the body can be "bathed in cold foul-smelling sweat" and that pneumonia is common. He also pointed out that suffocation can ensue, often with aspiration of excessive amounts of salivary secretions if the patient in status epilepticus turns on his face. In some series of patients studied, acute deaths have been related to the pulmonary complications of pneumonia associated with pulmonary congestion.

The important background of medical complications of status epilepticus and the grave prognosis in this condition are due to the state of coma accompanied by severe autonomic disturbances and the associated cumulative anoxia. Such status epilepticus must be regarded as a medical emergency. Table 1 presents an overview of such medical complications involving many bodily systems and altering the metabolic-biochemical internal homeostatic environment.

The cardiovascular system is particularly disturbed, with initial tachycardia and then possibly bradycardia. Cardiac arrest can occur. Cardiac arrhythmias are common. When these are present,

TABLE 1. *Status epilepticus: medical complications*

Interictal coma with severe autonomic disturbances
Cumulative anoxia: systemic and cerebral
Cardiovascular system complications and failure
    Tachycardia, bradycardia, cardiac arrest
    Cardiac failure
    Cardiac arrhythmias
    Hypertension, hypotension, shock
Respiratory system failure
    Apnea, polypnea (tachypnea, bradypnea),
      Cheyne-Stokes
    Pulmonary congestion (may be neurogenic)
    Pneumonia, aspiration effects, cyanosis
Kidney failure
    Oliguria, uremia
    Acute tubular necrosis
    Lower nephron nephrosis
    Contributing factor: rhabdomyolysis-myoglobinuria
Autonomic system disturbances (in addition to above)
    Hyperpyrexia
    Excessive sweating, vomiting, dehydration, electrolyte loss
    Hypersecretion (salivary, tracheobronchial)
    Airway obstruction
Metabolic-biochemical
    Acidosis (metabolic, respiratory, especially lactic acidosis)
    Anoxemia
    Hyperazotemia
    Hyperkalemia
    Hypoglycemia
    Hyponatremia
    Hepatic failure
Infections: pulmonary, bladder, skin

particular care must be taken if intravenous phenytoin is being used, for example, in an attempt to control the acute repetitive generalized convulsions in such status. Hypertension, then hypotension, and occasionally circulatory collapse and a shocklike state can ensue.

Respiratory system dysfunction and failure accompany the disturbances of the cardiovascular system. Disturbances in the rate of breathing are frequent, with apnea, hyperventilation, and occasionally Cheyne-Stokes respirations. Pulmonary congestion is frequent and is associated with cardiac failure. However, a neurogenic factor may be present, as recently studied by Simon et al. (13). In an investigation of experimentally induced severe generalized seizures, they found that such seizures transiently elevated pulmonary microvascular pressure and pulmonary lymphatic flow. There was an increase in pulmonary capillary permeability persisting after the microvascular pressure returned to base-line value. They indicated the possibility of two independent neuronally mediated events that such severe seizures can produce, related to transcapillary fluid movement in the lung, both by elevating the pulmonary capillary hydrostatic pressure and by altering capillary permeability. Pneumonia as a concomitant may be severe (8) and may also be related to the effects of aspiration.

These involvements of the cardiovascular and respiratory systems usually are associated in status epilepticus with cumulative anoxia, both systemic and cerebral, the latter contributing to the probability of further brain damage in particularly susceptible areas such as the limbic system (especially the hippocampus) and also the cerebellum. The effects (particularly increasing the cerebral venous pressure) associated with accumulations of carbon dioxide during respiratory failure often are associated with elevated cerebrospinal fluid pressure. Also associated with the anoxemia is acidosis of metabolic and respiratory origin. There is also a particularly marked lactic acidosis that is augmented by the severe exertional activity of the skeletal musculature in the generalized convulsions.

Kidney failure can occur and can be either mild or severe. The severe states of kidney failure are associated with oliguria and uremia, with hyperazotemia and hyperkalemia. In such patients, acute renal tubular necrosis and lower nephron nephrosis may be produced. A contributing factor that often is neglected is rhabdomyolysis (9). The generalized convulsive state is associated with massive muscular activity. In some patients this can cause muscle damage, with marked elevation of serum creatine phosphokinase. Also, it is known that patients in severe coma can undergo damage to certain muscles by virtue of various pressures on dependent muscle tissues (9). The phenomenon in status epilepticus is also enhanced because of the elevated body temperatures in the usual hyperpyretic state. Rhabdomyolysis then ensues, and associated with myoglobinuria it can produce the renal damage of lower nephron nephrosis and acute renal failure (9).

The various disturbances in cardiovascular, respiratory, and kidney functions, along with the severe autonomic system disturbances of hyperpyrexia, excessive sweating, often vomiting leading to dehydration and electrolyte loss, and hypersecretion of both salivary and tracheobronchial activities with airway obstruction, contribute to the severe metabolic disorders present in these patients. The prominence of acidosis and anoxemia has been mentioned, and the associated uremic state along with hyperkalemia may be severe. Hypoglycemia after initial hyperglycemia has been described in experimental status epilepticus (6,7,15), and it can be found in cases of repetitive generalized seizures in humans. The initial hyperglycemia probably is related to the early marked autonomic discharge, with release of epinephrine, and also probably an activation of hepatic gluconeogenesis (7). The later hypoglycemia has a number of likely causative factors (7): increased plasma insulin, enhanced cerebral glucose consumption, and excessive muscular activity. Hyponatremia also has been described as severe and as a complication that could be related to the various disturbances in fluid balance. Hepatic failure is unusual and is more likely to occur in association with cardiac and renal dysfunction. Of course, the differential diagnosis must include primary renal, cardiovascular, and other medical metabolic disorders complicated by secondary status epilepticus.

As already stated, certain infections may involve these patients and may contribute to the morbidity and mortality. Pneumonia is quite frequent, as are bladder infections and, eventually, infections of the skin associated with decubitus ulceration. These, of course, must be treated as rapidly as possible.

In summary, status epilepticus (grand mal) is a medical emergency, with all the complications of cerebral and generalized anoxia, elevated cerebrospinal fluid pressure, and concomitant coma. Cardiovascular, respiratory, and renal failures must be recognized and treated. The effects of vomiting may be severe and may enhance disturbances in water and electrolyte metabolism. Excessive muscle activity can produce myolysis and myoglobinuria and can lead to lower nephron nephrosis. Acidosis, particularly lactic, is prominent. Variations in blood sugar occur, especially hypoglycemia. The autonomic nervous system dysfunction may be marked, with hyperthermia, excessive sweating, further dehydration, hypertension and hypotension, and eventual shock. Uncontrolled, these complications can lead to high morbidity, further cerebral damage, and mortality.

REFERENCES

1. Aicardi, J., and Chevrie, J. J. (1971): Convulsive status epilepticus in infants and children: A study of 239 cases. *Epilepsia*, 11:187–197.
2. Calmeil, L. F. (1824): De l'épilepsie étudiée sous la rapport de son siège et de son influence sur la production de l'aliénation mentale. Thesis. Didot, Paris (cited in ref. 11).
3. Gowers, W. R. (1885): *Epilepsy and Other Chronic Convulsive Diseases*, pp. 160–161. William Wood, New York.
4. Hunter, R. A. (1959): Status epilepticus: History, incidence and problems. *Epilepsia*, 1:162–188.
5. Lennox, W. G. (1960): *Epilepsy and Related Disorders. Vol. 1*. Little, Brown, Boston.
6. Meldrum, B. S., and Horton, R. W. (1973): Physiology of status epilepticus in primates. *Arch. Neurol.*, 28:1–9.
7. Meldrum, B. S., Horton, R. W., Bloom, S. R., Butler, J., and Keenan, J. (1979): Endocrine factors and glucose metabolism during prolonged seizures in baboons. *Epilepsia*, 20:527–534.
8. Oxbury, J. M., and Whitty, C. W. M. (1971): Causes and consequences of status epilepticus in adults. *Brain*, 94:733–744.
9. Penn, A. S., Rowland, L. P., and Fraser, D. W. (1972): Drugs, coma and myoglobinuria. *Arch. Neurol.*, 26:336–343.
10. Rodin, E. A. (1968): *The Prognosis of Patients with Epilepsy*, pp. 156–171. Charles C Thomas, Springfield, Ill.
11. Roger, J., Lob, H., and Tassinari, C. A. (1974): Status epilepticus. In: *Handbook of Clinical Neurology, Vol. 15, The Epilepsies*, edited by P. J. Vinken and G. W. Bruyn, pp. 145–188. North-Holland, Amsterdam.
12. Rowan, A. J., and Scott, D. F. (1970): Major status epilepticus. A series of 42 patients. *Acta Neurol. Scand.*, 46:573–584.
13. Simon, R. P., Bayne, L. L., and Tranbaugh, R. F. (1980): Mechanisms of neurogenic pulmonary edema following seizures in sheep. *Ann. Neurol.*, 8:97 (abstract).

min. The plasma insulin concentration was initially unchanged but subsequently increased threefold to fivefold. In each animal there was a close reciprocal relationship between the glucose and insulin changes for both timing and amplitude (Fig. 2). The plasma GH concentration fluctuated initially but rose after 30 to 60 min. This increase did not correlate in timing with the changes in plasma glucose or insulin. Thus, changes in plasma GH concentration during seizures are the algebraic sum of abnormal neuronal activities (tending to increase or decrease GH release) and the influence of various systemic factors such as excessive motor activity and hypoglycemia. It may be questioned whether or not physiological factors remain effective in controlling GH release after hypothalamic neurosecretory cells, producing somatostatin and GH-releasing factor, have been subjected to a pathologically enhanced input for 60 min. A failure of somatostatin release might explain the variable late rise in plasma GH. Plasma cortisol showed a variable delayed increase, probably resulting from systemic consequences of seizure activity. Plasma prolactin also showed marked increases, but with a variable time relationship to seizure onset.

ENDOCRINE CHANGES AND THE OUTCOME OF STATUS EPILEPTICUS

The hormonal and metabolic changes described are likely to influence the outcome of status epilepticus.

Hyperglycemia has been shown in monkeys and rats to exacerbate the morbidity and mortality of cerebral ischemia (14,24), possibly because of the more severe lactic acidosis (13) or possibly because it facilitates postischemic epilepsy (23).

The combination of hyperglycemia with a raised plasma insulin concentration is accompanied by increased movement of glucose into the brain and accumulation of glycogen. This mechanism can be invoked to explain the otherwise surprising finding of an increasing brain glycogen content during the second hour of sustained seizure activity (4). The hypoglycemia observed late in seizures will impair brain energy metabolism (3). Its frequency of occurrence and severity in human status epilepticus are uncertain. Therapeutic administration of glucose during status epilepticus is probably appropriate, but the optimal blood sugar concentration during seizures is not known.

Corticosteroids influence ionic movements in the brain and the development of edema. Specific ef-

fects of glucocorticoids on hippocampal neuronal activity have been described (7,21). In aging Fischer rats there is a correlation between plasma corticosterone concentration and astrocytic hypertrophy in the hippocampus (6). Insufficient attention has been paid in both experimental and clinical studies to endocrine changes as important variables in determining the outcome of status epilepticus.

An additional complication is that patients with epilepsy may have abnormal endocrine regulation either as a consequence of repetitive seizures (8,11) or as a side effect of anticonvulsant therapy (25).

SUMMARY

Seizures are accompanied by increases in plasma hormones as a result of (a) spread of abnormal activity to the hypothalamus or other regulatory brain regions, (b) activation of a massive autonomic discharge, or (c) secondary systemic consequences of seizures (e.g., motor activity, hyperglycemia, hypoglycemia). During status epilepticus these changes can show complex sequential interactions. Endocrine changes may critically influence the activity and metabolism of neurons and glia and thus determine the outcome of status epilepticus.

ACKNOWLEDGMENT

The financial support of the Medical Research Council, The Wellcome Trust, and the National Fund for Research into Crippling Diseases is gratefully acknowledged.

REFERENCES

1. Abbott, R. J, Browning, M. C. K., and Davidson, D. L. W. (1980): Serum prolactin and cortisol concentrations after grand mal seizures. *J. Neurol. Neurosurg. Psychiatry*, 43:163–167.
2. Arató, M., Erdós, A., Kurcz, M., Vermes, I., and Fekete, M. (1980): Studies on the prolactin response induced by electroconvulsive therapy in schizophrenics. *Acta Psychiatr. Scand.*, 61:239–244.
3. Blennow, G., Brierley, J. B., Meldrum, B. S., and Siesjö, B. K. (1978): Epileptic brain damage. The role of systemic factors that modify cerebral energy metabolism. *Brain*, 101:687–700.
4. Chapman, A. G., Meldrum, B. S., and Siesjö, B. K. (1977): Cerebral metabolic changes during prolonged epileptic seizures in rats. *J. Neurochem.*, 28:1025–1035.
5. Havens, L. L., Zileli, M. S., DiMascio, L. A., Boling, L., and Goldfien, A. (1959): Changes in catecholamine response to successive electric convulsive treatments. *J. Ment. Sci.*, 105:821–828.

6. Landfield, P. W., Waymire, J. C., and Lynch, G. (1978): Hippocampal aging and adrenocorticoids: Quantitative correlations. *Science*, 202:1098–1102.

7. McEwen, B. S. (1976): Steroid receptors in neuroendocrine tissues: Topography, subcellular distribution, and functional implications. In: *Subcellular Mechanisms in Reproductive Neuroendocrinology*, edited by F. Naftolin, pp. 277–304. Elsevier, Amsterdam.

8. McWilliam, J. R., Meldrum, B. S., and Checkley, S. A. (1981): Enhanced growth hormone response to clonidine after repeated electroconvulsive shock in a primate species. *Psychoneuroendocrinology*, 6:77–79.

9. Meldrum, B. S. (1982): Pathophysiology. In: *A Textbook of Epilepsy*, edited by J. Laidlaw and A. Richens. pp. 456–487. Churchill Livingstone, Edinburgh.

10. Meldrum, B. S., and Horton, R. W. (1973): Physiology of status epilepticus in primates. *Arch. Neurol.*, 28:1–9.

11. Meldrum, B. S., Horton, R. W., Bloom, S. R., Butler, J., and Keenan, J. (1979): Endocrine factors and glucose metabolism during prolonged seizures in baboon. *Epilepsia*, 20:527–534.

12. Meldrum, B., and McWilliam, J. (1981): Hormone changes following seizures. In: *Advances in Epileptology: XII Epilepsy International Symposium*, edited by M. Dam, L. Gram and J. K. Penry, pp. 441–448. Raven Press, New York.

13. Myers, R. E. (1979): A unitary theory of causation of anoxic and hypoxic brain pathology. In: *Advances in Neurology, Vol. 26*, edited by S. Fahn, J. N. Davis, and L. P. Rowland, pp. 195–217. Raven Press, New York.

14. Myers, R. E., and Yamaguchi, M. (1976): Nervous system effects of cardiac arrest in monkeys. *Arch. Neurol.*, 34:65–74.

15. Naquet, R., Meldrum, B. S., Balzano, E., and Charrier, J. P. (1970): Photically-induced epilepsy and glucose metabolism in the adolescent baboon *(Papio papio)*. *Brain Res.*, 18:503–512.

16. Öhman, R., Walinder, J., Balldin, J., Wallin, L., and Abrahamsson, L. (1976): Prolactin response to electroconvulsive therapy. *Lancet*, 2:936–937.

17. Raskind, M., Orenstein, H., and Weitzman, R. E. (1979): Vasopressin in depression. *Lancet*, 1:164.

18. Riche, D. (1973): L'hypothalamus du singe *Papio papio* (Desm): Stereotaxie, cytologie et modifications neurosécrétoires liées aux crises d'épilepsie induites par la lumière. *J. Hirnforsch.*, 14:527–547.

19. Ryan, R. R., Swanson, D. W., Faiman, C., Mayberry, W. E., and Spadoni, A. J. (1970): Effects of convulsive electroshock on serum concentrations of follicle stimulating hormone, luteinising hormone, thyroid stimulating hormone and growth hormone in man. *J. Clin. Endocrinol.*, 30:51–58.

20. Schally, A. V. (1978): Aspects of hypothalamic regulation of the pituitary gland. *Science*, 202:18–28.

21. Segal, M. (1976): Interactions of ACTH and norepinephrine on the activity of rat hippocampal cells. *Neuropharmacology*, 15:329–333.

22. Seite, R., Picard, D., and Luciani, J. (1964): Effets précoces du choc pentetrazolique sur les noyaux neurosécrétoires hypothalamiques chez le chat. *Prog. Brain Res.*, 5:171–190.

23. Siemkowicz, E. (1980): Improvement of restitution from cerebral ischaemia in hyperglycemic rats by pentobarbital or diazepam. *Acta Neurol. Scand.*, 61:368–376.

24. Siemkowicz, E., and Hansen, A. J. (1978): Clinical restitution following cerebral ischaemia in hypo-, normo- and hyperglycemic rats. *Acta Neurol. Scand.*, 58:1–8.

25. Toone, B. K., Wheeler, M., and Fenwick, P. B. C. (1980): Sex hormone changes in male epileptics. *Clin. Endocrinol.*, 12:391–395.

26. Trimble, M. R. (1978): Serum prolactin in epilepsy and hysteria. *Br. Med. J.*, 2:1682.

27. Vigaš, M., Stowasserova, N., Németh, S., and Jurčovičová, J. (1975): Effect of electroconvulsive therapy without anticonvulsive premedication on serum growth hormone in man. *Horm. Res.*, 17:65–70.

28. Vigaš, M., Wiedermann, S., Németh, S., Jurčovičová, J., and Zigo, L. (1976): Alpha-adrenergic regulation of growth hormone release after electroconvulsive therapy in man. *Neuroendocrinology*, 21:42–48.

29. Weil-Malherbe, H. (1955): The effect of convulsive therapy on plasma adrenaline and noradrenaline. *J. Ment. Sci.*, 101:156–162.

Advances in Neurology, Vol. 34: Status Epilepticus, edited by A.V. Delgado-Escueta, C.G. Wasterlain, D.M. Treiman, and R.J. Porter. Raven Press, New York © 1983.

41

Status Epilepticus: Nursing Management

Gwendolyn H. Waddell

The patient suffering from status epilepticus presents a medical and nursing emergency. Constant supervision by a registered nurse skilled in neurological assessment and management is required; the nurse is the primary source of information for the physician and other health team members in developing the protocol or plan of care. Not only does the nurse collaborate in the diagnosis and treatment plan of the physician, the professional nurse also monitors the progress of the patient throughout the acute and recovery phases of status epilepticus. More specifically, nursing management is directed toward the goals of optimal functioning of physiological and psychological systems. The stressors to the patient are presented, with interventions that prevent or minimize them.

NURSING PROCESS

The nursing role during diagnosis and treatment of status epilepticus is that of assisting the patient throughout the procedures and administering the prescribed therapy. During the electroencephalographic, X-ray, and multiple blood and intravenous procedures (9) the nursing goals are threefold: (a) to assure that the patient and family have been informed of the nature and purpose of the procedure, as well as the associated risks and possible side effects (the patient must continue to be treated as though he can comprehend everything); (b) to see that serious untoward side effects have been prevented or immediately reversed; (c) to make

sure that the patient has successfully coped with the anxiety and discomfort attending the procedure (2). Therefore, the nurse combines the role of teacher and health care provider at this time. During the treatment phase of status epilepticus the medical goal is to control the condition quickly and to prevent its recurrence. A therapeutic serum concentration of a long-acting antiepileptic drug must be achieved quickly and maintained. The nurse must have anticonvulsant medications readily available and must have a thorough knowledge of pharmacokinetics. Vital signs and EKG should be monitored when any depressants are used, such as diazepam and phenytoin. The nurse should be aware of the adverse side effects of cardiac arrest and hypotension and should be alert to any indication of their occurrence (1).

The nurse uses the conceptual framework of the nursing process to meet the needs of the patient. The nursing process consists of assessment, intervention, evaluation, and planning (2). Assessment, the first step in the nursing process, requires the intensive care nurse to make an accurate neurological appraisal of the patient in status epilepticus. Because the patient does not fully recover from one seizure before having another, accurate, detailed, and continuous observations must be made in the four neurological areas: level of consciousness, vital signs, pupillary response, and movement (8). The nurse is observing not only for baseline assessment information but also for any sudden changes in physiological and behavioral responses. A second aspect of assessment specifically involves the observation and reporting of the continuous seizure state (4). The nurse is responsible for observing and reporting the following (6): (a) the duration of a seizure; the times it begins and ends; the durations of the tonic, clonic, flaccid, and postictal phases; (b) the presence and characteristics of an aura; (c) the changes in the patient's level of consciousness; (d) the motor activity during the episode, including where the activity begins and what parts of the body become involved; (e) the presence or absence of bowel or bladder incontinence; (f) the patient's response to the seizure; (g) the patient's response to drug therapy; (h) the frequency of seizures.

Interventions by the nurse are directed toward the goals of maintenance of normal body functions, prevention of complications that may prevent recovery or cause residual harm, and support to the patient during the alteration in functioning. In addition to those observational interventions related to assessment, the nurse is responsible for assisting the patient to progress in the activities of daily living, providing a comfortable and healthy environment, and supporting activities important to the patient's rehabilitation.

Maintenance of a safe environment is also essential. The patient is not capable of protecting himself from hazards in the health care setting. The patient's bed must be padded along side rails and headboards to prevent physical injury during the seizure activity. Side rails must be in place and secure whenever the nurse is not rendering direct care.

Evaluation is that part of the nursing process that determines the success of the constant nursing activities. Have the goals of maintenance, prevention, and support been met? All members of the health care team provide information that helps to answer the evaluation question. This process is carried out on an hour-by-hour, day-by-day basis, because the recovery of the patient depends on nursing care high in quality and quantity (5).

A fourth aspect, planning, is the most significant part of the nursing process. A protocol of procedures, therapies, and responsibilities specific for the patient in status epilepticus must be established. The intensive care nurse, other trained personnel, and physicians can then competently deliver the required health care. Following in this presentation are specific nursing interventions that are appropriate for inclusion in such a protocol.

PHYSIOLOGICAL STRESSORS

Specific physiological stressors cause the patient in status epilepticus to disrupt homeostasis and normal body functioning. The stressor may involve oxygenation, fluid and electrolytes, absorption and excretion of nutrients, or regulatory mechanisms (8).

Alterations in Oxygenation

The preservation of adequate ventilation is of primary importance. An oral airway device must be placed in the patient's mouth during a seizure, prior to the development of tonic-clonic movements. Positioning the patient to prevent aspiration, suffocation, and falls is also important. The anticonvulsant drugs used to treat status epilepticus may necessitate oral or nasal endotracheal intubation (4). The nurse must be experienced in performing this act or must have trained personnel present to act at the direction of the physician. Adequate oral and nasal suctioning is also necessary during seizures; this is best accomplished during the quiet phase of status. Careful monitoring of arterial blood gases will provide indications for the nursing interventions to correct alterations in oxygenation.

Alterations in Fluid and Electrolytes

Alterations in fluid and electrolyte balance can occur because of dysfunction of the cardiovascular system, respiratory system, or endocrine system. In the status patient, such alteration can be caused by a simple deficit in the intake of water or electrolytes. The extent of the imbalance is determined by blood electrolyte tests. Appropriate nursing interventions include placement of a large intravenous catheter to administer fluid that does not contain glucose. Precipitation of phenytoin has been documented when it has been mixed with intravenous glucose. Other nursing interventions include distribution of the intravenous fluid infusion over 12 to 24 hr, prevention of foreign objects in the intravenous solution, and restriction of hypertonic solutions to 200 cc/hr and isotonic solutions to 600 cc/hr (3). Comfort measures to be used may include proper positioning of the extremity containing the injection site, anchoring the tubing securely, providing sufficiently long tubing to allow freedom of movement, and maintaining a sterile dressing over the injection site. Observation of the mechanical infusion, such as checking the tube for patency, checking the solution for flow rate, and checking for infiltration of the solution, is important (7). Measurement of intake, output, and vital signs is also essential.

Alterations in Absorption and Excretion of Nutrients

An imbalance in the body fluid and electrolytes probably is accompanied by an alteration in the absorption and excretion of nutrients. The areas of the body that are concerned with this alteration are the digestive, respiratory, urinary, and integumentary systems.

The digestive system should be supported by providing regular mouth care, suctioning oral secretions, administering supplemental oral feedings via nasogastric tube, and observation and care of bowel elimination. Prevention of airway obstruction is the primary goal of nursing care related to the respiratory system. Maintenance by intermittent suctioning or removal of secretions, liquification of thick tenacious secretions, and positioning for maximum oxygenation is necessary. Inspection of the chest for respiratory rate, rhythm, and symmetry and auscultation for abnormal breath sounds are also duties of the nurse.

The urinary system ensures an adequate fluid and electrolyte balance for the body. When the patient is in status epilepticus, the urine output must be monitored and directly related to the fluid intake. Predisposing factors such as dehydration, profuse perspiration, diarrhea, and vomiting can be assessed by the nurse. Intravenous fluid adjustment over each 12- to 24-hr period will facilitate the balance in urinary output. In addition, the skin and integument of the patient need protection from physical injury during the period of continuous seizures. Appropriate interventions that provide for this protection are padding the bony prominences, using a sheepskin on the bed, and maintaining clean, dry, wrinkle-free linen. The patient will also need meticulous hair care, because numerous electroencephalograms will be needed. Generally, provision of adequate circulation, stimulation, cleanliness, and comfort to the skin will ensure that the patient's needs are met.

Alterations in Regulatory Mechanisms

Regulatory mechanisms preserve an organism's ability to adapt to stresses yet maintain its inner balance of homeostasis; failure of regulation is an inability of the organism to adapt appropriately to its environment. Homeostasis must then be assisted by the health care team. All of the foregoing interventions indirectly serve to preserve the homeostasis of the patient. Hypoxia, respiratory acidosis and alkalosis, and metabolic acidosis and alkalosis are all threats to the patient in status. Therefore, specific conditions require certain treatments as directed by the physician. The nurse then acts in a collaborative role, using her observational skills and following the specified drug and treatment plan.

PSYCHOLOGICAL STRESSORS

Once the acute phase of status epilepticus is over, the nurse must be aware of psychological stressors affecting the patient. The patient may suffer from immobility, sensory deprivation or overload, pain, or an altered support system (8).

Alterations in Mobility

The patient is confined to a supine or lateral position, at bedrest, throughout the status episode and may be restrained for safety or restricted in movement by EEG wires, intravenous catheters, or other tubes. This physical immobility, if prolonged, may be accompanied by emotional and social immobility. Emotional immobility exists when the patient cannot use the usual coping mechanisms effectively to meet the stress of this condition. Reactions may vary from overadapting or total withdrawal from the situation to disintegration of coping mechanisms. Social immobility exists when the patient's normal patterns of social interactions are interrupted. The quality and quantity of interactions are decreased because of the constant supervision and activities of the health team.

What can the nurse do to minimize the effects of this immobility? Frequent changes of position, support with pillows and other comfort measures, and releasing restraints whenever possible will decrease the patient's physical immobility. Even moving the bed to present another view can help. The nurse can share observations with the patient regarding this emotional immobility: "I notice that you seem to be withdrawing and not responding to us when you are awake." "Your emotions don't seem to fit what you're feeling." A recognition that the patient may not be able to cope may assist him in more successful coping later. Although there are restrictions on the interactions of family and significant others, the nurse must provide opportunities for social interactions to occur with the patient. This serves to orient the patient to reality and to fill in those "unknown" phases when the patient is unaware or unconscious. The unconscious patient often is talked about, over, around, and not to; the nurse and the health care team are responsible for talking to the patient as if he can hear, regardless of consciousness level. In summary, the nurse's interventions serve to prevent immobility, reduce the effects of immobility, and enhance the patient's ability to cope with immobility.

Alterations in Sensory Stimulation

The patient in status epilepticus immediately experiences a form of sensory deprivation. The senses of hearing, sight, smell, taste, and touch are reduced or obliterated. Perception is distorted after the acute phase, rendering the patient unable to distinguish reality or unable to maintain homeostasis. A state of sensory overload then occurs when the patient regains consciousness and perceives blurring lights, people busy doing things to him, and tubes and wires running across and into his body. The patient sinks into and out of sleep as the medications flow through his system. The deprivation in sensory ability can be minimized by these nursing interventions: (a) speak to the patient as if he can understand everything; (b) use two or more sensory modalities to communicate with the patient (i.e., touch and hearing); (c) increase environmental stimuli, such as lights, visitors, and sounds. Sensory overload can be minimized by decreasing the foregoing activities. A dim room, one voice speaking to the patient at a time, and limited visits all help to clarify the patient's perceptions.

Alterations in Sensory Perception

Pain from the frequent muscle tension of status epilepticus is a problem for most of these patients. They usually are exhausted after the acute episode, and muscle tenderness and fatigue are present. Because pain is a subjective experience and can be verified only by the person experiencing it, the nurse must first assess the presence of pain. Pain-relieving actions that may be used by the nurse consist of approaching the patient unhurriedly and handling gently, performing frequent range-of-motion exercises to extremities, positioning the patient comfortably, and having the patient ambulate as soon as possible.

Alterations in Support Systems

Support systems imply a pattern of continuous or intermittent ties that maintain psychological and physical integrity of the patient over time. An interruption in that pattern occurs when the status patient is hospitalized. Along with social immobility, changes in relationships with significant others may be a potential problem. Again, the nurse must assess the presence of changes in the patient's relationships with others close to him. Minimizing the effects of such changes may prevent later problems. Actions that serve this purpose may include provision of privacy for the patient and visitors, provision of time for emotional expression, expression of empathy for the patient, observing for signs of excessive stress, and encouraging the use of normal coping mechanisms. Planning has been identified as a mediating factor in the nursing process. A protocol of procedures, treatment, and responsibilities of the intensive care nurse should be established and made available to all trained personnel.

Because psychological stressors may manifest themselves in various ways in every patient, individualized nursing interventions must be planned to assist the patient in solving these problems. These interventions may be as simple as switching off a light or as complicated as a psychiatric referral. Therefore, equal attention is warranted by the nurse and health care team in decreasing or preventing the effects of stressors on the psychological being of the patient with status epilepticus.

SUMMARY

During the acute phase of status epilepticus, the intensive care nurse performs constant neurological assessment and collaborative interventions to complete the treatment regimen for the patient. Then the nursing goals are directed toward maintaining optimal physiological functioning and preventing psychological stress. Through the maintenance, prevention, and support of the health care team, the patient receives quality care in the context of status epilepticus, a medical and nursing emergency.

ACKNOWLEDGMENTS

Appreciation is expressed to Sandy T. Carwile, Patricia P. Miller, and A. V. Delgado-Escueta for their guidance and review of this manuscript.

REFERENCES

1. Browne, T. R. (1978): Drug therapy of status epilepticus. *Am. Hosp. Pharm.*, 35:915–922.
2. Campbell, C. (1978): *Nursing Diagnosis and Intervention in Nursing Practice.* John Wiley & Sons, New York.
3. Davis, J. E., and Mason, C. B. (1979): *Neurologic Critical Care.* D. Van Nostrand, New York.
4. Delgado-Escueta, A. V., Boxley, J., Stubbs, N., Waddell, G., and Wilson, W. A. (1974): Prolonged twilight state and automatisms: A case report. *Neurology (Minneap.)*, 24:331–339.
5. Delgado-Escueta, A. V., Nashold, B., Freedman, M., Keplinger, C., Waddell, G., Miller, P., and Carwile, S. (1979): Videotaping epileptic attacks during stereo-electroencephalography. *Neurology (Minneap.)*, 29: 473–489.
6. Korte, M. L. (1972): Intensive care of the neurologic patient. *Nurs. Clin. North Am.*, 7:335–348.
7. Lipe, H. (1979): Clinical evaluation of anticonvulsants: One role of the epilepsy nurse specialist in research. *J. Neurosurg. Nurs.*, 11:238–241.
8. Phipps, W. J., Long, B. C., and Woods, N. F. (editors) (1979): *Medical-Surgical Nursing: Concepts and Clinical Practice.* C. V. Mosby, St. Louis.
9. Plum, F., and Posner, J. B. (1970): *The Diagnosis of Stupor and Coma.* F. A. Davis, Philadelphia.

Advances in Neurology, Vol. 34: Status Epilepticus, edited by A.V. Delgado-Escueta, C.G. Wasterlain, D.M. Treiman, and R.J. Porter. Raven Press, New York © 1983.

42

A Monkey Model for Status Epilepticus: Carbamazepine and Valproate Compared to Three Standard Anticonvulsants

Joan S. Lockard, René H. Levy, Kevin M. Koch,
Donald O. Maris, and Patrick N. Friel

A review of clinical status epilepticus (8) has indicated that the condition is fatal in up to 20% of affected patients and that the likelihood of a fatal outcome co-varies with the frequency of severe seizures and the duration of the status epilepticus. A variety of anticonvulsants have been prescribed for the treatment of status, but there are still marked discrepancies regarding their efficacies (4). Moreover, status epilepticus is not a singular concept; there are as many types of status epilepticus as there are different seizure categories (see Chapter 2). Even the diagnoses of status are variant, with different interpretations of its definition depending on the particular circumstances. The World Health Organization has defined status epilepticus as an "epileptic seizure which is so prolonged or so frequently repeated as to create a fixed and lasting epileptic condition" (6). However, in the case of a series of seizures, unconsciousness between seizures may or may not be an essential component of its diagnosis. Also, in the case of a prolonged seizure, the prerequisite duration varies with the reference source; Dreyer (3) suggested 5 to 10 min, Matthes (21) suggested longer than 15 min, and Gastaut et al. (7) suggested a matter of hours.

Therefore, the general intent of the study reported here was to establish an experimental paradigm for status epilepticus—one in which the status was well defined and involved only a single seizure category—that could be used to compare the efficacies of different anticonvulsants to alleviate this precipitous and life-threatening disease state. The specific objective was to test the efficacies of carbamazepine and valproate, as compared with known effective anticonvulsants, in the treatment of status.

An exclusive seizure type was provided by our alumina-gel monkey model (14), which manifests only focal motor and secondarily generalized tonic-clonic seizures. Spontaneous status epilepticus in this model involves frequent discrete seizures, with an animal-specific, relatively fixed interseizure interval (Fig. 1, bottom two lines). In some monkeys the interval may be as short as 5 min, and in others, as long as an hour. In any event, if effective pharmacological intervention is not provided, death usually ensues within 24 hr.

The 4-deoxypyridoxine hydrochloride (4-DP) protocol described for monkeys by Meldrum and Horton (23) was used in an attempt to mimic spontaneous status epilepticus in our model (Fig. 2).

Monkey ⋆ 9

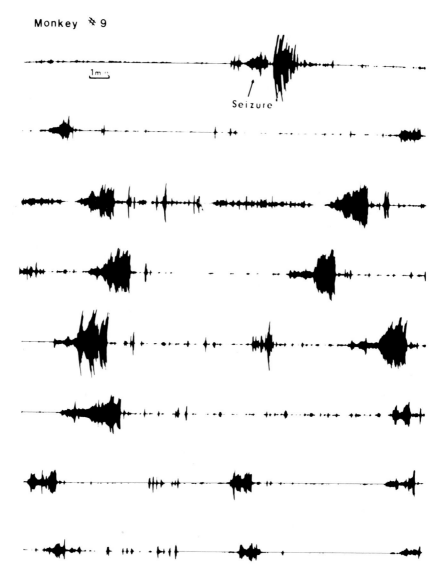

FIG. 1. Spontaneous status epilepticus in an alumina-gel monkey model. Note the largely invariant interseizure interval in the bottom two lines.

The rationale for this choice was based, first, on the fact that 4-DP elicits discrete serial seizures, the process of which may be easily reversed by an antagonist. Also, the proposed mechanism of action of 4-DP, namely, the blocking of the synthesis of glutamic acid decarboxylase (GAD) in synaptosomes (1), diminishes the production of the inhibitory neurotransmitter γ-aminobutyric acid (GABA) in critical midbrain regions. Brain GABA concentrations have been strongly implicated in the mechanisms of epilepsy and in its therapy (5,13,25),

although GABA concentrations in whole brain may not reflect such a relationship (2,22,26).

A 100- to 150-mg/kg dose of 4-DP elicits (usually within 30 min) paroxysms in the monkey model at the site of the alumina focus (left sensorimotor cortex, Fig. 3B) that culminate in a series of secondarily generalized tonic-clonic seizures, with a largely invariant (≤ 20%) interseizure interval. These seizures can be immediately inhibited (if it becomes necessary for the safety of the animal) by a 100- to 175-mg/kg intravenous injection of

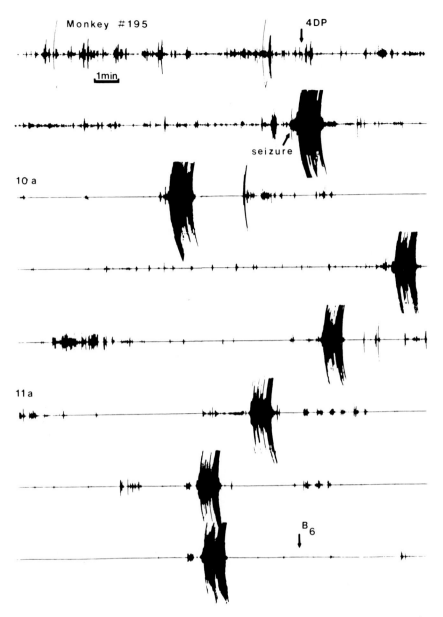

FIG. 2. Experimental status percipitated by administration of 4-DP. Note the largely invariant interscizure interval in the bottom two lines.

pyridoxine hydrochloride (vitamin B_6). The ability of carbamazepine or valproate, as compared with diazepam, phenobarbital, or phenytoin, to alleviate a series of 4-DP-induced seizures was tested by alternating experimental sessions (4-DP + an anticonvulsant) on different days with control sessions (either 4-DP alone or 4-DP + the vehicles of the treatment drugs). Analyses of seizure frequency and severity, interseizure interval, and plasma and CSF drug concentrations provided a relative comparison of the efficacies of the anticonvulsants.

METHODS

Animals. Eight male rhesus monkeys *(Macaca mulatta)* weighing 3.5 to 7.5 kg were used as sub-

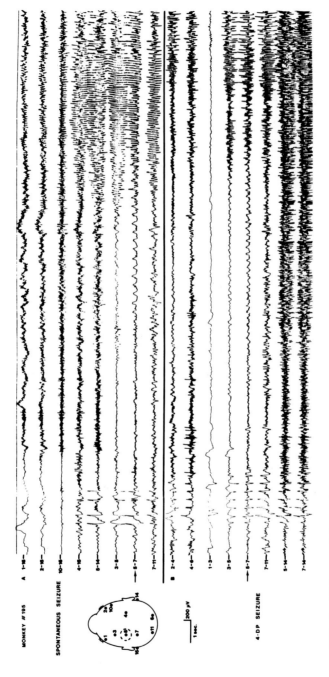

FIG. 3. EEG onset of siezures in an alumina-gel monkey model. **A:** Spontaneous seizures during night recording. **B:** 4-DP-elicited seizure during day recording. Both **A** and **B** show site of seizure onset at electrode 5, immediately over alumina focus.

jects. (Each test situation had an $N = 5$, except the saline control, which had an $N = 3$.) The epileptic preparation (under sterile conditions and halothane anesthesia) consisted of subpial injections of aluminum hydroxide (0.22 cc total) in the left precentral and postcentral gyrus, sensorimotor hand and face areas, as confirmed by physiological stimulation. EEG paroxysms and focal motor and secondarily generalized tonic-clonic seizures developed within 3 months. Seizure frequency was stable for 1 year prior to the conduct of this study. By means of the methods of Lockard (14), each monkey was implanted with a chronic EEG plug, a femoral catheter for drug delivery, a jugular catheter for blood sampling, and an intrathecal catheter (fourth ventricle) for CSF sampling of drug concentration, assayed by gas-liquid chromotography. The animals were housed in primate restraining chairs during the research period but were cage rested prior to and following the project.

Procedures. Seizures were monitored continuously for the duration of the study, as described by Lockard et al. (15), and standard EEG recordings were obtained prior to the administration of 4-DP and before, during, and after each control and experimental session. A session consisted of a 5-hr test day with 7 no-test days between sessions for each animal. After determining for each monkey the intravenous threshold dose of 4-DP that elicited a predictable series of seizures lasting 2 to 4 hr, a random sequence of two to four control and four to nine experimental sessions was scheduled individually for each animal.

The experimental sessions comprised two to three dose levels (low to medium) of diazepam (DZP), phenobarbital (PB), phenytoin (PHT), and carbamazepine (CBZ) and a single dose level (medium to high) of valproate (VPA), because infusion of a relatively high concentration of this drug involved little risk. If the initial dose of any of the first four drugs prevented 4-DP-initiated seizures for the duration of treatment, then no subsequent higher dose of that drug was administered. However, if seizures were manifested at the low dose, a higher dose (up to three dose steps) of the treatment drug was tested in a later session.

Each 5-hr session comprised a continuous EEG recording starting 1 hr (0830 hr) prior to the 4-DP bolus (0930 hr) and ending 1 hr after (1330 hr) a vitamin B_6 injection (1230 hr), which terminated the session. (Occasionally B_6 had to be administered earlier if the monkey was too fatigued by the seizures.) After the 4-DP bolus and immediately following the first seizure, one of five treatments was administered intravenously, first in a loading dose taking 10 to 20 min to infuse (< 1 min for VPA) and then at a constant-rate infusion for 50 to 60 min for a total treatment time of 70 min (60 min for VPA). Eight blood samples and up to four CSF samples were taken during each session, starting immediately after the 4-DP bolus.

Dosing regimen. The solubilizing agents for DZP, PB, PHT, and CBZ were 40% propylene glycol (PG) and 10% ethanol (ETOH); saline was the vehicle for VPA, because it is water-soluble. Following the first 4-DP-initiated seizure, each animal received for 60 to 70 min one of the following: saline alone; PG + ETOH alone; DZP, PB, PHT, or CBZ in PG + ETOH; VPA in saline. The total volumes of treatment solution were different among animals (depending on animal weight). The volume of solution administered ranged from 21 to 32 ml for saline alone, 3 to 32 ml for PG + ETOH, either alone or with drug, and 5 to 9 ml for VPA in saline. For the saline-alone treatment, a volume similar to that of PG + ETOH was given, rather than the usually smaller volume for the VPA-in-saline treatment, because the larger volume served as a more stringent control.

The PHT concentration ranges for the loading infusion and the 1-hr infusion were 12 to 80 mg/10 min and 23 to 84 mg/hr, respectively. The particular rates for each monkey determined the dose steps, based on earlier single-dose kinetic studies in the same animal. Similarly, the concentration ranges of CBZ were 23 to 84 mg/10 to 20 min (the larger concentrations were infused over a longer period) and 23 to 52 mg/hr; for VPA, 125 to 240 mg/< 1 min (VPA was given initially as a bolus and was not infused) and 125 to 200 mg/hr; for DZP, 4 to 7 mg/10 min and 0.5 to 0.9 mg/hr; for PB, 10 to 21 mg/min and 21 to 41 mg/hr.

RESULTS

Drug concentrations. Although plasma drug concentrations do not adequately reflect the amount of drug at the receptor site during the drug distribution phase, the low to medium dose range for the 1-hr treatment period produced mean plasma drug concentrations of 134 to 189 ng/ml for DZP, 152 to 238 ng/ml for its metabolite nordiazepam (nDZP), 4 to 7 µg/ml for PB, 2 to 11 µg/ml for PHT, 3 to 7 µg/ml for CBZ, and 70 to 104 µg/ml for VPA; peak concentrations of each drug were

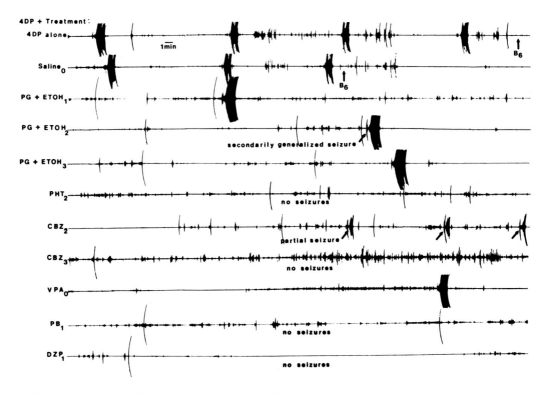

FIG. 4. Treatment of 4-DP serial seizures in monkey 195. Treatment followed an initial seizure (not shown) and usually continued for 60 min (the length of each polygraph line shown). In two instances the antagonist vitamin B_6 was given early (terminating the treatment period) because of animal fatigue from seizures. Subscripts 0, 1, 2, and 3 indicate increasing dose level and/or the volume of the vehicle used. PHT, CBZ, PB, and DZP were administered in a vehicle of PG + ETOH, comparable to the volume of PG + ETOH when given alone as a control solution. VPA was administered in saline at one-third the volume of saline when the latter was given alone as a control solution.

considerably higher. The convulsant 4-DP had a mean plasma drug concentration range during the treatment period of 6 to 43 μg/ml, but much higher immediately after its injection (113–256 μg/ml), some 7 to 30 min earlier. The CSF drug concentration ranges during treatment were 0.8 to 28 μg/ml for 4-DP, 2 to 20 ng/ml for DZP, 10 to 23 ng/ml for nDZP, 10 to 34 μg/ml for VPA, and 1 to 3 μg/ml for CBZ, PB, and PHT (there were too few CSF values to report means).

Seizure data. As shown in Figs. 4 and 5 (for 2 of 8 monkeys), CBZ compared favorably to DZP, PB, and PHT in reducing (low dose level) or eliminating (higher dose level) 4-DP seizures. The solvent PG + ETOH was itself efficacious at the larger volume of administration (Fig. 5, line 4), but it made seizures more severe (Fig. 5, line 3) at the smaller volume. Therefore, CBZ, DZP, PB, and PHT at their low dose levels were even more ef-

fective than indicated, because they compensated for the detrimental influence of PG + ETOH at that volume of administration. Saline alone was not effective against seizures, and VPA delayed seizures but did not prevent their occurrence in the treatment period.

The increases in mean interseizure interval for the five test drugs and the two vehicles as compared with 4-DP alone are shown in Table 1 for the highest treatment dose used, or greatest volume of vehicle in the case of control sessions. The mean latency for the second seizure (with 120 min taken as the upper limit) between the 4-DP and either CBZ, VPA, PHT, PB, DZP, or solvent (PG + ETOH given alone) sessions was significant ($p < 0.05$–0.001), but not that between either PG + ETOH and saline or saline and 4-DP alone ($p > 0.05$). There were also consistent differences between VPA and either CBZ, PHT, PB, or DZP

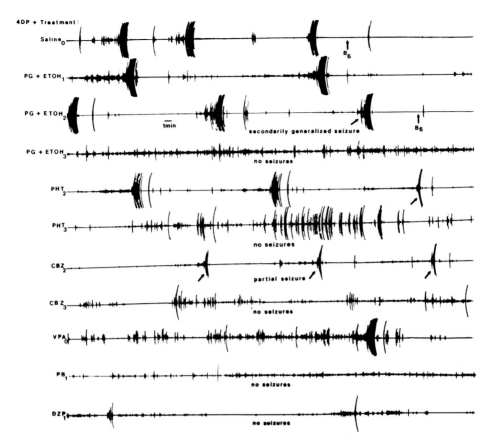

FIG. 5. Treatment of 4-DP serial seizures in monkey 568A. Treatment followed an initial seizure (not shown) and usually continued for 60 min (the length of each polygraph line shown). In two instances the antagonist vitamin B_6 was given early (terminating the treatment period) because of animal fatigue from seizures. Subscripts 0, 1, 2, and 3 indicate increasing dose level and/or the volume of the vehicle used. PHT, CBZ, PB, and DZP were administered in a vehicle of PG + ETOH, comparable to the volume of PG + ETOH when given alone as a control treatment. VPA was administered in saline at one-third the volume of saline when the latter was given alone as a control treatment.

(t = 3.60, 3.97, 2.19, and 7.34, respectively; p < 0.10–0.001), but not between any of the latter four drugs (p > 0.05).

DISCUSSION

The findings of this study, as summarized below, indicate that the 4-DP paradigm in our monkey model may be a viable method to test the potential efficacy of new anticonvulsants in the treatment of status epilepticus:

1. 4-DP-precipitated seizures were initiated at the epileptogenic focus, and in similarity to spontaneous status of partial epilepsy in monkeys, they had a largely invariant interseizure interval.

2. Anticonvulsants that are effective in clinical status epilepticus (DZP, PB, and PHT) were effective in this paradigm.

3. Newer anticonvulsants, such as CBZ, whose modes of action are similar to those of drugs currently used for status, were effective in this paradigm.

4. An anticonvulsant such as VPA, whose proposed mechanism of action dictates a different time course of effect, was, as expected, less efficacious than those with a more immediate action.

Starting with the last point, a recent study of seizure protection and GABA levels in mice (5) has indicated that VPA appears to affect nerve-terminal GABA only after other compartments of

Table 1. *Seizure latency during treatment compared to 4-DP alone[a]*

Treatment	Mean difference in interseizure interval (min)	SD	t	p
Saline	5.3	3.4	1.58	ns
Solvent	38.5	12.9	2.98	<0.05
Phenytoin	52.6	18.9	2.78	<0.05
Carbamazepine	61.6	12.2	5.07	<0.01
Valproate	23.8	5.9	4.04	<0.01
Phenobarbital	60.2	18.4	3.27	<0.05
Diazepam	84.2	10.9	7.72	<0.001

[a]Latency = mean time between first seizure and second seizure (with a maximum upper limit of 120 min); SD = standard deviation; t = Student's test for dependent mean differences; p = probability that the mean difference could have occurred by chance alone; ns = not statistically significant.

GABA have been elevated severalfold. Moreover, the time involved to accomplish this elevation is a matter of many hours. Therefore, it seems reasonable to assume that VPA may not be efficacious in a precipitous disease state such as spontaneous status epilepticus. Its effects on 4-DP status were consistent with this notion. The fact that VPA initially delayed the onset of seizures suggests that it may have an initial immediate effect of its own that is short-lived. We (16) have suggested this possibility on the basis of data gathered in the monkey model during chronic administration of VPA.

The finding that DZP (currently the drug of choice in clinical status) and PHT (an increasingly used drug for status in patients) were effective in 4-DP status lends support to the validity of this paradigm. Testing PHT also provided the most appropriate comparative data (in terms of assumed mechanism of action) for the effects of CBZ in experimental status. No parenteral formulation of CBZ is commercially available at present, but the results of this study predict its efficacy in clinical status. It is noteworthy that both PHT and CBZ at low dose levels did reduce the spread of secondarily generalized 4-DP seizures to partial seizures, as would be anticipated from their similar effects on posttetanic potentiation (9,24). Even at less than optimal plasma drug concentrations, these drugs behaved in terms of experimental status in a manner consistent with what is known clinically and from other animal models.

The fact that the solvent PG + ETOH was also active in this paradigm does not detract from its application but rather lends indirect support for its utility. We (17) have previously found polyethelene glycol 400 (PEG), another well-known solvent, to be both toxic and efficacious with respect to spontaneous seizures in the alumina-gel monkey model.

Whereas Meldrum and Horton (23) had shown that 4-DP seizures in *Papio papio* baboons and normal rhesus monkeys commenced over the occipital-parietal cortex, the seizure onset in our monkey model was specific to its epileptogenic focus (left motor strip) and was secondarily generalized to other cortical areas. The electroencephalographic similarities between spontaneous and 4-DP-elicited seizures in this model and the results obtained, particularly for CBZ, suggest that this paradigm would be useful in facilitating the therapeutic arsenal against status epilepticus.

ACKNOWLEDGMENTS

The authors wish to express their appreciation to William C. Congdon, Jr. (research associate) and Larry L. DuCharme (research technologist supervisor), to research technologists Barbara C. Kirkevold, Colleen Timmis, and Leonard D. Salonen, and to laboratory technician James C. Congdon, without whom this study could not have been accomplished.

This research was supported by NIH research contract NO1-NS-1–2282 and research grant NS-04053 awarded by the National Institute of Neurological and Communicative Disorders and Stroke, Department of Health, Education, and Welfare, U.S. Public Health Service.

REFERENCES

1. Abe, M. (1978): Relationship between γ-aminobutyric acid metabolism and antivitamin B_6-induced convulsions. *J. Nutr. Sci. Vitaminol. (Tokyo)*, 24:419–427.
2. Baxter, C. F., and Roberts, E. (1960): Demonstration of thiosemicarbazide-induced convulsions in rats with elevated brain levels of γ-aminobutyric acid. *Proc. Soc. Exp. Biol. Med.*, 104:426–427.
3. Dreyer, R. (1969): Die Behandlung des Status epilepticus. *Med. Welt*, 20:1211–1217.
4. Froscher, W. (1979): *Treatment of Status Epilepticus*. University Park Press, Baltimore.
5. Gale, K., and Iadarola, M. J. (1980): Seizure protection and increased nerve-terminal GABA: Delayed effects of GABA transaminase inhibition. *Science*, 208:288–291.

6. Gastaut, H. (1973): *Dictionary of Epilepsy, Part 1: Definition.* World Health Organization, Geneva.
7. Gastaut, H., Roger, L., and Lob, H. (1967): *Les états de mal epileptiques.* Masson, Paris.
8. Heintel, H. (1972): *Der Status epilepticus, Seine Atiologie, Klinik und Letalitat.* Fischer, Stuttgart.
9. Hernandez-Peon, R. (1964): Anticonvulsive action of G 32883. In: *Proceedings of the 3rd Collegium Internationale Neuro-Psychopharmacologicum Congress* (Munich, 1962), *Vol. 3*, edited by P. B. Bradley, F. Flugel, and P.H. Hoch, pp. 303–311. Elsevier, Amsterdam.
10. Koch, K. M., Ludwick, B. T., and Levy, R. H. (1981): Phenytoin–valproic acid interaction in rhesus monkey. *Epilepsia*, 22:19–25.
11. Kuriyama, K., Roberts, E., and Rubenstein, M. K. (1966): Elevation of γ-aminobutyric acid and susceptibility to convulsive seizures in mice: A quantitative re-evaluation. *Biochem. Pharmacol.*, 15:221–236.
12. Levy, R. H. (1980): CSF and plasma pharmacokinetics: Relationship to mechanisms of action as exemplified by valproic acid in monkey. In: *Epilepsy: A Window to Brain Mechanisms*, edited by J. S. Lockard and A. A. Ward, Jr., pp. 191–200. Raven Press, New York.
13. Levy, R. H., Lockard, J. S., and Ludwick, B. T. (1980): Plasma protein binding and CSF concentration of valproic acid in monkey. In: *Proceedings of Academy of Pharmaceutical Sciences Meeting* (Washington, D.C., April 19–24, 1980).
14. Lockard, J. S. (1980): A primate model of clinical epilepsy: Mechanisms of action through quantification of therapeutic effects. In: *Epilepsy: A Window to Brain Mechanisms*, edited by J. S. Lockard and A. A. Ward, Jr., pp. 11–49. Raven Press, New York.
15. Lockard, J. S., Congdon, W. C., DuCharme, L. L., and Finch, C. A. (1980): Slow-speed EEG for chronic monitoring of clinical seizures in monkey model. *Epilepsia*, 21:325–334.
16. Lockard, J. S., and Levy, R. H. (1976): Valproic acid: Reversibly acting drug? *Epilepsia*, 17:477–479.
17. Lockard, J. S., and Levy, R. H. (1979): Polyethylene glycol 400: Solvent and anticonvulsant? *Life Sci.*, 23:2499–2502.
18. Lockard, J. S., Levy, R. H., Congdon, W. C., DuCharme, L. L., and Patel, I. H. (1977): Efficacy testing of valproic acid compared to ethosuximide in monkey model: II. Seizure, EEG and diurnal variation. *Epilepsia*, 18:191–204.
19. Lockard, J. S., Levy, R. H., Uhlir, V., and Farquhar, J. A. (1976): Interactions of phenytoin and phenobarbital in terms of order and temporal spacing of administration in monkeys. *Epilepsia*, 17:481–485.
20. Lockard, J. S., Levy, R. H., Uhlir, V., and Farquhar, J. A. (1974): Pharmacokinetic evaluation of anticonvulsants prior to efficacy testing exemplified by carbamazepine in monkey model. *Epilepsia*, 15:351–359.
21. Matthes, A. (1975): *Epilepsie. Diagnostik und Therapie für Klinik und Praxis*, ed. 3. Thieme, Stuttgart.
22. Maynert, E. W., and Kaji, H. K. (1962): On the relationship of brain GABA to convulsions. *J. Pharmacol. Exp. Ther.*, 137:114–121.
23. Meldrum, B. S., and Horton, R. W. (1971): Convulsive effects of 4-deoxypyridoxine and of bicuculline in photosensitive baboons *(Papio papio)* and in rhesus monkeys *(Macaca mulatta). Brain Res.*, 35:419–436.
24. Toman, J. E. P. (1969): Further discussions on diphenylhydantoin. In: *Basic Mechanisms of the Epilepsies*, edited by H. H. Jasper, A. A. Ward, and A. Pope, pp. 682–688. Little, Brown, Boston.
25. Tower, D. B. (1976): GABA and seizures: Clinical correlates in man. In: *GABA in Nervous System Function*, edited by E. Roberts, T. N. Chase, and D. B. Tower, pp. 461–478. Raven Press, New York.
26. Wood, J. D., and Peesker, S. J. (1975): The anticonvulsant action of GABA-elevating agents: A re-evaluation. *J. Neurochem.*, 25:277–282.

Advances in Neurology, Vol. 34: Status Epilepticus, edited by A.V. Delgado-Escueta, C.G. Wasterlain, D.M. Treiman, and R.J. Porter. Raven Press, New York © 1983.

43

Clinical Pharmacokinetics of Drugs Used in the Treatment of Status Epilepticus

E. van der Kleijn, A. M. Baars, T. B. Vree, and A. van der Dries

Prolonged and continuous epileptic seizures and tonic-clonic status epilepticus require immediate management. In order to minimize bodily injuries and prevent brain damage, the airway and vital functions must be maintained and seizures controlled as rapidly as possible. For rational management of status epilepticus, the causes and immediate triggers of seizures must be determined. Next to structural brain lesions, withdrawal of antiepileptic treatment and consequent absence of effective serum concentrations of antiepileptic drugs is second in importance as a cause of status epilepticus. Rarely, the presence of toxic serum concentrations of phenytoin can precipitate status epilepticus. Other drugs such as lidocaine may also produce status when given in high dosages, and discontinuation of long-term use of certain hypnotics (e.g., glutethimide, barbiturates, and ataractics like meprobamate) may also be responsible.

One single but most important requirement that determines the choice of drug is that it acts rapidly. The intravenous route of administration usually is indicated. At home, in a family situation or in an environment of medically inexperienced attendants, intravenous injection of drugs may not be practical, and rectal administration may be the indicated route. The preferred route, however, is either intravenous bolus injection or continuous intravenous infusion or both. These routes of administration give the best predictable outcome, at least in terms of amount of drug in the body and the plasma concentration at any one time. Intramuscular injection of antiepileptic drugs is an uncertain route, because poorly soluble substances deposit at the site of injection and only slowly diffuse into the general circulation. In this chapter, only intravenous and rectal administration of the major agents used to stop status epilepticus will be discussed.

ANALYTICAL METHODS FOR DETERMINATION OF ANTIEPILEPTIC DRUGS IN BODY FLUIDS

After being administered to a patient, drugs are absorbed, distributed, metabolized, and excreted. The rates at which these processes occur are specific for each drug, although many interindividual and intraindividual variations have been identified. Whereas small tissue quantities of antiepileptic drugs are already biologically effective and stop seizures, their distribution in the course of time within a complex biological system will also lead to small concentrations in body fluids. These body fluids are available for sampling, such as blood plasma or serum, urine, saliva, tears, and wound exudates. The latter three body fluids rarely are reliable sample materials, but they contain the drugs and their metabolites at concentrations that correspond to the free (unbound to plasma proteins) concentration.

When 50 mg of phenytoin is given to a patient of 50 kg at a regimen of three times per day, a concentration of 7 mg/liter or 0.7 μg (0.7×10^{-6} g) per 100 μl (the mean volume for analysis) can be expected. This requires accurate analytical separation techniques from a bulk of water, protein, electrolytes, and organic biogenous substances (12).

Two major methods are currently in use for the determination of antiepileptic drugs in body fluids (Table 1).

1. In the heterogeneous methods, substances are extracted from the aqueous medium by an immiscible organic solvent from which the drug is separated after enrichment by chromatographic methods such as gas-liquid chromatography (GC) and high-pressure liquid chromatography (HPLC). The separated substances are detected by hydrogen flame ionization (FID), by alkali hydrogen flame (AFID), by electron capture (EC) or mass spectrometry (MS) in case of GC, and by spectrophotometry (Sp) or spectrofluorophotometry (Sfp) in case of HPLC.

2. The homogeneous methods are based on drug-specific antibody complexes in which the detection is realized either by a radiolabeled tracer in the radioimmunoassay (RIA) or by an enzyme, as in the enzyme-multiplied immunoassay technique (EMIT).

PHARMACOKINETIC LOGIC

In pharmacokinetics, one uses the understanding that amounts of drugs are homogeneously distributed in compartments of particular drug-specific volumes. The resulting concentrations are, subject to continuous changes as a result of mass input and output. The dominant driving forces are hemodynamics, secretion, and enzyme-substrate reactions. The analogies used are strongly simplified and have no direct relationship to the anatomy and physiology of living individuals. The models bear most resemblance to communicating vessels, where the flow rates are controlled by taps or connected electric condensers in which the charges and currents are controlled by potentiometers. Homogeneous distribution does not necessarily imply equal concentrations in all parts of the body. It does mean that absorption and distribution of the drug have no quantitative influence on the elimination process. A compartment is a volume of complete abstract entity. Several more or less complex models of parallel and serially connected compartments have been proposed and mathematically resolved

TABLE 1. *Analytical assay methods for determination of some antiepileptic drugs*

Drug	Assay method
Amobarbital	GC-(A)-FID
Carbamazepine	EMIT, HPLC-Sp
Clonazepam	GC-ECD, HPLC-Sp, GC-MS, RIA
Clorazepate	HPLC-Sp
Diazepam	GC-ECD, HPLC-Sp
Desmethyldiazepam	GC-ECD, HPLC-Sp
Lorazepam	GC-ECD, HPLC-Sp
Midazolam	HPLC-Sp
Pentothiobarbital	HPLC-Sp
Phenytoin	GC-(A)-FID, HPLC-Sp, RIA, EMIT
Phenobarbital	GC-(A)-FID, HPLC-Sp, EMIT
Valproate	GC-FID, EMIT

to fit experimentally or clinically acquired data. In the treatment of status epilepticus, three major methods of drug administration are practiced: (a) intravenous bolus injection; (b) rectal administration by suppository or microclysma; (c) intravenous infusion. The models most suitable to describe these methods of administration can be summarized as follows:

Intravenous Bolus Injection

One-compartment open model. When the curves of plasma concentrations follow a straight line on log-linear graph paper, distribution and elimination correspond to a one-compartment open model (Fig. 1A). In this model, the drug can be considered to be homogeneously distributed in a constant volume from which it is eliminated in an exponential manner, or, in mathematical terms, according to a first-order equation (Fig. 2). Although this model generally denies the existence of a much faster distribution phase, it predicts the time course of drug effects in cases where the minimum effective concentration is known.

Two-compartment open model. The mathematical equation that describes the curves of drug concentrations of a two-compartment open model (Fig. 1B) and fits most of the biphasic plasma concentration time curves of intravenously administered antiepileptic drugs, with the exception of phenytoin, has been extensively described in the literature (13,30):

$$C_1(t) = Ae^{-\alpha t} + Be^{-\beta t} \qquad (1)$$

$$Q_2(t) = Pe^{-\beta t} - Pe^{-\alpha t} \qquad (2)$$

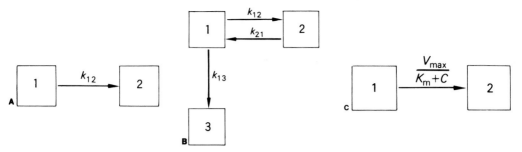

FIG. 1. Schematic descriptions of the one-compartment open model (**A**), the two-compartment open model (**B**), and the one-compartment model with enzyme capacity-limited elimination (**C**).

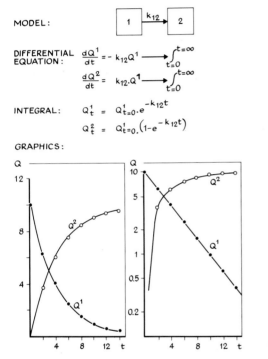

FIG. 2. Schematic and mathematical description of the one-compartment open model.

in which A, B, and P are hybrid factors with dimensions of concentration $(A \cdot B)$ or amount (P) describing the level of the curves, and α and β are hybrid reciprocal time constants composed of k_{12}, k_{21}, and k_{13} describing the directions of the curve in time. Depending on the values of these parameters, there may be rapid or slow distribution and/or elimination and small or large concentrations or quantities of the drug in the various compartments. For many antiepileptic drugs, with the exception of valproate, the amount of drug in compartment 2, often corresponding to the extravascular tissues

and organs, is much larger than that in compartment 1. It is likely that relatively high concentrations of antiepileptic drugs are found in the central nervous system (Fig. 3). The α and β factors are independent of dose and within certain limits are characteristic for every drug.

One-compartment model with enzyme capacity-limited elimination. When the capacity of the enzyme system(s) responsible for elimination of the drug is saturated, the result of the course of the plasma concentration is that a constant amount of drug is eliminated per time unit. This model (Fig. 1C) is valid for the period that the enzyme(s) is saturated. The course of the concentration is essentially different from that of the one-compartment open model, in which a constant fraction of

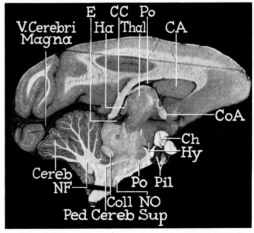

FIG. 3. Regional distribution of 2-^{14}C-desmethyldiazepam in the brain of a squirrel monkey when approximately 75% of the steady state has been reached. White areas correspond to the presence of radiolabeled drug. Note the relatively high concentration in the white matter, as compared with gray matter and blood.

the amount present in the body is eliminated. The equations describing the course of the concentration in such a system (24) read

$$\ln C = \ln A + \frac{A - C}{K_M} - k \cdot t \qquad (3)$$

in which k is the reciprocal time constant of the terminal part of the curve, A is the intercept of the curve with the ordinate, and K_M is the apparent Michaelis-Menten constant

$$\ln C = \ln A^* - kt \qquad (4)$$

in which A^* is the intercept of the extrapolated terminal (exponential) phase of the concentration curve with the ordinate: in practice when $C < 0.1K_M$. K_M can be calculated by the difference between intercept A^* of the regression line with the ordinate and a slope described by k and the real intercept of the curve, A.

$$K_M = \frac{\ln A^* - \ln A}{A} \qquad (5)$$

Another method to calculate K_M graphically is given by

$$K_M = \frac{A}{k \cdot \Delta t} \qquad (6)$$

in which Δt is the shift of the slope described by k and A^* parallel to a line described by k and A (Fig. 4). V_{max}, the maximum rate of metabolism, can be calculated as

$$V_{max} = k \cdot V \cdot K_M =$$
$$Cl \cdot K_M = \frac{Dose}{A^*} \cdot k \cdot K_M \qquad (7)$$

in which Cl is the clearance of the drug in the exponential phase ($C < 0.1K_M$), V is the apparent distribution volume, and Dose is the amount present at $t = 0$ or the amount given.

Open Two-Compartment Model with Exponential Absorption

This model has many similarities to the one-compartment open model (Fig. 1A). It has didactic value in that it demonstrates the possible courses of the drug in various body regions. For example, at a point where 40% of the drug still has to be absorbed from the gastrointestinal tract, the maximum concentration in the central compartment (e.g., the plasma) has already been reached. The maximum in the peripheral compartment is reached only when absorption is practically complete (Fig. 5). After repetitive drug administration, the drug keeps accumulating in the peripheral compartment, whereas accumulation in the central compartment is relatively small and can easily be overlooked and underestimated. The model also shows that a steady residue remains at the absorption site (Fig. 6). In practice, one has to watch variations in rate and extent of absorption, even in one individual, because, for example, the presence of feces, defecation, and antiperistaltic motility can cause differences.

Chain Model of Consecutive Compartments

In this model (Fig. 7), when the drug is continuously infused at a constant amount per unit time and biotransformation (e.g., by metabolism) to a pharmacologically active metabolite takes place, the metabolite having its own elimination rate, the set of equations reads

$$C_1(t) = \frac{k_0}{V_1 \cdot k_{12}} (1 - e^{-k_{12}t}) \qquad (8)$$

$$C_2(t) = \frac{k_0}{V_2 \cdot k_{23}} \cdot \frac{1 + (k_{23}e^{-k_{12}t} - k_{12}e^{-k_{23}t})}{k_{12} - k_{23}} \qquad (9)$$

When $t = \infty$, then equations 8 and 9 can be simplified to

$$C_1(t) = \frac{k_0}{k_{12} \cdot V_1} = \frac{k_0}{Cl_1} \qquad (10)$$

$$C_2(t) = \frac{k_0}{k_{23} \cdot V_2} = \frac{k_0}{Cl_2} \qquad (11)$$

in which Cl is the total body clearance (Fig. 8). This model can also be applied for describing chronic intermittent medication. When drugs show a small k_{12} (large $t_{1/2}$) and are given at a relative high frequency per day (small dosage interval, Δt), then

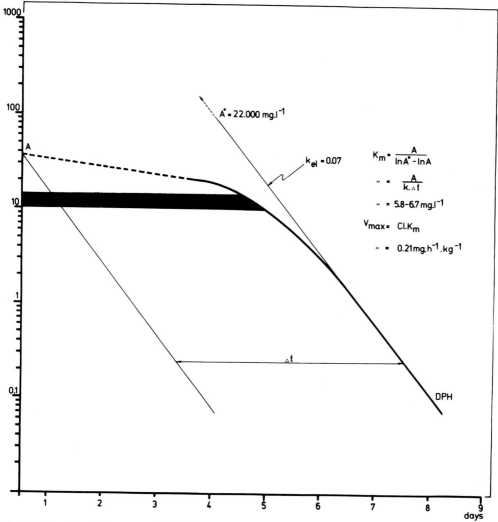

FIG. 4. Calculation of the apparent Michaelis-Menten parameters for phenytoin. Data come from a patient in status epilepticus (see Fig. 14).

$$k_0 = \frac{\text{Dose}}{\Delta t} \tag{12}$$

Usually one wants to limit the oscillation of the plasma concentration to a maximum of 20%. If so, and when practically feasible, one can apply the following rule of thumb for calculation of the dosage interval (27):

$$\Delta t \, (20\%) = \frac{1}{3} \cdot t_{1/2} \tag{13}$$

DOSAGE CALCULATION

When the minimum effective concentration of a drug needed to control the symptoms of status epilepticus is known approximately, one can roughly predict the required dosage or the dosing rate for the models described earlier. In the case of the one-compartment open model (Fig. 1A), dose and total body clearance determine the time course of the drug that will produce the desired therapeutic concentration. Although often this concentration is hardly exactly defined, one can retrospectively determine the minimum concentration required to produce a therapeutic effect (Table 2). To calculate the dose of the bolus injection required to produce effective brain tissue concentrations and a corresponding plasma concentration, one can use the following equation:

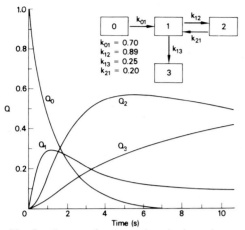

Fig. 5. Courses of concentrations in the various compartments following a single oral, rectal, or intramuscular dose, according to the open two-compartment model with exponential absorption.

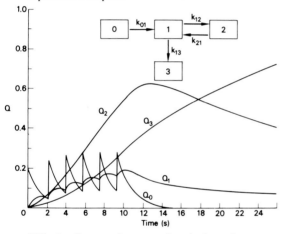

FIG. 6. Courses of concentrations in the various compartments, as in Fig. 5, but after repetitive doses in smaller amounts.

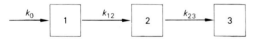

FIG. 7. Schematic description of the chain model of consecutive compartments.

$$D = C \cdot V \qquad (14)$$

in which C is the concentration that produces the effect at the highest probability. Often one accepts the risk of even severe adverse reactions in order to stop status epilepticus. V (liters) is the apparent distribution volume that can often be related to body weight (W). In this case one handles the

relative apparent distribution volume V' (liters/kilogram) (Table 2):

$$\text{Dose} = C \cdot V' \cdot W \qquad (15)$$

The time course of action (T), assuming well-defined and equal minimum effective concentrations for every indication, can be approached according to the equation

$$y = 1 + \frac{t_{1/2}}{0.7T} \cdot \ln x \qquad (16)$$

in which y is the extension factor for the time course of effectivity (T) at a certain initial dose and x is the factor by which this dose is multiplied (when $x = 2$, $\ln x = 0.7$; when $x = 3$, $\ln x = 1.1$; when $x = 4$, $\ln x = 1.4$). Thus, equation 16 reads

$$y_{D^1} = 2D = \frac{t_{1/2}}{T} + 1 = \frac{t_{1/2} + T}{T} \qquad (16a)$$

$$y_{D^1} = 3D =$$
$$\frac{1.586 \cdot t_{1/2}}{T} + 1 = \frac{1.586 \cdot t_{1/2} + T}{T} \qquad (16b)$$

$$y_{D^1} = 4D = \frac{2 \cdot t_{1/2}}{T} + 1 = \frac{2 \cdot t_{1/2} + T}{T} \qquad (16c)$$

The dosage calculation in a two-compartment model (Fig. 1B) is essentially the same, although the time course of activity is more complicated and depends to a large extent on the rate and volume parameters. Essentially, one can calculate the dose required from the apparent volume of distribution of the first or central compartment. Because of the biphasic distribution and elimination pattern, the time course of activity will be much more difficult to establish. Because the rate of distribution often is very high for the lipophilic drugs used in treatment of status epilepticus, one can practically rely on the one-compartment model (Fig. 1A) for the time course of activity. In other words, one can rely on the second phase of the elimination curve. Because a residue will remain in the body and will be eliminated more slowly, one will have to taper down the dose administered in the course of subsequent periods. Initially, one can administer a

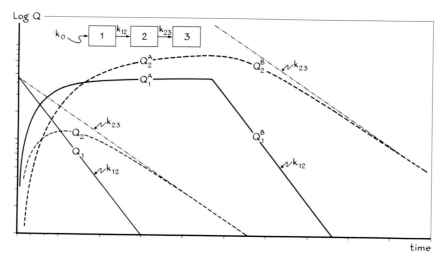

FIG. 8. Courses of a drug (Q_1) and its metabolite (Q_2) after a bolus injection and during *(A)* and following *(B)* intravenous infusion, according to the chain model of single consecutive compartments.

TABLE 2. *Pharmacokinetic parameters of some antiepileptic drugs*

Drug substance	k_{el} (per hr)	$t_{1/2}$ (hr)	V_d' (liter/kg)	Cl' (ml/hr/kg)	C_{mean} (mg/liter)	References
Amobarbital		25			10–20	4,8
Carbamazepine	0.07–0.017	10–40	1.3	91–23	7	27
Clonazepam	0.035–0.030	20–25	3.0	100	0.020–0.060	10
Clorazepate	—	—	—	—	—	
Desmethyldiazepam	0.007–0.015	40–100	1.13	20	0.5–4.5	2,18
Diazepam	0.023	30	1.3	30	0.4	7
Lorazepam	0.0462	15	1.3	60	0.050–0.100	5
Midazolam	0.92	0.75	0.8	740	0.4	29
Phenobarbital	0.0007	100	0.6	4.2	25	
Phenytoin	0.07	10	0.63	45	20	27
Valproate						
epilepticus	0.08	9	0.175	14	50–100	14–16,21
non epilepticus	0.055	12.5	0.147	8		
alone				11	50–100	21
+ comedication				16	50–100	21

dose that has been calculated according to the following equation:

$$D = C \cdot V' \qquad (17)$$

Preferably, this method should be combined with a simultaneous constant infusion (chain model, Fig. 7) in which the bolus injection serves as priming dose and the infusion as a maintenance regimen until the patient is well recovered and oral drug treatment can be started or continued.

In the case of the one-compartment model with enzyme capacity-limited elimination (Fig. 1C),

dosage calculation for a priming dose of phenytoin is essentially similar to that for the one-compartment model (Fig. 1A). Because the enzyme capacity expressed by K_M and V_{max} of the individual is seldom known, one has to rely on an average value for the apparent distribution volume and cannot accurately predict the time course of activity. It must be realized that when diazepam is simultaneously given, the K_M and V_{max} values for phenytoin may be substantially lower than when the drug is given alone (20). Therefore, a much longer time course of activity and possible toxicity can be anticipated (Fig. 17).

In the case of the two-compartment model with exponential absorption (Fig. 5), exact calculation of the dose for rectal administration is of little relevance, because the amount of drug that enters the general circulation depends on many factors, such as the state of the rectum in relation to feces contents, defecation stimulus, and surfactant quality of the suppository or clysma. Because this method will be used only in extraordinary emergency cases, one can apply an average dose that can be repeated at 1-hr intervals when no emergency care is directly available. Depending on the nature of the status epilepticus, a physician will be alerted and will take measures involving either bolus injection or infusion or both.

The chain model (Fig. 7) allows calculation of the infusion rate when severe convulsions with a drug-resistant history have to be treated. Equation 8 can be rearranged to

$$\overset{\bullet}{k_0} = \frac{C_t \cdot V \cdot k}{(1 - e^{-k \cdot t})} \tag{18}$$

When t becomes very large, equation 17 can be simplified like equation 10 to

$$k_0 = C_t \cdot V \cdot k \tag{19}$$

and

$$k_0 = C_t \cdot Cl \tag{20}$$

or

$$k_0 = C_t \cdot Cl' \cdot W \tag{21}$$

The mean relative clearance values (Cl') are given in Table 2.

Equation 21 combined with equation 12 can be used in chronic intermittent oral treatment for drugs with a relatively long half-life in relation to dosage interval (Δt). And because clearance is dependent on many variable factors such as comedication (M), age (A), and enzyme capacity limitation (N), one needs to correct the dose accordingly (27):

$$D = C \cdot Cl'(M \cdot A \cdot N) \cdot W \cdot \Delta t \tag{22}$$

MINIMUM AND MEAN EFFECTIVE CONCENTRATIONS

In order to calculate the dosage, it is essential to know what concentration will have the highest probability for successful interruption of seizures.

The plasma concentration will show high values following intravenous bolus injection. These high values will not necessarily reflect the effective concentration in the target organ. These high values are more associated with the concentration in the peripheral compartment or compartment 2 in the two-compartment model (Fig. 1B). Depending on the rate constant between the compartments, the concentration of the effective substance will sooner or later reach a maximum. In general, the higher the lipophilicity of the compound, the more rapidly the drug will reach the brain (25). This may explain why thiopental, amobarbital, and diazepam are frequently used in the acute treatment of status epilepticus, whereas these compounds either are not effective or are erratically effective in chronic oral intermittent treatment. In the clinical control of status epilepticus, when conservative measures are available, one will only secondarily be concerned about the toxic side effects. The benzodiazepines show negligible untoward effects on respiration and circulation. Their long-lasting muscle-relaxing effect may be initially an advantage and only secondarily a disadvantage for quickly remobilizing the patient. As will be explained later, care should be taken when diazepam and phenytoin are given simultaneously (20).

DRUGS OF FIRST CHOICE FOR TONIC-CLONIC STATUS EPILEPTICUS

Benzodiazepines

Intravenously administered diazepam is currently the most frequently used drug in treating tonic-clonic status epilepticus. None of the benzodiazepines is effective for chronic control of status epilepticus. However, their central effects (e.g., rapid suppression of seizures, sedation, muscle relaxation, and anxiolysis) make them the first choice for acute treatment of tonic-clonic status epilepticus. All benzodiazepines show similar spectra of activity. Small quantitative differences in intensity and time course of activity are observed among the various members of the group in respect to anxiolysis, muscle relaxation, anticonvulsant action, hypnosis, and anesthesia. The compounds are very lipophilic, which makes them penetrate the brain rapidly after intravenous injection. They are rapidly metabolized, mostly by liver microsomal mixed-function oxidases. They are poorly soluble in water, which means that the compounds have

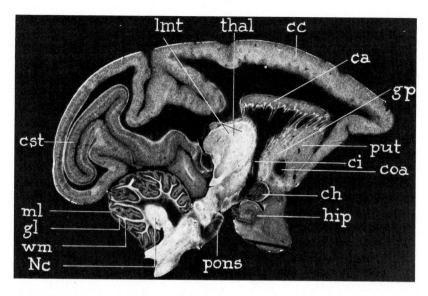

FIG. 9. Regional distribution of 2-¹⁴C-oxazepam in the brain of a squirrel monkey after 1 hr of intravenous infusion. Compared with Fig. 3, distribution is still incomplete. Highest concentrations are found in the gray matter structures and the thin myelin fibers.

to be dissolved in a water-miscible organic solvent such as propylene glycol. The exception to this rule is clorazepate, in which at the C-3 position a carboxyl group has been substituted, allowing formation of a salt that is easily water-soluble.

Two phases of the plasma concentration time profile can be distinguished after rapid intravenous bolus injection: a rapid distribution phase and a slower elimination phase. No large differences can be distinguished in this pattern between different compounds or between individual patients. The rates of elimination, however, can differ widely. Midazolam has the shortest biological half-life ($t_{1/2}$ = 1–2 hr), and desmethyldiazepam has the longest (Table 2). It seems rational to use a drug with a short half-life when rapid cessation of tonic-clonic status is desired. When seizures continue, infusion with a compound of longer half-life is indicated. Although benzodiazepines penetrate the blood-brain barrier rapidly, distribution equilibrium among all regions takes a longer period of time (Figs. 3 and 9).

Lipophilicity does not prevent the drugs from penetrating the placental barrier. Although the rate of penetration may be relatively low, equal concentrations in mother and child are found after subchronic administration of diazepam (28) (Fig. 10).

The benzodiazepines discussed in this chapter (Fig. 11) are metabolized by the following means:

1. N-oxidation and demethylation	diazepam	at position 1
2. Hydroxylation	diazepam	at position 3
	desmethyldiazepam	at position 3
	clonazepam	at position 3
	midazolam	at position 1,4
3. Decarboxylation	clorazepate	at position 3
4. Nitroreduction	clonazepam	at position 7
5. Glucuronidation	lorazepam	at position 3
	midazolam	at position 1,4
	hydroxy metabolites of step 2	

The first three metabolic routes lead to compounds that are pharmacologically active and protect against convulsions. The last two lead to compounds that are ineffective against seizures and are excreted via the kidneys.

Clonazepam

The pharmacokinetic rationale for dosage calculation is still little understood. The empirical dosage recommendation for clonazepam calls for an initial dose of 1 mg in adults with an additional 0.5 or 1 mg every 1 to 2 min until seizures stop or respiration or cardiovascular functions become depressed (3). Effective concentrations can differ

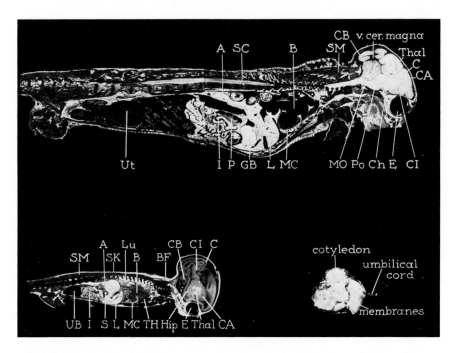

FIG. 10. Whole body distribution of 2-^{14}C-diazepam in a pregnant squirrel monkey 2 hr after intravenous injection. High concentrations are seen in the brain of the mother, whereas the concentration in the fetus is lower.

greatly, ranging from 0.020 to 0.080 mg/liter. Frequent, successive bolus injections will bring the clonazepam concentration rapidly above this level. After discontinuation of administration, the concentration declines to a much lower level, with a terminal biological half-life of 20 to 25 hr (Fig. 12). When 4 to 5 mg of clonazepam is administered within 10 min, one can initially expect a plasma concentration of over 0.100 mg/liter. Because the terminal phase has a longer half-life, residual effects can be long-lasting. Muscle relaxation is most notable, and patients can remain atactic for several days. Abundant production of saliva often prohibits extended use of the compound.

If the patient has received phenobarbital for a long period prior to the episode of status, the half-life of clonazepam is suggested by animal experiments to be much shorter, and more drug is required to sustain the anticonvulsant effect (Fig. 20). In dogs, it appeared that the half-life of clonazepam decreased during phenobarbital treatment; the phenomenon appeared to be dose-dependent at low doses, but the effect on half-life of clonazepam reached a maximum at high doses. Enzyme induction does not influence the initial distribution processes; so acute seizures are controlled by the same amount of drug in experimental status epilepticus. This phenomenon has not yet been confirmed in humans.

Clorazepate

Clorazepate is rapidly decarboxylated to desmethyldiazepam, especially in an acid medium; hence, there has been very little concern about the fate and action of the parent compound. Moreover, the concentration of the compound is difficult to determine. Clorazepate is dissociated at the physiological pH of the body, and rapid urinary excretion can be anticipated. The substance is water-soluble and can be given as an intravenous infusion. Figure 13 shows the course of desmethyldiazepam concentration, together with that of its metabolite oxazepam during and following 17 days of intravenous infusion. The drug was infused into a patient who had tetanus. Initially, diazepam was given, but because of the expected large requirement and the avoidance of large amounts of propylene glycol, diazepam was replaced by clorazepate. The steady-state concentration was maintained at 4.5 mg/liter and was occasionally supported by concomitant administration of the neuromuscular blocking agent pancuronium. After

R1
O
N
R2
H
R3
N
H
R4

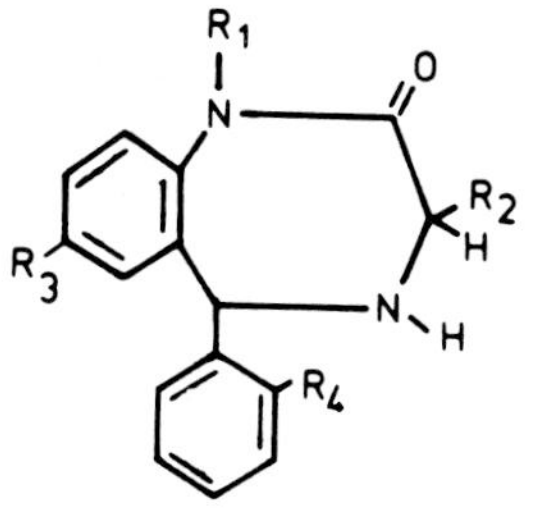

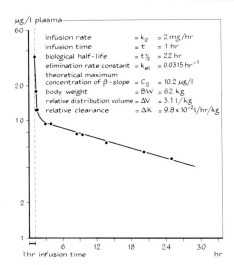

	R_1	R_2	R_3	R_4
Clonazepam			NO_2	H
Clorazepate	H	COOH	Cl	H
Desmethyldiazepam	H	H	Cl	H
Diazepam	CH_3	H	Cl	H
Lorazepam	H	OH	Cl	Cl

H3C
N
C
N
C
Cl
C
N
F

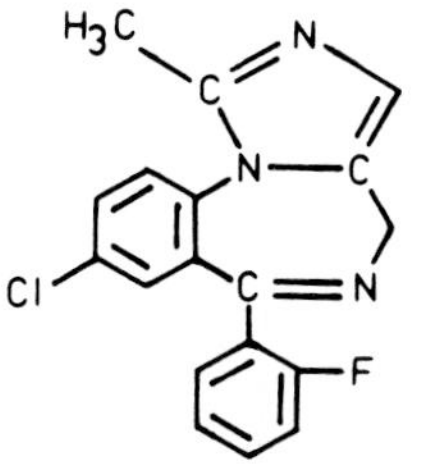

Midazolam

FIG. 11. Structural formulas of six benzodiazepines.

µg/l plasma
60
20
10
2
1
infusion rate = k0 = 2 mg/hr
infusion time = t = 1 hr
biological half-life = t½ = 22 hr
elimination rate constant = kel = 0.0315 hr⁻¹
theoretical maximum concentration of β-slope = C0 = 10.2 µg/l
body weight = BW = 62 kg
relative distribution volume = ΔV = 3.1 l/kg
relative clearance = ΔK = 9.8 x 10⁻² l/hr/kg
6
12
18
24
30
1 hr infusion time
hr

FIG. 12. Course of plasma clonazepam concentration after 1 hr of linear intravenous infusion of 2 mg of drug.

discontinuation of drug administration, the patient rapidly recovered and became fully conscious. At times when the desmethyldiazepam concentration was still high relative to the level it would have reached after normal dosages of diazepam, the patient requested a hypnotic or ataractic drug and reported a positive effect. Clorazepate has also been used to treat status epilepticus after phenytoin and thiopental injections have been unsuccessful in controlling seizures (Fig. 14). The clearance parameter appears stable.

Diazepam

Diazepam is the most commonly used anticonvulsant in all varieties of status epilepticus. High dosages are well tolerated (Fig. 15). Administration usually starts with 10 mg and is repeated every 2 to 5 min until the symptoms cease. In a severe case, this may require several hundred milligrams. As shown in Fig. 15, a preeclamptic patient received 1,300 mg during 3 days by infusion. Diazepam and desmethyldiazepam were further eliminated according to the normal pattern. After these high dosages, long-lasting residual and possibly effective concentrations can be observed for

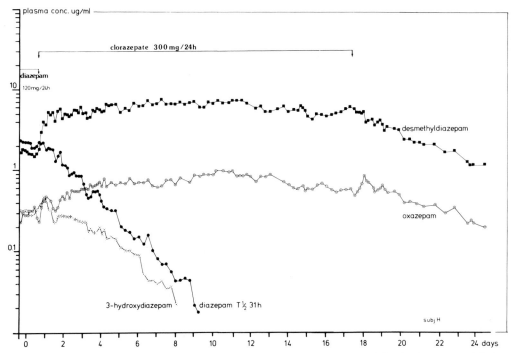

FIG. 13. Plasma concentrations of diazepam, desmethyldiazepam, and oxazepam following intravenous infusion of diazepam during 36 hr and subsequent infusion of clorazepate during 16.5 days in a patient with tetanus. Desmethyldiazepam was maintained at a steady-state concentration of 4 to 5 mg/liter throughout the treatment period. The oxazepam concentration, a compound with a much shorter intrinsic biological half-life, follows its precursor at a lower level. The half-life of desmethyldiazepam is 50 hr.

as long as 4 weeks. Rectal administration of diazepam has been successful in children suffering status epilepticus. Although the bioavailability accounts for about 50% (possibly because of incomplete bioavailability as a result of fecal loss), it appears that the mean maximum plasma concentration is rapidly reached within 20 min following administration. Doses up to 1 mg/kg lead to plasma concentrations of 270 to 320 mg/ml within 5 min and peak concentrations of 600 to 1,300 mg/kg after 10 to 60 min (11).

Lorazepam

Lorazepam has been reported to have efficacy similar to that of diazepam for treatment of status epilepticus (31). It may have advantages over diazepam because of its shorter biological half-life (mean $t_{1/2} = 15$ hr) and the absence of active metabolites. It has been reported that even high dosages of lorazepam did not cause side effects such as the respiratory depression, bradycardia, and sudden hypotension that have been reported for other benzodiazepines (9).

Midazolam

Midazolam has only recently been introduced as a hypnotic and possibly as an anesthetic agent. It is mentioned here because of its extremely short half-life, which may prove advantageous in the rapid interruption of seizures. It may allow more rapid reinstitution or continuation of oral medication. Intravenous infusion would rapidly lead to a steady state. When necessary, it can be combined with one or more bolus injections. After infusion is stopped, the drug is rapidly eliminated.

Phenytoin

Intravenous phenytoin, given simultaneously with intravenous diazepam, constitutes the first line of pharmacological defense against tonic-clonic status epilepticus.

Phenytoin depresses respiration less than barbiturates. Because phenytoin is poorly soluble in water, it is dissolved in a mixture of water and propylene glycol. From this solvent, it may still precipitate when diluted in large volumes of par-

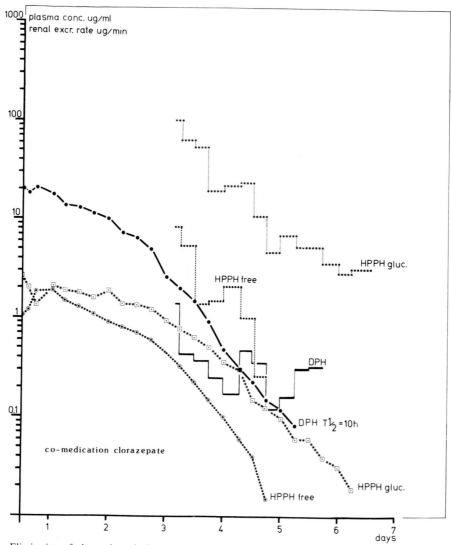

Fig. 14. Elimination of phenytoin, *p*-hydroxyphenytoin, and its conjugate in an epileptic patient with severe status epilepticus. Initially treated with phenytoin (500 mg i.v.), followed by thiopental (50 mg i.v.), the seizures were finally controlled by intravenous infusion of clorazepate (3 mg/hr).

enteral fluids. Unfortunately, propylene glycol may cause cardiovascular difficulties when given rapidly in the large quantities often required; the amount of drug necessary to control status epilepticus often exceeds 15 mg/kg. When given intramuscularly, the substance precipitates at the site of injection and is absorbed slowly and at an unpredictable rate.

The drug is rapidly distributed throughout the body water. Its relative apparent volume of distribution is about 0.6 liter/kg, corresponding to the total-body water space. The drug is distributed in the brain with only small differences between regions. Higher concentrations are measured in white matter than in gray matter, with a ratio of 1.3 in humans (6).

Like phenobarbital and most other lipophilic drugs, phenytoin is metabolized by the mixed-function oxidases of the liver microsomes to the *p*-hydroxy derivative (HPPH). This compound is conjugated with glucuronic acid and is predominantly excreted as such into the urine. Other hy-

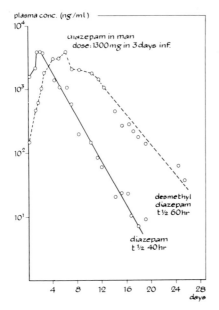

FIG. 15. Intravenous infusion of 1,300 mg of diazepam during a 3-day period in a preeclamptic patient.

droxy metabolites are detected in other species. HPPH can be determined with the same analytical technique as used for phenytoin (Fig. 14). The amount of phenytoin given for therapeutic efficacy is such that the enzymes responsible for the hydroxylation become saturated. This means that the rate of metabolism becomes constant at increasing amounts in the body. This phenomenon of capacity-limited metabolism can be described by apparent Michaelis-Menten kinetics. Large interindividual variations have been observed in the K_M and V_{max} values among patients (19): $K_M = 1$ to 25 mg/liter (mean 6 mg/liter), and $V_{max} = 0.15$ to 0.30 mg/hr/kg (mean 0.20 mg/hr/kg). Thus, careful monitoring of the concentration of the drug in body fluids is urged, especially because high concentrations of the drug may be responsible for seizures. Rogers et al. (20) reported 2 patients treated with diazepam showing unusually low phenytoin K_M values, thus causing extended high concentrations of phenytoin that could be held responsible for sustained toxicity (Fig. 16). At low concentrations, the rate of elimination will regain the same exponential-nature first-order elimination kinetics as for most other drugs with an elimination half-life of approximately 10 hr (Fig. 17).

The renal clearance values are 0.90 ml/min for phenytoin, 26 ml/min for the metabolite HPPH, and 100 ml/min for HPPH glucuronide.

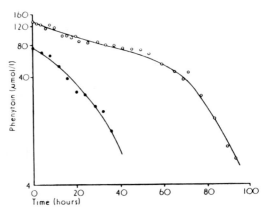

FIG. 16. Influence of diazepam on elimination of phenytoin, thus being responsible for the extended time course of intoxication (20).

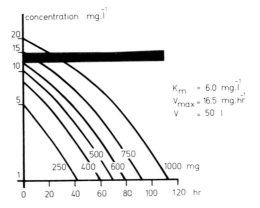

FIG. 17. Patterns of elimination of phenytoin at various amounts in the body. Note the decrease in rate of elimination at higher concentrations.

DRUGS OF SECOND CHOICE FOR TONIC-CLONIC STATUS EPILEPTICUS

Barbiturates

Amobarbital and Thiopental

Barbiturates are no longer considered drugs of first choice for treatment of status epilepticus. However, they are still indicated in cases refractory to benzodiazepines and when anesthesia remains the only method left. Because benzodiazepines have already been given, it is not necessary to suppress the restlessness of the patient by curarizing agents, although they may be added when muscle jerking does not stop. The drugs are given as repetitive boluses or as a slow injection over 10 to 15 min at 0.5 to 1.5 mg/kg/min to a

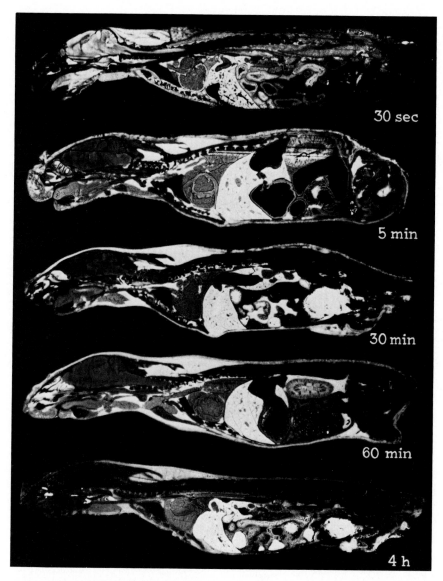

FIG. 18. Whole-body autoradiography of ^{32}S-thiopental (i.v. injection) in mice. Note the extremely rapid uptake of the compound into the brain and subsequent rapid elimination. Accumulation in body fat can be observed.

maximum of 7 mg/kg. Respiratory depression is the major risk, and special caution should be taken when high concentrations of barbiturates and hydantoin derivatives are already present. Amobarbital and thiopental are unstable in solution and must be constituted instantly.

Thiopental is an extremely lipophilic substance. After intravenous injection, the compound is rapidly taken up into the brain but also rapidly eliminated, while accumulation in body fat continues (Fig. 18). The compound is also rapidly metabolized to pentobarbital, with a much longer biological half-life. When the drug is repeatedly given, this pharmacologically effective substance may reach a considerable concentration and may thus account for delayed effect and sustained risk for respiratory depression. The compounds are also available in tablets and could be considered to be given as suppositories.

Phenobarbital

Phenobarbital is seldom considered a drug of first choice in status epilepticus. Its solubility in

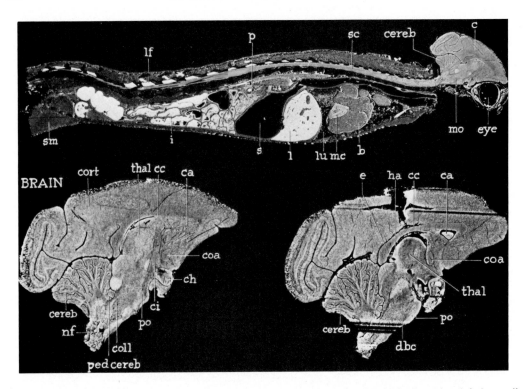

FIG. 19. Regional distribution of ¹⁴C-phenobarbital in squirrel monkey brain after 31 hr linear i.v. infusion until practically steady-state conditions have been established. Note the homogeneous distribution, with slightly higher concentrations in colliculi and white matter of the cerebellum than in the other regions of the cerebrum.

water is poor, and a solvent of glycerol, ethanol, and water is used. It can be given intravenously and may replace amobarbital and thiopental when the seizures have already stopped. The patient may then be loaded by the intravenous route when phenobarbital is used as a chronic antiepileptic agent.

Phenobarbital is much less lipophilic than amobarbital and thiopental and accumulates at a much slower rate into the brain. The distribution is much more uniform. In the brain, only very small concentration differences can be observed between white and gray matter. The colliculi and the white matter of the cerebellum show only slightly higher concentrations (Fig. 19).

The drug is hydroxylated by the liver microsomal mixed-function oxidases and conjugated to presumably ineffective compounds. Its biological half-life has been reported as 60 to 150 hr and thus is extremely variable. Its clearance is influenced by other drugs (26), whereas (sub)chronic treatment can enhance the clearance of other drugs (Fig. 20). Young children require relatively more phenobarbital per kilogram of body weight during chronic treatment because their relative clearance is higher, depending on their ages. When the drug is combined with other drugs, the clearance becomes unpredictable, and the age-clearance relationship may disappear (27).

Valproate

Sodium valproate is used at increasing frequency for chronic oral treatment of absence seizures, generalized tonic-clonic seizures, and myoclonic epilepsy. Only seldom has it been reported as a useful agent in status epilepticus.

In laboratory animals it is immediately effective against chemically induced seizures; it is less effective against electroshock seizures. Valproate has been used successfully in predelirium states in alcoholics. It is administered by intravenous infusion in high dosages of 1,200 to 1,400 mg (1). In chronic treatment of epilepsy, valproate administered orally demonstrates its efficacy 2 to 4 weeks after institution of treatment. This is in sharp contrast to the 2 days (4–5 times $t_{1/2}$ = 40–50 hr) it takes to reach steady state. To explain this phenomenon,

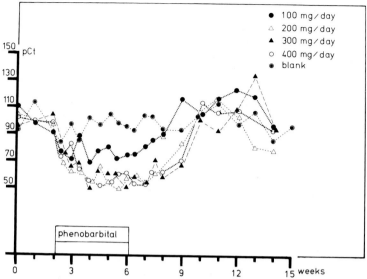

FIG. 20. Decreases in the biological half-life of clonazepam in the course of concomitant treatment with phenobarbital in dogs. The induction phenomenon appears saturable at high dosage regimens.

it has been postulated that valproate acts through a biologically active metabolite. Alternatively, it is suggested that the drug itself or one or more of its metabolites accumulate slowly in the target site of activity. Nevertheless, after intravenous injection of 5.3 to 28 mg/kg (mean 14.8 ± 6.4 mg/kg) in experimental animals, the effect on the electroencephalogram appears 8 to 10 min after administration, whereas the effect on clinical status is already apparent within 5 min and is stabilized at 15 min. In a study reporting on a small number of patients, valproate appeared most effective in partial seizures and photosensitive myoclonic epilepsy (22). In another study, valproate was administered rectally when patients with status epilepticus appeared refractory to parenteral barbiturates and benzodiazepines (23). The concentration able to control the symptoms appeared to range between 35 and 60 mg/kg. The dosages required to reach these concentrations accounted for 800 to 3,200 mg/day.

The kinetics of valproate after oral administration have been extensively studied. Although intraindividual and interindividual differences in rates of oral absorption have been noticed, there is no reason to assume incomplete absorption (15). Because the drug may cause paralytic ileus, nausea, and vomiting, oral valproate is not indicated in status epilepticus, even when a nasal intragastric

tube can be used. No data are available on the efficiency of rectal administration, although, based on daily concentration recordings, absorption appears complete (23).

Being a fairly acidic small-chain fatty acid, valproate reaches a small distribution volume (0.15–0.25 liter/kg). The drug shows high concentrations in plasma, liver, and excretory organs such as kidney, bile bladder, intestines, and skin. Surprisingly, low concentrations are found in the brain (Fig. 21). In the cerebrum, the olfactory bulb appears to accumulate drug and metabolites (21), and relatively high concentrations are found in the white matter of the cerebellum and the optic lobe. High concentrations are found in the ligaments (e.g., ligamentum flavum) but not in the myocardium. The drug rapidly crosses the placenta.

Valproate is rapidly metabolized to a multitude of oxidative products, of which γ-valprolactone and 2-propyl-3-hydroxypropene acetate can be analyzed in human blood plasma (Fig. 22) (21). It has not been determined if these compounds have antiepileptic effects, even though their biological half-lives appear to be longer. It appears that valproate can reduce the total body clearance of phenobarbital, for example, by 25% to 40% (27). This means that the phenobarbital concentration will increase when the same dosage regimen is continued.

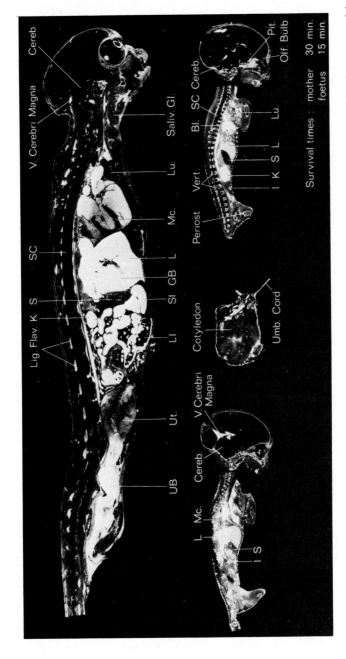

FIG. 21. Distribution of ^{14}C-carboxy valproate in a pregnant squirrel monkey 4 hr after i.v. infusion. White areas correspond to the presence of the drug. Note the low concentration in the cerebrum and high concentrations in liver, intestines, and yellow ligaments. Complete distribution can also be observed in the fetus.

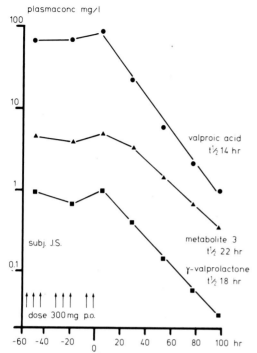

FIG. 22. Course of valproate concentration and its two main metabolites detectable in plasma of a patient whose treatment had been discontinued.

In the case of status epilepticus, one can best start with a bolus injection that can be calculated by

$$Dose = C \cdot V' \cdot W$$

in which V' is the relative distribution volume (0.25 liter/kg)

$$= 50 \times 0.25 \times W$$
$$Dose' = 12.5 \text{ mg/kg}$$

in which the prime stands for "relative," referring to body weight (W). Simultaneously, an intravenous infusion can be started. Based on the parameters given by Perucca et al. (14–16), this intravenous infusion rate (k_0) can be calculated as follows:

$$k_0 = C \times V' \times W$$
$$k_0 = 50 \times 0.012 \times W$$
$$k_0 = 0.6 \text{ mg/hr/kg}$$

When other drugs are or have been given simultaneously, the clearance appears an average of 0.016

liter/hr/kg, and thus the infusion rate will be 0.8 mg/hr/kg.

Carbamazepine

Carbamazepine is an extremely poorly soluble drug and therefore cannot be brought into solution suitable for intravenous solution. Intramuscular suspension would place an only slowly absorbed depot in the gluteal muscle. An incidental report has shown that carbamazepine has been compounded in 200-mg suppositories with good success. No pharmacokinetic studies are known to us demonstrating the rate and extent of absorption and their relevance for this therapeutic effect. The drug has peculiar pharmacokinetic characteristics, e.g., its autoinduction and heteroinduction phenomena during subchronic treatment, which have been reported in detail elsewhere (17,27). Because the drug is only seldom used for this purpose, distribution and metabolism will not be discussed (32).

Paraldehyde, Chlormethiazole, and Lidocaine

Paraldehyde, a cyclic polymer of acetaldehyde, chlormethiazole, a sedative-hypnotic drug with pharmacological properties that place it in the alcohol-barbiturate group, and lidocaine are frequently resorted to when the drugs of first choice (phenytoin and diazepam) fail to stop status epilepticus. Their efficacy and pharmacology are described in Chapter 54.

SUMMARY

Pharmacokinetics as the basis for dosage calculation for acute and subacute treatment of status epilepticus have been discussed. Bolus injection and intravenous infusion are the most common forms of drug administration in these cases. Rectal administration may be a good alternative in certain conditions. Intravenous diazepam and phenytoin are the first-line drugs against status epilepticus. Diazepam and sodium valproate have been reported to be effective by the rectal route. Depending on its pharmacokinetic parameters, each drug effect has a different onset, intensity, and time course.

REFERENCES

1. Brasseur, R. (1981): Depakine bei der Behandelung des chronischen Alkoholimus. *Therapie Woche*, 28:9981.

2. Carrigan, P. J., Chao, G. C., Barker, W. M., Hoffman, D. J., and Chum, A. H. C. (1977): Steady state bioavailability of two clorazepate dipotassium dosage forms. *J. Clin. Pharmacol.*, X:18–28.

3. Eadie, M. J., and Tyrer, J. H. (1980): *Anticonvulsant Therapy*, ed. 2. Churchill Livingstone, Edinburgh.

4. Garrett, E. R., Bres, J., Schnelle, K., and Rolf, L. L. (1974): Pharmacokinetics of saturably metabolized amobarbital. *J. Pharmacokinet. Biopharm.*, 2:43–103.

5. Greenblatt, D. J., Shader, R. J., Frank, K., MacLaughlin, D. S., Harmatz, J. S., Allen, M. D., Werner, A., and Woo, E. (1979): Pharmacokinetics and bioavailability of intravenous, intramuscular and oral lorazepam in humans. *J. Pharm. Sci.*, 68:57–63.

6. Harvey, C. D., Sherwin, A. L., and van der Kleijn, E. (1977): Distribution of anticonvulsant drugs in grey and white matter of human brain. *Can. Sci. Neurol.*, 4:89–92.

7. Hillestad, L., Hansen, T., Melsom, H., and Drivenes, A. (1974): Diazepam metabolism in normal man. Serum concentrations and clinical effects after intravenous, intramuscular and oral administration. *Clin. Pharmacol. Ther.*, 16:479–484.

8. Kadar, D., Inaba, T., Endrenyi, L., Johnson, G. E., and Kalow, W. (1973): Comparative drug elimination capacity in man—glutethimide, amobarbital, antipyrine and sulfinpyrazone. *Clin. Pharmacol. Ther.*, 14:552–560.

9. Knapp, R. B., and Fierro, L. (1974): Evaluation of the cardiopulmonary safety and effects of lorazepam as a premedicant. *Anesth. Analg. (Cleve.)*, 53:122–124.

10. Knop, H. J., van der Kleijn, E., and Edmunds, L. C. (1975): The determination of clonazepam in plasma by gas-liquid chromatography. *Pharm. Wkbl.*, 110:297–309.

11. Magnussen, J., Oxlund, H. R. W., Alsbirk, K. E., and Arnold, E. (1979): Absorption of diazepam in man following rectal and parenteral administration. *Acta Pharmacol. Toxicol. (Kbh.)*, 45:87–90.

12. Merkus, F. W. H. M. (editor) (1980): *The Serum Concentrations of Drugs*. Excerpta Medica, Amsterdam.

13. Notari, R. (1971): *Biopharmaceutics and Pharmacokinetics*. Marcel Dekker, New York.

14. Perucca, E., Gatti, G., Frigo, G. M., Crema, A., Calzette, S., and Visintini, D. (1978): Pharmacokinetics of sodium valproate in epileptic patients and normal volunteers. In: *Advances in Epileptology 1977*, edited by H. Meinardi and A. J. Rowan, pp. 245–248. Swets and Zeitlinger, Amsterdam.

15. Perucca, E., Gatti, G., Frigo, G. M., and Crema, M. (1978): Pharmacokinetics of valproic acid after oral and intravenous administration. *Br. J. Clin. Pharmacol.*, 5:313–328.

16. Perucca, E., Gatti, G., Frigo, G. M., Crema, A., Calzetti, S., and Visintini, D. (1978): Disposition of sodium valproate in epileptic patients. *Br. J. Clin. Pharmacol.*, 5:495–499.

17. Pitlick, W. H., and Levy, R. (1977): Time dependent kinetics, exponential autoinduction of carbamazepine in monkeys. *J. Pharm. Sci.*, 66:647–649.

18. Post, C., Lindgren, S., Bertler, A., and Malmeren, H. (1977): Pharmacokinetics of N-desmethyldiazepam in healthy volunteers after single daily doses of dipotassium chlorazepate. *Psychopharmacology*, 53:105–109.

19. Richens, A. (1979): Clinical pharmacokinetics of phenytoin. *Clin. Pharmacokinet.*, 4:153–169.

20. Rogers, H. J., Haslam, R. A., Longstreth, J., and Lietman, P. S. (1977): Phenytoin intoxication during concurrent diazepam therapy. *J. Neurol. Neurosurg. Psychiatry*, 40:890–895.

21. Schobben, A. F. A. M. (1979): Pharmacokinetics and therapeutics in epilepsy. Ph.D. thesis, Catholic University of Nijmegen, The Netherlands.

22. Sorel, L., and de Ridder-Vanderdeelen, P. (1979): Rapport sur l'utilization du depakine par voie intraveineuze Center William Lennox, 1340 Ottignies, Belgium.

23. Vajda, F. J. E., Mihaly, G. W., Miles, J. L., Doman, G. A., and Bladin, P. F. (1978): Rectal administration of sodium valproate in status epilepticus. *Neurology (Minneap.)*, 28:897–899.

24. Van Ginneken, C. A. M., van Rossum, J. M., and Fleuren, H. L. J. M. (1974): Linear and non linear kinetics of drug elimination. *J. Pharmacokinet. Biopharm.*, 2:395–415.

25. van der Kleijn, E., van Rossum, J. M., Muskens, T. J. M., and Rijntjes, N. V. M. (1971): Pharmacokinetics of diazepam in dog, mice and humans. *Acta Pharmacol. [Suppl. 3]*, 29:109–127.

26. van der Kleijn, E., Vree, T., Guelen, P., Schobben, F., Westenberg, H., and Knop, H. (1978): Kinetics of drug interactions in the treatment of epilepsy. *Int. J. Clin. Pharmacol.*, 16:467–473.

27. van der Kleijn, E., Schobben, F., and Vree, T. B. (1980): Clinical pharmacokinetics of antiepileptic drugs. *Drug Intell. Clin. Pharm.*, 14:674–685.

28. van der Kleijn, E., Vree, T. B., Baars, A. M., Wijsman, R., Edmunds, L. C., and Knop, H. J. (1981): Factors influencing the activity and fate of benzodiazepines in the body. *Br. J. Pharmacol.*, 11:85S–98S.

29. Vree, T. B., Baars, A. M., Booy, L. H. D., and Driessen, J. J. (1981): Simultaneous determination and pharmacokinetics of midazolam and its hydroxymetabolites in plasma and urine of man and dog by means of HPLC. *Arzneim. Forsch.*, 31:2215–2219.

30. Wagner, J. C. (1975): *Fundamentals of Clinical Pharmacokinetics*. III 62341. Drug Intelligence Publications, Hamilton.

31. Walker, J. E., Homan, R. W., Vasko, M. R., Crawford, J. L., Bell, R. D., and Tasker, W. G. (1979): Lorazepam in status epilepticus. *Ann. Neurol.*, 6:207–213.

32. Westenberg, H. G. M. (1980): Bioanalysis and pharmacokinetics of carbamazepine. Ph.D. thesis, Department of Pharmacy, State University of Groningen, The Netherlands.

Advances in Neurology, Vol. 34: Status Epilepticus, edited by A.V. Delgado-Escueta, C.G. Wasterlain, D.M. Treiman, and R.J. Porter. Raven Press, New York © 1983.

44

Efficacy of Phenytoin in Treatment of Status Epilepticus

B. J. Wilder

Status epilepticus is defined as a fixed and continuous state of prolonged seizures that persists for more than 30 min. It is most commonly exemplified by a series of convulsions occurring without recovery of consciousness during intervals between convulsions. Status epilepticus is a medical emergency that requires immediate treatment to prevent permanent brain damage or death. Treiman and Delgado-Escueta (17) reported mortality of 8% in the acute phase of status epilepticus.

The causes of status epilepticus are varied. Janz (9,10) reported that generalized tonic-clonic status is six times more common in epileptic patients with complex or simple partial seizures than in patients with primary generalized seizures. A significant portion of patients who present in status epilepticus have structural brain lesions, such as a mass lesion (neoplasm, subdural) or the residua of old head trauma or stroke. Status epilepticus may accompany acute injuries to the brain, such as infections, hypertensive encephalopathy, intracerebral or subarachnoid hemorrhage, head trauma with brain contusion, anoxic or metabolic encephalopathy, and recent cerebral infarction.

In known epileptic patients, status epilepticus is often precipitated by withdrawal from antiepileptic drugs, therapeutic drug manipulation, systemic febrile illnesses, electrolyte imbalance, and hypoglycemia. Withdrawal from alcohol or sedative drugs may cause status epilepticus in nonepileptic persons as well as epileptic patients. Often the precipitating factor for status epilepticus is not apparent in epileptic patients.

Thus, patients who present with status epilepticus in the emergency room may be classified into two broad categories: type A, patients known to have epilepsy and patients whose status epilepticus is eventually diagnosed as the first manifestation of a partial or generalized seizure disorder; type B, patients with acute cerebral insults or encephalopathy. Patients experiencing drug or alcohol withdrawal who present in status epilepticus are categorized as type A patients. This separation of patients with status epilepticus is similar to that presented by Cranford et al. (2).

Regardless of its cause, status epilepticus may induce life-threatening pathophysiological changes. Acidosis may be severe (pH < 7.2), requiring immediate correction. Cyanosis, if present, should be managed by intubation and administration of oxygen. Dehydration should be treated with appropriate intravenous solutions (normal or 0.5-N saline and bicarbonate or Ringer's lactate solution). Acute treatment of status epilepticus should be directed toward restoring central nervous system homeostasis and controlling convulsions.

A general principle in the management of status epilepticus is to give a major antiepileptic drug in a dose to load brain tissues sufficiently to stop seizures. In special situations, anticonvulsant drug selection may depend on the cause of status epilepticus. If second-line anticonvulsant agents are added concurrently with or following the first-line antiepileptic drug, the second drug ideally should potentiate the antiepileptic effects of the first agent. Drugs that potentiate central nervous system or cardiorespiratory depression should be avoided whenever possible.

Ideally, a drug for the treatment of status epilepticus should (a) be available for intravenous administration, (b) penetrate the blood-brain barrier rapidly and accumulate quickly at its site of action, (c) effectively stop status in a high percentage of cases, (d) have a span of activity (half-life) that permits institution of oral dosing of the desired antiepileptic drug before the anticonvulsant effect declines, (e) produce little or no cardiorespiratory depression, (f) not produce additional somnolence or deepen coma, (g) not produce major changes in the neurological examination, and (h) not potentiate central nervous system depression of other antiepileptic agents that might be required.

PHENYTOIN AS THE FIRST-LINE DRUG IN STATUS EPILEPTICUS

Of the antiepileptic drugs used for treatment of status, only phenytoin fulfills most of the criteria outlined. In 1972 we began to standardize the treatment of status epilepticus at the Gainesville Veterans Administration Medical Center and the Shands Teaching Hospital of the University of Florida with the use of intravenous phenytoin as the single drug of choice. We have used intravenous phenytoin in more than 200 patients with type A status and have verified the efficacy and safety of this drug (19). We have also reported the stability of phenytoin mixed in normal saline and have described the pharmacokinetic and clinical effects of intravenously administered loading doses of 15 mg/kg (14,15). The timed brain uptake of phenytoin following intravenous loading has been measured in humans and animals and compared with the uptake of phenobarbital and diazepam in animals (13,19).

Our protocol for treatment of status epilepticus is directed toward restoration of normal physiological homeostasis and termination of convulsions. Patients who presented in the emergency room with type A status epilepticus or who developed type A status epilepticus during hospitalization were treated in the manner outlined in Table 1. Phenytoin was administered intravenously at a rate of 50 mg/min using a dose of 15 mg/kg. More than 80% of the patients stopped convulsing within 20 min of commencing the administration of phenytoin (Fig. 1). The anticonvulsant effect of phenytoin was evident as early as 10 min after the start of intravenous infusion. By that time, approximately 400 mg (7.5 mg/kg) of phenytoin had been administered, and about 30% of patients had stopped convulsing. After 15 min of intravenous phenytoin, almost 50% of patients stopped having seizures. Maximal effects were seen 20 min after the start of intravenous infusion. At that time, approximately 1,000 mg of phenytoin (10–12 mg/kg) had been administered, and more than 80% of the patients had stopped convulsing. Thus, if a favorable response to phenytoin was to occur (i.e., the

TABLE 1. *Treatment of status epilepticus with intravenous phenytoin*

1. Airway management to ensure adequate ventilation; oral airway device or intubation and assisted ventilation with oxygen if cyanosis is present
2. Immediate arterial pH determination and correction of acidosis with bicarbonate if arterial pH < 7.2
3. Correction of fluid and electrolyte imbalance
4. Administration of B-complex vitamins, pyridoxine, and glucose by a separate intravenous route
5. Intravenous administration of phenytoin (15 mg/kg) mixed in normal saline at a concentration of 10 mg/ml at a rate of 50 mg/min
6. Electrocardiogram monitoring desirable, but not necessary during phenytoin administration
7. Blood pressure monitoring during phenytoin administration
8. Intravenous administration of other drugs if seizures persist for 30 min following infusion of phenytoin

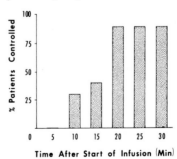

FIG. 1. Control of generalized convulsive status epilepticus with intravenous phenytoin (mean dose 13 mg/kg; mean infusion time 17.8 min).

disappearance of seizures), it occurred by the time the complete dose of phenytoin (15 mg/kg) had been administered. This took a minimum of 10 to 20 min.

No severe adverse reactions occurred as a result of intravenous phenytoin administered at the rate and in the dose recommended. Approximately 50% of patients treated were observed to have mild transient decreases in blood pressure ($< 10\%$ of pretreatment systolic blood pressure). Mild slowing of the pulse ($< 10\%$) occurred in less than 25% of patients. The cardiac arrhythmias that were observed were believed to have existed prior to administration of phenytoin.

Several patients awoke following cessation of seizures and reported vertigo, and nystagmus was observed in some patients. However, in general, the neurological examinations were unchanged by the intravenous phenytoin, and respiratory and cardiovascular depressions were not deepened or induced. False-positive pathological neurological signs did not appear to be induced by the treatment.

Initially, when setting up the protocol for treating status, phenytoin was administered at rates up to 100 mg/min, and mild hypotension and bradycardia were induced. Respiratory arrest and asystole can be produced in experimental animals by bolus intravenous injection of phenytoin.

After treatment, the patients were transferred to the neurology ward or medical intensive care unit for follow-up management. Single daily doses of oral or, rarely, intravenous phenytoin (5–6 mg/kg) were commenced within 6 to 10 hr after the initial phenytoin treatment of status. This resulted in the maintenance of therapeutic plasma concentrations of phenytoin.

Patients who have type B status epilepticus respond poorly to anticonvulsant therapy. We have used intravenous phenytoin in these patients with generally poor results. In these rare cases of refractory status epilepticus, phenobarbital was the second drug chosen; it was administered intravenously in a dose of 10 mg/kg at a rate of 100 mg/min. Some 50% of these patients treated with phenytoin have required extensive additional treatment with phenobarbital, lidocaine, or other barbiturates. Often the use of multiple therapies is unsuccessful. Cranford et al. (2,3) have reported on the results of phenytoin therapy in both types of status epilepticus.

PLASMA AND BRAIN CONCENTRATIONS OF PHENYTOIN, PHENOBARBITAL, AND DIAZEPAM

Phenytoin, diazepam, and phenobarbital are the drugs most commonly used for treatment of convulsive (generalized tonic-clonic, focal motor, or unilateral) status epilepticus. All three drugs are considered first-line drugs for treatment of status epilepticus and are effective in terminating convulsions. Various combinations of these drugs have been recommended (17).

Diazepam was first shown by Gastaut et al. (5) to be highly effective in rapidly stopping seizures. In reviewing diazepam treatment of status epilep-

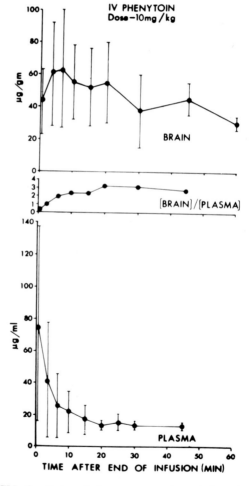

FIG. 2. Brain and plasma concentrations of phenytoin following intravenous infusion of phenytoin (10 mg/kg at 50–100 mg/min) in experimental animals. Brain-to-plasma ratios are shown in the middle graph.

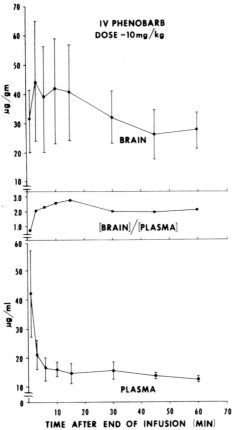

FIG. 3. Brain and plasma concentrations of phenobarbital following intravenous infusion of phenobarbital (10 mg/kg at 100 mg/min) in experimental animals. Brain-to-plasma ratios are shown in the middle graph.

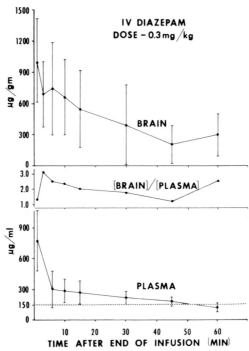

FIG. 4. Brain and plasma concentrations of diazepam following intravenous infusion of diazepam (0.3 mg/kg at 1 mg/min) in experimental animals. Brain-to-plasma ratios are shown in the middle graph.

ticus, Browne and Penry (1) found that seizures responded to the drug in 88% of patients but recommenced after 20 to 40 min in a high percentage of patients. Only 9 of 20 patients were reported by Prensky et al. (12) to be seizure-free 2 hr after administration of diazepam for status epilepticus. Primarily because of its short duration of action, diazepam is not considered an ideal drug for status epilepticus.

Phenobarbital is also highly effective in terminating status epilepticus. However, large doses are required, coma is deepened, and severe cardiorespiratory depression may result, especially if diazepam has been used prior to phenobarbital. Moreover, little is known of the pharmacokinetics of intravenous phenobarbital in status. For these reasons, phenobarbital also is not considered an ideal drug for status.

To better understand the pharmacology of intravenous diazepam, phenobarbital, and phenytoin in status, we measured plasma and brain concentrations in experimental animals. All three drugs penetrate the central nervous system rapidly following intravenous infusion (13). Figures 2, 3, and 4 show the brain and plasma concentrations of the three drugs and brain-to-plasma ratios in experimental animals after loading with intravenous doses comparable to those that would be used in humans.

Following intravenous infusion of diazepam, phenobarbital, or phenytoin, the brain parenchyma behaves as a component of the shallow or rapidly equilibrating compartment, because all three drugs rapidly enter and concentrate in brain tissue. Peak brain concentrations of phenobarbital and phenytoin occur 3 to 6 min after completion of the intravenous dose. No significant differences were found between brain concentrations measured at 1 min and at 1 hr after infusion. This observation indicates that substantial binding of phenobarbital and phenytoin occurs in the brain. Similar findings have been reported in studies on brain lipid binding (7,8). This is also reflected in the brain-to-plasma ratio, which peaked at 15 min for phenobarbital and 20 min for phenytoin. A stable brain concentration persists even as plasma concentrations fall. In contrast to the situation with phenytoin, brain concentrations of diazepam decline from maximal levels 1 min after completion of intravenous infusion and are significantly lower 45 min later. Brain concentrations decline in parallel with plasma concentrations.

Figure 5 shows brain and plasma concentrations of phenytoin in humans. They confirm the animal studies and show stable and therapeutic brain phenytoin concentrations (15–20 μg/ml). The plasma-to-brain ratio decreases (reciprocal of brain-to-plasma ratio illustrated in Figs. 2, 3, and 4) during the first hour after intravenous infusion (19).

CONCLUSION

Prior to the late 1960s, intravenous phenobarbital, paraldehyde, and more rapidly acting barbiturates were used in the management of status epilepticus. Intravenous diazepam was introduced in the mid-1960s and has been used extensively until the present time. In 1958, McWilliams and Leeds (11) reported on the efficacy of intravenous phenytoin for treatment of status in children. This work was largely ignored until the reports of Easton (4) and Wallis et al. (18). Although Goldberg (6) and Simpson (16) challenged Easton's report, our initial investigation of intravenous phenytoin was encouraging and led to the additional studies reported earlier. Based on our experience, we have concluded that intravenous phenytoin is the drug of choice for treatment of type A status and should also be the initial drug used for treatment of type B status. Because administration of the total dosage of intravenous phenytoin takes about 10 to 20 min, a second drug that acts within seconds can be given.

Except for its transient and short duration of action, diazepam is an excellent, rapid-acting anticonvulsant for treatment of status epilepticus. However, increasing doses of the drug frequently are required to maintain the seizure-free state, and diazepam in large doses produces respiratory and cardiac depression and even cardiac arrest. For these reasons, it is not an ideal first-line drug. It can, however, be used as a second drug for status, if given as a single bolus injection.

Thus, we have recently modified our treatment protocol for status epilepticus to include simultaneous administration of diazepam at 0.1 mg/kg at a rate of 1 mg/min (not to exceed a total dose of 10 mg) and intravenous administration of phenytoin (15 mg/kg at a rate of 50 mg/min). Diazepam should be given under constant supervision and should not be used in patients who have previously received barbiturates or other central nervous system depressants. Also, diazepam should not be used in status epilepticus patients who have chronically received any of the benzodiazepines.

REFERENCES

1. Browne, T. R., and Penry, J. K. (1973): Benzodiazepines in the treatment of epilepsy: A review. *Epilepsia*, 14:277–310.
2. Cranford, R. E., Leppik, I. E., Patrick, B., Anderson, C. B., and Kostick, B. (1979): Intravenous phenytoin in acute treatment of seizures. *Neurology*, 29:1474–1479.
3. Cranford, R. E., Patrick, B., Anderson, C. B., and Kostick, B. (1978): Intravenous phenytoin: Clinical and pharmacokinetic aspects. *Neurology*, 28:874–880.
4. Easton, J. D. (1972): DPH and epilepsy management. *Ann. Intern. Med.*, 77:421–423.
5. Gastaut, H., Naquet, R., Poire, R., and Tassinari, C. A. (1965): Treatment of status epilepticus with diazepam (Valium). *Epilepsia*, 6:167–182.
6. Goldberg, M. A. (1973): Use of DPH. *Ann. Intern. Med.*, 78:305.
7. Goldberg, M. A., and Crandall, P. H. (1978): Human brain binding of phenytoin. *Neurology*, 28:881–885.
8. Goldberg, M. A., and Toderoff, T. (1976): Diphenylhydantoin binding to brain lipids and phospholipids. *Biochem. Pharmacol.*, 25:2079–2083.
9. Janz, D. (1961): Condition and causes of status epilepticus. *Epilepsia*, 2:170–177.
10. Janz, D. (1964): Status epilepticus and frontal lobe lesions. *J. Neurol. Sci.*, 1:446–457.
11. McWilliams, P. K. A., and Leeds, M. B. (1958): IV phenytoin sodium in continuous convulsions in children. *Lancet*, 2:1147–1149.

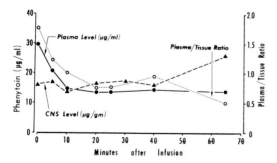

FIG. 5. Simultaneous plasma (solid line) and brain (dash line) phenytoin concentrations following intravenous infusion of 8.1 to 16.7 mg/kg in three patients during surgery. Note that the plasma-to-brain ratio (dotted line) is the reciprocal of the brain-to-plasma ratios shown in Figs. 2, 3, and 4.

12. Prensky, A. L., Raff, M. C., Moor, M. J., and Schwab, R. S. (1967): Intravenous diazepam in the treatment of prolonged seizure activity. *N. Engl. J. Med.,* 276:779–784.

13. Ramsay, R., Hammond, E. J., Perchalski, R. J., and Wilder, B. J. (1979): Brain uptake of phenytoin, phenobarbital and diazepam. *Arch. Neurol.,* 36:535–539.

14. Salem, R. B., Yost, R. L., Torosian, G., Davis, F. T., and Wilder, B. J. (1980): Investigation of the crystallization of phenytoin in normal saline. *Drug Intell. Clin. Pharm.,* 14:605–608.

15. Salem, R. B., Wilder, B. J., Yost, R. L., Doering, P. L., and Lee, C. C. (1981): Rapid phenytoin infusion for administration of loading doses. *Am. J. Hosp. Pharm.,* 38:354–357.

16. Simpson, J. F. (1973): Use of DPH. *Ann. Intern. Med.,* 78:305.

17. Treiman, D. M., and Delgado-Escueta, A. V. (1980): Status epilepticus. In: *Critical Care of Neurologic and Neurosurgical Emergencies,* edited by R. A. Thompson and J. R. Green, pp. 53–99. Raven Press, New York.

18. Wallis, W., Kutt, H., and McDowell, F. (1968): IV DPH in treatment of acute repetitive seizures. *Neurology (Minneap.),* 18:513–525.

19. Wilder, B. J., Ramsay, R. E., Willmore, L. J., Feussner, G. G., Perchalski, R. J., and Shumate, J. B. (1977): Efficacy of intravenous phenytoin in the treatment of status epilepticus. *Ann. Neurol.,* 1:511–518.

Advances in Neurology, Vol. 34: Status Epilepticus, edited by A.V. Delgado-Escueta, C.G. Wasterlain, D.M. Treiman, and R.J. Porter. Raven Press, New York © 1983.

45

Treatment of Acute Seizures and Status Epilepticus with Intravenous Phenytoin

Ilo E. Leppik, Barbara K. Patrick, and Ronald E. Cranford

Many drugs have been used in the treatment of status epilepticus, but no single agent has been universally successful (6). Diazepam often terminates seizures shortly after infusion (12,15), but the duration of its antiepileptic activity is brief (2). Phenytoin enters the brain rapidly following intravenous infusion in experimental animals (13), and its anticonvulsant properties are present immediately on attaining adequate concentrations (11). In this chapter we shall review our experience with large doses of phenytoin administered intravenously to adult patients presenting at an acute care hospital.

METHODS

Population

During a 3-year period, phenytoin was administered intravenously on 159 occasions to 139 adult patients referred to us for acute treatment of seizures. The 74 male and 65 female patients ranged in age from 17 to 94 years (mean 52 years) and weighed 37 to 113 kg (mean 65 kg). Phenytoin (Dilantin Steri-Vial®) was infused at 50 mg/min or less, as previously described (4). During the initial 35 infusions, standard doses were given, but subsequently 69 infusions of 15 mg/kg and 55 infusions of 18 mg/kg were administered. Total doses ranged from 650 mg to 2,000 mg. On 52 occa-

sions, diazepam (mean dose 0.18 ± 0.09 mg/kg) had been administered prior to referral. Other conditions such as hyponatremia were treated concomitantly when present. Phenytoin was used for status epilepticus, serial seizures, isolated seizures when withdrawal from antiepileptic drugs was suspected ($N = 137$ infusions), and prophylaxis after subarachnoid hemorrhage ($N = 22$).

Classification

Patients were classified as having generalized status epilepticus only if seizures were continuous for 30 min or if there was a decrease in the level of consciousness between recurrent seizures. Patients with acute encephalopathy severe enough to decrease consciousness were classified as being in status if they had four or more generalized seizures in 1 hr. The diagnosis of electroencephalographic (EEG) status was based on continuous epileptiform abnormality. There were no cases of generalized absence status. Partial, simple, or complex status was diagnosed by clinical or EEG observations. Persons not in status were listed as having serial seizures if three or more seizures occurred during the 24 hr preceding phenytoin infusion. Most partial seizures were simple motor, but there was 1 patient with complex partial status.

Each episode requiring phenytoin infusion was classified by the precipitating factor (Table 1). Pa-

TABLE 1. *Precipitation factors for seizures for which large doses of phenytoin were administered intravenously*

Precipitating factors	No. of infusions
Medication withdrawal	
By serum phenytoin concentration[a]	40
By history[b]	9
Cause undetermined	
By serum phenytoin concentration[c]	18
By history[d]	9
Atypical alcohol withdrawal	6
Miscellaneous	17
Anoxic encephalopathy	6
Metabolic encephalopathy	8
Acute vascular	14
CNS neoplasm	5
Trauma	4
Meningitis	1
Total (for seizures)	137
Subarachnoid hemorrhage (no seizures)	22
Total	159

[a] Preinfusion serum phenytoin concentration <5 µg/ml.
[b] Definite history of recent noncompliance.
[c] Preinfusion serum phenytoin concentration ≥ 5 µg/ml.
[d] Definite denial of recent noncompliance.

tients were considered to be withdrawing from antiepileptic drugs if (a) the preinfusion serum phenytoin concentration was less than 5µg/ml or concentrations of other prescribed antiepileptic drugs were below "therapeutic" concentrations, (b) a definite history of recent noncompliance was obtained, or (c) no other cause of exacerbation was evident. Epileptic patients with concomitant medical problems sufficient to account for exacerbation of seizures were classified under the specific condition (e.g., trauma, metabolic). Where none of these conditions applied, patients were listed in the category of "cause undetermined."

Antiepileptic drug concentrations were measured by standard GLC procedures (4).

RESULTS

Adverse Effects

Hypotension was the most common adverse effect of phenytoin infusion, especially in patients with anoxic or metabolic encephalopathy, but it was always reversible by decreasing the rate of infusion. The occurrence of hypotension was age-related: No one under age 40 developed a decrease in blood pressure greater than 20 mm Hg, systolic, whereas 2 of 3 patients 80 years or older had this

degree of hypotension. Reversible nonfatal EKG abnormalities occurred during three infusions. Temporary respiratory depression was observed in only 1 patient whose preinfusion phenytoin concentration had been 32 µg/ml and reached a peak of 61 µg/ml. The level of consciousness was not significantly altered by these large doses of phenytoin. Other side effects were noted only occasionally (4).

Pharmacokinetics

Doses of 18 mg/kg were associated with a mean phenytoin concentration of 15.0 ± 2.9 µg/ml 24 hr after infusion in patients whose preinfusion concentrations were less than 1 µg/ml. Concentrations over the 24-hr period are presented in Fig. 1 The volume of distribution was relatively constant, but clearance and half-life varied considerably (Table 2). There was a trend toward shorter half-lives and larger clearances among patients previously treated

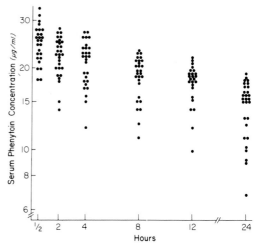

FIG. 1. Serum phenytoin concentrations following intravenous administration of 18 mg/kg in 28 patients whose preinfusion concentrations were < 1 µg/ml.

TABLE 2. *Volume of distribution (V_d), clearance (C), and half-life ($t_{1/2}$) calculated from 53 intravenous phenytoin infusions (preinfusion concentration 1 µg/ml; mean dose 16.6 ± 1.8 mg/kg*

Parameter	Mean ± SD
V_d (liter/kg)	0.78 ± 0.11
C (liter/kg/hr)	0.0157 ± 0.0132
$t_{1/2}$ (hr)	51.2 ± 31.6

with antiepileptic drugs, but interindividual variability was so large that no significant difference was observed between previously treated patients and those receiving phenytoin for the first time.

Seizure Control

Seizures occurred during the approximately 30 min required for phenytoin infusion in 10 patients. Six of these had been in status epilepticus prior to treatment, and two had severe anoxic or metabolic encephalopathy.

Evaluation of the effects of phenytoin was based on the 24-hr observation period commencing with completion of phenytoin infusion. No other antiepileptic drugs were given during this period unless seizures recurred.

There were clear relationships between the causes of seizures and the results of treatment. Few patients listed in Table 3 (group I) had isolated seizures following infusion. Those in group II

TABLE 3. *Results of antiepileptic drug treatment in patients with preexisting epilepsy, atypical alcohol withdrawal, and miscellaneous condition (group I)*[a]

Initial seizure frequency	No. of patients	Patients with seizures after phenytoin	
		(No.)	(%)
Status	14	3	21
Serial seizures	59	5	8
Two or less	17	1	10
Not recorded	9	1	11
Total	99	10	10

[a]Observation period after treatment was 24 hr.

TABLE 4. *Results of antiepileptic drug treatment in patients with anoxic or metabolic encephalopathy, acute vascular event, CNS neoplasm, and trauma (group II)*[a]

Initial seizure frequency	No. of patients	Patients with seizures after phenytoin	
		(No.)	(%)
Status	11	4	36
Serial seizures	15	10	67
Two or less	9	5	56
Not recorded	2	2	100
Total	37	21	57

[a]Observation period after treatment was 24 hr.

continued to have multiple seizures following phenytoin, although overall seizure frequency was reduced (Table 4).

Classified by precipitating factors, the seizure frequencies in group I following phenytoin infusion were as follows: antiepileptic drug withdrawal, 3 of 49 patients, or 6% (one with partial epilepsy, one with myoclonic seizures, and one with seizures on the EEG); epilepsy, cause undetermined, 3 of 27, or 11% (one with generalized seizures, one with partial seizures, one with both); atypical alcohol withdrawal, 1 of 6, or 17%; miscellaneous causes, 3 of 17, or 18%. In general, seizures were more likely to recur in group I if status epilepticus existed prior to treatment (Table 3).

In contrast to group I, the seizure frequencies in group II were higher after phenytoin infusion: patients with anoxic encephalopathy, 4 of 6, or 66%; with metabolic diseases, 5 of 8, or 63%; with acute vascular disorders, 6 of 14, or 43%; with central nervous system (CNS) neoplasm, 2 of 5, or 40%; with trauma, 4 of 4, or 100%. Those who continued to have seizures often had reductions in seizure severity; in three instances, generalized seizures were followed by only partial seizures, and in 2 patients the numbers of generalized seizures were reduced by 50% or more. Various treatments, including additional phenytoin, phenobarbital, and other drugs, were administered to patients who continued to have seizures, often with little success.

In patients treated prophylactically following subarachnoid hemorrhage, no seizures occurred.

The single patient with meningitis had no further seizures following phenytoin infusion, but was not included in either group.

The most obvious difference between group I and group II was the nature of the disease process. Patients in group II were generally severely ill with acute involvement of the CNS. This was reflected in their mortality: 14 of 37 patients (38%) in group II died within 1 month after treatment. Only 1 patient (1%) in group I died. Deaths in group II included 4 of 6 patients with anoxic encephalopathy, 4 of 8 with metabolic encephalopathy, 2 of 5 with tumor, and 4 of 14 with acute vascular lesions. There was little difference in group II between initial seizure frequency and mortality, as 7 of 11 patients (64%) initially in status died, compared with 7 of 15 patients (47%) with serial seizures.

Serum phenytoin concentrations were obtained 30 min after infusion in 93 patients and 24 hr after infusion in 106 patients. The mean serum phenytoin concentrations in patients having no seizures following infusion in both groups I and II were $26.2 \pm 6.6 \mu g/ml$ ($N = 76$) 30 min after infusion and $15.9 \pm 4.6 \mu g/ml$ ($N = 87$) 24 hr after infusion. Patients continuing to have seizures in either group had similar levels: The mean 30-min and 24-hr levels were $25.1 \pm 10.6 \mu g/ml$ ($N = 17$) and $15.0 \pm 6.6 \mu g/ml$ ($N = 19$), respectively. Therefore, recurrence of seizures appeared to be related to seizure threshold rather than to phenytoin concentration during the observation period. Phenytoin infusion affected the type of seizure. Prior to infusion, 116 seizures (85%) were generalized; after infusion, 17 of 26 (65%) were partial.

Diazepam had been administered prior to referral on 52 occasions. In group I, 16 of the 37 patients initially treated with diazepam had subsequent seizures. In contrast, only 7 of 62 initially treated with phenytoin loading had further seizures. For patients in group II, there was no difference between phenytoin alone and initial treatment with diazepam (5).

DISCUSSION

Patients presenting with status epilepticus or acute seizures may be divided into two categories; those with preexisting epilepsy and those with acute brain lesions ("symptomatic status") (1,3,14). Our results indicate that administration of large doses of phenytoin intravenously is associated with marked reductions in the numbers of seizures in patients showing no evidence of acute CNS disease. This would suggest that prompt treatment of seizures in adults would be associated with good control of seizures and low mortality (1,3,14). In contrast, patients with encephalopathy, tumors, acute vascular disease, or recent trauma may continue to have seizures after phenytoin, additional antiepileptic drugs, and other interventions (1,3,14,17). Patients who died within the study period had severe abnormalities that were sufficient to account for death without implicating seizures (1,14).

Considering the low risk of phenytoin infusion, we believe that treatment is indicated before status develops. Furthermore, because antiepileptic drug withdrawal may precipitate status epilepticus (9,10,16), infusion of phenytoin should be given for exacerbation of seizures in any epileptic outpatient in whom drug concentrations are low. When antiepileptic drug concentrations are not available at the time of infusion, use of an 18-mg/kg dose of phenytoin is recommended. Because the volume of distribution of phenytoin is 0.78 liter/kg, a dose of 18 mg/kg increases the plasma concentration by approximately 23 $\mu g/ml$ (4). This increase is not associated with toxic effects unless the preinfusion concentration is more than 20 $\mu g/ml$. Furthermore, even though one-third of our epileptic patients had "therapeutic" concentrations prior to infusion, the increase in phenytoin concentration was effective in suppressing seizures.

Most previous reports have focused on the effectiveness of drugs in treating status epilepticus rather than dealing with the full spectrum of acute seizures (1,17). Our study indicates that seizure frequency prior to treatment is less important than the cause of the acute seizures. Thus, patients with focal or diffuse encephalopathy had poor results, regardless of seizure frequency prior to treatment.

Although diazepam has been widely used for treatment of status epilepticus, our results and those of others indicate that this drug has a brief duration of action (2,8,15). It has often been suggested that status initially be treated with diazepam, followed by phenytoin (6). However, our results indicate that many patients may be successfully treated with phenytoin alone. If diazepam is used initially, phenytoin loading should be performed immediately to prevent recurrent seizures.

Following intravenous administration, phenytoin distributes rapidly to the brain (7,18). Anticonvulsant activity of phenytoin in rats is present as soon as 3 min after infusion (11), and the major limiting factor in clinical application is the slow rate of administration required to avoid cardiovascular complications (17).

ACKNOWLEDGMENTS

The assistance provided by Ruth Lowenson in statistical analysis of data and the advice given by Ronald Sawchuck regarding pharmacokinetic aspects is gratefully acknowledged.

This study was supported by contract NO1-NS-5–2327 from the National Institute for Neurological and Communicative Disorders and Stroke.

REFERENCES

1. Celesia, C. G. (1976): Modern concepts of status epilepticus. *J. A. M. A.*, 235:1571–1574.
2. Celesia, C. G., Booker, H. E., and Sato, S. (1974): Brain and serum concentrations of diazepam in experimental epilepsy. *Epilepsia*, 15:417–425.

3. Celesia, C. G., Messert, B., and Murphy, M. J. (1972): Status epilepticus of late adult onset. *Neurology (Minneap.)*, 22:1047–1055.

4. Cranford, R. E., Leppik, I. E., Patrick, B., Anderson, C. B., and Kostick, B. (1978): Intravenous phenytoin: clinical and pharmacokinetic aspects. *Neurology*, 28:874–880.

5. Cranford, R. E., Leppik, I. E., Patrick, B. K., Anderson, C. B., and Kostick, B. (1979): Intravenous phenytoin in acute treatment of seizures. *Neurology*, 29:1474–1479.

6. Duffy, F. H., and Lombroso, C. T. (1978): Treatment of status epilepticus. In: *Clinical Neuropharmacology, Vol. 3*, edited by H. L. Klawans, pp. 41–56. Raven Press, New York.

7. Firemark, H., Barlow, C. F., and Roth, L. J. (1963): The entry, accumulation and binding of diphenylhydantoin-2-C[14] in brain. *Int. J. Neuropharmacol.*, 2:25–38.

8. Howard, F. M., Jr., Seybold, M. E., and Reihr, J. (1968): The treatment of recurrent convulsions with intravenous injection of diazepam. *Med. Clin. North Am.*, 52:977–987.

9. Hunter, R. A. (1959/60): Status epilepticus: History, incidence and problems. *Epilepsia*, 4:162–188.

10. Janz, D. (1961): Conditions and causes of status epilepticus. *Epilepsia*, 2:170–177.

11. Leppik, I. E., and Sherwin, A. L. (1979): Intravenous phenytoin and phenobarbital anticonvulsant action, brain content and plasma binding in rat. *Epilepsia*, 20:201–207.

12. Naquet, R., Soulayrol, R., Dolce, G., Tassinari, C. A., Broughton, R., and Loeb, H. (1965): First attempts at treatment of experimental status epilepticus in animals and spontaneous status epilepticus in man with diazepam (Valium). *Electroencephalogr. Clin. Neurophysiol.*, 18:427.

13. Noach, E. L., Woodbury, D. M., and Goodman, L. S. (1958): Studies on the absorption, distribution, fate and excretion of 4-C[14] labeled diphenylhydantoin. *J. Pharmacol. Exp. Ther.*, 122:301–314.

14. Oxbury, J. M., and Whitty, C. W. M. (1971): Causes and consequences of status epilepticus in adults. *Brain*, 94:733–744.

15. Prensky, A. L., Raff, M. C., Moore, M. J., and Schwab, R. S. (1967): Intravenous diazepam in the treatment of prolonged seizure activity. *N. Eng. J. Med.*, 276:779–784.

16. Rowan, A. J., and Scott, D. F. (1970): Major status epilepticus: A series of 42 patients. *Acta Neurol. Scand.*, 46:573–584.

17. Wallis, W., Kutt, H., and McDowell, F. (1968): Intravenous diphenylhydantoin in treatment of acute repetitive seizures. *Neurology (Minneap.)*, 18:513–525.

18. Wilder, B. J., Ramsay, E., Wilmore, L. J., Feussner, G. F., Perchalski, R. J., and Shumate, J. B. (1977): Efficacy of intravenous phenytoin in the treatment of status epilepticus. *Ann. Neurol.*, 1:511–518.

Advances in Neurology, Vol. 34: Status Epilepticus, edited by A.V. Delgado-Escueta, C.G. Wasterlain, D.M. Treiman, and R.J. Porter. Raven Press, New York © 1983.

46

A New Phenytoin Infusion Concentrate for Status Epilepticus

H.-H. von Albert

Intravenous infusion of phenytoin has been reported as the best method of controlling and preventing repetitive seizures, restoring consciousness, and stabilizing respiratory exchange in status epilepticus (3,8,10,11). These reports were confirmed in the study (10) briefly summarized here.

METHODS

A total of 84 patients with status epilepticus or repeated seizures, ages 15 to > 70 (Table 1) were treated with an infusion concentrate of phenytoin (Phenhydan®), now available only in Germany, Austria, and Switzerland (Desitin-Werke, Hamburg, West Germany). This is a 50-ml solution containing 750 mg of phenytoin; it was diluted with 500 ml of saline or dextrose solution for intravenous administration. Infusions were given as rapidly as possible, usually within 5 to 20 min. The infusion was slowed if the status epilepticus was broken. Serum phenytoin concentrations were estimated before and after infusion.

RESULTS

Rapid intravenous infusion of this phenytoin preparation was extremely effective in controlling status epilepticus and repeated seizures. Status epilepticus was broken during infusion in 75% of the patients (Fig. 1) and ended some minutes after infusion in 10% of them. The treatment had minimal or no effect in 15%, the persistence of status epilepticus being associated with conditions such as delirium tremens or severe encephalitis.

Serum phenytoin concentrations were determined in 49 patients with status epilepticus (Table 2), ranging from 11.6 to 41.0 μg/ml (mean 19.9 μg/ml) in patients not pretreated with phenytoin. With phenytoin premedication, concentrations ranged from 3.9 to 24.8 μg/ml (mean 8.7 μg/ml) before infusion and from 9.6 to 39.0 μg/ml (mean 23.6 μg/ml) afterward, the increase ranging from 7.1 to 30.9 μg/ml (mean 15.7 μg/ml).

TABLE 1. *Age distribution of patients with status epilepticus*

Age (yr)	No. of patients
≧70	6
65–69	2
60–64	8
55–59	5
50–54	1
45–49	2
40–44	11
35–39	24
30–34	5
25–29	6
20–24	8
15–19	6

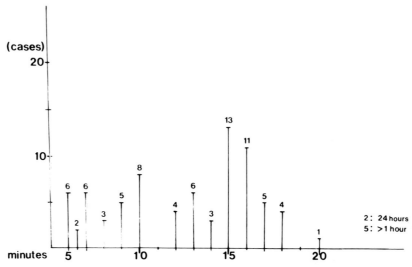

FIG. 1. Time to cessation of status epilepticus after initiation of phenytoin infusion in 84 patients. Status epilepticus was controlled in 5 to 20 min in 77 patients, in more than 1 hr in 5 patients, and in 24 hr in 2 patients. Numbers over bars indicate numbers of patients.

TABLE 2. *Serum phenytoin concentrations in patients with status epilepticus treated by phenytoin infusion (N = 49)*

Without phenytoin premedication (N = 19)	
After infusion	19.9 (11.6–41.0) μg/ml
With phenytoin premedication (N = 30)	
Before infusion	8.7 (3.9–24.8) μg/ml
After infusion	23.6 (9.6–39.0) μg/ml
Increase	15.7 (7.1–30.9) μg/ml

Serum and CSF phenytoin concentrations were estimated in 1 patient (Fig. 2). Status epilepticus was under control 11 min after treatment.

In another 34 patients, the phenytoin infusion was used to reach therapeutic concentrations of phenytoin rapidly in patients with repeated seizures (two to four seizures within a few hours). In these patients the infusions were given over a period of 30 min to 3 hr.

Local and systemic tolerances to the infusions were good. A few patients experienced nystagmus or drowsiness after the status epilepticus was controlled, but there was no respiratory depression or hypotension.

Mortality due to status epilepticus in this group was 4.1%; 4 patients with hemorrhagic encephalitis and 1 patient with hematoma also died.

DISCUSSION

The diluted phenytoin concentrate can be infused either rapidly or over a period of hours. The phenytoin is solubilized in tetraglycol (Glycofurol®) with a small amount of Tris buffer, and there is no danger of crystallization. After mixing, the solution has a pH of approximately 10 and is stable for hours (5,6).

A survey of the pharmacological and toxicological characteristics of injectable phenytoin solutions has been made by Leuschner et al. (4). According to Anschel (1) and Spiegel and Noseworthy (7), the phenytoin solution produced with tetraglycol and Tris buffer has both pharmacological and toxicological advantages over the customary phenytoin solutions (e.g., with propylene glycol/ethanol/water as solvent). The latter are not without danger of minor crystallization (2).

Of special interest in this study is the fact that the rapidly given phenytoin infusion concentrate was effective in 3 patients who had failed to respond to intravenous doses of 750 to 1,000 mg of phenytoin in divided doses of 250 mg each within 2 to 5 hr before admission to our hospital.

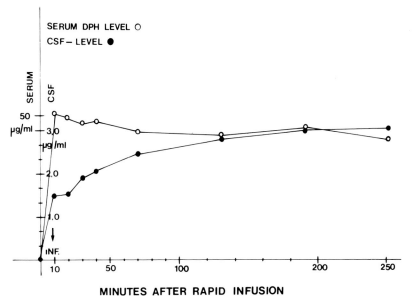

FIG. 2. Serum and CSF concentrations of phenytoin (DPH) after phenytoin infusion (750 mg within 6 min) in 1 patient.

There were no severe or long-lasting side effects in our patients. The contraindications to intravenous phenytoin therapy, however, are well known: severe arteriosclerotic heart disease, cardiac dysrhythmias, or cardiac block.

It should be noted that the effectiveness of this treatment does not depend on the type of convulsion,[1] but the lack of effectiveness does depend on the type of cerebral lesion. Further, status epilepticus in patients with a history of alcoholism is best treated with controlled infusion of clomethiazole (Distaneurine®).

This same phenytoin infusion concentrate, administered over a period of 30 min to 4 hr, was used to treat trigeminal neuralgia (9). Again, crystallization was no problem, and the infusion was well tolerated.

CONCLUSION

The medical emergency of status epilepticus is best dealt with by rapid intravenous administration of phenytoin. The phenytoin infusion concentrate used in this study effectively controls status epi-

lepticus and repeated seizures, poses no danger of crystallization, can be given within minutes, and is well tolerated. Less effective methods may take hours or days to control the status epilepticus.

REFERENCES

1. Anschel, J. (1965): Lösungsmittel und Lösungsvermittler in Injektionen. *Pharm. Indust.*, 27:781–787.
2. Cloyd, J. C., Gumnit, R. J., and McLain, L. W., Jr. (1980): Status epilepticus. The role of intravenous phenytoin. *J. A. M. A.*, 244:1479–1481.
3. Cranford, R. E., Leppik, I. E., Patrick, B., Anderson, C. B., and Kostick, B. (1978): Intravenous phenytoin: Clinical and pharmacokinetic aspects. *Neurology*, 28:874–880.
4. Leuschner, F., Neumann, W., and Reith, H. (1977): Beitrag zur Pharmakologie und Toxikologie injizierbarer Phenytoin-Lösungen. *Arzneim. Forsch.*, 27:811–819.
5. Reith, H. (1979): German phenytoin formulation compatible with intravenous fluids. *Am. J. Hosp. Pharm.*, 36:1317.
6. Reith, H. (1979): Availability of phenytoin infusion concentrate. *Drug Intell. Clin. Pharm.*, 13:783.
7. Spiegel, A. J., and Noseworthy, M. M. (1963): Use of nonaqueous solvents in parenteral products. *J. Pharm. Sci.*, 52:917–927.
8. Sutton, G. G. (1980): Emergency management of seizures in adults. In: *Neurologic Emergencies: Recognition and Management*, edited by M. Salcman, pp. 165–179. Raven Press, New York.
9. von Albert, H.-H. (1978): Infusionsbehandlung der akuten Trigeminus-neuralgie mit Phenytoin i.v. *Munch. Med. Wochenschr.*, 120:529–530.

---

[1]The editors disagree; available evidence shows that intravenous phenytoin and diazepam are more effective in primary generalized convulsive status epilepticus, such as tonic-clonic, clonic-tonic-clonic, and clonic status epilepticus.

10. von Albert, H.-H. (1980): Die Therapie des Status
    epilepticus. Neue Entwicklungen, Phenytoin-Schnel-
    linfusion. In: *Anästhesie bei zerebralen Krampfan-
    fällen und Intensivtherapie des Status epilepticus*, edited
    by A. Opitz and R. Degen, pp. 209–215. Perimed,
    Erlangen.

11. Wilder, B. J., Ramsay, R. E., Willmore, L. J., Feuss-
    ner, G. F., Perchalski, R. J., and Shumate, J. B., Jr.
    (1977): Efficacy of intravenous phenytoin in the treat-
    ment of status epilepticus: Kinetics of central nervous
    system penetration. *Ann. Neurol.*, 1:511–518.

Advances in Neurology, Vol. 34: Status Epilepticus, edited by A.V. Delgado-Escueta, C.G. Wasterlain, D.M. Treiman, and R.J. Porter. Raven Press, New York © 1983.

48

Benzodiazepines: Efficacy in Status Epilepticus

C. A. Tassinari, O. Daniele, R. Michelucci, M. Bureau, C. Dravet, and J. Roger

As it became evident that paroxysmal generalized spike or multiple spike-and-wave discharges were immediately abolished by intravenous injection of certain benzodiazepines (26,27), the next predictable step was to use these drugs in the treatment of status epilepticus. Consequently, first diazepam (13,22) and then clonazepam (12) gained wide recognition as extremely effective drugs for this purpose. It is now evident, however, that benzodiazepines obviously do not provide unique and definitive treatment for status epilepticus of all kinds. In this chapter we shall first review the literature on benzodiazepine efficacy in status epilepticus and then present complementary data from our own studies.

BENZODIAZEPINES AND ROUTES OF ADMINISTRATION

The benzodiazepines most used in the treatment of status epilepticus are diazepam (Valium®) and clonazepam (Rivotril®, Clonopin®). Nitrazepam (Mogadon®) has also been used to a limited extent (3,19,29), and, most recently, lorazepam (Ativan®) has been considered for treatment of status epilepticus (1,37,38). These drugs are administered intravenously or intramuscularly, and some, mainly diazepam, can also be used rectally, with absorption and efficacy analogous to or superior to that of the intramuscular route. The following discussion will concentrate on diazepam and clon-

azepam, which, by slow (1–2 min) intravenous injection at variable dosages (10–20 mg and 1–2 mg, respectively), have quite similar effectiveness, rapidity of action, and side effects *(vide infra)*.

PREVIOUS STUDIES

The use of benzodiazepines in the treatment of epilepsy was comprehensively reviewed by Browne and Penry (9), who dealt mainly with diazepam, by Pinder et al. (25), who dealt with clonazepam, and by Fröscher (11) in an excellent monograph on the treatment of status epilepticus. The effectiveness of clonazepam in status epilepticus was also considered in 1972 at a symposium in Marseille (30). Also available are general reviews of status epilepticus that refer specifically to treatment with benzodiazepines as well as other drugs (10,29,34).

Diazepam

In Browne and Penry's review of 35 articles on the use of benzodiazepines in 439 cases of status epilepticus, diazepam was considered "to be very effective in grand mal, secondarily generalized grand mal, focal motor, absence, myoclonic and hemiclonic status epilepticus. In patients with these types of status epilepticus, lasting control was achieved in 63–83% and temporary control in 10–27%. Absence status was the most sensitive to diazepam, temporary or lasting control being obtained in 93% of these cases" (Table 1). These authors concluded that "a large body of evidence shows diazepam to be extremely effective in a wide range of types of status epilepticus. Intravenous diazepam is probably the drug of choice in this condition" (9).

Clonazepam

From the review of Pinder et al. (25) on the effectiveness of clonazepam in 417 cases of status epilepticus (Table 2), it would appear that it may not be fair to compare the mean positive results achieved with clonazepam (84.5%) with the "lasting control" achieved with diazepam (70.4%). It can safely be assumed, however, that clonazepam has a quite large spectrum of effectiveness, similar to that of diazepam, and that the higher percentage of positive results in this review pertains to the use of clonazepam in status epilepticus with tonic-clonic seizures or in cases of petit mal or absence status, the latter probably encompassing various conditions. Even so, more than half the cases of status epilepticus involved chronic, mostly generalized, epilepsy. The remaining cases were status epilepticus with partial seizures and 27 cases with hemiclonic status. Of the 21 cases of status epilepticus with tonic seizures, one-third did not respond to treatment.

Data on 194 patients (49 children, 128 adults, 17 aged patients) collected from 20 French laboratories by Beck and Tousch (4) seem generally to agree with the findings of other studies. These

data showed that clonazepam was effective in 80% of cases after a single injection of approximately 1 mg; in the remaining cases, clonazepam had to be given repeatedly up to a daily dose of 13 to 18 mg in order to control the status. It was also found that clonazepam, like other drugs, had its lowest rate of success in status epilepticus symptomatic of acute brain lesions (e.g., vascular, anoxic). The occurrence of side effects (namely, hypotension and respiratory disturbances) was also relatively greater in such cases, owing partly to the large doses of benzodiazepines required and partly, and above all, to the severe underlying brain lesion.

Side Effects of Benzodiazepine Injections

The hope and fear attending the introduction of a new drug lead to overemphasis of both its effectiveness and its dangers. Fear of the dangers of benzodiazepine injection constitutes, in our opinion, an example of such overemphasis, as evidenced by case reports from 1967 to 1971, mainly concerning diazepam. The side effects of benzodiazepines can be divided into three major groups related to (a) respiratory function and hypotension, (b) local adverse effects, and (c) paradoxical effects (precipitation of tonic status).

Respiratory Depression and Hypotension

In the study of Browne and Penry (9), 16 cases of respiratory depression and 10 cases of hypotension were associated with the injection of diaze-

TABLE 1. *Efficacy of diazepam in the treatment of status epilepticus*

Type of status epilepticus	No. of patients	No effect	Temporary control[a]	Lasting control[b]
Grand mal (all types)	188	23 (12%)	37 (20%)	128 (68%)
Secondary generalized grand mal	38	4 (10%)	6 (16%)	28 (74%)
Focal motor	103	13 (13%)	15 (15%)	75 (73%)
Absence	30	2 (7%)	3 (10%)	25 (83%)
Myoclonic	28	4 (14%)	4 (14%)	20 (71%)
Partial (temporal lobe)	8	2 (25%)	1 (13%)	5 (62%)
Tonic	8	3 (38%)	0	5 (62%)
Clonic	9	1 (11%)	0	8 (89%)
Hemiclonic	22	2 (9%)	6 (27%)	14 (63%)
Infantile myoclonic	5	0	4 (80%)	1 (20%)
Total	439	54 (12.3%)	76 (17.3%)	309 (70.4%)

Adapted from Browne and Penry (9).

[a]Status epilepticus was not controlled for more than 24 hr with three or fewer injections of diazepam, or more than three injections were required for control of status epilepticus within 24 hr.

[b]Uninterrupted control of status epilepticus for more than 24 hr with three or fewer injections.

TABLE 2. *Efficacy of clonazepam in the treatment of status epilepticus*

Ref.	No. of cases	Type of status epilepticus	Positive response (%)
Bergamini et al. (6)	12	6 Tonic-clonic 2 Absence 2 Jacksonian 1 Temporal 1 Tonic	88
Papini (23)	5	3 Myoclonic 1 Hemiconvulsive 1 Unclassified	60
Giménez-Roldán et al. (14)	17		97
Kruse and Blank-enhorn (17)	40	26 Absence 4 Tonic-clonic 4 Psychomotor 2 Epilepsia partia-lis continua 2 Myoclonic 2 "Electrical"	75
Tridon and Weber (35)	30	10 Tonic-clonic 2 Tonic 8 Absence 9 Partial motor 1 Partial adversive	84
Bladin (8)	8		100
Martin and Hirt (20)	13	7 Absence 2 Tonic-clonic 3 Partial focal 1 Psychomotor	77
Ketz et al. (16)	65	13 Tonic-clonic 9 Absence 1 Hepatic coma 39 Corticofocal 3 Psychomotor	83
Beck and Tousch (4)[a]	194	33 Tonic-clonic 18 Tonic 16 Clonic and myo-clonic 29 Absence status 58 Partial 26 Hemiclonic 2 Hemitonic 12 Unclassified	81
Gregoriades and Frangos (15)	31	22 Tonic-clonic 9 Absence	100

Adapted from Pinder et al. (25).

[a]Comprising 36 cases of Gastaut et al. (12) and unpublished observations from 20 French neurological departments.

pam. Respiratory depression followed the injection of clonazepam in 5 patients reported by Beck and Tousch (4) and in 3 patients of Tridon and Weber (35). A detailed review of these 34 cases allows the following remarks:

1. More than two-thirds of the patients who showed cardiorespiratory distress had also received large doses of barbiturates prior to the benzodiazepines, a situation also noted in the often quoted series of Bell (5).

2. Thirty-one of the cases had clear-cut evidence of severe acute brain lesions (trauma, hemorrhage, infections, anoxia, or metabolic disturbances, mainly diabetic encephalopathies). Such pathological conditions were responsible for the fatal outcome in half of the patients and could also have accounted per se for the cardiorespiratory disturbances (24). Obviously, benzodiazepines could have been a factor rendering more evident the impending cardiorespiratory failure in such conditions.

3. In the 3 patients without evidence of such acute brain lesions, the benzodiazepine injection provoked only a transient, never fatal, depression of respiration. In some instances, it could have been only a matter of sleep-related apnea (21,36).

4. Cardiorespiratory distress could hardly be related to a previous benzodiazepine injection when the distress occurred several minutes or even hours after the injection, as, for example, after 10 min (36), after 45 min in a 2.5-year-old boy with a bleeding glioma (39), and after 3 hr in a patient with diabetic coma (21).

Local Complications

Local complications, mainly venous thrombosis, may occur at the site of the benzodiazepine injection. However, in a review provoked by a startling article on the loss of a limb following intravenous diazepam, not one significant local vascular complication was found in a total of 15,813 injections (33). Overall, the dangers of local complications from intravenous or intramuscular injections of benzodiazepines seem irrelevant.

Paradoxical Effects

Paradoxical effects, such as the precipitation of tonic status epilepticus, have been reported with the use of nitrazepam and diazepam (28,31,32) and also with clonazepam (7). These effects have been observed in 7 patients so far and usually occur in patients with Lennox-Gastaut syndrome, in whom benzodiazepine injections, as well as other antiepileptic drugs or anesthetics, can induce brief bouts of tonic status epilepticus. More frequently observed, albeit still rare, is a transient increase in subclinical paroxysmal discharges immediately after injection of diazepam (18) or clonazepam (6). It should also be noted that high plasma concentrations of orally administered clonazepam can also increase tonic seizures to the extent of status epilepticus (2).

In conclusion, after reviewing the efficacy and side effects of benzodiazepines, we agree with Browne and Penry (9) that "the benefits of careful intravenous administration probably outweigh the possible hazards." Furthermore, after 15 years of worldwide use of benzodiazepines, we can safely substitute "certainly" for "probably."

PERSONAL EXPERIENCE

Patients and Methods

These findings concern patients treated from 1965 to 1980 in the Centre St. Paul, Marseille, where benzodiazepines were largely used by the intravenous route or, less frequently, the intramuscular route in epileptic and nonepileptic conditions. By 1974, more than 900 benzodiazepine injections had been given, usually under polygraphic control, i.e., electroencephalography, electrocardiography, pneumoencephalography, and electromyography.

We shall discuss only those patients in whom status epilepticus was treated by single or repeated injections of benzodiazepines with continuous polygraphic monitoring for hours up to several days and nights. We shall not include cases of partial status epilepticus, because considerable data on this type of status have been reported. Also excluded are those cases of status epilepticus previously reported by Gastaut et al. (12,13).

Table 3 shows our population of 78 patients, mostly children, who had frequently repeated status epilepticus for a total of 129 episodes. They were treated with single or repeated injections of 10 to 20 mg of diazepam or 2 to 3 mg of clonazepam (diazepam was used 81 times and clonazepam 66 times).

Results

The effectiveness of benzodiazepines on status epilepticus varied greatly, depending on the type of epilepsy (see Conclusions). Our findings in children with secondary generalized epilepsy (Table 4) complement the findings of other studies (Tables 1 and 2) dealing mostly with status epilepticus in patients with primary generalized epilepsy or partial epilepsies. We considered that the benzodiazepines were ineffective when status epilepticus was not at all modified electroclinically (no effect), when changes were evident but were of little relevance, such as a relative decrease in amplitude of the EEG discharges or a transitory decrease, disappearance, or modification of the motor modifications (no effect), or when changes were only of short duration (temporary control). In 100 episodes of status epilepticus, benzodiazepines were effective in only 38%. Such an extremely low rate of benzodiazepine effectiveness calls for two comments:

1. Such poor results should be viewed in the context of the severe epileptic conditions of our patients, as evidenced by the high incidence of repeated status.

2. The episodes of tonic status and absence status with or without myoclonias deserve special mention.

In other studies, *tonic status* was consistently resistant to treatment, lasting control being achieved

TABLE 3. *Efficacy of benzodiazepines in 129 episodes of status epilepticus in 78 patients from Centre St. Paul, Marseille (1965–1980)*

No. of patients	Episodes of status epilepticus	Type of status epilepticus[a]	Type of epilepsy	Lasting control
5	5	Absence status	Primary generalized	100%
6	6	Hemiclonic[b]		100%
55	100	Various (see Table 4)	Secondary generalized	38%
12	18	Various	Various causes in non-epileptics	0%–100%

[a]Partial status epilepticus is excluded.
[b]In children without focal brain lesions.

TABLE 4. *Efficacy of benzodiazepines in status epilepticus in 55 patients with secondary generalized epilepsy, mainly Lennox-Gastaut syndrome, from Centre St. Paul, Marseille*

| Type of status epilepticus | Episodes of status epilepticus | Ineffective | | Effective |
		No effect	Temporary control	
Tonic-clonic	1		1 (100%)	
Hemiclonic	2			2 (100%)
Clonic and myoclonic	10			10 (100%)
Tonic	38	25 (65.8%)	8 (21.1%)	5 (13.1%)
Absence status	20	16 (80%)	1 (5%)	3 (15%)
Absence status with myoclonic components	29	5 (17.2%)	6 (20.7%)	17 (58.7%)
Total	100	46	16	38

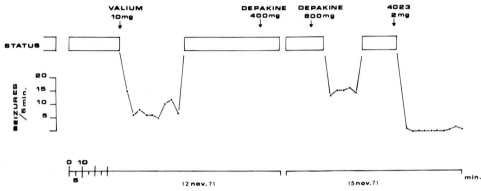

FIG. 1. Effect of diazepam (Valium®) versus valproate (Depakine®) and clonazepam (4023) in a 10-year-old patient with Lennox-Gastaut syndrome during the two episodes of status epilepticus illustrated in Figs. 2 and 3. **Left:** In status of November 12, diazepam (10 mg i.v.) effectively interrupted the status, but some seizures persisted; the control was only partial and temporary; valproate (400 mg i.v.) was ineffective. (The record was prolonged several hours and is not represented here.) **Right:** 3 days later. Valproate (800 mg i.v.) had a partial and transitory effect, whereas clonazepam was definitely effective.

in approximately 62% of patients treated with diazepam (Table 1) and in 65% of patients treated with clonazepam (Table 2). The resistance was even greater in our 38 cases of tonic status epilepticus; repeated injections of benzodiazepines achieved complete and lasting control in only 13% of cases (Table 4). In the remaining cases, the electroclinical features of the status were not modified at all or were only temporarily suppressed or decreased.

Absence status is a condition characterized essentially by clinically evident decreases in vigilance and performance ranging from mild to severe impairment of consciousness, usually accompanied by subcontinuous or continuous diffuse slow spike or multiple spike-and-wave discharges. Such absence status, with or without occasional muscle twitching, was successfully treated with benzodiazepine injections in only 15% of cases (Table 4). In absence status with frequent, well-evident asynchronous or arrhythmic myoclonia or with rhythmic synchronous clonia, the benzodiazepines achieved lasting control in 59% of cases (Table 4), a significantly higher rate than with absence status without evident clonic components. Such results are somewhat at variance with those in the literature, but these discrepancies will not be discussed here.

A most important conclusion stems from our data on absence status occurring in patients with secondary generalized epilepsy. Such absence status with or without myoclonic components should be definitively distinguished from other apparently similar electroclinical absence status occurring in

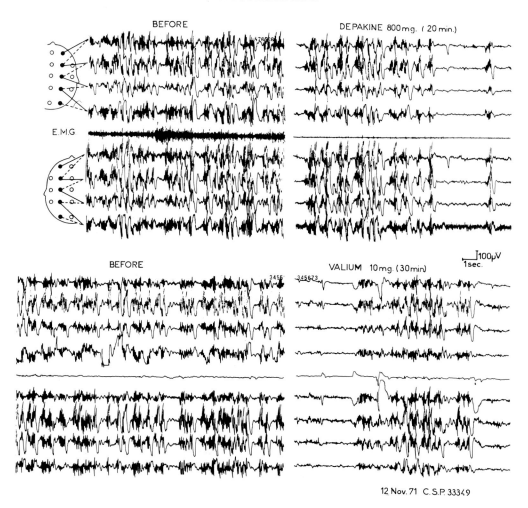

FIG. 2. Polygraphic record of the partial effects of valproate *(top)* and diazepam *(bottom)* in the patient from Fig. 1. Status was a combination of absence status and tonic seizures, with variable impairment of consciousness. **Left:** Before treatment. **Right:** After treatment.

patients with primary generalized epilepsy. The use of benzodiazepine injections in absence status occurring in secondary epilepsy has a very low percentage (15%–59%) of definite arrest of the status. Contrarily, absence status in patients with primary epilepsy is successfully treated with benzodiazepines in significantly higher percentages (90%–100%) of cases (see Conclusions).

Diazepam versus Clonazepam

Our patients with secondary generalized epilepsy and persistent status epilepticus offered a unique opportunity to compare the effectiveness of diazepam and that of clonazepam under continuous polygraphic and clinical control. There are

obvious difficulties in comparing various drugs for effectiveness in controlling status epilepticus, particularly when the drugs are similarly efficacious in the different types of status epilepticus, as is the case with diazepam and clonazepam. Furthermore, a patient can have more than one type of status (e.g., tonic status coexisting with absence status), or different episodes of an apparently single type of status in a patient can behave differently in response to a given treatment, depending on the chronic oral treatment, the general condition of the patient, the factors that precipitated the status, and so on.

During a single episode of status epilepticus in a given patient, how can we appreciate the effec-

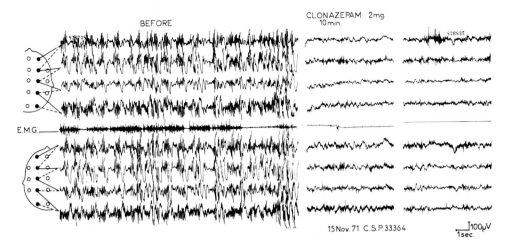

FIG. 3. Same patient as in Figs. 1 and 2. Clonazepam was definitely successful in controlling the status.

tiveness or the side effects of a drug when it is given after a previously administered one? We have seen that the side effects of benzodiazepines are enhanced by previous barbiturate treatment. In addition, if, for example, an injection of clonazepam is successfully given after a previously unsuccessful diazepam injection, how can we be sure that a second diazepam injection would not have had the same results?

Notwithstanding such limitations, it can be of some interest to compare the effects of diazepam and clonazepam in 17 of the 55 patients with secondary generalized epilepsy. These 17 patients had 28 episodes of status epilepticus. We can distinguish two subgroups:

1. The first subgroup consisted of 6 patients who during a given episode of status epilepticus (four of the tonic type, two of the absence type) received large doses of diazepam and clonazepam repeatedly and in various successions. Both drugs achieved only temporary control in 1 patient and were totally ineffective in 5 patients, the status continuing for hours and days.

2. The second subgroup consisted of the remaining 11 patients, each patient having two status episodes (total of 22 episodes) with similar electroclinical features. Either diazepam or clonazepam was given repeatedly in one or the other of the episodes. The drugs were equally ineffective in 7 patients (14 episodes), had similar temporary effects in 2 patients (4 episodes), and were equally effective in 1 patient (2 episodes). In 1 patient, clonazepam was more effective than diazepam (Figs. 1–3).

Overall, in our population of patients with Lennox-Gastaut syndrome, we can say that the effectiveness of diazepam and that of clonazepam in the control of status epilepticus were quite similar.

Benzodiazepines and Other Drugs

In 14 patients with Lennox-Gastaut syndrome (16 episodes of status epilepticus), both benzodiazepines and barbiturates were given during the evolution of a given episode. The results were the same regardless of whether the barbiturates were given before (3 patients with 3 episodes) or after (11 patients with 13 episodes) the benzodiazepines. The drugs were equally ineffective in 13 patients (14 episodes) and equally partially and temporarily effective in the remaining patient.

Benzodiazepines were compared with valproate (Depakine®) in 10 patients with Lennox-Gastaut syndrome (11 episodes of status epilepticus). The doses of valproate ranged from 20 to 43 mg/kg, which may have been too low. During a given episode of status epilepticus, valproate was given as the first drug in 4 patients (5 episodes) and after previously unsuccessful treatment with benzodiazepines in 6 patients (6 episodes). Valproate was ineffective in 9 of these 10 patients; in the remaining patient, the status progressively subsided when valproate was given after a previous benzodiazepine injection. The benzodiazepine treatment was effective in 4 patients, but it had no significant effect in the remaining 6 patients.

Benzodiazepine and phenytoin were given to 2 patients with Lennox-Gastaut syndrome (3 epi-

EPILEPSIA PARTIALIS CONTINUANS

sodes). Phenytoin, at intravenous doses ranging from 7 to 10 mg/kg, was as ineffective as the benzodiazepine.

Partly from these results and partly from our general experience, we can generally conclude that status of the tonic or absence type occurring in patients with Lennox-Gastaut syndrome is as resistant to other drugs as it is to the benzodiazepines. In these patients, excessive antiepileptic drug therapy should be avoided as ineffective or dangerous, and treatment should focus on general, cardiorespiratory, and metabolic care.

CONCLUSIONS

From the findings of others, and our own experience as well, it seems fair to conclude that benzodiazepines are among the most effective and safe drugs for the treatment of status epilepticus. Nevertheless, important distinctions can and should be made. Based on the efficacy of benzodiazepines, it seems possible to distinguish status epilepticus according to the *type of epilepsy* when the status occurs in patients with chronic epilepsy and to distinguish it according to the *etiological and neurological conditions* when the status occurs in nonepileptic patients.

Status Epilepticus in Patients with Chronic Epilepsy

1. Status epilepticus occurring during the evolution of primary generalized epilepsy, i.e., in patients with tonic-clonic seizures, typical 3/sec absences, or myoclonic jerks, and usually without neurological and psychic deficits, is successfully treated in 90% to 100% of cases with a benzodiazepine injection (Tables 1–3) (34).

2. In our experience, hemiclonic status epilepticus, when occurring in the context of febrile convulsions in neurologically normal children, responds successfully to benzodiazepine treatment. Unfortunately, the reported data make it impos-

sible to distinguish true hemiclonic status in neurologically normal children from other status, erroneously termed "hemiclonic," that probably is composed of partial motor seizures due to focal brain lesions.

3. Status epilepticus in patients with secondary generalized epilepsy occurs mainly in those with Lennox-Gastaut syndrome. The most frequent status is of the tonic type or the absence type, with or without myoclonic or clonic components. Tonic status epilepticus is particularly resistant to treatment (complete control being achieved in 63% of the reported cases and in only 13% of cases in our experience). Absence status occurring in Lennox-Gastaut syndrome is also resistant to treatment, complete control being achieved in 15% to 59% of our cases. This constitutes a very low control rate compared with the efficacy of benzodiazepines in absence status occurring in primary epilepsy. For this reason, any statistical data on the effectiveness of benzodiazepines in absence status should take into account precisely the kind of epilepsy (primary or secondary) in which the absence status occurred. Unfortunately, such distinction was not made in the majority of previous reports.

In fact, in order to predict the effectiveness of benzodiazepines in status epilepticus among patients with chronic epilepsy, it would seem more relevant to know the type of epilepsy than the semiology of the status itself. This is particularly so for the various types of absence status, which are quite similar electroclinically whether occurring in patients with primary or secondary epilepsy (and at times when they result from a secondary generalization in partial epilepsy).

4. In partial status epilepticus (motor status, "temporal lobe" or "psychomotor" status), benzodiazepines give uniformly good results in 62% to 73% of cases (9). However, intravenous phenytoin, or some other drug, can be used as an alternative to benzodiazepines in partial status,

FIG. 4. Effect of benzodiazepines on epilepsia partialis continua. **Left:** Transitory effectiveness of clonazepam (Rivotril®), diazepam (Valium®), and valproate (Depakine®). The numbers of spikes were counted for 5 min before, immediately after, and 15 min after the injection. **Right:** Hemispheric and central spikes before clonazepam (A), after 1 mg of clonazepam (B), and after 2 mg of clonazepam (C,D). Myoclonias were recorded on the extensor muscles of the wrist (EMG Ext. WL) contralateral to the spikes. Benzodiazepines effectively but only temporarily suppressed the myoclonias and decreased the diffusion of the discharge. The myoclonias and discharges progressively reappeared as the effects of the drug abated.

particularly if phenytoin is to be the chronic oral treatment. Epilepsia partialis continua is obviously a separate consideration. In such cases, benzodiazepines achieve only symptomatic, temporary control of the status (Fig. 4).

Status Epilepticus in Nonepileptic Patients

We are in substantial agreement with other investigators on the treatment of status epilepticus occurring in previously nonepileptic patients as a result of a usually sudden and severe brain insult. In these instances, neither benzodiazepines nor any other antiepileptic drug can solve the problem. Benzodiazepines can give temporary, symptomatic relief, decreasing the motor manifestations of the seizures. Obviously, the important matter is not the status itself but the clinical conditions related to its cause (e.g., degree and site of the brain lesion, metabolic factors). In this context, benzodiazepines are certainly useful symptomatically.

When status epilepticus occurs in nonepileptic patients under "good" general conditions (e.g., petit mal status in the aged, particularly women; occasional status related to hormonal factors), it is our experience that benzodiazepines can be helpful, but reports on the subjects, unfortunately, are scarce.

SUMMARY

Both our personal experience and the findings of others indicate that the benzodiazepines (a) are the drugs of first choice for control of status epilepticus occurring in patients with primary generalized epilepsy (90%–100% effective) or control of hemiclonic convulsions in children without brain lesions, (b) are effective in approximately 60% of cases of status epilepticus occurring in partial epilepsy, (c) are effective in only 15% to 59% of cases of tonic status or various types of absence status occurring in secondary generalized epilepsy (but no other drug is more effective), (d) are helpful in status epilepticus occurring in nonepileptic patients if there is no overt brain lesion (but give only temporary relief when status is the result of a severe organic brain lesion), and (e) are generally safe drugs.

REFERENCES

1. Amand, G., and Evrard, P. (1976): Injectable lorazepam in epilepsy. *Rev. Electroencephalogr. Neurophysiol. Clin.*, 6:532–533.
2. Baruzzi, A., Bordo, B., Bossi, L., Castelli, D., Gerna, M., Tognoni, G., and Zagnoni, P. (1977): Plasma levels of di-*n*-propylacetate and clonazepam in epileptic patients. *Int. J. Clin. Pharmacol. Biopharm.*, 15:403–408.
3. Baruzzi, A,. Michelucci, R., and Tassinari, C. A. (1982): Benzodiazepines: Nitrazepam. In: *Antiepileptic Drugs*, ed. 2, edited by D. M. Woodbury, J. K. Penry, and C. E. Pippenger, pp. 753–770. Raven Press, New York.
4. Beck, H., and Tousch, C. (1973): Management of status epilepticus by clonazepam. *Sem. Hop. Ther. (Paris)* [Supp.,], 49:21–27.
5. Bell, D. S. (1969): Dangers of treatment of status epilepticus with diazepam. *Br. Med. J.*, 1:159–161.
6. Bergamini, L., Mutani, R., Fariello, R., and Liboni, W. (1970): Elektroenzephalographische und klinische Bewertung des neuen Benzodiazepin Ro 5/4023. *EEG-EMG*, 1:182–188.
7. Bittencourt, P. R. M., and Richens, A. (1981): Anticonvulsant-induced status epilepticus in Lennox-Gastaut syndrome. *Epilepsia*, 22:129–134.
8. Bladin, C. F. (1973): The use of clonazepam as an anticonvulsant—clinical evaluation. *Med. J. Aust.*, 1:683–688.
9. Browne, T. R., and Penry, J. K. (1973): Benzodiazepines in the treatment of epilepsy: A review. *Epilepsia*, 14:277–310.
10. Duffy, F. H., and Lombroso, C. T. (1978): Treatment of status epilepticus. In: *Clinical Neuropharmacology, Vol. 3*, edited by H. L. Klawans, pp. 41–56. Raven Press, New York.
11. Fröscher, W. (1980): *Treatment of Status Epilepticus*. University Park Press, Baltimore.
12. Gastaut, H., Courjon, J., Poiré, R., and Weber, M. (1971): Treatment of status epilepticus with a new benzodiazepine more active than diazepam. *Epilepsia*, 12:197–214.
13. Gastaut, H., Naquet, R., Poiré, R., and Tassinari, C. A. (1965): Treatment of status epilepticus with diazepam (Valium). *Epilepsia*, 6:167–182.
14. Giménez-Roldán, S., Peraita, P., López Agreda, J. M., and Martin, J. F. (1972): Un nuevo medicamento eficaz en el tratamiento del "status" epilepico (Ro 5–4023). *Med. Clin. (Barcelona)*, 58:133–140.
15. Gregoriades, A. D., and Frangos, E. G. (1977): Clinical observations on clonazepam in intractable epilepsy. In: *Epilepsy: The Eighth International Symposium*, edited by J. K. Penry, pp. 169–175. Raven Press, New York.
16. Ketz, E., Bernouilli, C., and Siegfried, J. (1973): Clinical and EEG study of clonazepam (Ro 5–4023) with particular reference to status epilepticus. *Acta Neurol. Scand.* [Suppl. 53], 49:47.
17. Kruse, R., and Blankenhorn, V. (1973): Zusammenfassender Erfahrungsbericht über die klinische Anwendung und Wirksamkeit von Ro 5–4023 (Clonazepam) auf verschiedene Formen epileptischer Anfalle. *Acta Neurol. Scand.* [Suppl. 53], 49:60.
18. Lombroso, C. T. (1966): Treatment of status epilepticus with diazepam. *Neurology (Minneap.)*, 16:629–634.

19. Martin, D. (1970): The intravenous application of nitrazepam (Mogadan) in the treatment of epilepsy. *Neuropaediatrie*, 2:27–37.

20. Martin, D., and Hirt, H. R. (1973): Klinische Erfahrungen mit Clonazepam (Rivotril) in der Epilepsiebehandlung bei Kindern. *Neuropaediatrie*, 4:245.

21. McMorris, S., and McWilliam, P. K. A. (1969): Status epilepticus in infants and young children treated with parenteral diazepam. *Arch. Dis. Child.*, 44:604–611.

22. Naquet, R., Soulayrol, R., Dolce, G., Tassinari, C. A., Broughton, R., and Loeb, H. (1965): First attempt at treatment of experimental status epilepticus in animals and spontaneous status epilepticus in man with diazepam (Valium). *Electroencephalogr. Clin. Neurophysiol.*, 18:427.

23. Papini, M. (1971): The treatment of epilepsy in childhood and of status epilepticus with Ro 5–4023. *Electroencephalogr. Clin. Neurophysiol.*, 31:528.

24. Parsonage, M. J., and Norris, J. W. (1967): Use of diazepam in treatment of severe convulsive status epilepticus. *Br. Med. J.*, 3:85–88.

25. Pinder, R. M., Brogden, R. N., Speight, T. M., and Avery, G. S. (1976): Clonazepam: A review of its pharmacological properties and therapeutic efficacy in epilepsy. *Drugs*, 12:321–361.

26. Poiré, R., and Beck, L. (1973): Compared experimental electrographic assessment of anticonvulsant properties of clonazepam (Ro–05–4023), a new benzodiazepine derivative. *Sem. Hop. Ther. (Paris)* [Suppl.], 49:7–20.

27. Poiré, R., Roger, J., Lob, H., Regis, R., and Gastaut, H. (1963): Traitement des états de mal epileptiques pour le diazepam (Valium). In: *C. R. Congrès de Psychiatrie et de Neurologie de Langue Française, LXIII Session, Lausanne, 13–18 September 1965*, pp. 1259–1270. Masson, Paris.

28. Prior, P. F., Maclaine, G. N., Scott, D. F., and Laurance, B. M. (1972): Tonic status epilepticus precipitated by intravenous diazepam in a child with petit mal status. *Epilepsia*, 13:467–472.

29. Roger, J., Lob, H., and Tassinari, C. A. (1974): Status epilepticus. In: *Handbook of Clinical Neurology, Vol. 15, The Epilepsies*, edited by O. Magnus and A. M. Lorentz de Haas. North-Holland, Amsterdam.

30. Symposium on Ro–05–4023, Marseille, 1972 (1973): *Sem. Hop. Ther. (Paris)* [Suppl.], 49:1–76.

31. Tassinari, C. A., Dravet, C., Roger, J., Cano, J. P., and Gastaut, H. (1972): Tonic status epilepticus precipitated by intravenous benzodiazepine in five patients with Lennox-Gastaut syndrome. *Epilepsia*, 13:421–435.

32. Tassinari, C. A., Gastaut, H., Dravet, C., and Roger, J. (1971): A paradoxical effect: Status epilepticus induced by benzodiazepines. *Electroencephalogr. Clin. Neurophysiol.*, 31:182.

33. Tassinari, C. A., Roger, J., Dravet, C., and Gastaut, H. (1975): Comments on a startling article: Loss of limb following intravenous diazepam. *Pediatrics*, 6:898–899.

34. Treiman, D. M., and Delgado-Escueta, A. V. (1980): Status epilepticus. In: *Critical Care of Neurological and Neurosurgical Emergencies*, edited by R. A. Thompson and J. R. Green, pp. 55–99. Raven Press, New York.

35. Tridon, P., and Weber, M. (1973): How to conduct the treatment of status epilepticus with clonazepam. *Sem. Hop. Ther. (Paris)* [Suppl.], 49:29–31.

36. Van Melkebeek, A., and de Barsy, A. M. (1970): À propos d'un inconvénient rare, mais dramatique de l'utilisation du Diazépam intraveineux. *Acta Neurol. Belg.*, 70:286–294.

37. Walker, J. E., Homan, R. W., Vasco, M. R., Crawford, J. L., Bell, R. D., and Tasker, W. G. (1979): Lorazepam in status epilepticus. *Ann. Neurol.*, 6:207–213.

38. Waltregny, A., and Dargent, J. (1975): Preliminary study of parenteral lorazepam in status epilepticus. *Acta Neurol. Belg.*, 75:219–229.

39. Wilson, P. J. E. (1968): Treatment of status epilepticus in neurosurgical patients with diazepam (Valium). *Br. J. Clin. Pract.*, 22:21–24.

Advances in Neurology, Vol. 34: Status Epilepticus, edited by A.V. Delgado-Escueta, C.G. Wasterlain, D.M. Treiman, and R.J. Porter. Raven Press, New York © 1983.

49

Combination Therapy for Status Epilepticus: Intravenous Diazepam and Phenytoin

Antonio V. Delgado-Escueta and F. Enrile-Bacsal

Intravenous diazepam became the drug of choice in convulsive status epilepticus after initial reports on its efficacy by Gastaut et al. (7), Naquet et al. (13), and Bamberger and Matthes (1). According to Roger et al. (17), diazepam was effective in 85% of 350 cases of status epilepticus. Smith and Masotti (20) observed that diazepam was also effective in 87% of children with status epilepticus. Kaeser (11) and Tassinari (22) considered diazepam more effective than phenytoin in acutely stopping the continuing convulsions of status epilepticus. However, recurrence of seizures after temporary control of convulsions was frequently noted by several investigators. Reviewing the literature in 1973, Browne and Penry (2) noted that intravenous diazepam controlled convulsions of status epilepticus permanently in 63% to 83% of cases, and it controlled seizures temporarily in 10% to 27% of cases. Bamberger and Matthes (1) controlled 16 of 30 patients with status by using a single bolus injection of 10 mg diazepam. In the other 14 cases, seizures recurred after 15 to 120 min. A second injection produced definite control in 6 of these 14 cases. Prensky et al. (16) also reported on temporary control of convulsive status by intravenous diazepam. Seizures were interrupted for as long as 2 hr in only 9 of 20 patients. More recently, recurrences of seizures have been explained by the fast redistribution of intravenously administered diazepam into a large distribution volume. Thus,

initial high serum concentrations of diazepam rapidly drop to negligible serum concentrations in 15 min, and convulsions reappear.

Phenytoin was first used intravenously in the treatment of epilepsy by Murphy and Schwab (12). Wallis et al. (24) were the first investigators to use high doses of intravenous phenytoin (1,000–1,500 mg) in status epilepticus. In 1965, they reported a high failure rate; only 4 of 10 patients responded to phenytoin. They related the failure to the presence of active progressive neurological lesions as subdural hematoma and brain abscess. Most recently, Wilder et al. (25) and Cranford et al. (3,4) have shown the effectiveness of phenytoin in status epilepticus, demonstrating that it can be rapidly and safely administered intravenously without depressing respiration and level of alertness. These authors have, independently, shown that intravenous phenytoin stops 60% to 70% of convulsive status epilepticus.

However, if intravenous phenytoin is administered at the recommended maximum rate of 50 mg/min, it will take approximately 20 min to administer a full loading dose to an adult, and peak brain and cerebrospinal fluid concentrations may not be reached until another 30 min after completion of infusion. Thus, if a loading dose of phenytoin is infused as the only medication, seizures may continue during the infusion and for as long as 30 min after the infusion is completed.

In order to circumvent the disadvantages of the rapid decrease in serum diazepam concentration after its intravenous injection and the delay in intravenous phenytoin effects, we devised a combination treatment protocol for the management of convulsive status epilepticus. We combined an intravenous bolus of diazepam with intravenous phenytoin. In some instances, continuous infusion of diazepam was also used.

PATIENT SELECTION AND TREATMENT PROTOCOL

Patients were included in the protocol when they had at least two tonic-clonic seizures or two clonic-tonic-clonic seizures with no recovery of conciousness between seizures. Unconscious patients with generalized clonic jerks that continued for at least 30 min were also considered to have convulsive status epilepticus.

An endotracheal tube was inserted in each patient to assure an adequate airway and oxygenation. Intravenous fluids were started with normal saline (0.9% sodium chloride), and blood was withdrawn for measurement of antiepileptic drug concentration, glucose, blood urea nitrogen, electrolytes, and red and white blood cells. Blood pressure, respiration, and electroencephalogram were recorded. The EEG was recorded for at least two consecutive seizures. At the start of the second seizure, treatment was started. The EEG recording ensured that the patient was truly in status epilepticus.

A bolus injection of diazepam was given intravenously by a house officer or a nurse specialist at the rate of 2 mg/min for a total dose of 10 to 20 mg. Simultaneously, intravenous phenytoin was started in the opposite arm. In the first 28 patients, phenytoin was given at a rate of 50 mg every 2 min for a total of 300 mg. This was repeated every hour until a total dose of 15 mg/kg was administered over a span of 3 to 4 hr. In the remaining 22 patients, intravenous phenytoin was continuously administered at 50 mg/min to a total dose of 15 mg/kg. Phenytoin was given as a secondary drug in order to prevent recurrence of seizures.

If seizures recurred within 20 to 30 min after the initial bolus injection of diazepam, intravenous bolus injection of 20 mg diazepam was repeated or intravenous infusion of diazepam was started; 50 mg of diazepam in 500 ml of dextrose/water (D/W) was infused intravenously at a rate of 100 ml or 8 mg/hr for 3 hr.

Fifty patients were enrolled in the protocol. Fifteen patients had primarily generalized convulsions, as denoted by clinical and EEG patterns. Thirty-five patients had secondarily generalized tonic-clonic seizures (Table 1).

The EEGs of patients with primarily generalized seizures showed one of three patterns: (a) diffuse 8- to 10-Hz sharp waves (2 patients), (b) diffuse 1.5- to 5-Hz spike-and-slow-wave complexes (12 patients), (c) diffuse 16-Hz spikes (1 patient).

Of the 35 patients with secondarily generalized seizures, 29 showed focal 12- to 18-Hz spikes spreading diffusely, and 6 showed focal spikes repeating at 1/sec spreading diffusely.

EEG suppression bursts occurred in 26 patients during and after intravenous diazepam.

Of 35 patients with secondarily generalized tonic-clonic seizures, 7 patients had old cerebral infarctions, and 5 patients had acute infarctions (Table 2). Six cases were due to antiepileptic drug withdrawal. Four patients had CNS infections, of which two were pneumococcal meningitis and one was a presumed viral form of encephalitis. There were 4 patients with cerebral anoxia secondary to cardiorespiratory arrest and 3 patients with brain tumors. Two patients had seizures after craniotomy for evacuation of subdural hematoma, and 2 patients had a previous history of head injury. One case was attributed to a metabolic disorder suspected to be hyperosmolar nonketotic hyperglycemic coma.

Diazepam and desmethyldiazepam concentrations in the serum were measured by the laboratories of Hal Booker using electron-capture gas-liquid chromatography and double internal standardization according to the method of Greenblatt (8). Figure 1 shows the serum concentrations of diazepam in 2 patients whose seizures were controlled after single intravenous injections of 10 and 20 mg. The continuous line shows serum concentrations of diazepam in a patient whose seizures responded to a single injection of 10 mg. During the first 3 min, diazepam was measured at 0.5 μg/ml in serum. At 10 min, diazepam measured 0.4 μg/ml, and at 25 min diazepam measured 0.275 μg/ml. At 30 min, the diazepam concentration had decreased to 0.175 μg/ml.

The broken line in Fig. 1 shows serum concentrations of diazepam in a patient who received two bolus injections intravenously. Soon after the first bolus of 20 mg diazepam, the serum concentration measured 0.95 μg/ml. Twenty minutes later, the

TABLE 1. *Electroclinical patterns and causes of generalized convulsive status epilepticus*

Clinical and EEG features	Cause (proven or presumed)	No. of patients
Primary generalized		
Generalized clonic with diffuse 8–10-Hz	Lafora's disease	1
sharp waves	Kuf's disease	1
Clonic-tonic-clonic with diffuse 1.5–5-Hz	Positive family history	1
spike-wave complexes	Renal encephalopathy	1
	Multiple metabolic disorders	2
Tonic-clonic with diffuse 1.5–5-Hz spike-	Positive family history	3
slow-wave complexes	Encephalopathy associated with renal disease	3
	Kuf's disease	2
Tonic-clonic with diffuse 16-Hz spikes	No proven cause, but drug noncompliance	1
Secondary generalized		
Secondary tonic-clonic with focal 12–18	Diffuse or focal structural lesions	24
Hz spikes spreading diffusely	Diffuse focal structural lesions and drug non-compliance	5
Secondary tonic-clonic with focal 1 Hz	Focal structural lesion	6
spikes spreading diffusely		
Total		50

TABLE 2. *Causes of secondary generalized tonic-clonic seizures*

Proven or presumed cause	No. of patients
Acute meningitis	
Pneumococcal	2
Meningococcal	1
Encephalitis	1
Cerebral infarction, acute	5
Post cerebral infarction	7
Brain tumor	3
Cerebral anoxia (cardiac or respiratory arrest)	4
Antiepileptic drug withdrawal	6
Metabolic disorders	1
Post craniotomy (evacuation of subdural hematoma)	2
Posttraumatic	2

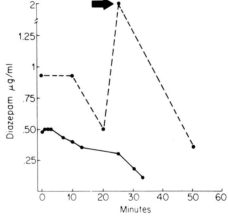

FIG. 1. Diazepam serum concentrations after intravenous bolus injections of 10 mg (solid line) and 20 mg (dash line).

plasma concentration dropped to 0.50 µg/ml. Seizures recurred a few minutes later, and a second intravenous bolus of 20 mg was given. This resulted in a rapid rise in serum concentration to 2 µg/ml. Twenty-five minutes after the second injection, diazepam was measured at 0.35 mg/ml in the serum.

To determine the amount and rate of diazepam infusion necessary to stop convulsive status, we studied 5 patients whose seizures recurred after intravenous injections of diazepam (Fig. 2). In these patients we established that diazepam serum con-

centrations varied from 0.3 µg/ml to 0.55 µg/ml when 50 mg of diazepam in 500 cc of 5% D/W was continuously infused at a rate of 8 mg/100 cc/hr. Hence, in the remaining patients requiring intravenous infusion, we used the same method (Fig. 2).

Nineteen patients were enrolled in our protocol without prior treatment (Table 3). Thirty-one patients received various forms of treatment that had failed prior to intravenous diazepam. Eight patients received 700 to 1,000 mg of phenobarbital at a slow rate. Twelve patients received 5 to 10 mg of

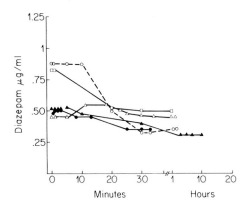

FIG. 2. Diazepam serum concentrations during intravenous infusions of 50 mg of diazepam in 500 cc of 5% D/W at 8 mg/100 cc/hr. Serum concentrations from five separate patients are represented.

TABLE 3. *Treatment failure before diazepam-phenytoin protocol*

I.	20 patients:	wrong rate of i.v. administration
	8 patients:	i.v. phenobarbital 700–1,000 mg (slow rate)
	12 patients:	i.v. diazepam 5–10 mg (slow rate)
II.	6 patients:	wrong drugs or wrong route
	1 patient:	i.m. Thorazine
	1 patient:	i.m. Librium
	3 patients:	i.m. diazepam
	1 patient:	i.m. phenobarbital
III.	5 patients:	unresponsive to i.v. phenytoin and/or barbiturates
	5 patients:	i.v. phenytoin 900 mg (50 mg/min); in 3 patients, combined with 700 to 1,000 mg of i.v. amobarbital or phenobarbital

diazepam, also at an extremely slow rate (2 mg/10 min). Five patients had received 900 mg of intravenous phenytoin.

In 3 of these patients, phenytoin treatment was combined with 700 to 1,000 mg of intravenous amobarbital or phenobarbital. Six patients either had received the wrong drug or had been given the drugs intramuscularly (Table 3).

RESULTS

Bolus intravenous injections of diazepam stopped convulsions in 32 patients. In another 18 patients, a single bolus injection temporarily stopped convulsions. When seizures recurred, intravenous infusion of diazepam stopped convulsions in 12 of

these patients. Six patients did not respond to our regimen and required intravenous paraldehyde and/or were placed under general anesthesia. Of these 6 unresponsive patients, 4 died. Two had pneumococcal meningitis, and 2 had cerebral anoxia secondary to cardiorespiratory arrest. Thus, we achieved long-lasting seizure control in 88% of our patients; 12% (6 patients) were resistant to diazepam and phenytoin.

Figure 3 depicts the rapidity of diazepam action. Convulsions stopped in 10% of patients 2 min after the start of intravenous bolus injections when 4 mg had been administered. Three minutes after the start of intravenous injection, seizures were controlled in 32% of patients. Five minutes after the start of intravenous diazepam, 68% of patients had their seizures controlled. Ten minutes after the start of intravenous treatment, seizures stopped in 80% of patients. Interestingly, seizures stopped in 4 patients 15 to 60 sec after completion of drug administration.

In our series of 50 patients, 18 patients received continuous infusion of diazepam for at least 3 hr, after one to three separate intravenous bolus injections failed to permanently control seizures. Table 4 lists the proven or presumed causes of status in these patients. Most commonly, progressing structural lesions were present, and there were 4 cases of metabolic disorders; acute cerebral infarctions, cerebral anoxia secondary to cardiorespiratory arrest, meningitis, encephalitis, cerebral

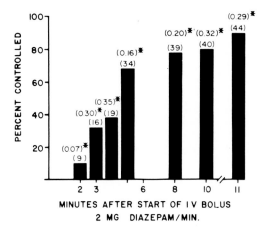

FIG. 3. Clinical responses to intravenous diazepam. Convulsions stopped in 32% of patients after 3 min, in 68% of patients after 5 min, and in 80% of patients after 10 min. * = average dose in mg/kg for the number of patients represented by the bar.

metastasis, and glioblastoma multiforme were also observed (Table 4).

The electroclinical patterns of status epilepticus and their responses to diazepam are depicted in Table 5. Patients with primarily generalized seizures responded quickly to bolus injections and rarely required intravenous infusion of diazepam. When intravenous infusions were necessary, patients with primarily generalized seizures usually had severe metabolic encephalopathies. As outlined in Table 4, the most common reason for requiring intravenous diazepam drip was the presence of a rapidly progressing CNS disease, e.g., acute infectious encephalopathies and severe cerebral anoxia.

Of the 12 patients who had previously received intravenous diazepam at an unusually slow rate (2 mg/10 min), as administered by physicians outside of our unit, 7 patients responded to a single 20-

mg bolus of intravenous diazepam. Seizures did not recur in these patients, suggesting that the rate of infusion of intravenous diazepam is an important factor in successful control of status. Four other patients responded to 20 mg of intravenous diazepam, but seizures recurred, requiring an intravenous drip. One other patient required intravenous paraldehyde infusion in spite of intravenous infusion of diazepam.

DISCUSSION AND OUTLOOK

Only since the nineteenth century has status epilepticus been a problem to neurologists. Status epilepticus occurred with more frequency after bromides were introduced as a form of treatment for chronic seizures in 1861. In 1959, Hunter (9) suggested that the use of effective antiepileptic drugs had, in fact, led to the increasing incidence of status epilepticus, because drug withdrawal and acute CNS infections constituted the most frequent precipitating factors. Although subsequent authors have questioned these conclusions, Hunter succeeded in provoking interest in the subject. It is generally estimated that 1% to 8% of epilepsy patients will develop status epilepticus during the course of their disorders.

In spite of the importance and frequency of status epilepticus, there have been few reports on this matter in recent years (3,4,25). Although two excellent prospective studies on treatment using phenytoin were recently published, the varieties of convulsive status epilepticus were not verified by

TABLE 4. *Eighteen patients: required i.v. drip of diazepam*

Proven or presumed cause	No. of patients
Metabolic disorders	4
Acute cerebral infarction	4
Post CVA	1
Meningitis	2
Encephalitis	1
Metastatic lesions	1
Cerebral anoxia (cardiorespiratory arrest)	4
Glioblastoma multiforme	1

TABLE 5. *Convulsive status epilepticus: response to i.v. diazepam*

Clinical	EEG	No. of patients	Needed i.v. drip	Response to diazepam: i.v. bolus or drip	Recurrence
Generalized tonic-clonic	Diffuse 1.5–3-Hz spike wave complexes	8	1[a]	8	0
Generalized tonic-clonic	Diffuse 16-Hz spikes	1	0	1	0
Generalized clonic	Diffuse 8–10-Hz sharp waves	2	0	2	0
Generalized clonic-tonic-clonic	Diffuse 1.5–4-Hz spike-wave complexes	4	3[b]	4	0
Secondary generalized	Focal rhythmic 12–18-Hz spikes spreading diffusely	29	11	23	6[c]
Secondary generalized tonic-clonic	Focal 1-Hz spikes and sharp waves spreading diffusely	6	3	6	0
Total		50		44	6

[a] Renal encephalopathy.
[b] One case of renal encephalopathy and 2 cases of multiple metabolic encephalopathies.
[c] Two cases of pneumococcal meningitis, 2 cases of cerebral anoxia secondary to cardiorespiratory arrest, 1 case of encephalitis, presumably viral, and 1 case of meningococcal meningitis.

CCTV or EEG, nor were the subvarieties of convulsive status correlated with treatment results. In the study reported here we attempted to relate the electroclinical subvarieties of status to drug responses; however, our report does not pretend to answer most of the questions on status epilepticus. The EEGs in all our cases were studied with or without CCTV videotaping as we classified the subvarieties of convulsive status. By clearly defining the electroclinical subvarieties of status, we were better able to identify unresponsive status epilepticus (unresponsive to diazepam and phenytoin). We also attempted to control status in progressing neurological lesions by infusing diazepam and maintaining therapeutic serum concentrations.

In a sense, we verified previous reports that showed the extremely fast action of intravenous diazepam and its potency in status epilepticus, especially in primary generalized convulsive status (1,7,11,13,20,22). Primarily generalized convulsive status was extremely sensitive to serum concentrations of diazepam of 0.3 to 0.8 μg/ml (4). However, even secondarily generalized convulsive status responded to intravenous diazepam as long as therapeutic serum concentrations were maintained. Intravenous bolus injections or infusions of diazepam stopped convulsions in 23 of 29 patients with secondarily generalized convulsive status. Most important, intravenous infusion of diazepam stopped convulsions in 7 of 13 patients with progressing neurological lesions. Sawyer et al. (18) and Prensky et al. (16) independently reported on the failure of intravenous diazepam to control convulsive status in patients with acute, rapidly progressive cerebral disorders. Sawyer et al. (18) emphasized that only 5 of 15 patients with acute neurological diseases experienced good seizure control for more than 24 hr. Prensky et al. (16) pointed out that only 9 of 20 patients with acute cerebral disorders had interrupted seizure activity for periods of more than 2 hr. We believe one explanation why convulsive status in progressing cerebral lesions does not stop after intravenous diazepam is because serum concentrations drop below 3 μg/ml. Infusing diazepam and ensuring therapeutic serum concentrations should stop convulsive status in most of these patients.

Our studies indicated a higher percentage of control in convulsive status than in studies previously reported by authors who used diazepam alone (7,13,16,18) or phenytoin alone (3,4,25). We achieved better results because we used intravenous diazepam infusion for at least 3 hr when seizures recurred, and we prevented the recurrence of seizures with intravenous phenytoin. With this combination treatment, we stopped convulsive status in 88% of patients, including some who had acutely progressing CNS lesions. Thus, aside from achieving a higher control rate, our studies further suggest that our combination treatment regimen decreases the percentage of intractable or drug-resistant status epilepticus usually seen in acute and progressing CNS disease. Understandably, our failures were also caused by acute infections and metabolic encephalopathies, but this accounted for only 12% of all our patients, in contrast to the usually reported incidence of 25% to 30% (3,4,25).

Another possibly important reason why a higher percentage of control was achieved, in contrast to previous studies that had used phenytoin alone (3,4,25), is the extremely fast action of intravenous diazepam. Whereas the anticonvulsant effects of intravenous phenytoin become evident 10 to 20 min after the start of its infusion, intravenous diazepam stops convulsions as early as 2 min in 10% of patients and as early as 3 min in 32% of patients. Ten minutes after the start of intravenous diazepam, seizures had stopped in 80% of patients. With phenytoin, only 30% of patients have convulsions controlled 10 min after the start of its infusion. The maximal antiepileptic effects of intravenous phenytoin occur 20 to 30 min after the start of its intravenous infusion (25).

The moderately slow rate we used in injecting diazepam intravenously should also be noted. Intravenous diazepam has been administered at rates faster than that used in our protocol. Gastaut et al. (7), Naquet et al. (13), Bamberger and Matthes (1), Sawyer et al. (18), Prensky et al. (16), and Smith and Masotti (20) in 1971 all administered intravenous diazepam at a rate of 5 mg/min. Because diazepam crosses the blood-brain barrier within 10 sec of intravenous administration (23), control of seizures was achieved by these authors almost immediately, or within 20 sec of completing the injection (when diazepam was effective). We elected to administer intravenous diazepam at the slower rate of 2 mg/min because of the reports of respiratory depression and hypotension. In the 50 patients we studied, we did not encounter hypotension induced by diazepam. We are unable to comment on the depressive effects of diazepam on respiration, because we elected to artificially ventilate the patients at the start of the treatment.

Whereas the main disadvantage of diazepam is the short duration of its effects, one of the main advantages of intravenous phenytoin is the long duration of its antiepileptic action. The use of an intravenous loading dose of phenytoin therefore avoids a therapeutic gap, prevents recurrence of seizures, and starts chronic antiepileptic drug treatment. During treatment with intravenous diazepam drip, Parsonage and Norris (15) observed that patients developed tolerance 24 hr after initiation of infusion. For this additional reason, intravenous phenytoin should be administered in addition to intravenous diazepam infusion.

The suggestion that diazepam and phenytoin be used in combination and that diazepam be administered as an intravenous infusion for status epilepticus did not originate in our unit. Whereas we started our studies as early as 1970, Sutherland and Tait (21) recommended intravenous diazepam and intravenous phenytoin in 1969; Janz (10) did the same in 1975, as did Wellhorner (26). Other investigators, notably Scheid and Gibbels (19) in 1969 and Niedermeyer (14) in 1974, recommended combining diazepam and phenobarbital. *We do not recommend this combination.* These drugs potentiate sedative effects and depress respiratory and cardiovascular systems. Diazepam-phenobarbital combination therapy is especially contraindicated when a patient has to be transferred to another hospital and will therefore be exposed to a period of limited supervision. We have also observed that respiratory and cardiovascular complications are particularly frequent in July and August of each academic calendar year, when new house officers arrive. Patients with status epilepticus receive barbiturates or paraldehydes before intravenous injections of diazepam, and these combinations lead to respiratory depression.

Whereas the combination of phenobarbital and diazepam is particularly bad for the respiratory centers, intravenous diazepam, by itself, can produce varying degrees of respiratory depression. Some cases with fatal results have been reported by Doose (5). In newborns and infants, this is particularly frequent. For this reason, we inserted an oropharyngeal tube in each of our patients and supported artificial respiration.

Interestingly, intravenous diazepam has been reported to trigger tonic status epilepticus in Lennox-Gastaut syndrome (5,22); however, this is a rare event.

Eisenberg (6) reported that diazepam may produce cholestasis with inflammatory reactions, and Parsonage and Norris (15) described a patient who developed reversible liver disturbance. These are also rare events, and intravenous diazepam usually is recommended as the initial therapy for patients with status epilepticus and liver disease. Intravenous diazepam can also be used as the initial treatment in patients with status epilepticus and renal disease.

As mentioned previously, intravenous diazepam may also have depressive effects on the cardiovascular system, producing hypotension. In rare cases, cardiac asystole can result. These complications occur mainly after too-fast injections in older patients with cardiovascular disease. These cardiovascular complications apparently are produced by the solvent propylene glycol. However, the positive effects of intravenous diazepam (namely, its fast and effective action) outweigh the extremely rare occurrences of respiratory and cardiovascular complications.

When diazepam is used as an infusion, a maximum of 20 mg of diazepam should be dissolved and thoroughly mixed in a minimum of 250 ml of solvent. This solution will not precipitate in a 5% to 10% glucose solution or in a 0.9% saline solution. The infusion solution should be used immediately after mixing, using a large-caliber vein. Diazepam may produce thrombophlebitis when injected into veins of small caliber.

Table 6 summarizes the main advantages and disadvantages of the first-line drugs (diazepam, phenytoin, and phenobarbital) used against convulsive status epilepticus. Most authors now consider diazepam and phenytoin to be more effective than phenobarbital or amytal. In general, when the repeating convulsions of status epilepticus confront the physician, either in the outpatient clinic or in the hospital wards, we recommend artificial respiration and the use of a fast-acting drug (diazepam) combined with a medication of relatively slow action (phenytoin), adequate for preventing the recurrence of seizures. Thus, we recommend the combination of diazepam and phenytoin, because convulsions should be interrupted in 10 to 20 min, and occurrences of serious side effects are extremely rare with the reduced speed of intravenous injection of either drug. Ideally, artificial respiration should be administered at the start of treatment in order to prevent the serious metabolic consequences of status and irreversible cell dam-

TABLE 6. *Treatment of tonic-clonic status epilepticus*

	Diazepam	Phenytoin	Barbiturates (amytal or phenobarbital)
Effectiveness	+ + + +	+ + + +	+ +
Latency of antiepileptic action	Acts immediately	Delayed (10–20 min after i.v. administration)	Delayed (5–15 min after i.v. administration)
Duration of effects	Short	Relatively long	Relatively long
Depression of conscious-ness	+ (10–30 min)	Minimal to none	+ +
Depression of respiration	+ (0.5–1 min)	Minimal to none	+ +
Hypotension	None to rare	In 2/3	+ +
Atrial fibrillation	None	+	None
Cardiac arrest	None to rare	+ (mainly after fast injections)	+ (2 g or more)
Indicated as primary-choice drug	In almost all cases as i.v. bolus injections, including status with renal and liver disease	In suspected subdural hematoma and in subarachnoid hemorrhage as i.v. bolus injection or i.v. infusion	No longer considered a first-choice drug, except barbiturate withdrawal
Indicated as secondary drug to prevent recurrence	Intravenous diazepam drip, 50 mg/500 cc D/W	250 mg i.v. q. hr × 3; rate of 50 mg per 5 min	
Indicated as maintenance treatment	No	Yes	Yes (phenobarbital)
Contraindications	In patients who have received high doses of barbiturates and par-aldehyde	(1) Severe arteriosclerotic heart disease; (2) 60 years of age and over; (3) bradycardia; (4) A-V dissociation, especially 3rd-degree block	

age in the cerebral cortex, hippocampus, amygdala, and cerebellum.

When convulsions of status recur in patients with rapidly progressing cerebral disease, intravenous infusions of diazepam will effectively control another 25% of these patients. If the foregoing regimen is not effective and status has continued for an hour, general anesthesia and muscle relaxants should be administered. Stopping muscle contraction diminishes cardiovascular demands and prevents progressive acidosis. Adequate oxygenation prevents damage due to cerebral or cardiac hypoxia. General anesthesia should stop the damaging effects of sustained and continuous neuronal depolarizations.

REFERENCES

1. Bamberger, P., and Matthes, A. (1966): Eine neue Therapiemoglichkeit des Status Epilepticus in Kinde salter mit Valium I. V. *Z. Kinderheilkd.*, 95:155–163.
2. Browne, T. R., and Penry, J. (1973): Benzodiazepines in the treatment of epilepsy. *Epilepsia*, 14:277–310.
3. Cranford, R. E., Leppik, I. E., Patrick, B. K., Anderson, C. B., and Kostick, B. (1978): Intravenous phenytoin: Clinical and pharmacokinetic aspects. *Neurology (Minneap.)*, 28:874–880.
4. Cranford, R. E., Leppik, I. E., Patrick, B. K., Anderson, C. B., and Kostick, B. (1979): Intravenous phenytoin in acute treatment of seizures. *Neurology,* 29:1474–1479.
5. Doose, H. (1970): Spezielle Probleme antikonvulsiver Therapie. In: *Epilepsy*, edited by E. Niedermeyer, pp. 195–234. Karger, Basel.
6. Froescher, W., ed. (1979): *Treatment of Status Epilepticus*, translated by H. Luders, p. 25. University Park Press, Baltimore.
7. Gastaut, H., Naquet, R., Poire, R., and Tassinari, C. A. (1965): Treatment of status epilepticus with diazepam (Valium). *Epilepsia (Amst.)*, 6:167–182.
8. Greenblatt, D. J. (1978): Simultaneous gas chromatographic analysis of diazepam and its major metabolite, desmethyldiazepam with use of double internal standardization. *Clin. Chem.*, 24:1838–1841.
9. Hunter, R. A. (1959): Status epilepticus: History, incidence, and problems. *Epilepsia*, 1:62–88.
10. Janz, D. (1975): Discussion remark, seminar on Bestimmung von Antiepileptika in Korperflussigkeiten, Berlin. In: *Treatment of Status Epilepticus*, edited by W. Froescher, translated by H. Luders, p. 7. University Park Press, Baltimore.
11. Kaeser, H. E. (1967): Der Status Epilepticus. *Praxis*, 56:750–751.
12. Murphy, J. T., and Schwab, R. S. (1956): Diphenylhydantoin (Dilantin sodium) used parenterally in the control of convulsions. A five year report. *J.A.M.A.*, 160:385–388.

13. Naquet, R., Soulayrol, R., Dolce, G., Tassinari, C. A., Broughton, R., and Loeb, H. (1965): First attempt of treatment of experimental status epilepticus in animals and spontaneous status epilepticus in man with diazepam (Valium). *Electroencephalogr. Clin. Neurophysiol.*, 18:427.

14. Niedermeyer, E. (1974): *Compendium of the Epilepsies.* Charles C Thomas, Springfield, Ill.

15. Parsonage, M. J., and Norris, J. W. (1967): Use of diazepam in treatment of severe convulsive status epilepticus. *Br. Med. J.*, 11:85–88.

16. Prensky, A. L., Raff, M. C., Moore, M. J., and Schwab, R. S. (1967): Intravenous diazepam in the treatment of prolonged seizure activity. *N. Engl. J. Med.*, 276:779–784.

17. Roger, J., Lob, H., and Tassinari, C. A. (1974): Status epilepticus. In: *Handbook of Clinical Neurology, Vol. 15, The Epilepsies*, edited by O. Magnus and A. M. Lorentz de Haas, pp. 145–188. North-Holland, Amsterdam.

18. Sawyer, G. T., Webster, D. D., and Schut, L. L. (1968): Treatment of uncontrolled seizure activity with diazepam. *J.A.M.A.*, 203:913–918.

19. Schied, W., and Gibbels, E. (1969): *Therapie in der Neurologie und Psychiatrie einschlieblich Rehabilitation.* Thieme, Stuttgart.

20. Smith, B. T., and Masotti, E. (1971): Intravenous diazepam in the treatment of prolonged seizure activity in neonates and infants. *Dev. Med. Child Neurol.*, 13:630–634.

21. Sutherland, J. M., and Tait, H. (1969): *The Epilepsies. Modern Diagnosis and Treatment.* Livingstone, Edinburg.

22. Tassinari, C. A. (1972): A paradoxical effect. Benzodiazepine induced status epilepticus. In: *Antiepileptic Drugs*, edited by D. M. Woodbury, J. K. Penry, and R. P. Schmidt, p. 518. Raven Press, New York.

23. Van der Kleijn, E. (1969): Kinetics of distribution and metabolism of diazepam and chlordiazepoxide in mice. *Arch. Int. Pharmacodyn.*, 178:193–215.

24. Wallis, W., Kutt, H., and McDowell, F. (1968): Intravenous diphenylhydantoine in treatment of acute repetitive seizures. *Neurology (Minneap.)*, 18:513–525.

25. Wilder, B. J., Ramsay, R. E., Wilmore, L. J., Faussner, G. F., Perchalski, R. J., and Shumate, J. B., Jr. (1977): Efficacy of intravenous phenytoin in the treatment of status epilepticus. *Ann. Neurol.*, 1:511–518.

26. Wellhorner, H. (1975): Epileptische Erkrankungen. In: *Pharmakotherapie—Klinische Pharmacologie*, edited by G. Fulgraff and D. Palm, p. 24. Fischer, Stuttgart.

Advances in Neurology, Vol. 34: Status Epilepticus, edited by A.V. Delgado-Escueta, C.G. Wasterlain, D.M. Treiman, and R.J. Porter. Raven Press, New York © 1983.

50

Diazepam Versus Lorazepam: Relationship of Drug Distribution to Duration of Clinical Action

David J. Greenblatt and Marcia Divoll

Clinical studies of the actions of diazepam and lorazepam in the treatment of seizure disorders or in anesthetic practice have indicated that the duration of action of an intravenous single dose of lorazepam is much longer than that of diazepam (1,2,9,11,14). These differences appear paradoxical in light of comparative pharmacokinetic studies of the two drugs, which clearly indicate that the elimination half-life of diazepam is much longer than that of lorazepam (4,5,8). The study reported here suggests that the clinical differences between these two drugs are in fact not paradoxical, but rather logical consequences of their differing properties of distribution.

METHODS

Eight healthy volunteers, ages 21 to 78 years, participated after giving written informed consent (Table 1). On two occasions, separated by at least 1 month, they received single intravenous doses of diazepam (5–10 mg) and of lorazepam (2–3 mg). Following the dose of diazepam, multiple venous blood samples were drawn over the next 5 to 10 days. After the lorazepam dose, samples were drawn over the next 48 to 72 hr.

Concentrations of diazepam and its major metabolite, desmethyldiazepam, in all plasma sam-

ples were determined by electron-capture gas-liquid chromatography (3). Lorazepam concentrations in all samples were similarly determined (6). The extent of drug binding to plasma protein for each drug in each subject was determined by equilibrium dialysis (15).

Pharmacokinetic parameters of drug distribution, elimination, and clearance for both diazepam and lorazepam were determined by iterative nonlinear least-squares regression techniques, as described in detail previously (8). Because inferences about volume of distribution (V_d) and clearance are strongly influenced by the extent of drug binding to plasma protein (10), values of V_d and clearance for each subject were corrected for individual differences in binding, yielding corresponding values of unbound V_d and unbound clearance. Differences in kinetic parameters between diazepam and lorazepam were analyzed using Student's paired t test.

RESULTS

The apparent elimination half-life of diazepam $(t_{1/2})$ averaged 51.2 hr, as compared with 15.7 hr for lorazepam. The difference was highly significant (Table 1, Figs. 1 and 2).

The two drugs differed greatly in terms of extent of drug binding to plasma protein. Diazepam was

TABLE 1. *Comparative kinetics of diazepam and lorazepam*

Subject	Age/Sex	Diazepam kinetics				Lorazepam kinetics			
		$t_{1/2}$ (hr)	Free fraction (%)	Unbound V_d (liter/kg)	Unbound clearance (ml/min/kg)	$t_{1/2}$ (hr)	Free fraction (%)	Unbound V_d (liter/kg)	Unbound clearance (ml/min/kg)
WN	27/F	63.0	1.15	178.3	32.6	19.1	10.2	11.5	7.0
LG	21/F	26.6	1.30	164.6	71.5	13.3	9.7	13.2	12.6
LM	34/M	21.1	1.30	53.8	29.5	12.6	9.2	17.3	16.4
ED	61/F	60.8	1.50	160.7	30.5	15.0	9.4	9.5	7.3
HK	78/F	64.8	2.00	111.0	19.8	18.7	11.2	8.8	5.4
EJH	72/M	60.1	1.40	127.1	24.1	17.9	8.2	14.7	9.5
HM	70/M	84.5	2.65	78.5	10.7	19.5	12.1	9.3	5.5
DB	31/F	28.3	0.90	187.8	76.7	9.5	10.4	12.0	14.6
Mean (± SE)		51.2 (±8.1)	1.53 (±.20)	132.7 (±17.2)	36.9 (±8.5)	15.7 (±1.3)	10.1 (±.43)	12.0 (±1.0)	9.8 (±1.5)
Paired t for diazepam vs. lorazepam		5.10 ($p < 0.001$)	25.4 ($p < 0.001$)	6.88 ($p < 0.001$)	3.56 ($p < 0.01$)				

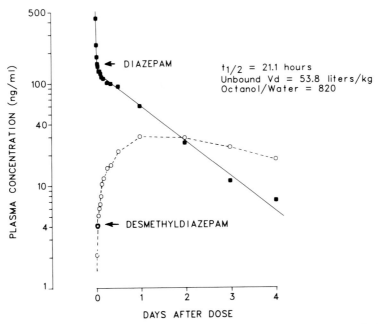

FIG. 1. Plasma concentrations of diazepam and its major metabolite, desmethyldiazepam, in a healthy 34-year-old male volunteer (subject L.M., Table 1) following a single 7.5-mg intravenous injection of diazepam. Solid line represents the pharmacokinetic function of best fit for diazepam determined by nonlinear least-squares regression analysis.

much more extensively bound, with a mean free fraction of 1.53% of the total amount present in plasma. In the case of lorazepam, the mean free fraction was 10.1% of the total plasma concentration. After correction of V_d values for these differences in binding, unbound V_d for diazepam was found to average 133 liter/kg, as compared with 12.0 liter/kg for lorazepam. This difference was highly significant. Likewise, clearance of unbound diazepam averaged 37 ml/min/kg, as compared with 9.8 ml/min/kg for lorazepam ($p < 0.01$).

DISCUSSION

Our study confirmed that the apparent elimination half-life for diazepam is considerably longer than that for lorazepam. However, the two drugs differed greatly in terms of extent of distribution. The apparent volume of distribution of unbound diazepam among these 8 subjects averaged more than 10-fold greater than that of lorazepam. This very large difference is at least partly explained by the difference in lipid solubilities of the two drugs. The *in vitro* octanol/water partition coefficient is considered to be a reasonably good predictor of a drug's lipid solubility and of its extent of distribution within the living organism. The par-

tition coefficient of diazepam is 840, as compared with 240 for lorazepam (13). Thus, although both drugs are lipid-soluble, the lipophilicity of diazepam is greater than that of lorazepam, thereby accounting for its more extensive distribution *in vivo*.

The clinical action of intravenous diazepam is of short duration because of its very rapid and extensive distribution into fatty tissues. Clinically effective concentrations in the brain following a single intravenous injection are rapidly terminated as the drug exits from the central compartment into peripheral sites in fat. In the case of lorazepam, this peripheral tissue uptake is less extensive, allowing clinically effective concentrations in the central compartment to persist for much longer after a single dose.

The longer elimination half-life of diazepam as compared with lorazepam is not due to slower clearance of the unbound drug by the liver. In fact, clearance of unbound diazepam is considerably higher than clearance of unbound lorazepam. The observed half-life depends on both distribution and clearance and can be prolonged as a result of either increased distribution or reduced clearance. In the case of diazepam, its higher clearance as compared with lorazepam is more than offset by the larger unbound volume of distribution, causing its elim-

SIDE EFFECTS

In addition to effectiveness, the second concern in evaluating an anticonvulsant is its safety. Animal studies suggested that lorazepam was relatively safe, and clinical studies thus far appear to bear that out. Drowsiness was the most common side effect reported by Sorel et al. (9), who also noted 3 cases of agitation and confusion (Table 3). DeOliveira (5) noted tremors, vomiting, agitation, somnolence, and hallucinations but did not indicate the frequencies at which these complications occurred. Hallucinations were noted in 2 patients in our study (10), and 1 patient experienced mild ataxia for approximately 12 hr. Ataxia and confusion were also reported by Amand and Evrard (2,3). Two types of major complications have been noted. Three cases of paradoxical tonic seizures have occurred in patients being treated for atypical absence associated with the Lennox-Gastaut syndrome. One patient experienced a transient respiratory arrest, with return to normal respiratory function following a few minutes of assisted ventilation (10). No other cases of respiratory arrest have been reported, either in patients being treated for status epilepticus or in the more common situation of administration of lorazepam as a surgical premedicant. The basis for this episode of respiratory arrest is uncertain. The patient did not have chronic respiratory disease, and no other anticonvulsants had been administered prior to the use of lorazepam. In addition, the lorazepam concentration at 15 min was only 40.5 mg/ml, a concentration well below that attained in several other patients without untoward consequences. Finally, no cases of cardiovascular collapse have been attributed to lorazepam.

TABLE 3. *Complications of lorazepam in status epilepticus*

Amand and Evrard (2,3)	Tonic seizure (1), ataxia, confusion
Griffith and Karp (8)	None
DeOliveira (5)	Tremors, vomiting, agitation, hallucinations, somnolence
Sorel et al. (9)	Drowsiness, agitation, confusion
Walker et al. (10)	Respiratory arrest (1), hallucinations, ataxia
Waltregny and Dargent (11)	Tonic seizures (2)

CLINICAL PHARMACOLOGY

The doses of lorazepam administered for status epilepticus have ranged from 2.5 to 10 mg administered in a single intravenous injection. Although in our study (10) we administered 4 mg of lorazepam over a 2-min period, most investigators have injected the lorazepam more rapidly. Amand and Evrard (2,3) indicated that 5 mg of lorazepam was given over 15 sec, DeOliveira (5) employed rapid repeated injection of 2 mg, and Sorel et al. (9) reported rapid injection of up to 10 mg of lorazepam. Because the only major respiratory complication occurred in our series, where slow administration was employed, there is currently no evidence that the rate of administration of lorazepam is a critical factor. Sorel et al. (9) provided the only data with regard to dosing in terms of milligrams per kilogram body weight. They reported 7 patients with doses ranging from 0.05 to 0.23 mg/kg.

Despite the facts that the peak effect of lorazepam occurs at 45 to 60 min (4,6) and that lorazepam penetrates the blood-CSF barrier slowly and incompletely (1), the rapidity of its onset of action is quite satisfactory in the clinical setting of status epilepticus. Most workers have found that the usual latency of onset of effective action is under 3 min. Control in 1 min or less was reported for 3 patients by Waltregny and Dargent (11) and in 2 patients in our series (10). In our study (10), the longest latency for control by a single 4-mg injection was 15 min, beyond which time a second 4-mg injection was given. Thus, although somewhat slower in its onset of effect than diazepam, lorazepam nevertheless produces effects rapidly enough to be acceptable for use in status epilepticus. The duration of seizure control following administration of lorazepam appears to be a primary advantage of this medication. Lorazepam, when effective, was found to prevent the recurrence of seizures for from 2 hr to longer than 72 hr. Table 4 shows the duration of control following administration of lorazepam in our series of 25 patients. However, in many instances, if not the majority, patients were receiving oral anticonvulsants either before or after the control of status epilepticus by lorazepam. Ethical medical practice would not permit the withholding of these medications following a bout of status epilepticus in most cases; so it is not possible to assess the duration of action of lorazepam administered alone.

TABLE 4. *Duration of control following lorazepam*

Seizure type	Number of patients	Immediate control	Duration of control				
			2 hr	6 hr	12 hr	24 hr	48 hr +
Partial seizures	12	11	11	10	10	8	8
Generalized tonic-clonic convulsions	9	9	8	8	7	7	7
Myoclonus epilepsy	3	2	2	2	2	2	1
Absence seizures	1	0	0	0	0	0	0

Nevertheless, the studies clearly indicate that one or at most two injections of lorazepam have a sufficiently prolonged duration of action to allow termination of the status epilepticus. This is in contrast to the findings with diazepam, where frequent intravenous administration or intravenous drip may be necessary to terminate an episode of status epilepticus.

Plasma concentrations of lorazepam have been correlated with clinical effectiveness in our study (10) and that of Sorel et al. (9). We found, in 10 patients whose seizures ceased following a single 4-mg injection, a mean lorazepam concentration of 60.1 ng/ml 15 min after the injection and 51.7 ng/ml 120 min after the injection. The range in concentrations at 15 min was 30.5 to 100.2 ng/ml, and the range at 120 min was 28.3 to 93.1 ng/ml. Sorel et al. (9) reported lorazepam concentrations at shorter intervals than we studied. In 2 patients successfully treated with 5 mg of lorazepam, they found lorazepam concentrations of 920 and 350 ng/ml at 30 sec following the initial injection. At 20 min these concentrations had fallen to 50 and 84 ng/ml, respectively. In our series (10) we found that the 15-min lorazepam concentrations in 3 patients who failed to respond to a single 4-mg intravenous injection exceeded effective concentrations, with values of 55.4, 89.5, and 116.6 ng/ml. We also found a similar overlap between patients experiencing adverse side effects and those who did not. The 15-min concentrations in patients with adverse side effects were 40.5, 71.3, and 100.2 ng/ml.

SUMMARY

The collective clinical data support the concept that lorazepam is highly effective for a broad range of seizure types, with the major inadequacy being in myoclonus, a seizure type typically highly resistant to other anticonvulsants as well. In addition to its effectiveness, lorazepam appears to have two other major advantages: a prolonged duration of action, which makes frequent or continuous administration unnecessary, and a high degree of freedom from serious side effects involving either the respiratory or cardiovascular system. Although experience at this time is insufficient to allow a firm statement concerning effective concentrations, such concentrations appear readily achievable in most patients with injections of 4 to 5 mg. Lorazepam appears to meet all the requirements of an anticonvulsant useful for treatment of status epilepticus and should prove to be a major drug in the treatment of this condition.

REFERENCES

1. Aaltonen, L., Kanto, J., and Salo, M. (1980): Cerebrospinal fluid concentrations and serum protein binding of lorazepam and its conjugate. *Acta Pharmacol. Toxicol. (Kbh.)*, 46:156–158.
2. Amand, G., and Evrard, P. (1975): Le lorazepam injectable dans les etats de mal epileptique rebelles. In: *Journees de Pediatrie*, pp 17–18 (abst). Proceedings of the Belgium Society for Pediatrics.
3. Amand, G., and Evrard, P. (1976): Le lorazepam injectable dans etats de mal epileptiques. *Rev. Electroencephalogr. Neurophysiol. Clin.*, 6:532–533.
4. Bobon, J., Bourdauxhe, S., Breulet, M., Parent, M., and Bobon, D. P. (1973): Pilot clinical trial of parenteral lorazepam (Temesta) in anxiety states. *Psychopharmacology*, 33:377–384.
5. DeOliveira, R. S. P. (1978): Treatment of convulsive seizures with a new benzodiazepine, lorazepam. *Rev. Bras. Clin. Terap.*, 7:295–298.
6. Elliott, H. W. (1976): Metabolism of lorazepam. *Br. J. Anaesth.*, 48:1017–1023.
7. Greenblatt, D. J., and Shader, R. I. (1974): *Benzodiazepines in Clinical Practice*. Raven Press, New York.
8. Griffith, P. A., and Karp, H. R. (1980): Lorazepam in therapy for status epilepticus. *Ann. Neurol.*, 7:493.
9. Sorel, L., Mechler, L., and Harmant, J. (1980): Comparative trial of intravenous lorazepam and clonazepam in status epilepticus. *Acta Neurol. Belg.*, 80:368–379.

10. Walker, J., Homan, R., Vasko, M., Crawford, I., Bell, R., and Tasker, W. (1979): Lorazepam in status epilepticus. *Ann. Neurol.*, 6:207–213.

11. Waltregny, A., and Dargent, J. (1975): Preliminary study of parenteral lorazepam in status epilepticus. *Acta Neurol. Belg.*, 75:219–229.

12. Waltregny, A., and Dargent, J. (1976): Preliminary report: Parenteral lorazepam in induced epileptic states in man. *Acta Neurol. Belg.*, 76:173–179.

*Advances in Neurology, Vol. 34: Status
Epilepticus*, edited by A.V. Delgado-Escueta,
C.G. Wasterlain, D.M. Treiman, and R.J. Porter.
Raven Press, New York © 1983.

52

Barbiturates in the Treatment of Status Epilepticus

Mark A. Goldberg and Hugh B. McIntyre

Barbiturates were introduced into clinical medicine at the beginning of the twentieth century and were quickly recognized as a significant improvement over bromides for treatment of epilepsy. Phenobarbital (PB) was first used in 1912 and soon became the drug of choice for long-term treatment of most types of seizures. Although its popularity diminished as newer agents were developed, it remains one of the most widely used antiepileptic drugs. When a soluble preparation became available, PB was introduced as a treatment for status epilepticus and was used as a replacement for ether and chloroform, which had previously been the only agents available for status that did not require oral or rectal administration. The use of PB increased steadily until the mid-1960s, when the introduction of diazepam and an improved understanding of the pharmacokinetics of phenytoin offered alternative forms of parenteral therapy. Nevertheless, many neurologists consider PB a safe and effective drug in status, and it is still used extensively for this condition in infants, children, and adults.

PHARMACOLOGY

PB (5-ethyl-5-phenylbarbituric acid) is a weak acid with a pKa of 7.2. As a consequence, it is approximately 50% ionized at physiological pH (2). Its partition coefficient against organic sol-vents is 3.5. By comparison, pentobarbital has a partition coefficient of 40 and thiopental 580. The sodium salt of PB is soluble in water (1 g/ml). PB is a potent inducer of hepatic microsomal enzymes, but it is not known to affect the function of tissues outside of the nervous system when administered in conventional doses.

ACTIONS ON THE CENTRAL NERVOUS SYSTEM

At low doses, barbiturates may activate the EEG, producing low-voltage, fast (15–25 Hz) activity. At higher doses there is slowing, and characteristic spindles may be seen. At toxic levels, marked slowing (1–3 Hz), burst suppression, and even electrocortical silence may occur. PB can depress cortical spread of electrical discharges originating from direct stimulation or from an epileptogenic lesion. It raises the threshold of most neuronal pathways to direct and indirect stimulation, and the reticular activating system appears especially sensitive to barbiturates. As a result of this general CNS depressant activity, barbiturates are effective in most forms of experimental epilepsy, including those induced by drugs, cortical lesions, and kindling.

The biochemical actions of barbiturates are poorly understood. Inhibition of energy metabolism, especially oxidative metabolism, occurs at toxic concentrations. There is little evidence that PB anticonvulsant actions are related to membrane permeability or ion movements, although inhibition of Na^+, K^+, and Ca^{2+} fluxes has been observed by a few investigators. There is also a paucity of evidence implicating an effect on release, reuptake, or degradation of synaptic transmitters to explain its actions. In summary, there is abundant evidence for the effectiveness of PB as an anticonvulsant, but little evidence to explain the mechanism of this action.

SPECIFIC ACTIONS OF PB

Although PB shares all of the actions of other barbiturates, and all are potentially anticonvulsants, there are several quantitative differences that help to explain why PB is a relatively selective anticonvulsant in clinical use. In 1931, Keller and Fulton (11) reported that PB elevated the threshold of the motor cortex in monkeys for electrical stimulation. PB was relatively specific in this regard in that it completely abolished the response to direct stimulation at doses that did not produce surgical anesthesia. This was unlike pentobarbital, amobarbital, and several depressant drugs that required anesthetic doses in order to block cortical spread. Aston and Domino (1) confirmed these differences many years later using more sophisticated electrophysiological techniques. They found pentobarbital to be six times more potent as an anesthetic, but when PB and pentobarbital were compared on the basis of threshold to cerebral cortical stimulation, pentobarbital was only slightly more effective than PB. Next, they studied the effect on the threshold for reticular activation, and pentobarbital was four times more potent than PB. In summary, pentobarbital was 2.5 times more potent as a depressant of the reticular activating system than of the cortex, as compared with PB. Similar differences have been noted by others. These findings explain the well-recognized clinical experience that PB can suppress cortical seizure activity at doses that do not produce excessive sedation.

A recent report by Macdonald and Barker (13) is an important contribution to an understanding of the possible synaptic mechanisms that account for the differential actions of anticonvulsant and anesthetic barbiturates and suggests a possible cellular basis for the anticonvulsant action itself. Using cultured spinal cord neurons, they found that barbiturates enhanced GABA effects and increased membrane conductance, an action that was suppressed by GABA antagonists. Quantitatively, pentobarbital was far more potent in these actions than PB. The latter, however, was able to abolish picrotoxin-induced paroxysmal activity at concentrations that did not affect spontaneous activity. Picrotoxin is a GABA antagonist that is known to produce experimental seizures through interference with GABA-sensitive synaptic mechanisms. An excellent review of the literature on the mechanism of anticonvulsant actions of PB has recently been published (6).

PHARMACOKINETICS

Numerous published studies have described the clinical pharmacokinetics of oral PB, but data on the disposition of intravenously administered drug are scarce. In the treatment of status epilepticus, intravenous administration is required, and it is possible that the accompanying changes in blood pressure, acid-base balance, and cerebral blood flow may influence the drug's distribution and elimination.

Distribution

In monkeys, maximum blood concentrations of PB occur 20 min after intravenous administration (16), and in cats 60 min are required (5). In addition to the delay in peak serum concentrations, there is clinical and experimental evidence for a delayed onset of maximum pharmacological action. The delayed sedative effect of PB was first noted by Hauptmann in 1912 (2) and subsequently by many other investigators. This correlates with the slow penetration of PB into brain, as reported by Domek et al. (5). In their detailed study these investigators noted peak cortical concentrations 60 min after administration; white matter penetration was slower, requiring 180 min to maximum. There are several possible explanations for the delay in brain penetration. As a consequence of its pKa, approximately 50% of PB in blood is in the ionized form, and only the un-ionized form can penetrate the blood barrier. Studies in which the degree of ionization has been manipulated have shown that this is an important variable (9). PB is not very lipid-soluble as compared with phenytoin and the rapidly acting barbiturates, and lipid solubility is critical in determining rate of penetration into brain. Furthermore, 40% to 50% of PB in serum is bound to plasma proteins, and only unbound drug enters brain, as indicated by CSF concentrations that correspond to free concentrations in plasma. In contrast to phenytoin, relatively little PB is bound to brain, and brain concentrations are only slightly higher than CSF concentrations (7). Degree of ionization, protein binding, and poor lipid solubility are therefore important factors contributing to the slow entry of PB into brain. Leppik and Sherwin (12) found maximal protective effect against electroshock in 3 min in rats, but it is unlikely that maximal brain concentrations were present in the short interval. However, maximum concentration may not be necessary for the onset of anticonvulsant activity.

Human Studies

There has been only one published report on the intravenous pharmacokinetics of PB in humans. Wilensky et al. (17) administered 130 mg of PB intravenously to volunteers. They found a distribution half-life of 0.25 hr and a volume of distribution of 0.54 liter/kg. The elimination half-life was similar to that found after oral administration, and the volume of distributuion was slightly less than that usually reported for PB.

In order to determine the intravenous pharmacokinetics of PB in patients in status epilepticus, we have begun a preliminary study using a single dose of 250 mg administered over 150 sec (8). Our results indicate a very brief distribution half-life of less than 5 min, with a maximum serum concentration of 8.4 µg/ml and a volume of distribution of approximately 0.5 liter/kg. All patients in this study ceased convulsing within a few minutes after administration of PB. Although quite preliminary, these data indicate a rapid distribution phase, possibly as a consequence of hypermetabolic activity in the convulsing patient, and a peak serum concentration below the 15 µg ml, usually considered the therapeutic concentration for PB.

TREATMENT OF STATUS EPILEPTICUS

It is surprising how little has been published about the use of PB in status epilepticus in adults. The widespread use of PB in this condition can be appreciated from Table 1. In a survey of 318 American neurologists, 25% indicated that PB was their preferred drug in status (8).

We have used the following procedure extensively in tonic-clonic status and believe it to be similar to that used at many hospitals. Initially,

TABLE 1. *Most useful drugs in status epilepticus[a]*

Diazepam	47%
Phenytoin	19%
PB	25%
Others	9%

[a]Based on a written survey of 318 U.S. neurologists in 1978 (8).

the patient's ventilation is assured, and an adequate intravenous line is placed. A sample of blood is withdrawn for determination of anticonvulsant drug concentration, and 250 to 300 mg of PB is given at a rate of 100 mg/min. The patient is then observed for 20 to 30 min, and if seizures have not stopped, then a second similar dose is administered. Rarely, a third dose may be necessary. This treatment program is effective in most patients and appears to be particularly useful in patients with anoxic encephalopathy and other metabolically induced seizures. Respiratory depression may occur, but usually this is a relatively slow process. These patients usually are under careful observation and may have been intubated earlier. In any case, ventilatory assistance must be immediately available to any patient in status epilepticus. We have not encountered sudden respiratory failure with the use of PB, as has occurred with other forms of therapy. We have had only 1 patient out of a large group who has had circulatory collapse. This patient was extremely hypercapneic, and hypercapnia is associated with increased brain penetration of PB (9). It is more likely that respiratory or circulatory collapse may occur in patients who have been treated previously with diazepam or short-acting barbiturates.

We have found this method of treatment to be both effective and safe. Post-treatment sedation occurs but rarely interferes with patient management. In fact, many patients tolerate relatively large doses of PB with minimal sedative effects.

In a patient suspected of having active intracranial disease, a CT scan is extremely useful. Among the advantages of PB for treatment of status epilepticus is the relatively rapid rate of infusion that can be employed, in contrast to the extreme caution necessary in using intravenous phenytoin. In addition, PB is soluble in all of the commonly used intravenous solutions and may be mixed with them without concern for precipitation. In summary, we find PB to be both safe and effective for treatment of status epilepticus of almost any course.

The treatment of status is a controversial subject, and other chapters in this volume suggest other forms of treatment. The underlying basis for this lack of agreement is the lack of carefully controlled clinical trials comparing various agents for effectiveness in status epilepticus of different causes. Such clinical studies are extremely difficult to carry out and may in fact be impossible under current regulations pertaining to human experimentation. Selection of the best drug will depend on the personal experience of the treating physician as well as the circumstances under which treatment is carried out. Controversy also exists as to how much of the various agents to use. Some authors have recommended a dose that will achieve a serum concentration that has been found therapeutically useful in long-term management of epilepsy. The dose of PB that we have used will not achieve the so-called therapeutic serum concentration in most patients.

We are, in effect, recommending undertreatment of a few patients in order to avoid a possibly greater incidence of toxicity. In so doing, we may be delaying effective treatment in those patients in order to avoid a greater incidence of toxicity in the majority. It appears likely, however, that generalized tonic-clonic seizures can be controlled acutely at serum concentrations well below those associated with the prophylactic use of this agent.

BARBITURATE ANESTHESIA

There is abundant information on preliminary treatment and "first-line" drugs for treatment of status epilepticus. In contrast, the management of major motor status epilepticus that has failed to respond to the usual emergency room treatment is a therapeutic problem that has received little investigative attention. Guidelines for treating such patients are inconsistent. Many standard texts and articles do not mention the subject, and those that do advocate the use of little more than general anesthesia. The choice of anesthetic agent, length of anesthesia, stage of anesthesia, and monitoring considerations generally are not specified. However, a method for the use of thiopental has been described by Brown and Horton (3). They used a continuous infusion for an average duration of 48 hr. All of their 117 patients in status epilepticus were "controlled," and no side effects were encountered. We would like to propose a protocol

using pentobarbital for the treatment of resistant generalized status epilepticus. We have used the method presented here on a pilot basis and have found it both expedient and successful.

The key factors in the method to be described are the administration of pentobarbital anesthesia by the neurologist and the use of continuous electroencephalographic monitoring. In view of the recent findings on barbiturate protection in cerebral hypoxia (4,10,14,15), the selection of pentobarbital as the anesthetic agent may have some theoretical basis beyond just that of the depression of seizure activity. Often patients experiencing major motor status epilepticus will have suffered periods of hypoxia due to respiratory insufficiency. Furthermore, continued convulsive activity creates systemic and local brain metabolic alterations that might, like those of hypoxia, be ameliorated by administration of barbiturate anesthesia.

The patients admitted to the pilot study were those in major motor status epilepticus who did not respond to initial emergency room treatment. Such treatment was not specified other than being that of the prevailing and usual emergency room practice. Most often this consisted of intravenous administration of PB, diazepam, and phenytoin, alone or in combination. All patients had failed to respond to the initial therapy for a minimum of 2 hr. Major motor status epilepticus was taken as the presence of continuous generalized seizures or the occurrence of generalized seizures in such rapid succession that full recovery between seizures did not take place.

According to the protocol, all patients are admitted to an intensive care unit, undergo tracheal intubation, and receive respiratory assistance. Therapy appropriate to the correction of any existing metabolic disturbances is given. Electrocardiogram, blood pressure, and temperature are monitored on a continuous or frequent basis. The electroencephalogram is continuously available and is monitored on an as-needed basis. Patients receive an intravenous pentobarbital infusion in amounts sufficient to achieve an EEG pattern that is alternately isoelectric ("burst suppression"). Therapy might begin with maintenance of pentobarbital anesthesia without interruption for 4 hr. Following the period of initial anesthesia, the patients are tested for reappearance of seizure activity by reducing the amount of pentobarbital infused. If there is reappearance of clinical seizures and/or generalized EEG seizure discharges, then the pentobarbital is increased to the prior level and held there for a period of another 2 to 4 hr. This procedure is then repeated as necessary. If there is no reappearance of clinical or EEG generalized seizure activity, or if there are only occasional brief, focal, clinical seizures or EEG transients, the pentobarbital is reduced and withdrawn over 12 to 24 hr. Simultaneously with the pentobarbital administration, the patients are given a maintenance anticonvulsant medication judged appropriate to their circumstances such that therapeutic blood concentrations are achieved by the time the pentobarbital is withdrawn. If possible, blood concentrations of pentobarbital can be measured at the time intervals indicated in the foregoing procedure. This may provide some guide to future initial selection of pentobarbital concentration and infusion rate. At the present time, such determinations must be a matter of individual judgment based on the EEG pattern and the amount of PB or similar drug the patient may already have received. In general, an initial intravenous dose of 5 mg/kg may be considered for both children and adults. Thereafter, the amount infused hourly is on the order of 1 to 3 mg/kg.

REFERENCES

1. Aston, R., and Domino, E. F. (1961): Differential effects of phenobarbital on motor cortical and reticular thresholds in the rhesus monkey. *Psychopharmacologia*, 2:304–317.
2. Bluter, T. (1978): Some quantitative aspects of the pharmacology of phenobarbital. In: *Antiepileptic Drugs: Quantitative Analysis and Interpretation*, edited by C. E. Pippenger, J. K. Penry, and H. Kutt, pp. 261–271. Raven Press, New York.
3. Brown, A., and Horton, J. (1967): Status epilepticus treated by intravenous infusions of thiopentone sodium. *Br. Med. J.*, 1:27–28.
4. Corkill, G., Silvalingam, S., Reitan, J. A., Gilory, B., and Helphrey, M. (1978): Dose dependency of the post-insult protective effect of pentobarbital in the canine experimental stroke model. *Stroke*, 9:10.
5. Domek, N., Barlow, C., and Roth, L. (1960): An ontogenic study of phenobarbital-C^{14} in cat brain. *J. Pharmacol. Exp. Ther.*, 130:285–293.
6. Glaser, G. H., Penry, J. K., and Woodbury, D. M. (editors) (1980): *Antiepileptic Drugs: Mechanisms of Action*, pp. 473–562. Raven Press, New York.
7. Goldberg, M. A. (1980): Phenobarbital binding. In: *Antiepileptic Drugs: Mechanisms of Action*, edited by G. Glaser, J. K. Penry, and D. Woodbury, pp. 501–504. Raven Press, New York.
8. Goldberg, M. A. (1978): unpublished observations.
9. Goldberg, M. A., Barlow, C., and Roth, L. (1961): The effects of carbon dioxide on the entry and accumulation of drugs in the central nervous system. *J. Pharmacol. Exp. Ther.*, 131:308–318.
10. Hoff, J. T., Smith, A. L., Hankinson, H. L., and Nielsen, S. L. (1975): Barbiturate protection from cerebral infarction in primates. *Stroke*, 6:28.
11. Keller, A., and Fulton, J. (1931): The action of anesthetic drugs on the motor cortex of monkeys. *Am. J. Physiol.*, 47:537.
12. Leppik, I., and Sherwin, A. (1979): Intravenous phenytoin and phenobarbital anticonvulsant action, brain content, and plasma binding in rat. *Epilepsia*, 20:201–207.
13. Macdonald, R., and Barker, J. (1978): Different actions of anticonvulsant and anesthetic barbiturates revealed by use of cultured mammalian neurons. *Science*, 200:775–777.
14. Smith, A. L. (1975): Barbiturate protection in cerebral hypoxia. *Anesthesiology*, 47:285.
15. Smith, A. L., Hoff, J. T., Nielsen, S. L., and Larson, C. P. (1975): Barbiturate protection in acute focal cerebral ischemia. *Stroke*, 5:1.
16. Snead, O. C. (1978): Gamma hydroxybutyrate in the monkey. *Neurology*, 28:1173–1178.
17. Wilensky, A., Levy, R., Friel, P., and Comfort, C. (1979): Phenobarbital pharmacokinetics after single IV, IM, and oral doses. *Proc. Am. Epilepsy Soc. Abstr.*, 23:37.

Advances in Neurology, Vol. 34: Status Epilepticus, edited by A.V. Delgado-Escueta, C.G. Wasterlain, D.M. Treiman, and R.J. Porter. Raven Press, New York © 1983.

53

Phenobarbital Dosage for Neonatal Seizures

Lawrence A. Lockman

Seizures occur in at least 0.5% of all live-born infants (2) and in as many as 20% of infants who weigh less than 2,500 g at birth (10). These seizures take a variety of clinical forms because of the immature pattern of dendritic connections and the small amount of myelin present in the newborn's brain (12). The types of seizures seen in older patients, such as tonic-clonic, absence, and partial complex, are unusual in the neonate. Ictal events that would be classified as partial seizures are more common; the symptoms include sucking, random eye movements, stretching, yawning, and bicycling. These seizures are frequently referred to as subtle. So-called convulsive apnea is also seen at this age.

Of overriding concern is the observation that neonatal seizures often accompany serious underlying disease. Although the convulsion itself may be subtle, the threat to the infant's life and the risk of permanent nervous system damage are well known (5). Therefore, it must be stressed that drugs are used for symptomatic management of seizures in the newborn only after an appropriate search for underlying pathological disease has been initiated. The infants considered in the study reported here had neonatal seizures without an identifiable, specifically treatable metabolic cause.

The majority of infants who have neonatal seizures are premature infants who have suffered subependymal or subarachnoid hemorrhage, infants who have been asphyxiated during labor and delivery, and infants who have serious congenital cardiac defects requiring surgery, during which embolization or decreased perfusion has caused injury to the brain. Wasterlain and Plum (13) have shown experimentally that permanent damage to the brain results from uncontrolled seizures in immature animals, even though the animals are adequately oxygenated and maintain normal blood glucose concentrations. These studies raise the possibility that neonatal seizures may cause permanent future brain damage in humans. On the other hand, it has been argued that the brain damage antedates the onset of seizures and that further damage cannot be demonstrated. Operationally, it seems reasonable to assume that neonatal seizures are not beneficial and should be stopped or controlled.

It is likely that exposing the newborn infant to commonly used anticonvulsant agents poses problems of another kind. Not only is there risk of direct and immediate toxic effects, such as sedation and respiratory depression, but also there is evidence accruing from tissue culture and animal studies (3,11) that exposure to anticonvulsants is detrimental to the structure and function of the developing neuron.

We have been investigating the use of phenobarbital in newborn infants with seizures in an attempt to define an effective nontoxic loading dose, an appropriate maintenance dose, and an appropriate duration of symptomatic anticonvulsant treatment.

PATIENTS AND METHODS

We studied infants in two neonatal intensive care units. The decision to treat infants for seizures was made by the director of the unit at each hospital, either St. Paul-Ramsey or the University of Minnesota. The route of drug administration was also determined by the director. Intravenous medication was given routinely at St. Paul-Ramsey Hospital, and either intravenous or intramuscular medication was administered at the University of Minnesota. We decided to study every infant who received phenobarbital regardless of gestational age, birth weight, clinical condition, or etiological diagnosis. In practice, treatment proceeds regardless of these factors. Although the directors of the units selected the patients and the route of administration, the study protocol determined the dose. Repeat doses were not to be given within 18 hr of the initial dose, if possible. Although infants could be withdrawn from the study at any time if the requirements of the study seemed to jeopardize their well-being, no infant had to be withdrawn. We assumed at the outset that a blood concentration of 20 µg/ml was therapeutic, and we wished to reach this concentration after the loading dose. The Committee on the Use of Human Subjects in Research approved the study design and the consent form; appropriate consent was obtained.

Blood phenobarbital concentrations were determined in one of three laboratories. All used gas-liquid chromatography; one used on-column methylation after the method of Kupferberg, and two used underivatized extracted plasma. During the course of the study, the EMIT assay became available, allowing determination of phenobarbital concentrations in much smaller blood samples. The agreement among these methods was excellent, as we have previously reported (7). The loading dose was increased as the study progressed. Following entry of the 40th infant, we initiated a protocol to study recalcitrant seizures of the newborn. This new protocol, which is still in effect, enrolls patients more slowly and will require larger numbers for analysis.

RESULTS

The ratio of dose to peak phenobarbital concentration was not significantly influenced by the method of administration, gestational age, or body weight. This ratio, reported as volume of distribution, was 0.81 liter/kg for intravenous admin-

istration and 0.91 liter/kg for intramuscular administration. The difference was not statistically significant ($p > 0.60$). However, there was a statistically significant difference between the variabilities, the standard deviation for intramuscular administration being 0.33 liter/kg. This observation suggests that absorption from intramuscular sites is less predictable and may result in more variation in serum concentrations.

There was a statistically significant relationship between the theoretical concentration at time zero and the dose, with a correlation coefficient of 0.805 (Fig. 1). Sixty-four percent of the variation in concentration can be explained by the change in dose. Ninety percent of the infants had a volume of distribution between 0.6 and 1.2 liter/kg (Fig. 2). Although this represents a twofold variation, it nonetheless is a relatively small intersubject variation for this type of administration. Thus a standard loading dose can be expected to lead to fairly consistent blood concentrations.

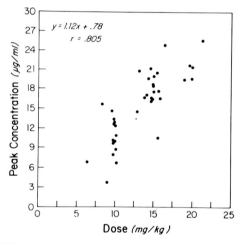

FIG. 1. Relationship of peak concentration to dose of phenobarbital.

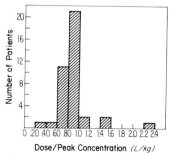

FIG. 2. Frequency distribution of the dose/peak-concentration ratio.

We recognized from the outset that there would be some infants in whom seizures would not be controlled with this or any other regimen. Therefore we attempted to establish a base-line concentration of phenobarbital below which seizures were not controlled in any infant. This turned out to be 16.9 µg/ml, as shown in Fig. 3. During the course of the study, the highest blood concentration achieved was 25.8 µg/ml, and no sedation was noted. As part of the study of recalcitrant seizures, blood concentrations of 40 µg/ml have been reached in several infants without sedation.

The phenobarbital doses and blood concentrations were significantly higher in patients who were successfully controlled than in those who continued to have seizures. The mean dose was 12.3 mg/kg for uncontrolled patients and 16.2 mg/kg for controlled patients. The mean blood concentration in the controlled patients was 19.8 µg/ml, as compared with 14.3 µg/ml in the uncontrolled patients.

Asphyxiated patients have been reported to be among the most difficult to control. We could demonstrate no such resistance in the 7 asphyxiated infants who had blood concentrations equivalent to those of the 13 nonasphyxiated infants.

Phenobarbital kinetics were determined in 15 infants who received the drug intramuscularly. Their gestational ages ranged from 31 to 40 weeks and their weights from 1,220 to 2,820 g. The doses ranged from 12.9 to 21.4 mg/kg. A one-compartment model adequately characterized the disposition of the phenobarbital during the postabsorption phase. The apparent volume of distribution was 0.81 ± 0.12 liter/kg. The mean half-life was 103.4 ± 49.1 hr, and the elimination rate constant was 0.0081 ± 0.0036 per hour. Median half-life was 83.0 hr. Apparent total body clearance was 6.4 ± 2.3 ml/hr/kg (Fig. 4).

Thus, to achieve and maintain a plasma phenobarbital concentration of 20 µg/ml would require a loading dose of 16.2 mg/kg and a daily maintenance dose of 3.1 mg/kg. A plasma phenobarbital concentration of 25 µ/ml would require a loading dose of 20.2 mg/kg and daily maintenance dose of 3.8 mg/kg.

DISCUSSION

Our findings generally are in agreement with those of others on the use of phenobarbital in neonatal seizures. Jalling (6), for example, reported that phenobarbital, in loading doses of 5 to 20 mg/kg, controlled seizures in 8 of 18 neonates (44%). Plasma concentrations ranged from 5.4 to 19.5 µg/ml, but seizures were controlled only with blood concentrations above 12 µg/ml. Painter et al. (8) used phenobarbital in 59 neonates; seizures stopped in 21 infants (36%). An intravenous loading dose of 15 to 20 mg/kg led to a mean plasma concentration of about 21 µg/ml. Brachet-Liermain et al. (1) used intramuscular phenobarbital, approximately 10 mg/kg, in 39 infants. A mean peak concentration of 13.28 µg/ml was reached in

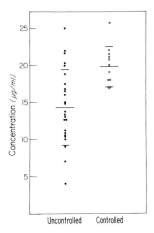

FIG. 3. Relationships of phenobarbital concentrations in patients whose seizures were controlled and those whose seizures were not controlled.

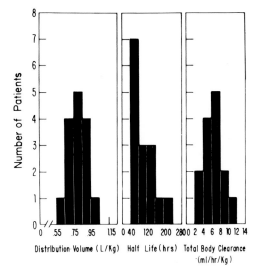

FIG. 4. Distribution, volume, half-life, and total body clearance in 15 patients who received intramuscular phenobarbital.

most cases within 2 hr. Seventy percent of the maximum blood concentration could be achieved within 30 min by this route. Pippenger and Rosen (9) used traditional doses of 5 mg/kg/day in 4 patients by the intravenous route. It took 4 to 5 days to achieve levels above 10 μg/ml. With doses of 10 mg/kg/day, concentrations exceeded 10 μg/ml within 24 to 48 hr.

Loading doses of phenobarbital can be safely given to premature and full-term newborn infants who have seizures. Our study has shown that doses between 20 and 25 mg/kg are safe and that smaller doses are unlikely to yield minimal therapeutic concentrations quickly. If seizures are injurious to the brain in the developing human, then rapid control is desirable. The use of incremental doses of 5 to 10 mg/kg/day will delay seizure control for several hours or days and eventually will lead to excessive blood phenobarbital concentrations. The data from this study indicate that dosage recommendations frequently underestimate the size of the initial dose and overestimate the maintenance dose (4).

Our current recommendations for symptomatic management of neonatal seizures are as follows:

1. An initial phenobarbital loading dose of 20 mg/kg is given intravenously if a line is in place or intramuscularly if it is not.

2. Clinical seizure activity is monitored carefully over the next 6 hr.

3. If seizures do not remit, an additional phenobarbital loading dose of 10 mg/kg is given intravenously.

4. If, in another 6 hr, seizures continue, then an initial loading dose of phenytoin of 20 mg/kg is given intravenously.

5. Phenobarbital maintenance with a daily dose of 3.5 mg/kg is begun 24 hr after the loading is completed.

6. Phenobarbital concentrations are determined daily so that concentrations in the therapeutic range can be maintained.

ACKNOWLEDGMENT

This study was supported in part by the Comprehensive Epilepsy Program, state of Minnesota.

REFERENCES

1. Brachet-Liermain, A., Goutieres, F., and Aicardi, J. (1975): Absorption of phenobarbital after the intramuscular administration of single doses in infants. *J. Pediatr.*, 87:624–626.
2. Craig, W. S. (1960): Convulsive movements in the first 10 days of life. *Arch. Dis. Child.*, 35:336–344.
3. Diaz, J., and Schain, R. J. (1978): Phenobarbital: Effects of long-term administration on behavior and brain of artificially reared rats. *Science*, 199:90–91.
4. Fisher, J. H., Lockman, L. A., Zaske, D., and Kriel, R. L. (1981): Phenobarbital maintenance dose requirements in the treatment of neonatal seizures. *Neurology*, 31:1042–1044.
5. Holden, K. R., Freeman, J. M., and Mellits, E. D. (1980): Outcomes of infants with neonatal seizures. In: *Advances in Epileptology, The Tenth Epilepsy International Symposium*, edited by J. A. Wada, and J. K. Penry, p. 155. Raven Press, New York.
6. Jalling, B. (1975): Plasma concentration of phenobarbital in the treatment of seizures in newborns. *Acta Paediatr. Scand.*, 64:514–524.
7. Lockman, L. A., Kriel, R., Zaske, D., Thompson, T., and Virnig, N. (1979): Phenobarbital dose for control of neonatal seizures. *Neurology*, 29:1445–1449.
8. Painter, M. J., Pippenger, C. E., MacDonald, H., and Pitlick, W. (1978): Phenobarbital and diphenylhydantoin levels in neonates with seizures. *J. Pediatr.*, 92:315–319.
9. Pippenger, C. E., and Rosen, T. S. (1975): Phenobarbital plasma levels in neonates. *Clin. Perinatol.*, 2:111–115.
10. Seay, A. R., and Bray, P. F. (1977): Significance of seizures in infants weighing less than 2500 grams. *Arch. Neurol.*, 34:381–382.
11. Swaiman, K. F., Schrier, B. K., Neale, E. A., and Nelson, P. G. (1980): Effects of chronic phenytoin and valproic acid exposure on fetal mouse cortical cultures. *Ann. Neurol.*, 8:230 (abstract).
12. Volpe, J. J. (1977): Neonatal seizures. *Clin. Perinatol.*, 4:43–63.
13. Wasterlain, C. B., and Plum, F. (1973): Vulnerability of developing rat brain to electroconvulsive seizures. *Arch. Neurol.*, 29:38–45.

Advances in Neurology, Vol. 34: Status Epilepticus, edited by A.V. Delgado-Escueta, C.G. Wasterlain, D.M. Treiman, and R.J. Porter. Raven Press, New York © 1983.

54

Paraldehyde, Chlormethiazole, and Lidocaine For Treatment of Status Epilepticus

Thomas R. Browne

PARALDEHYDE

Chemistry and Methods of Determination

Paraldehyde (PA), a cyclic polymer of acetaldehyde (Fig. 1), is a colorless liquid with a strong

Paraldehyde

Lidocaine

Chlormethiazole

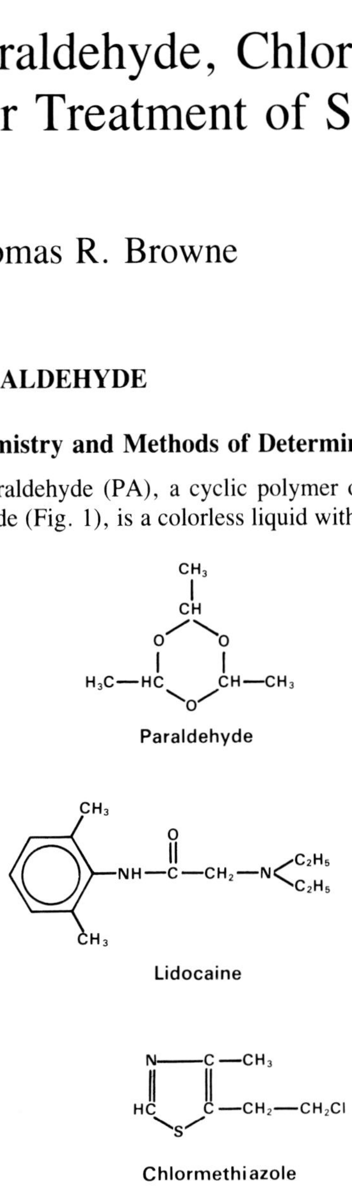

FIG. 1. Structural formulas for paraldehyde, chlormethiazole, and lidocaine.

aromatic odor and a burning disagreeable taste. PA is miscible with oils and has a molecular weight of 132.16.

The water solubility of PA is greatest (12.8%) at 12°C and decreases as the temperature rises above or falls below this point (63). At 37°C the water solubility of PA is 7.8% (63). Unawareness of these crucial facts has led to the practice of intravenous injection of PA in its pure form or as a 10% solution. In either event, the solubility of PA at 37°C would be exceeded, and one might expect droplets of pure PA to be formed in the bloodstream, resulting in pulmonary embolization *(vide infra)*.

In the presence of air, acetaldehyde oxidizes to acetic acid, which then acts as a catalyst for further depolymerization of PA to acetaldehyde (74). Improper storage of PA has resulted in some samples containing 40% to 98% acetic acid (11,32), and as little as 7 ml of such decomposed PA has proved fatal (3,4). A survey of 42 PA samples collected from hospital wards in 1957 revealed that only 11% were within U.S.P. standards (32).

In 1965, U.S.P. specifications were altered to state that PA must be preserved "in well-filled, tight, light resistant containers...not exceeding 30 ml" and that "the user...discard the unused contents of any container that has been opened more than 24 hours." Such procedures should reduce (but may not completely eliminate) the hazards of decomposed PA (74).

Methods for determining the concentration of PA in biological fluids have been reported using gas-liquid chromatography (5), enzymatic analysis (73), spectrophotometry (19,32), and dichromate titration (50).

Clinical Pharmacology

Absorption

The times to peak plasma concentration of PA are as follows: i.v. route, immediately after infusion (24); i.m. route, 20 to 60 min (73); p.o. route (in water), 30 min (5); p.o. route (in olive oil), 2 to 4 hr (23); p.r. route, 2 to 4 hr (5,23) (Fig. 2). The data in Fig. 2 are based on different studies employing different patients and different protocols. The data from these four different studies are therefore not strictly comparable, although the relationships shown probably are qualitatively correct.

Distribution

PA is rapidly distributed to the brain. Following an i.v. injection, drowsiness ensues within 2 to 5

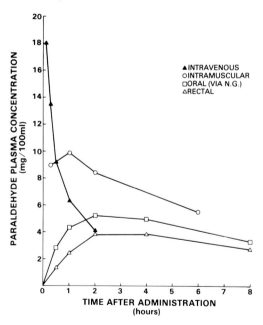

FIG. 2. Plasma-concentration-versus-time relationships for PA following administration of 0.1-ml/kg doses via the i.v., i.m., p.o., and p.r. routes. (Based on data from Gardner et al. (23,24) and Thurston et al., ref. 73.)

sec, and anesthesia occurs within less than 2 min (5,24,65). The steady-state volume of distribution of PA is 890 ml/kg (5). PA readily crosses the placental barrier and may cause delayed respirations in neonates (46).

Biotransformation and Excretion

PA is 70% to 80% metabolized by the liver, 20% to 30% exhaled by the lungs, and excreted unchanged by the kidney in very small amounts (6,31). In patients with liver disease, the rate of elimination of PA and the percentage of PA eliminated by the liver decrease, and the percentage of PA eliminated by the lungs increases (10,31,51).

On the basis of indirect evidence (34,43) it has been widely assumed that PA is depolymerized to acetaldehyde by the liver and that acetaldehyde is then oxidized to acetic acid, which is ultimately metabolized to CO_2 and H_2O. Gessner (25) has recently cited indirect evidence that acetaldehyde may not be formed from PA in $vivo$.

Elimination Half-Life

The elimination half-life of PA is 3.4 to 9.8 hr (mean 6.1–7.4 hr) (5,73). The plasma disposition kinetics of PA fit an open two-compartment model after i.v. injection (5).

Plasma Concentration

The therapeutic range of plasma concentrations of PA necessary to control seizures is unknown. Plasma concentrations of 12 to 33 mg/dl produce anesthesia (23). The minimum lethal plasma concentration of PA is 50 mg/dl (19,32).

Indications

Alcohol-withdrawal Syndrome and Delirium Tremens

When given by the p.o. or i.m. route, PA (or PA in combination with chloral hydrate) has proved significantly ($p < 0.05$) more effective than promazine or chlordiazepoxide in preventing the occurrence of alcohol-withdrawal seizures and delirium tremens and in reducing the complications of delirium tremens once the condition has begun (25,71) (Fig. 3). In the only comparison of PA with diazepam for treatment of delirium tremens, i.v. diazepam had a significantly ($p < 0.05$) shorter

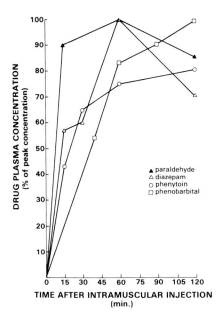

FIG. 3. Plasma-concentration-versus-time relationships for PA, diazepam, phenytoin, and phenobarbital following intramuscular injections. Based on data from Hillestad et al. (33), Jalling (39), Kostenbauder et al. (45), and Thurston et al. (73).

induction time and a significantly ($p < 0.001$) smaller incidence of untoward reactions than p.r. paraldehyde (72). However, this study has been widely criticized (25) because absorption of rectally administered PA is slow *(vide supra)* and the dosage of PA far exceeded that used in other studies.

Status Epilepticus

Evidence for efficacy of PA in status epilepticus consists of 36 case reports in two uncontrolled trials (56,79) and two widely quoted testimonials (17,77). These reports contained few details but indicated the following: (a) PA probably can control status epilepticus in the majority of patients, both adults and children; (b) PA may control status epilepticus when other agents fail; (c) PA may be more effective for tonic-clonic status epilepticus than for partial status epilepticus.

Comparison of PA with other agents for status epilepticus has never been done in a controlled clinical trial. Comparison of reported evidence for efficacy and toxicity of antiepileptic drugs leads to the conclusions that for most patients i.v. diazepam is preferable to i.v. PA when immediate control of seizures is necessary and that for most

patients a loading dose of phenytoin or phenobarbital followed by maintenance doses is preferable to continued PA therapy for longer-term control of status epilepticus (12). There are four special situations in which PA may be indicated for control of status epilepticus:

(a) When initial therapy must be given intramuscularly (e.g., no physician immediately available, suitable vein cannot be found, resuscitation equipment not available), i.m. PA is a very effective drug for status epilepticus. PA absorption via the i.m. route produces near-peak plasma concentrations in 15 to 20 min (73). Diazepam, phenytoin, and phenobarbital require significantly longer times for absorption via the i.m. route (Fig. 4) and do not produce therapeutic plasma concentrations within 15 to 20 min when given in usual doses via the i.m. route (33,39,40,44,45,68).

(b) In status epilepticus that is believed to be due entirely or chiefly to alcohol withdrawal, PA may be the drug of choice. Such patients would include patients with no history of seizures except during alcohol withdrawal and patients with true seizure disorders and therapeutic blood concentrations of antiepileptic drugs who have seizures only when withdrawing from alcohol. PA may be the drug of choice for the following reasons: (a) PA is very effective for control of alcohol-withdrawal symptoms and prevention of delirium tremens *(vide supra)*; thus PA might be administered regardless of the status epilepticus, and the use of one drug avoids the dangers of polypharmacy; (b) the preponderance of experimental and clinical evidence suggests that phenytoin is not an effective drug for

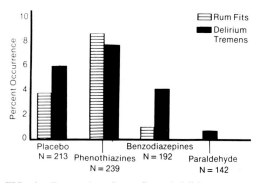

FIG. 4. Frequencies of rum fits and delirium tremens among patients in early alcohol withdrawal treated with placebo, phenothiazines, benzodiazepines, or PA (in some cases with chloral hydrate). (From Thompson, ref. 71, with permission. Copyright 1978, American Medical Association.)

alcohol-withdrawal seizures (25); (c) barbiturates are not generally used for treatment of alcohol-withdrawal symptoms in the United States because of concern about habituation to barbiturates as well as ethanol (25).

(c) When status epilepticus continues after full loading doses of phenytoin and phenobarbital have been administered, PA will sometimes stop the seizures (13,77).

(d) When the patient is allergic to safer agents used to treat status epilepticus (diazepam, phenytoin, phenobarbital), PA may be an effective alternative.

PA is now seldom used as a hypnotic, as an anesthetic agent, or in treatment of intractable pain because of the availability of safer agents.

Toxicity

Since PA was introduced in 1882, there have been at least 95 reports of death associated with PA use (6,32). These reports have led to widespread disrepute and infrequent use of PA. However, many (probably most) of these deaths were due to suicidal overdose, use of decomposed drug, use of doses larger than those currently recommended, or use of improperly diluted PA. The incidences of death and serious side effects with the use of U.S.P.-quality PA at recommended doses and following recommended administration procedures are unknown but probably are less than is generally supposed.

Overdosage

Overdosage with PA produces coma, right-sided heart failure, and pulmonary edema and hemorrhages (6,14,25).

Side Effects

PA administered by any route may cause disagreeable breath odor (from exhaled PA), right-sided heart failure, pulmonary edema and hemorrhages (especially if in excessive dosage) (6, 14,28,66), rash, irritability, toxic hepatitis (55), or toxic nephritis (46). With chronic administration, PA may produce metabolic acidosis (32,76). Chronic PA use may produce tolerance and/or physical dependence, with a withdrawal syndrome similar to that for alcohol (32,57).

Intravenous Route

Three studies (7,24,65) (totaling 181 patients) in which i.v. PA was used as an anesthetic agent reported no serious complications, although many patients experienced coughing, choking, pharyngeal irritation, tachycardia, or pain at the site of infusion. On the other hand, there have been case reports of i.v. PA suddenly producing apnea, coughing, cyanosis, hypotension, and clinical and X-ray signs of pulmonary edema (66). All the foregoing studies involved injection of undiluted or 10% solutions of PA and thus failed to properly dilute PA so that it would remain soluble after intravenous injection *(vide supra)*. Gessner (25) postulated that the previously cited pulmonary-cardiac complications were the result of pulmonary embolism of precipitated droplets of pure PA in the bloodstream due to improper dilution, and he cited two studies (5,62) in which properly diluted PA (4–8% solution) was administered i.v. without complications.

Oral and Rectal Routes

PA can cause irritation and corrosion of the mouth and stomach when given orally and of the rectum and large intestine when given rectally (2,31,67). Rectal administration of decomposed PA has resulted in large intestine perforation (2). The drug should be properly diluted before administration by these routes *(vide infra)*.

Intramuscular Route

Severe and permanent sciatic nerve damage may result if PA is injected too close to the nerve (32,80). Skin sloughing and sterile abscesses have also been caused by i.m. PA (32,80). This complication is rare in adults and older children but is not uncommon in neonates and young children.

Decomposed PA

Decomposed PA may contain very high concentrations of acetic acid. Acetic acid is a highly toxic substance, and PA containing acetic acid appears to be considerably more toxic than U.S.P.-quality PA (2–4,32,37).

Dosage and Administration

The dose of PA in treating status epilepticus is 0.1 to 0.15 ml/kg. This dose may be repeated every

2 to 4 hr if necessary. Before any PA is administered, it should be checked for purity and conformity with U.S.P. standards for storage *(vide supra)*.

Intravenous Route

The safety of i.v. PA is controversial *(vide supra)*. If possible, one should probably use another drug (e.g., diazepam) whose safety via the i.v. route has been better documented when immediate control of seizures with an i.v. medication is indicated. If i.v. PA is given, it must be diluted to a 4% solution and infused slowly.

PA can decompose plastic syringes and tubing within less than 2 min (1,18). Only glass syringes should be used, and PA should not be infused via plastic tubing.

Intramuscular Route

PA should be injected deep into the buttocks, taking care to avoid the sciatic nerve, and administering a maximum of 5 ml per injection site.

Oral Route

Absorption via the p.o. route is slower than via the i.m. route *(vide supra)*. There is also a risk of aspiration of PA, which is highly noxious to the lungs. The p.o. route is best avoided in patients with status epilepticus.

Rectal Route

The ease of administration of PA via the p.r. route probably accounts for its frequent administration this way. However, absorption of PA via the p.r. route is considerably slower than via the i.m. or p.o. route, making the p.r. route particularly undesirable for treating status epilepticus *(vide supra)*.

Furthermore, the slow absorption of PA via the p.r. route can result in administration of very large doses of rectal PA in order to obtain a plasma concentration high enough to control seizures. When the large rectal reservoir of PA is eventually absorbed, toxic plasma PA concentrations may result (15,25,26).

If rectal PA is administered, it should be diluted 2:1 in oil (olive or cottonseed) or diluted in 200 ml of 0.9% NaCl.

CHLORMETHIAZOLE

Chemistry and Methods of Determination

Chlormethiazole (chlormethazole, CTZ) is structurally similar to the thiazole part of thiamine (Fig. 1). CTZ is a sedative-hypnotic drug with pharmacological properties placing it in the alcohol-barbiturate group (25). CTZ is a white crystalline powder with a characteristic odor and a molecular weight of 513.5. CTZ is freely soluble in water, and concentrated solutions are quite acid.

GLC and GC-MS methods are available for determining the concentration of CTZ in biological fluids (22,38,41,42,58,59,61).

Clinical Pharmacology

Absorption, Distribution, and Elimination

Maximum plasma concentrations of CTZ occur 15 to 70 min after oral administration (20, 21,38,59,61). The bioavailability of CTZ by the oral route is 15% to 42% (41,59). CTZ is 60% to 69% protein-bound (41,61). Moore et al. (59) have identified four urinary metabolites of CTZ.

Pharmacokinetics

Following i.v. injection, plasma CTZ concentrations appear to follow the kinetics of an open two- or three-compartment model (41,59,61). The distribution half-life of CTZ is 30 min (59). The elimination half-life is 3.4 to 5.0 hr in healthy young adults (41,59), 2.6 to 4.7 hr in alcoholics (42), and 8.5 hr in normal aged subjects (61). The plasma concentration of CTZ necessary to control seizures is unknown; the minimum fatal concentration is 2.5 mg/dl (1 mg/dl in the presence of ethanol) (35).

Indications

CTZ is not an F.D.A.-approved drug. Evidence for the efficacy of CTZ in status epilepticus derives from 198 cases in eight reported series (8, 16,30,36,47,48,52,53). None of these series compared CTZ with other therapies, and almost every patient received several drugs. These studies indicated that i.v. CTZ had efficacy against tonic-clonic, partial, and absence status epilepticus in both children and adults and that i.v. CTZ sometimes stopped status epilepticus when diazepam, phenytoin, and phenobarbital (often given suboptimally) failed. However, these studies also revealed the following shortcomings of CTZ: (a) large bolus doses of CTZ cannot be given i.v. because of the danger of apnea (48); (b) i.v. CTZ must be given by slow infusion, and status epilepticus often is not controlled for 1 hr or several hours after beginning an infusion (30,36); (c) CTZ infusion (with attendant risks and need for intensive monitoring) often must be continued for several hours after the seizures stop to prevent their return (30,48); (d) CTZ may produce drowsiness, which interferes with evaluation of the patient's mental status; (e) there are other risks associated with i.v. CTZ (vide infra). The slowness with which i.v. CTZ often works is especially disconcerting because of the hazards of continued status epilepticus.

Overall, CTZ has some efficacy in status epilepticus, but it appears to have no advantage (and to have several disadvantages) when compared with diazepam, phenytoin, phenobarbital, and PA. Other indications for CTZ are reviewed elsewhere (21, 25,54).

Toxicity

Intravenous CTZ can cause respiratory depression, heart block, and death (64). Patients with respiratory, cardiac, liver, or CNS disease or other sedatives in the bloodstream are particularly susceptible to the respiratory depressant effects of CTZ (64). Infusion of solutions of CTZ more concentrated than 0.8% may result in hemolysis and/or thrombophlebitis (69).

Other side effects of CTZ include drowsiness, dizziness, tingling sensation in the nose, sneezing, conjunctival irritation, headache, fever, hypotension, increased bronchial secretions, dyspepsia, nausea, vomiting, rash, hiccups, elevated SGOT, physical dependence, and withdrawal syndrome (8,25,47,48,52,69).

Dosage and Administration

There is no agreement among the previously cited reports on the proper dosage of CTZ for status epilepticus. The manufacturer recommends an initial infusion of 20 to 60 mg/min, followed by a maintenance infusion of 4 to 8 mg/min using a 0.8% solution. CTZ reacts with, and is absorbed by, plastic tubing (52).

LIDOCAINE

Exhaustive reviews of lidocaine (Xylocaine®) (Fig. 1) are available elsewhere (27). This section will deal only with the use of lidocaine in status epilepticus.

Evidence for Efficacy

The evidence for efficacy of lidocaine in status epilepticus derives from 148 cases contained in eight reports (9,29,49,60,70,75,78,81). In the only one of these studies that was controlled (70), lidocaine proved superior to placebo in all 3 patients studied. In almost every case, the patients received multiple drugs in addition to lidocaine. Nevertheless, these studies indicate the following: (a) i.v. lidocaine is effective against tonic-clonic and simple partial status epilepticus (Fig. 5); (b) there are too few case reports to judge the efficacy of lidocaine in other types of status epilepticus; (c) lidocaine may sometimes control status epilepticus when varying combinations of diazepam, phenytoin, phenobarbital, and PA fail; (d) the antiepileptic effect of an i.v. bolus of lidocaine is rapid, with a decrease in seizures often noted in 20 to 30 sec; (e) the antiepileptic effect of lidocaine is often transient, lasting 20 to 30 min; (f) it is sometimes necessary to start a continuous lidocaine infusion in order to keep the seizures under control; (g) lidocaine does not cause drowsiness.

Dosage, Administration, and Precautions

The dosage of lidocaine for status epilepticus is not precisely known. Bernhard and Bohm (9) have the largest experience. They recommend initiating i.v. lidocaine with a single dose of 2 to 3 mg/kg. If the seizures do not stop, they may be refractory to lidocaine. If the seizures stop and then recur, one should begin a lidocaine infusion at a rate of 3 to 10 mg/kg/hr.

Before administering i.v. lidocaine for seizures, one should be aware of the following precautions: (a) Epilepsy is not an F.D.A.-approved indication for lidocaine; (b) in high doses, lidocaine may cause convulsions; (c) constant EKG and blood pressure monitoring is necessary to detect possible cardiovascular complications; (d) lidocaine should not be injected faster than 25 to 50 mg/min; (e) the dosage recommended by Bernhard and Bohm (9) may exceed the maximum recommended by the manufacturer (200–300 mg/hr); (f) evidence for proper usage in children is limited.

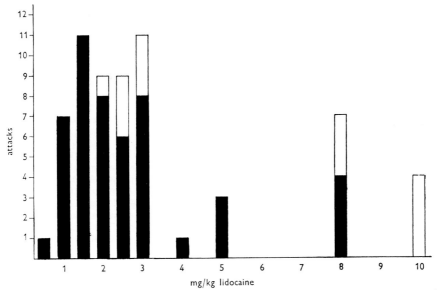

FIG. 5. Effects of single i.v. injections of lidocaine on 64 episodes of tonic-clonic and "Jacksonian" status epilepticus. Filled bars = "full effect." Open bars = no effect. (From Bernhard and Bohm, ref. 9, with permission.)

ACKNOWLEDGMENT

This work was supported in part by the Veterans Administration.

REFERENCES

1. Addy, D. P., Alestory, P., and Winter, L. (1978): Paraldehyde and plastic syringes. *Br. Med. J.*, 2:1434.
2. Agranat, A. L., and Trubshaw, W. H. D. (1955): The danger of decomposed paraldehyde. *S. Afr. Med. J.*, 29:1021–1022.
3. Anonymous (1954): Death from decomposed paraldehyde. *Br. Med. J.*, 2:1114–1115.
4. Anonymous (1954): Deteriorated paraldehyde. *Lancet*, 2:912.
5. Anthony, R. M., Andorn, A. C., Sunshine, I., and Thompson, W. L. (1977): Paraldehyde pharmacokinetics in alcohol abusers. *Fed. Proc.*, 36:285.
6. Baratham, G., and Tinckler, L. F. (1964): Paraldehyde poisoning: A little-known hazard of post-operative sedation. *Med. J. Aust.*, 2:877–878.
7. Beaucheim, J. A., Springer, R. G., and Elliot, G. A. (1935): Intravenous anesthesia with paraldehyde. *Med. Times*, 63:179–184.
8. Bently, G., and Mellick, R. (1975): Chlormethiazole in status epilepticus: Three cases. *Med. J. Aust.*, 1:537–538.
9. Bernhard, C. G., and Bohm, E. (1965): *Local Anesthetics as Anticonvulsants.* Almqvist and Wiksell, Uppsala.
10. Bodansky, M., Jinkins, J. L., Levine, H., and Gilbert, A. J. (1941): Clinical and experimental studies on paraldehyde. *Anesthesiology*, 2:20–27.
11. Bowles, G. C. (1964): Tighter system of drug control needed to prevent drug thefts. *Mod. Hosp.*, 103:120–127.
12. Browne, T. R. (1979): Drug therapy of status epilepticus. *Drug. Ther. Rev.*, 2:449–468.
13. Browne, T. R. (1980): unpublished data.
14. Burstein, C. L. (1943): The hazard of paraldehyde administration: Clinical and laboratory studies. *J.A.M.A.*, 121:187–190.
15. Colvin, E. D., and Bartholomew, R. A. (1935): Advantages of paraldehyde as basic amnesic agent in obstetrics. *J.A.M.A.*, 104:362–367.
16. Cvetanovic, V., and Mikic, D. (1971): Clomethiazole in the management of status epilepticus. *Neuropsihijatrija*, 19:61–64.
17. De Elio, F. J., De Jalon, P. G., and Obrador, S. (1949): Some experimental and clinical observations on the anticonvulsive action of paraldehyde. *J. Neurol. Neurosurg. Psychiatry*, 12:19–24.
18. Fenton-May, V., and Lee, F. (1978): Paraldehyde and plastic syringe. *Br. Med. J.*, 2:1166.
19. Figot, P. P., Hine, C. H., and Way, E. L. (1952): The estimation and significance of paraldehyde levels in blood and brain. *Acta Pharmacol. Toxicol. (Kbh.)*, 8:290–304.
20. Fischler, M., Frisch, E. P., and Ortengren, B. (1973): Plasma concentrations after oral administration of different pharmaceutical preparations of chlormethiazole. *Acta Pharm. Suec.*, 10:483–492.
21. Frisch, E. P. (1966): Chlormethiazole. *Acta Psychiatr. Scand. (Suppl. 192)*, 42:1–233.
22. Frisch, E. P., and Ortengren, B. (1966): Plasma concentration of chlormethiazole following oral intake of tablets and capsule. *Acta Psychiatr. Scand. [Suppl.]*, 192:35–40.

Advances in Neurology, Vol. 34: Status
Epilepticus, edited by A.V. Delgado-Escueta,
C.G. Wasterlain, D.M. Treiman, and R.J. Porter.
Raven Press, New York © 1983.

55

Valproic Acid in the Treatment of Status Epilepticus

F. J. E. Vajda

The discovery of valproic acid followed the accidental demonstration that compounds dissolved in this short-chain fatty acid exhibited anticonvulsant properties. Meunier et al. (30) first used valproic acid in France, and it has been used increasingly, worldwide over the past 5 years. Valproic acid differs from other anticonvulsants in that it is an eight-carbon, branched, short-chain fatty acid lacking the conventional heterocyclic ring structure of the barbiturates, phenytoin, succinimides, or carbamazepine.

For chronic treatment of epilepsy, valproate is available as either valproic acid or its sodium salt. It is not available for intravenous or intramuscular administration.

PHARMACOKINETIC PROPERTIES

The pharmacokinetic properties of valproic acid have been described in various reports (12, 21,23,35,41). Absorption of valproate is complete in both stomach and small intestine. Peak plasma concentrations are reached 1 to 4 hr after administration (41,52). Autoradiographic studies in rodents have shown that valproate is distributed rapidly, reaching the brain in a few minutes (11). Its distribution is more restricted than that of other anticonvulsants. Its apparent volume of distribution is 0.15 to 0.4 liter/kg body weight, corresponding to extracellular fluid volume (40).

Valproate does not appear to be bound to intracellular proteins in brain nor taken up selectively by brain tissue (14).

Valproate has an elimination half-life of 12 to 15 hr in healthy subjects and 8 to 10 hr in epileptic patients on long-term treatment (6,23,37,41). Its elimination is enhanced by enzyme inducers such as carbamazepine (31). After oral treatment, the rise in plasma concentration is linear and is related to dose, and peak levels occur 1.5 to 2 hr after the last dose. Plasma concentration fluctuations of 50% to 120% are common, and concentrations return to base line after 6 to 8 hr on a divided-dose regimen (52). Unlike phenytoin, valproate does not exhibit saturation kinetics, and the explosive clinical toxicity accompanied by high plasma concentrations on minor increases of dosage seen with phenytoin is not a therapeutic problem with valproate.

Binding of valproate in plasma is of the order of 85% to 95% (4,19), and the drug is capable of displacing other drugs from albumin binding sites in plasma (33).

Elimination is partly by β-oxidation like that of other short-chain fatty acids, and valproate shares microsomal enzyme pathways for the hydroxylation of its metabolites with other anticonvulsants. The metabolites of valproate are 2-propylhydroxypentanoic acid, propylglutaric acid, and glucocuranide conjugates (12,22).

PLASMA CONCENTRATION MEASUREMENTS

The most widely used method of plasma assay for valproic acid is gas-liquid chromatography (7, 50). Studies by various workers (15,39) have indicated lack of precise correlation between clinical and electroencephalographic effects and plasma concentration assay results. Others have used the presumed therapeutic ranges of 50 to 100 μg/ml and have shown that control of seizures is improved when plasma valproate concentrations fall within this range (27,34,43).

It is critical with a drug such as valproate, which has a short half-life and exhibits marked fluctuations in plasma concentrations between doses, to standardize sampling times and to take blood samples for drug assays at a time when the lowest concentrations prevail, which means sampling immediately before the next dose.

Recent work has shown that brain concentrations of valproate, unlike brain phenytoin and phenobarbital concentrations, do not represent an approximation to plasma concentrations (42,54). Valproate is not bound to brain fractions (14), and its concentration in human brain is of the order of 15% of its value in plasma, which corresponds quantitatively to the free, unbound, component in plasma (49). This information may be used to measure salivary concentration, which may give a closer approximation to brain concentrations than plasma concentration monitoring.

CLINICAL TRIALS

The first clinical trial of valproate was carried out by Meinardi (28), who demonstrated that 50% of refractory epileptic patients suffering from different types of seizures experienced 33% reduction in seizure frequency during valproate treatment, as compared with placebo, when either of these was added to preexisting medication. Richens and Ahmad (36) studied 20 patients with chronic refractory epilepsy, and Suzuki et al. (46) evaluated responses in 37 children with different types of seizures, mainly absences. Simon and Penry (43) and Pinder et al. (34) reviewed the evidence for efficacy of sodium valproate in various forms of epilepsy and collated the results in 41 trials, of which the majority were open evaluations.

The evaluations show that the drug is most effective in typical absences, myoclonic atypical absences, and common generalized seizures. No consistent benefit was obtained with treatment of all forms of partial seizures, tonic seizures, or infantile spasms.

The effects of valproic acid on spike-and-wave discharge in patients with absence seizures were studied by Villareal et al. (55). There was no correlation between plasma valproic acid concentration and EEG change, but clinical improvement occurred when valproic acid concentrations reached 50 to 60 μg/ml. Gram et al. (15) reported essentially similar results. Rowan et al. (39) studied the effects of sodium valproate in 4 patients by means of serial 24-hr EEG recordings. Valproate appeared to reduce diurnal paroxysmal discharges and clinical seizures. Redenbaugh et al. (35) and Bruni et al. (5) also assessed the control of absence attacks by 12-hr and 6-hr electroencephalograms and found a significant decrease in total duration and number of spike-and-wave discharges.

TOXICITY

The toxicity of valproate has been reviewed by Browne (3) and Bruni and Wilder (4). The gastrointestinal side effects of nausea, vomiting, and diarrhea may be minimized by gradual increases in dosage. Drowsiness and sedation may occur, especially with higher doses, and may be related to the effects of other anticonvulsants given simultaneously. Sedation is more common than behavior alteration and clouding of intellect, but these have also been reported.

Hepatotoxicity appears to be encountered more commonly in the United States than in Europe or Australia. Browne (3) reported 14 cases of death in association with valproate. Transient asymptomatic rises in transaminase are common. These are maximal 10 to 12 weeks after treatment and may represent the vast majority of adverse hepatic effects. The incidence may be as high as 15% to 30% in patients treated with valproate.

Adverse effects on coagulation have been reported, but they appear to be rare unless excessive doses are given. Alopecia usually is transient and reversible. Weight gain is common. A tremor that is electrophysiologically similar to essential tremor may occur, but it is reversible on reduction of dose. Occasionally, sexual problems may occur. In animals, selective uptake of the drug by cells of the testis, small litter size, and loss of reproductive function have been reported, but these have not been documented in humans. Teratogenicity has been shown to occur in rats on treatment with high doses, but no clear evidence is available to show that valproate causes teratogenicity in humans when used as a sole drug.

MECHANISM OF ACTION

Valproate is believed to act partly by elevation of γ-aminobutyric acid (GABA) concentrations by inhibition of GABA transaminase and succinic semialdehyde dehydrogenase, and it may also affect the rate of formation of GABA from glutamic acid by glutamic acid decarboxylase (13,22). It also has a possible direct cellular effect on neurons, and this may link its mechanism of action with the ketogenic diet. Harvey (16) proposed that valproic acid may inhibit GABA reuptake by glial cells and axonal terminals.

Turner and Whittle (48) have shown that sodium valproate is a potent inhibitor of the enzyme aldehyde reductase and will block its activity at therapeutic concentrations. The physiological significance of aldehyde reductase inhibition has not been established, but the enzyme may be involved in the formation of succinic semialdehyde to γ-hydroxybutyrate. This metabolite of GABA has been shown to cause an epilepsy-like stupor when administered to animals (45). Thus, valproate may be involved in the inhibition of an enzyme required to produce an epileptogenic metabolite of GABA. Alternative methods of action of valproate have been postulated, including an increase in GABA-mediated postsynaptic inhibition and modification of the receptor-ionophore complex or the lipid environment of the receptor (25).

Another possible effect of valproate may be to decrease levels of cyclic GMP in brain that may act as a second messenger for other neurotransmitters (24).

Slater and Johnston (44) found that valproic acid causes a dose-related increase in potassium membrane conductance that leads to hyperpolarization of the resting membrane potential. All the foregoing may be partly involved in the action of valproate, but the exact mechanism is unknown.

VALPROIC ACID IN STATUS EPILEPTICUS: EARLY STUDIES

Although valproic acid has been shown to be effective in human epilepsy, its use as a single drug has not been satisfactorily demonstrated. It is used frequently in combination with other drugs whose actions it may potentiate. Similarly, in sta-

tus epilepticus, which is a potentially life-threatening condition, sodium valproate has a potential role, not as a single drug but rather as an adjuvant drug intermediate in onset and duration of action between the immediately acting benzodiazepines and drugs with a more delayed onset of action and of longer duration, such as phenytoin.

Manhire and Espir (26) in 1974 first described the use of valproate in status epilepticus, given orally in a dose of 600 mg four times daily. In 1976, Barnes et al. (1) reported the good recovery of a further patient treated successfully for 5 days with sodium valproate (2,400 mg daily) by intragastric drip.

In 1976, we administered valproate as an enema to 2 patients (53). Plasma valproate concentrations indicated effective absorption and were related to reduction in seizure frequency. One patient with tonic seizures recovered 5 days after commencement of treatment with valproate enemas. The second patient also ceased having seizures 5 days after start of valproate treatment but subsequently died from staphyloccoccal sepsis.

The reason for the rectal route was the unavailability of parenteral valproate. In status epilepticus, paralytic ileus and vomiting prevent orally administered drugs from becoming therapeutically effective because of irregular absorption (1,17). Animal studies of drug absorption from the rectum have demonstrated that the rectal membrane is lipoidal and that the un-ionized form of the drug is rapidly absorbed (20).

In 1978, we reported the use of rectal valproate in a series of 6 patients with status epilepticus who were refractory to conventional anticonvulsant therapy (51). Five patients had generalized tonic-clonic seizures, and 1 patient had complex partial seizures (temporal lobe focus). The daily doses of valproate ranged from 21.6 to 45 mg/kg administered as lipid-based suppositories.

The mean daily frequency of seizures prior to sodium valproate treatment was 12.8 ± 3.7. Five patients experienced complete control of seizures, and the sixth patient obtained a 75% reduction. The plasma concentrations of valproate rose to values within the presumed therapeutic range of 50 to 100 μg/ml within 36 hr of starting therapy (44). Four patients were later switched to oral valproate at the same dose, with no significant changes in plasma valproate concentrations. These results, in addition to an effective clinical adjuvant action, indicated similar bioavailabilities of rectal and oral preparations of valproate (51).

VALPROIC ACID IN STATUS EPILEPTICUS: RECENT STUDIES

Since 1978, we have continued to evaluate sodium valproate in status epilepticus using rectal administration. Suppositories were prepared in a fatty base (Massupol) containing sodium valproate 200 mg per unit dose. Tablets of sodium valproate (200 mg) were crushed and incorporated into molten Massupol base at 50°C. The mixture was poured into suppository molds lubricated by spirit soap and allowed to set. To prepare 30 suppositories, 33.3 g of Massupol base were used and mixed with 30 tablets.

Patients and Methods

Of 23 patients suffering from status epilepticus, 11 were treated at the Austin Hospital, Melbourne, 9 at St. Vincent's Hospital, Melbourne, and 3 in Adelaide. The group of patients at St. Vincent's Hospital received rectal valproate and high doses of phenytoin; the other groups received benzodiazepines initially, followed by rectal valproate and conventional doses of phenytoin and other anticonvulsants as indicated.

The diagnosis of status epilepticus was based on a clinical diagnosis, as defined by the International League against Epilepsy, as a condition characterized by an epileptic seizure that is so prolonged or so frequently repeated as to create a fixed or lasting epileptic condition. EEG recordings were used in confirming and supporting the diagnosis and as a guide to progress in 11 patients.

The mean age of the 13 males and 10 females was 37.9 ± 4.4 years. Seventeen patients had status epilepticus with tonic-clonic seizures. One patient had tonic status, 3 patients had focal status, and 2 patients had myoclonic status. The associated illnesses in 23 patients comprised infection (7 cases), trauma (3 cases), mental retardation (7 cases), vascular accidents and peripheral venous thrombosis (5 cases), renal failure (1 case), cardiac valve surgery (1 case), diabetes and cardiac arrest (1 case), and hepatic cirrhosis (1 case). Seventeen patients were known epileptics with a variety of types of seizures. Eleven patients had common generalized epilepsy, 3 patients had temporal lobe epilepsy, 1 patient had Lennox-Gastaut syndrome, and 1 patient had myoclonic epilepsy. One patient

with cerebrovascular disease had a history of focal seizures. Six patients had epilepsy as a result of a vascular or metabolic disorder or trauma. Status epilepticus in this group was associated with vascular disease in 4 patients (stroke, abdominal aneurysm, cardiac disease, cardiac surgery), hypoglycemia in 1 patient, and trauma in another.

Concurrent Medication

The doses of concurrently administered drugs are shown in Table 1. Concurrent medication was given intravenously, intramuscularly, or nasogastrically (Table 1). Valproate was given as rectal suppositories in all cases in the dose range of 600 to 4,800 mg/day. The mean dose was 2,134 ± 225 mg. The most frequently used dosage regimen was 600 mg q.i.d.

Laboratory Measurements

Plasma concentrations of valproate and phenytoin were measured by gas-liquid chromatography (50,54). Plasma concentrations of valproate were monitored more closely than those of phenytoin because of the knowledge that steady-state plasma concentrations of phenytoin generally require 5 to 7 days of treatment to become stabilized.

Electroencephalograms

EEG recordings were performed by standard techniques in 11 patients from the Austin Hospital. Because continuous monitoring equipment was not available during this period, EEG recordings were performed on admission and at various intervals, depending on the duration of illness. The mean number of EEG recordings was 3.4 in this group of patients.

TABLE 1. *Concurrent medication*

Drug	No. of patients	Dose range
Sodium amylobarbital, i.v.	5	50–100 mg/hr
Phenytoin, i.v.	20	200–1000 mg/day
Carbamazepine, nasogastric	2	600–800 mg/day
Clonazepam, i.v.	5	3–12 mg/day
Diazepam, i.v.	8	10–120 mg/day
Thiopental, i.v.	1	50 mg
Paraldehyde, i.m.	1	2 cc
Phenobarbital, i.m.	1	150 mg
Chlormethiazole, i.v.	2	0.8% solution

Results

The overall response to treatment is shown in Table 2. Status epilepticus was controlled in 74% of the patients, with 56% recovering within 24 hr. Of the 6 patients (26%) who failed to respond to treatment, 3 patients died as a direct result of status epilepticus in spite of all available therapy.

Primary and Secondary Epilepsy

Analysis of the results in relation to whether patients had primary epilepsy or had a secondary cause of seizures is shown in Table 3. Seventeen patients were known epileptics or had no underlying medical illness causing secondary seizures. The majority had common generalized epilepsy.

Four patients had focal (temporal lobe) epilepsy, and 1 patient suffered from Lennox-Gastaut syndrome. The latter condition was characterized by slow 1.5- to 2-Hz spike-and-wave abnormalities, multiple symptoms, including motor and tonic seizures, mental retardation, and a poor prognosis. One infant developed myoclonic status epilepticus without an apparent cause. In this group of 17 patients with known epilepsy, 10 patients were readily controlled, 1 patient was controlled after a delay, and 6 patients failed to respond. Three died after prolonged illness of several weeks. Two patients recovered with multiple therapy but continued to have occasional seizures. One patient in whom withdrawal of phenytoin led to myoclonic status failed to respond to valproate and phenytoin had to be restarted to achieve control. Thus, 11 of the patients (64%) with primary epilepsy were controlled, and 6 patients were not helped (36%).

In the group of 6 patients with secondary epilepsy, 3 patients were controlled with treatment, including valproate, and recovered. Status epilepticus was well controlled in 2 patients, but they died 5 to 15 days later of complications associated with diabetes, infection, and vascular disease. Another patient died after a cerebrovascular accident and bronchopneumonia. This was the only patient whose seizures failed to be controlled.

Time of Valproate Administration

The effectiveness of valproate in relation to the time it was first used (on admission or after a variable delay) is shown in Table 4. Of the 14 patients given valproate rectally as the initial treat-

TABLE 2. *Results of treatment of status epilepticus (23 patients)*

Results	No. of patients
Control of seizures within 24 hr; patients recovered	13
Control of seizures after prolonged period of seizures (range 7–9 days); patients recovered	2
Control of seizures within 24 hr; patient died 5–15 days later	2
Prolonged seizures, failure to control; patients died of sepsis or metabolic complication	3
Seizures refractory to all therapy, including valproate; eventual control with multiple drugs	2
Induction of myoclonic status	1

TABLE 3. *Clinical results in relation to primary and secondary epilepsy*

Diagnosis	No. of patients	Control	Delayed control	Control, but later death	Failure to control	Failure and death
Primary epilepsy						
Common generalized epilepsy	11	6	1	—	2	2
Focal	4	4	—	—	—	—
Lennox-Gastaut	1	—	—	—	—	1
Myoclonic	1	—	—	—	1	—
Secondary epilepsy (metabolic group)						
C.V.A., chest infection	1	—	—	—	—	1
Aortic aneurysm, renal failure	1	1	—	—	—	—
Diabetes, cardiac arrest	1	—	—	1	—	—
Hypoglycemia, alcohol	1	—	—	1	—	—
Cardiac surgery	1	1	—	—	—	—
Cirrhosis, head trauma	1	1	—	—	—	—

TABLE 4. *Effectiveness of valproate in relation to time first administered*

Time of administration	No. of patients	Control	Delayed control	Control, but later death	Failure to control	Failure and death
Valproate given on admission	14	10	1	2	1	—
Valproate given ≤1 week later	7	3	1	—	2	1
Valproate given >1 week later	2	—	—	—	—	2

ment, 13 patients (93%) were controlled (12 patients within 24 hr and 1 patient after a delay). Two patients later died of their underlying medical conditions. When valproate was given during the first week, complete control occurred in 4 patients (57%) and failure in 3 patients (43%). Valproate given later in the illness was totally ineffective; 2 patients given the drug after 1 week failed to respond and died.

Number of Seizures on Presentation

The clinical outcome of status epilepticus was analyzed in relation to the number of seizures on presentation. Among 16 patients who had continuous seizures or more than six seizures when they presented, 11 patients achieved adequate control, but 1 patient died later as a result of metabolic complications of underlying disease. There were 5 therapeutic failures (31%), with 3 of these patients dying.

Among 7 patients who had fewer than six seizures on presentation, 5 patients were controlled, although 1 patient experienced a delay of several days, and 1 patient whose seizures were controlled later died of nonneurological complications. One patient failed to respond to all drugs, including valproate.

Single or Multiple Drug Therapy

The results were analyzed in relation to the drugs used in combination with valproate (Table 5). Valproate was used as sole therapy in only 2 patients; status epilepticus was controlled in both, but 1 patient subsequently died of the underlying medical illness. The combination of valproate and a benzodiazepine appears to be significantly less effective for control and subsequent outcome of the seizures than the combination of valproate and phenytoin. Ten patients were treated with valproate and diazepam or clonazepam; only 4 patients achieved immediate control; 1 patient had delayed control, and 5 patients (including 3 who died) did not respond. These results were similar even if phenytoin was used additionally, which occurred in the majority of cases. In contrast, when valproate and phenytoin were used without prior or simultaneous use of benzodiazepines, 9 of 12 patients were readily controlled, 1 patient was controlled after delay, and seizures in 1 patient were controlled, although the patient died later of nonneurological complications. There was one failure to control seizures in this group.

EEG Changes

Three patients with bilateral synchronous spike and spike-wave activity were rapidly controlled, with ablation of EEG abnormalities. One patient with bilateral temporal activity and right-hemisphere flattening who was semicomatose on presentation recovered adequately. Two patients who showed continuous bilateral activity but predominantly theta and delta waves recovered on treatment.

One patient with severe long-standing epilepsy had bilateral synchronous paroxysmal activity and failed to respond to treatment for 7 days. Her seizures eventually decreased in frequency, but she was discharged still subject to daily seizures. There were three deaths; 1 patient with Lennox-Gastaut syndrome had uncontrolled continuous paroxysmal activity throughout his illness over 10 weeks in spite of all treatment, including anesthetic doses of sodium amylobarbital and all other available medication. He was kept alive by supporting techniques in intensive care. The second patient who succumbed had short bursts of paroxysmal activity, even in circumstances when clinical seizures were not evident. The third patient had low-amplitude slow activity with occasional spikes more on the left than on the right, although he had generalized tonic-clonic seizures, poorly controlled.

One patient developed tonic-clonic status epilepticus on withdrawal of phenytoin. Sodium valproate

TABLE 5. *Clinical outcome in relation to drugs used in combination with valproate*

Drugs	No. of patients	Control	Delayed control	Control, but later death	Failure to control	Failure and death
Valproate alone	2	1	—	1	—	—
Valproate + benzodiazepine	10	4	1	—	2	3
Valproate + benzodiazepine + phenytoin	9	3	1	—	2	3
Valproate + phenytoin	12	9	1	1	1	—

was given, and her EEG showed spikes every 10 sec. Clinically, she lapsed into myoclonic status, and this was ablated only when phenytoin was restarted, and the EEG recording became normal.

Plasma Drug Concentrations

Mean plasma valproate and phenytoin concentrations 24, 48, and 72 hr after starting treatment are shown in Fig. 1. Plasma valproate concentrations were just within the postulated therapeutic range within 24 hr, and these continued to rise with further treatment.

Plasma phenytoin concentrations were in the lower reaches of the therapeutic range and subtherapeutic at 48 hr. The results include concen-

trations from patients who had been receiving long-term phenytoin therapy as well as those patients who were started on phenytoin on admission and were given a high dose parenterally.

The rise in plasma valproate concentrations following rectal administration is illustrated in Fig. 2. Plasma concentrations of valproate reached peak levels 3 to 4 hr after a single rectal dose of 400 mg of valproate, and on a 6-hr schedule of administration plasma valproate concentrations rose sharply to values close to the postulated therapeutic range.

DISCUSSION

It is difficult to compare the results of treatment of status epilepticus between different series be-

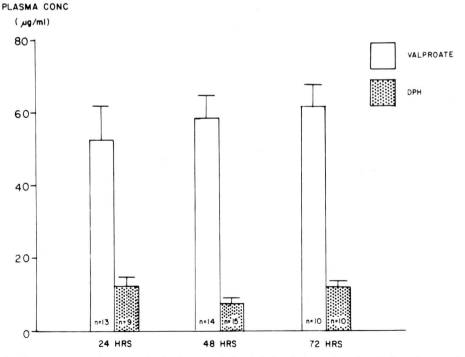

FIG. 1. Plasma concentrations (μg/ml) of valproate and phenytoin in relation to time elapsed after valproate administration. Times of measurement were 24, 48, and 72 hr (n indicates number of patients).

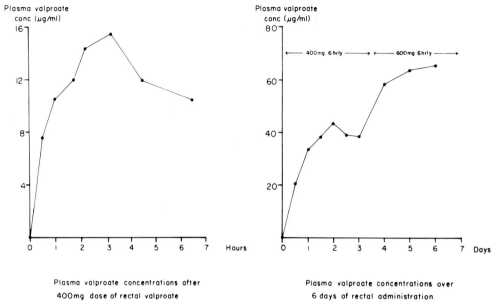

Plasma valproate concentrations after
400mg dose of rectal valproate

Plasma valproate concentrations over
6 days of rectal administration

FIG. 2. Left: Increases in plasma valproate concentrations (μg/ml) over 7 hr after single doses of 400 mg of rectal sodium valproate. **Right:** Change in valproate concentration (μg/ml) over a period of 6 days of rectal administration; doses are indicated in the body of the graph.

cause of variations in composition of patient groups and variations in EEG documentation. This study may be validly criticized for lack of EEG data in 12 of 23 patients. Such data in expert hands would greatly enhance the accuracy of diagnosis and would allow greater precision in treatment (10). The overall mortality of 22% in this series is comparable to quoted figures, but the series contains 2 patients with myoclonic status, which has lower mortality (38).

The overall results of treatment indicate prompt response in 15 patients (65%), two of whom died subsequently. All patients with primary epilepsy survived after their status epilepticus was controlled; the patients who died after their seizures were controlled belonged to the metabolic group and developed status epilepticus as a result of diabetes or vascular disease. The prognosis for this group is reported to be unfavorable (9).

Patients who failed to respond to valproate and subsequently died were given valproate as well as all available anticonvulsants and succumbed after prolonged illnesses of 5 to 11 weeks. It is unlikely that valproate, although ineffective, contributed adversely to their prognoses.

Two patients who failed to respond to valproate and continued to have seizures for several days after valproate withdrawal were severely disabled chronic epileptics.

Induction of myoclonic status in a patient following phenytoin withdrawal and substitution of phenytoin by valproate was unexpected and was terminated by recommencing phenytoin.

Valproate given on admission and combined with phenytoin produced the most favorable results. Patients who were given valproate later in the course of their illnesses fared badly, and this may be attributable to the use of valproate as a last resort in these severely afflicted patients.

In an earlier report, the use of phenytoin alone, without benzodiazepines, was shown to produce more satisfactory results in controlling recurrent seizures than phenytoin preceded by benzodiazepines (9).

In this study, the high percentage of patients (92%) responding to sodium valproate and phenytoin without benzodiazepines is an unexpected finding, especially because benzodiazepines have been regarded for many years as the most effective immediate short-term agents for treatment of status epilepticus. Their limitations with respect to short duration of action and a tendency to be associated with seizure recurrence are increasingly being recognized. On the basis of this small series, it is not possible to say that the combination of benzodiazepines and valproate is definitely contraindicated, because patients given both drugs were more refractory to all treatment. However, there is evidence that clonazepam and valproate may interact adversely and lead to absence status (18), and benzodiazepines even without valproate have been reported to have a potential for activating grand mal seizures (29,47).

The only suggestion that may be offered is that if rectal valproate is used, it should be used immediately, combined with intravenous phenytoin in high doses. Although benzodiazepines may have some adverse influence in long-term control, their dramatic immediate effect may counteract the suggestion that an interaction between valproate and benzodiazepines may be undesirable. If valproate is used, repeated injections of benzodiazepines may be unrewarding or unnecessary.

The plasma valproate concentrations shown in this study are within previously reported acceptable limits. These concentrations were obtained readily in 24 to 48 hr with rectal valproate.

The adequacies of absorption rate and bioavailability of valproic acid and its sodium salt in rectal dosage forms were recently confirmed by Moolenaar et al. (32). Fatty suppositories, aqueous solutions, and single oral doses were compared in volunteers. Rectal absorption was rapid and complete, and the free acid was absorbed more rapidly than the sodium salt. Changes in body position and composition of the suppository base had no influence on the bioavailability.

Plasma phenytoin concentrations in patients whose concentrations were monitored showed values in the lower part of the therapeutic range, and this highlights the difficulty of administering a sufficiently high dose of phenytoin to reach therapeutic plasma concentrations. Administration of phenytoin presents some technical problems, and significant cardiovascular side effects have been described (8,9).

The use of sodium valproate appears safe. No significant adverse side effects were noted in this study except induction of myoclonic status, which failed to respond until valproate was withdrawn.

The combination of a single dose of a benzodiazepine and subsequent use of valproate and phenytoin appears to offer advantages in attempting to cover both the immediate presentation of status epilepticus and the period of transition up to the time when phenytoin concentrations become stabilized. Valproate may enable small doses of phenytoin to become therapeutically effective.

The mechanism of action of valproate in status epilepticus is uncertain. The various postulated mechanisms of action were described earlier. Patsalos and Lascelles (33) reported that when a comparison was made between the brain/plasma ratios of phenytoin that was administered either alone or in combination with sodium valproate in animals, the brain/plasma ratios of phenytoin were significantly higher when sodium valproate was given as well as phenytoin. The brain/plasma ratios of phenytoin were 1.4 when phenytoin was used alone and 2.0 when phenytoin and valproate were given together. Valproate has been widely reported to displace phenytoin from plasma albumin binding sites. This displacement results in liberation of the active free moiety of phenytoin, which may enter the brain and bind to specific brain fractions. Valproate in status epilepticus may act by potentiating the action of phenytoin and thus enable earlier attainment of higher brain phenytoin concentrations than would otherwise be achieved. The rapid absorption and distribution of valproate may produce its own anticonvulsant effect, additionally. Thus, the use of valproate in status epilepticus is rational but needs controlled studies for further evaluation.

ACKNOWLEDGMENTS

I wish to thank Dr. P. F. Bladin, Dr. J. Currie, and Dr. Beran for support and permission to study patients under their care, Dr. G. Mihaly for support, and Miss J. Phillips, Miss J. Papanicolaou, and Miss D. Moore for technical assistance.

REFERENCES

1. Barnes, S. E., Bland, D., Cole, A. P., and Evans, A. R. (1976): The use of sodium valproate in a case of status epilepticus. *Dev. Med. Child Neurol.*, 18:236–238.
2. Bladin, P. F., Vajda, F. J., and Symington, G. R. (1977): Therapeutic problems related to tonic status epilepticus. *Clin. Exp. Neurol.*, 14:203–207.
3. Browne, T. R. (1980): Valproic acid. *N. Engl. J. Med.*, 302:661–666.
4. Bruni, J., and Wilder, B. J. (1979): Valproic acid: Review of a new antiepileptic drug. *Arch. Neurol.*, 36:393–398.
5. Bruni, J., Wilder, B. J., Bauman, A. W., and Wilmore, L. J. (1980): Clinical efficacy and long-term effects of valproic acid therapy spike-and-wave discharges. *Neurology*, 30:42–46.

6. Bruni, J., Wilder, B. J., Willmore, L. J., Perchalski, R. J., and Villareal, H. J. (1978): Steady-state kinetics of valproic acid in epileptic patients. *Clin. Pharmacol. Ther.*, 24:324–332.

7. Chard, C. R. (1975): A simple method for the determination of Epilim in serum. In: *Clinical and Pharmacological Aspects of Sodium Valproate (Epilim) in the Treatment of Epilepsy*, edited by N. J. Legg, pp. 88–91. MCS Consultants, Tunbridge Wells, England.

8. Conn, R. D. (1965): Diphenylhydantoin sodium in cardiac arrhythmias. *N. Engl. J. Med.*, 272:277–282.

9. Cranford, R. E., Leppik, I. E., Patrick, B., Anderson, C. B., and Kostick, B. (1979): Intravenous phenytoin in acute treatment of seizures. *Neurology*, 29:1474–1479.

10. Delgado-Escueta, A. V. (1979): Epileptogenic paroxysms: Modern approaches and clinical correlations. *Neurology*, 29:1014–1022.

11. Eymard, P., Simiand, J., Teoule, R., Polverelli, M., Werbenee, J. P., and Broll, M. (1971): Etude de la repartition et de la resorption de dipropylacetate de sodium marque au ^{14}C chez le rat. *J. Pharmacol. (Paris)*, 2:359–368.

12. Ferrandes, B., and Eymard, P. (1977): Metabolism of valproate sodium in rabbit, rat, dog and man. *Epilepsia*, 18:169–182.

13. Godin, Y., Heiner, L., Mark, J., and Mandel, P. (1969): Effects of di-*n*-propylacetate, an anticonvulsant compound, on GABA metabolism. *J. Neurochem.*, 16:869–873.

14. Goldberg, M. A., and Todoroff, T. (1980): Brain binding of anticonvulsants: Carbamazepine and valproic acid. *Neurology*, 30:826–831.

15. Gram, L., Wulff, K., Rasmussen, K. E., Flachs, H., Wuertz-Jorgensen, A., Sommerbeck, K., and Lohren, V. (1977): Valproate sodium: A controlled clinical trial including monitoring of blood levels. *Epilepsia*, 18:141–147.

16. Harvey, P. K. P. (1976): Some aspects of the neurochemistry of Epilim. In: *Clinical and Pharmacological Aspects of Sodium Valproate (Epilim) in the Treatment of Epilepsy*, edited by N. J. Legg, pp. 130–135. MCS Consultants, Tunbridge Wells, England.

17. Harvey, S. C. (1975): Hypnotics and sedatives. In: *The Pharmacological Basis of Therapeutics*, edited by L. S. Goodman and A. Gilman, pp. 102–136. Macmillan, New York.

18. Jeavons, P. M., Clark, J. E., and Maheshwari, M. C. (1977): Treatment of generalized epilepsies of childhood and adolescence with sodium valproate (Epilim). *Dev. Med. Child Neurol.*, 19:9–25.

19. Jordan, B. M., Shillingford, J. S., and Steed, K. P. (1975): Preliminary observations on the protein binding and enzyme inducing properties of sodium valproate (Epilim). In: *Clinical and Pharmacological Aspects of Sodium Valproate (Epilim) in the Treatment of Epilepsy*, edited by N. J. Legg, pp. 112–117. MCS Consultants, Tunbridge Wells, England.

20. Kakemi, K., Arila, T., and Muranishi, S. (1965): Absorption and excretion of drugs XXV-XXVII: Rectal absorption of sulphonamides. *Chem. Pharm. Bull. (Tokyo)*, 13:861–869, 969–985.

21. Klotz, U., and Antonin, K. H. (1977): Pharmacokinetics and bioavailability of sodium valproate. *Clin. Pharmacol. Ther.*, 21:961–964.

22. Kupferberg, H. J. (1980): Sodium valproate. In: *Antiepileptic Drugs, Mechanisms of Action*, edited by G. H. Glaser, J. K. Penry, and D. M. Woodbury, pp. 643–653. Raven Press, New York.

23. Loiseau, P., Brachet, A., and Henry, P. (1975): Concentration of dipropylacetate in plasma. *Epilepsia*, 16:609–615.

24. Lust, W. D., Kupferberg, H. J., Passonneau, J. V., and Penry, J. K. (1976): On the mechanism of action of sodium valproate: The relationship of GABA and cyclic GMP levels to anticonvulsant activity. In: *Clinical and Pharmacological Aspects of Sodium Valproate (Epilim) in the Treatment of Epilepsy*, edited by N. J. Legg, pp. 123–129. MCS Consultants, Tunbridge Wells, England.

25. Macdonald, R. L., and Bergey, G. K. (1979): Valproic acid augments GABA mediated postsynaptic inhibition in cultured mammalian neurons. *Brain Res.*, 170:558–562.

26. Manhire, A. R., and Espir, M. (1974): Treatment of status epilepticus with sodium valproate. *Br. Med. J.*, 3:808.

27. Mattson, R. (1979): Valproic acid and management of seizures. In: *Current Neurology, Vol. 2*, edited by H. R. Tyler and D. M. Dawson, pp. 229–248. Houghton Mifflin, Boston.

28. Meinardi, H. (1971): Clinical trials of anti-epileptic drugs. *Psychiatr. Neurol. Neurochir. (Amst.)*, 74:141–151.

29. Meinardi, H., and Stoel, L. M. K. (1974): Side effects of antiepileptic drugs. In: *Handbook of Clinical Neurology*, edited by P. J. Vinken and G. W. Bruyn, pp. 720–738. North-Holland, Amsterdam.

30. Meunier, G., Carraz, G., Meunier, Y., Eymard, P., and Aimard, M. (1963): Properties pharmacodynamiques de l'acide *n*-dipropylacetique. *Therapie*, 18:435–438.

31. Mihaly, G. W., Vajda, F. J. E., Miles, J. L., and Louis, W. J. (1979): Single and chronic dose pharmacokinetic studies of sodium valproate in epileptic patients. *Eur. J. Clin. Pharmacol.*, 16:23–29.

32. Moolenaar, F., Greving, W. J., and Huizinga, T. (1980): Absorption rate and bioavailability of valproic acid and its sodium salt from rectal dosage forms. *Eur. J. Clin. Pharmacol.*, 17:309–315.

33. Patsalos, P. N., and Lascelles, P. T. (1977): Valproate may lower serum phenytoin. *Lancet*, 1:50–51.

34. Pinder, R. M., Brogden, R. N., Speight, T. M., and Avery, G. S. (1977): Sodium valproate: A review of its pharmacological properties and therapeutic efficacy in epilepsy. *Drugs*, 13:81–123.

35. Redenbaugh, J. E., Sato, S., Penry, J. K., Dreifuss, F. E., and Kupferberg, H. J. (1980): Sodium valproate: Pharmacokinetics and effectiveness in treating intractable seizures. *Neurology*, 30:1–6.

36. Richens, A., and Ahmad, S. (1975): Controlled trial of sodium valproate in severe epilepsy. *Br. Med. J.*, 4:255–256.

37. Richens, A., Scoular, I. T., Ahmad, S., and Jordan, B. J. (1978): Pharmacokinetics and efficacy of Epilim in patients receiving long term therapy with other an-

tiepileptic drugs. In: *Clinical and Pharmacological Aspects of Sodium Valproate (Epilim) in the Treatment of Epilepsy*, edited by N. J. Legg, pp. 78–88. MCS Consultants, Tunbridge Wells, England.

38. Roger, J., Lob, H., and Tassinari, C. A. (1974): Status epilepticus. In: *Handbook of Clinical Neurology*, edited by P. J. Vinken and G. W. Bruyn, pp. 145–188. North-Holland, Amsterdam.

39. Rowan, A. J., Binnie, C. D., de Beer-Pawlikowski, N. K. B., Goedhart, D. M., Gutter, T., van der Geest, P., Meinardi, H., and Meijer, J. W. A. (1979): Sodium valproate: Serial monitoring of EEG and serum levels. *Neurology*, 29:1450–1459.

40. Schobben, F., and van der Kleijn, E. (1974): Pharmacokinetics of distribution and elimination of sodium di-*n*-propylacetate in mouse and dog. *Pharm. Weekbl.*, 109:30–33.

41. Schobben, F., van der Kleijn, E., and Gabreels, F. J. M. (1975): Pharmacokinetics of di-*n*-propylacetate in epileptic patients. *Eur. J. Clin. Pharmacol.*, 8:97–105.

42. Sherwin, A., Eisen, A., and Sokolowiski, C. (1973): Anticonvulsant drugs in human epileptogenic brain. *Arch. Neurol.*, 29:73–77.

43. Simon, D., and Penry, J. K. (1975): Sodium di-*n*-propylacetate (DPA) in the treatment of epilepsy. A review. *Epilepsia*, 16:549–573.

44. Slater, G. E., and Johnston, D. (1978): Sodium valproate increases potassium conductance in *Aplysia* neurons. *Epilepsia*, 19:379–384.

45. Snead, O. C. (1978): Gamma hydroxybutyrate in the monkey. II. Effect of chronic oral anticonvulsant drugs. *Neurology*, 28:643–648.

46. Suzuki, M., Maruyama, H., Ishibashi, Y., Ogawa, S., Seki, T., Hoshino, M., Maekawa, K., Yo, T., and Sato, Y. (1972): A double-blind comparative trial of sodium dipropylacetate and ethosuximide in epilepsy in children, with special emphasis on pure petit mal seizures (in Japanese). *Med. Prog. (Jpn.)*, 82:470–488.

47. Tassinari, C. A., Gastaut, H., Dravet, C., and Roger, J. (1971): A paradoxical effect: Status epilepticus induced by benzodiazepines (Valium and Mogadon). *Electroencephalogr. Clin. Neurophysiol.*, 31:182.

48. Turner, A. J., and Whittle, S. R. (1980): Sodium valproate, GABA and epilepsy. *TIPS*, 2:257–260.

49. Vajda, F. J. E., Donnan, G. A., Phillips, J., and Bladin, P. F. (1981): Human brain plasma and cerebrospinal fluid concentration of sodium valproate after 72 hours of therapy. *Neurology*, 31:486–487.

50. Vajda, F. J. E., Drummer, O. H., Morris, P. M., McNeil, J. J., and Bladin, P. F. (1978): Gas chromatographic measurement of plasma levels of sodium valproate: Tentative therapeutic range of a new anticonvulsant in the treatment of refractory epileptics. *Clin. Exp. Pharmacol. Physiol.*, 5:67–73.

51. Vajda, F. J. E., Mihaly, G. W., Miles, J. L., Donnan, G. A., and Bladin, P. F. (1978): Rectal administration of sodium valproate in status epilepticus. *Neurology*, 28:897–899.

52. Vajda, F. J. E., Mihaly, G. W., Miles, J. L., Morris, P. M., and Bladin, P. F. (1978): Sodium valproate: Dose-level relationship and interdose fluctuations. *Clin. Exp. Neurol.*, 15:145–153.

53. Vajda, F. J. E., Symington, G. R., and Bladin, P. F. (1977): Rectal valproate in intractable status epilepticus. *Lancet*, 1:359–360.

54. Vajda, F., Williams, F. M., Davidson, S., Falconer, M. A., and Breckenridge, A. M. (1974): Human brain, cerebrospinal fluid and plasma concentration of diphenylhydantoin and phenobarbital. *Clin. Pharmacol. Ther.*, 15:597–603.

55. Villareal, H. J., Wilder, B. J., Willmore, L. J., Bauman, A. W., Hammond, E. J., and Bruni, J. (1978): Effect of valproic acid on spike and wave discharges in patients with absene seizures. *Neurology*, 28:886–891.

Advances in Neurology, Vol. 34: Status Epilepticus, edited by A.V. Delgado-Escueta, C.G. Wasterlain, D.M. Treiman, and R.J. Porter. Raven Press, New York © 1983.

56

General Anesthesia in Patients with Epilepsy and Status Epilepticus

A. Opitz, M. Marschall, R. Degen, and D. Koch

The objective of this study was to find a consensus concerning the best possible anesthetic technique for patients with cerebral convulsive disorders and to address the use of general anesthetic agents and techniques in the management of status epilepticus.

PATIENTS AND METHODS

This study evaluated the use of general anesthesia in 1,172 epileptic patients from 1972 to the present. These patients had had at least two seizures per month. The anesthetic techniques used were inhalation anesthesia with halothane (642 patients) or enflurane (345 patients), regional anesthesia (132 patients), intravenous anesthesia (43 patients), and balanced anesthesia with droperidol and fentanyl (10 patients). Methohexital (913 patients), etomidate (39 patients), ketamine (20 patients), and thiopental (5 patients) were used for intravenous induction.

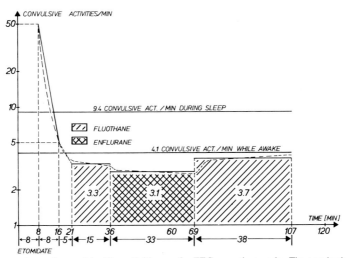

FIG. 1. Average numbers of convulsionlike activities on the EEG on a time scale. The two horizontal lines represent the average numbers of convulsionlike activities per minute in sleep and awake EEGs recorded preoperatively. Occurrences of convulsive potentials were higher after injection of etomidate, but significantly lower under halothane or enflurane anesthesia.

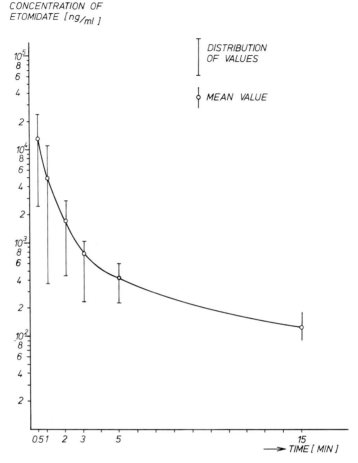

FIG. 2.   Concentration-time curve for etomidate in human serum during inhalation anesthesia.

We evaluated a series of 61 patients (inhalation anesthesia with enflurane or halothane in 45 patients, balanced anesthesia with droperidol and fentanyl in 10 patients, spinal anesthesia in 6 patients), all of whom had been hospitalized and had had detailed EEG history and neurological examination. All patients had received anticonvulsant therapy. Anesthesia with enflurane or halothane was induced with intravenous doses of methohexital or etomidate or through inhalation. Etomidate was used exclusively for induction of balanced anesthesia with intravenous droperidol and fentanyl and nitrous oxide/oxygen.

We used general anesthesia with EEG recording in 3 patients whose status epilepticus could not be managed successfully with intravenous antiepileptic drugs.

All patients were premedicated with diazepam and atropine 45 min prior to induction of anesthesia. Respiration was monitored during anesthesia in patients ventilated mechanically. In all patients, EEG recording was started prior to induction and continued to the end of the anesthetic procedure. The EEG changes were evaluated visually, and epileptiform paroxysms were counted per minute.

RESULTS AND DISCUSSION

Convulsionlike potentials or epileptiform paroxysms recorded during anesthesia were compared with those found in previous sleep and awake EEGs. The frequency of epileptiform potentials during anesthesia was much less. This was true in patients given inhalation anesthesia induced with metho-

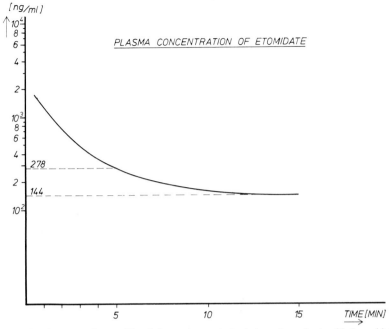

FIG. 3. Concentration-time curve for etomidate in human serum during balanced anesthesia with droperidol and fentanyl.

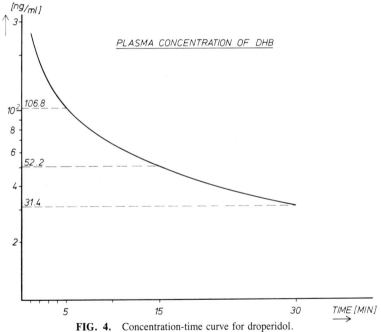

FIG. 4. Concentration-time curve for droperidol.

hexital. When anesthesia was induced with etomidate, convulsionlike potentials were found 24 sec after induction and occurred more frequently than in sleep and awake EEGs. However, when anesthesia was maintained with enflurane or halothane for 10 min, epileptiform potentials disappeared quickly, and their rate became less than in sleep or awake EEGs (Fig. 1). We can assume that these changes were due to etomidate, because convulsionlike potentials disappeared at the same time

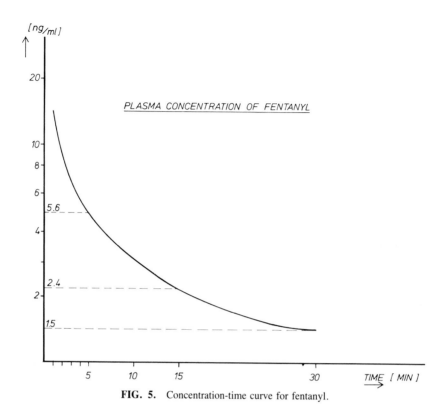

FIG. 5. Concentration-time curve for fentanyl.

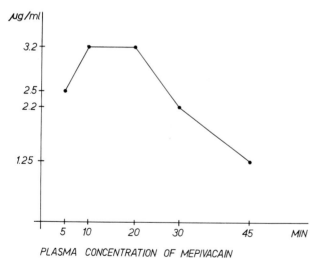

PLASMA CONCENTRATION OF MEPIVACAIN

FIG. 6. Plasma mepivacaine concentration in a patient showing convulsionlike activities during spinal anesthesia.

the serum concentration of etomidate fell to one-sixth its initial value (Fig. 2). We can therefore conclude that convulsionlike activity on the EEG occurs much less frequently during anesthesia maintained with enflurane or halothane than in awake or sleeping patients. Induction with etom-idate is an exception. Thus, in epileptic patients, waking activity or physiological sleep provokes epileptiform discharges more than anesthesia with enflurane or halothane.

To differentiate the effects of various drugs, balanced anesthesia with droperidol and fentanyl was divided into three phases: (a) injection of etomidate, (b) administration of droperidol and fentanyl, muscle relaxation with succinylcholine, intubation and mechanical ventilation with nitrous oxide/oxygen, and (c) start of surgery. We observed convulsive potentials following injection of etomidate, but they disappeared rather quickly and were not seen during the third phase, which was approximately 15 min after induction. At this point, the serum concentration of etomidate was one-tenth the initial concentration (Fig. 3).

The serum concentrations of both droperidol and fentanyl (Figs. 4 and 5) corresponded with the amounts usually found in neuroleptic anesthesia with these same agents. We can conclude, therefore, that except for induction with etomidate, anesthesia with droperidol and fentanyl provokes convulsionlike activity on the EEG less than physiological sleep.

In 1 patient with status epilepticus (male, 14 years of age), 6 g of hexobarbital given intravenously resulted in immediate burst suppression on the EEG. Intubation and controlled ventilation were necessary to overcome respiratory depression. Halothane or enflurane was used in children to treat status epilepticus resistant to other forms of therapy. Muscle relaxants were used concomitantly, and disappearance of spikes and waves was evident 20 min after induction of inhalation anesthesia. No convulsions were noted after recovery.

For the 6 patients with spinal anesthesia, the EEG was recorded throughout the whole duration of anesthesia. All patients were given 2 mg of mepivacaine intrathecally. Comparison of EEG patterns during anesthesia with those recorded while the patients were awake and asleep showed no differences in 5 patients. In 1 patient, however, convulsionlike potentials were recorded in the form of 3- to 4-Hz spikes and waves. Serum mepivacaine concentration measured 1.25 ng/ml, which is less than 10% of the toxic level (Fig. 6). It is important to emphasize that the patient had no convulsions and was alert and cooperative.

CONCLUSIONS

1. General anesthesia with either halothane or enflurane provokes convulsionlike activity on the EEG less than does physiological sleep.

2. Intravenous injection of etomidate can provoke convulsionlike potentials; however, other investigators have described successful therapy of status epilepticus with etomidate.

3. Doses of barbiturates used for intravenous induction of anesthesia are 10 times higher than those used for diagnostic provocation of convulsions.

4. It is important to provide adequate anticonvulsant therapy in the perioperative period.

5. General anesthetic techniques can and should be used in the treatment of severe status epilepticus that does not respond to intravenous antiepileptic agents.

6. Regional anesthesia can be given safely to epileptic patients; however, premedication should contain diazepam.

We have not seen clinical convulsions in any of these 1,172 patients during induction of anesthesia, while under anesthesia, or during emergence from anesthesia. A postoperative follow-up protocol, extended up to 6 weeks, did not show any increase in the frequency of convulsions as compared with the preoperative period.

In spite of our experience with this large number of epileptic patients, however, we cannot determine whether or not convulsionlike activity on the EEG is to be regarded as equal to an epileptic attack.

Advances in Neurology, Vol. 34: Status Epilepticus, edited by A.V. Delgado-Escueta, C.G. Wasterlain, D.M. Treiman, and R.J. Porter. Raven Press, New York © 1983.

57

Status Epilepticus: Summary

A. V. Delgado-Escueta, C. Wasterlain, D. M. Treiman, and R. J. Porter

> "There are times when as soon as one seizure is over, another starts, one following the other in succession, so that one may count 40, 60 seizures without interruption; the patients call this "état de mal" (status epilepticus). The danger is imminent; many patients die."
>
> L. F. Calmeil
> *De l'épilepsie*
> University of Paris, 1824

In 1824 Calmeil first described "grand mal" status epilepticus as part of his thesis *De l'épilepsie* (6). He observed as patients had repeated tonic-clonic seizures and did not recover consciousness between attacks. Thirty-two years later, Bourneville mentioned status epilepticus as "état de mal" in his book published in 1876 (1). The full meaning of status epilepticus, however, was not fully appreciated until 1962, when the Marseille conference extended the meaning of status epilepticus to "epileptic seizures that are so frequently repeated or so prolonged as to create a fixed and lasting epileptic condition" (13). The term was applied to continuous seizures lasting at least 30 min, even when consciousness was not impaired. Thus, as discussed in the section on electroclinical correlations, status epilepticus is presently classified as: (a) convulsive status epilepticus, in which the patient does not recover to a normal alert state between repeated tonic-clonic attacks; (b) nonconvulsive status epilepticus, such as absence status and complex partial status, in which the clinical presentation is a prolonged "twilight" state; and

(c) continuous partial seizures as "epilepsia partialis continuans," in which consciousness is preserved (2). Today, it is estimated that 60,000 to 160,000 Americans will have at least one bout of convulsive status epilepticus. We do not know how frequent nonconvulsive status is (10).

The risks of status epilepticus, its neuropathology, and the molecular events that are suspected to lead to cell death as a result of convulsive status were all discussed in the section on mechanisms of brain damage. Collectively, these chapters provide clinical and experimental studies that dictate that tonic-clonic status epilepticus be stopped as soon as possible. Convulsive status should not be allowed to progress beyond 60 min if severe, permanent brain damage or death is to be prevented (7,16,19,20,23, chapters 22 and 24). Mortality rates of 5 to 50% after tonic-clonic status epilepticus have been reported in both children and adults. More recently, mortality rates have not exceeded 10 to 12% (19,21,23).

Clinicians have long known that the longer tonic-clonic status continues, the more difficult it is to control and the higher the incidence of mortality and morbidity (19,21,23). The mean duration of convulsive status in patients who do not develop neurologic sequlae is 1½ hr (7,19,21,23). On the other hand, patients who develop neurologic sequelae have convulsive status that lasts an average of 10 hr. The mean duration of convulsive status in patients who die is 13 hr (7,19,21,23).

Experimental studies provide even more compelling arguments that convulsive status be terminated as soon as possible. Meldrum and Seisjö independently showed that permanent cell damage in the hippocampus, amygdala, cerebellum, thalamus, and middle cerebral cortical layers develops after 60 min of convulsive status (2,3,4,5,8,9,16, chapters 12, 22, and 40). Such selective cell damage continues (except in the cerebellum and amygdala) even in artificially ventilated animals whose metabolic side effects are corrected. Since vulnerable neurons can succumb in convulsive status in spite of adequate cerebral oxygenation and sufficient glucose and energy supply, cell death is suspected to result from excessively increased metabolic demands by the continuously firing neurons. Kreisman et al. demonstrated, in addition, that after 20 min of convulsive status, cerebral corticol Po_2 and cytochrome a,a^3 reductions decrease and regional oxygen insufficiency adds to further cell damage (the "transitional period of status") (chapter 22). Convulsive status should be stopped as soon as possible, however, because the molecular events that lead to selective cell death are already operational during the first two to three convulsions. Neuronal calcium concentrations rise as arachidonic acid, arachidonoyl diglycerols, prostaglandins, and leucotrienes accumulate to toxic amounts, causing brain edema and cell death in selected brain regions (8,9, chapters 40 and 56). Another reason why convulsive status should not be allowed to progress beyond 60 min is the appearance of secondary metabolic complications (16, chapters 39 and 40). After 60 min of status, lactic acidosis becomes prominent and cerebrospinal fluid pressure rises. Initial hyperglycemia is followed by hypoglycemia, and autonomic dysfunctions, consisting of hyperthermia, excessive sweating, dehydration, and hypertension followed by hypotension and eventual shock, appear. Excessive muscle activity can produce myolysis and myoglobinuria and lead to lower nephron nephrosis. Cardiovascular, respiratory, and renal failure may result (16).

Because the ideal drug for treating convulsive status epilepticus does not exist, more attention should be paid to the guiding principles that govern its rational management. The first principle of rational management demands the accurate identification of the subvarieties of status epilepticus. Convulsive status epilepticus requires immediate vigorous treatment. Moreover, subtypes of convulsive status have different responses to existing antiepileptic drugs. Primarily generalized tonic-clonic status and clonic-tonic-clonic status are extremely sensitive to diazepam or phenytoin. Ninety-five percent of patients with these types of status are easily controlled. In contrast, tonic-clonic status with partial onset may not always respond to treatment because an acute and active structural lesion may be present.

The second principle of rational management requires the treatment and correction of the causes and immediate trigger of status epilepticus. Tonic-clonic status most frequently results from acute central nervous system insults, e.g., acute cerebral infarctions, meningitis, encephalitis, head trauma, and cerebral anoxia from cardiorespiratory difficulties. Less frequently, convulsive status results from metabolic and fluid electrolyte disturbances associated with old cerebral infarctions, withdrawal from antiepileptic drugs, and metabolic diseases such as renal failure (7,19,21). Janz (14), Janz and Kautz (15), and Oxbury and Whitty (chapter 56) report that 22 to 25% of tonic-clonic status results from a cerebral neoplasm.

The third principle of rational management requires the stopping of convulsions as soon as possible to prevent selective neuronal cell damage and serious secondary metabolic consequences. Convulsive status must not be allowed to progress beyond 20 min, the so-called "transitional period." If convulsive status epilepticus continues beyond 60 min in spite of antiepileptic drug treatment, the patient should be placed under general anesthesia. Adequate cardiorespiratory function and brain oxygenation must be ensured to prevent selective cell damage in the cerebellum and amygdala, and, when present, secondary metabolic complications, such as hypoglycemia, electrolyte imbalance, lactic acidosis, dehydration, and hyperpyrexia must be corrected.

Table 1 shows a protocol for the treatment of convulsive status epilepticus. It is desirable to act deliberately and follow the protocol in a step-wise fashion to avoid unnecessary complications. Once

TABLE 1. *Management of tonic-clonic status epilepticus*

Time from initiation of observation and treatment (min)	Procedure
0	1. Assess cardiorespiratory function as the presence of tonic-clonic status is verified. If unsure of diagnosis, observe one tonic-clonic attack and verify the presence of unconsciousness after the end of the tonic-clonic attack. Insert oral airway and administer O_2 if necessary. Insert an indwelling intravenous catheter. Draw venous blood for anticonvulsant levels, glucose, BUN, electrolyte, and CBC stat determinations. Draw arterial blood for stat pH, Po_2, Pco_2, HCO_3. Monitor respiration, blood pressure, and electrocardiograph. If possible, monitor electroencephalograph.
5	2. Start intravenous infusion through indwelling venous catheter with normal saline, containing vitamin B complex. Give a bolus injection of 50 cc 50% glucose.
10	3. *Infuse diazepam intravenously* no faster than 2 mg/min until seizures stop or to total of 20 mg. *Also start infusion of phenytoin* no faster than 50 mg/min to a total of 18 mg/kg. If hypotension develops, slow down infusion rate. (Phenytoin 50 mg/ml in propylene glycol may be placed in a 100-ml volume control set and diluted with normal saline. The rate of infusion should then be watched carefully.) Alternately, phenytoin may be injected slowly by intravenous push.

30–40	4. If seizures persist, two options are available: iv phenobarbital *or* diazepam iv drip. The two drugs should *not* be given in the same patient, and an endotracheal tube should be inserted.
	    iv phenobarbital option: Start infusion of phenobarbital no faster than 100 mg/min until seizures stop or to a loading dose of 20 mg/kg.
	    diazepam iv drip option: 100 mg of diazepam is diluted in 500 cc D5/W and run in at 40 cc/hr. This ensures diazepam serum levels of 0.2 to 0.8 μg/ml.

50–60	5. If seizures continue, general anesthesia with halothane and neuromuscular junction blockade is instituted. If an anesthesiologist is not immediately available, start infusion of 4% solution of paraldehyde in normal saline; administer at a rate fast enough to stop seizures, *or* 50 to 100 mg of lidocaine may be given by intravenous push. If lidocaine is effective, 50 to 100 mg diluted in 250 cc of 5% D/W should be dripped intravenously at a rate of 1 to 2 mg/min.
80	6. If paraldehyde or lidocaine has not terminated seizures within 20 min from start of infusion, general anesthesia with halothane and neuromuscular junction blockade must be given.
	7. If status epilepticus reappears when general anesthesia is stopped, a neurologist who has expertise in status epilepticus should be consulted. Advice from a regional epilepsy center should also be sought on the management of intractable status epilepticus.

the diagnosis of tonic-clonic status is established, vigorous treatment should be instituted. To control seizures as soon as possible, diazepam is administered intravenously (12,18,21, chapter 49). Intravenous diazepam stops convulsions within 3 min in 33% of patients with status and within 5 min in 80% of patients (chapter 49). Ten to twenty minutes after cessation of intravenous diazepam administration, seizures may recur because diazepam is distributed quickly and widely to various organs and tissues. To prevent recurrence of seizures, phenytoin is given simultaneously in another intravenous line (11,23, chapter 44). The slow intravenous administration of phenytoin results in equally slow results. Anticonvulsant effects are not evident until 10 to 20 min after the start of phenytoin infusion (chapter 44). Phenytoin

stops status epilepticus in 30% of patients after approximately 400 mg has been administered, i.e., approximately 10 min after start of its infusion. Maximal anticonvulsant effects appear only after the full dose of phenytoin is administered, i.e., approximately 20 to 30 min after start of its infusion (chapter 44). Thus, to terminate convulsions rapidly, intravenous diazepam is administered simultaneously with phenytoin.

Both intravenous diazepam and phenytoin stop seizures in almost all patients with primarily generalized tonic-clonic, myoclonic, and clonic-tonic-clonic status (12, chapter 49). Both drugs arrest convulsive status resulting from alcohol and drug withdrawal. They also stop seizures in more than half (65%) of patients with tonic-clonic status with partial onset (21).

When intravenous diazepam and phenytoin fail to control status, a third drug must be used. The most commonly used third drug is intravenous phenobarbital. However, no prospective study has analyzed the effectiveness of phenobarbital in status epilepticus. Moreover, its use together with or after diazepam should be discouraged, since this drug combination causes respiratory depression. A more acceptable option is to administer diazepam by intravenous drip. In either case, an endotracheal tube must be inserted in the event of respiratory depression.

One study suggests that additional use of diazepam by intravenous drip controls another 22% of patients with convulsive status and effectively diminishes the number of patients with intractable status epilepticus from 35 to 12% (chapter 49). A continuing diazepam serum level of 0.2 to 0.8 µg/ml maintained by intravenous drip combined with a phenytoin serum level of 15 to 20 µg/ml stops convulsive status in 88% of patients who may or may not have acute destructive brain lesions (chapter 49).

By the time the first-line drugs (diazepam and phenytoin) and second-line agent (phenobarbital) have proved unsuccessful, convulsive status shall have continued for 60 min. General anesthesia with halothane and artificial respiration with neuromuscular junction blockade should be administered (chapter 56). While waiting for the anesthesiologist, alternative drugs considered third lines of defense, such as paraldehyde and lidocaine, can be used.

The protocol outlined in Table 1 may be modified by the patient's history. For instance, phenytoin is indicated as the initial and sole drug in the management of status epilepticus associated with head trauma or other neurosurgical disorders in which alteration of the patient's state of consciousness is contraindicated. Intravenous phenytoin is also used to treat partial motor status or serial tonic-clonic seizures. If seizures do not stop after a loading dose of 15 to 18 mg phenytoin/kg, then phenobarbital therapy can be initiated.

Complex partial status epilepticus should be treated vigorously following the protocol outlined above. It may be necessary to monitor the EEG prior to initiation of therapy if the diagnosis of complex partial status is uncertain. Complex partial status epilepticus can lead to serious sequelae. The more prolonged and uncontrolled these attacks are, the more likely they will cause chronic loss

of recent memory and symptoms like the Kluver-Bucy syndrome (2). Absence status or petit mal status is best managed by intravenous diazepam followed by oral administration of ethosuximide and/or valproic acid.

There remains a need for the development of an ideal drug for treating tonic-clonic status—one that would promptly stop status, remain in the brain long enough to prevent recurrence of seizures, and yet be free from undesirable side effects such as deep coma, hypotension, and respiratory depression (21).

Lorazepam, a 5-hydroxy-1,4-benzodiazepine, is similar in structure to diazepam and approximately five times more potent than diazepam in stopping status in experimental animals. Early clinical studies indicate that it effectively stops tonic-clonic status in humans and has relatively little effect on cardiac or respiratory functions. Tissue distribution of lorazepam is less rapid and less extensive than of diazepam, and its elimination half-life is 12 to 16 hr. The clinical effects of an intravenous bolus injection would therefore be more prolonged than diazepam. Available clinical studies, however, indicate that it is effective mainly in status epilepticus not associated with acute structural lesion, i.e., the "responsive type" of status epilepticus. It has been of limited benefit in the treatment of intractable status epilepticus (22). More clinical evaluation is needed to determine if lorazepam can replace diazepam and/or phenytoin in the treatment of status epilepticus.

REFERENCES

1. Bourneville, D. (1876): Recherches cliniques et thérapeutiques. In: L'épilepsie et l'hystérie, edited by Delahaye and Lacrosnier. Paris.
2. Brierly, J. B. (1976): Cerebral hypoxia. In: Greenfield's Neuropathology, edited by Blackwood, W., and Corsellis, J. A. N., pp. 43–85. Edward Arnold, London.
3. Brierley, J. B., Brown, A. W., Excell, B. J., and Meldrum, B. S. (1969): Brain damage in the rhesus monkey resulting from profound arterial hypotension. I. Its nature, distribution and general physiological correlates. Brain Res., 13:68–100.
4. Brierly, J. B., Brown, A. W., and Meldrum, B. S. (1971): The nature and time course of the neuronal alterations resulting from oligaemia and hypoglycaemia in the brain of Macaca mulatta. Brain Res., 25:483–499.
5. Brown, A. W., and Brierley, J. B. (1973): The earliest alterations in rat neurones after anoxia-eschaemia. Acta Neuropathol. (Berl)., 23:9–22.
6. Calmeil, L. (1824): De l'épilepsie. Thesis, University of Paris.

Subject Index

543